Oral Cavity Reconstruction

Oral Cavity Reconstruction

edited by

TERRY A. DAY

Medical University of South Carolina
Charleston, South Carolina, U.S.A.

DOUGLAS A. GIROD

University of Kansas Medical Center,
Kansas City, Kansas, U.S.A.

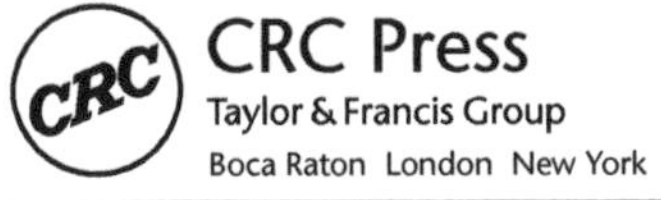

CRC Press is an imprint of the
Taylor & Francis Group, an **informa** business

CRC Press
Taylor & Francis Group
6000 Broken Sound Parkway NW, Suite 300
Boca Raton, FL 33487-2742

First issued in paperback 2019

ISBN-13: 978-1-57444-892-4 (hbk)
ISBN-13: 978-0-367-39200-0 (pbk)

Visit the Taylor & Francis Web site at
http://www.taylorandfrancis.com

and the CRC Press Web site at
http://www.crcpress.com

This book was completed through the love, support, and patience of my wife, Millie, and my children, Austen and Meredith. They became all too knowledgeable about the "Oral Cavity Textbook" but in an entirely different way than we as clinicians view this text! Additionally, I would like to give credit to the authors and all physicians, dentists, and health care professionals who have sacrificed their lives to help the lives of others stricken with head and neck cancers through patient care, research, and education.

Terry Day

I would like to dedicate my efforts on this text to my wife Susan Girod who strives to keep me sane and grounded through my many projects and has done such a wonderful job with our children Katelyn, Callie and Jimmy. I thank them all for their patience and love. I would like to thank my professional mentor Dr. Charles Cummings for his inspiration, insight, humor and support throughout my career and during this endeavor. Thanks also to Heather Barnhart, RN for her tireless support and endless compassion for the many cancer patients we have worked with over the last 11 years who have served as the motivation for this text. Lastly, I would like to thank the faculty, residents, students and staff of the Department of Otolaryngology—Head and Neck Surgery at the University of Kansas for the years of dedication and hard work for the sake of our patients.

Doug Girod

Foreword

It is my distinct pleasure to make comment about this well-timed text regarding oral cavity reconstruction. That this book has evolved is a testimonial to the evolution of medical understanding, enhancement, and therapeutic planning in the multidisciplinary approach to complex problems. What was once an arena of extirpation followed by modest attempts at reconstruction, management has been transformed (through the wonders of imaging, miniaturization, and visual magnification) to selective extirpation and functional as well as cosmetic reconstruction. Questions heretofore unasked, or at least unanswered, have in many instances fallen to resolution. This excellent work chronicles the breadth of understanding and implementation which now exists, such that the bottom line focus of the surgical rehabilitative team focuses on quality of life for the patient. I commend the editors for their creativity and all of the authors for their contribution thus enhancing the welfare of our patients. For those of us involved in treatment of advanced head/neck malignancy, this contribution comes at the right time.

Charles W. Cummings, MD
Distinguished Service Professor
Department of Otolaryngology—
Head and Neck Surgery

Preface

The twilight of the 20th century was a time of many advances in the management of head and neck cancer, but perhaps none have been so dramatic as those found in the reconstruction of defects of the oral cavity. The incidence of oral cavity carcinoma remains tied to the usage of tobacco and alcohol products, and thus, although preventable, is still quite prevalent. While radiotherapy has made advances as well, surgery remains the mainstay of management of oral cavity carcinoma. Unfortunately, surgical extirpation of oral cancers may result in significant functional and aesthetic compromise unless appropriate reconstructive and rehabilitative approaches are utilized. This text provides a comprehensive and detailed summary of these methods.

Unfortunately, the oral cavity is a major component of personal, professional, and social interaction through speech, deglutition, respiration, and cosmesis. It also serves in many aspects as a dividing line between dental and medical specialists related to appropriate oral and dental health. These specialists from a variety of backgrounds must collaborate in providing the optimal care for oral cancer patients. Additionally, the impact of surgical treatment of oral cavity carcinoma can be very profound for an individual. The success of reconstructive efforts in the oral cavity may be the difference between the retention of an individual as a productive member of society or complete social isolation.

Reconstructive management of oral cavity defects has now progressed beyond primary closure and skin grafts to a variety of pedicled flaps and, more recently, to microvascular free tissue transfers of composite flaps that can be tailor designed to match the missing tissues. These advances arm the reconstructive surgeon with a wide variety of options to consider when faced with an oral cavity defect. Additionally, the oncologic surgeon may now consider the resection of large debilitating tumors, which would have previously been deemed unresectable without the current options for complex reconstruction.

With the wide variety of reconstructive techniques for the oral cavity now available, the surgeon is faced with making choices for the repair of individual defects. Each patient and defect of the oral cavity is unique and requires a multidisciplinary approach to optimal function and cosmesis. The successful reconstructive surgeon relies heavily on experience in making these difficult decisions, taking a multitude of factors unique to a given situation into consideration.

Thus, the genesis of this text was to draw upon some of the most active and experienced oral and head and neck reconstructive surgeons to outline their approach to managing very site-specific defects of the oral cavity. A review of (i) oral cavity anatomy and physiology, (ii) benign and malignant pathology, (iii) reconstructive history with patient evaluation and, (iv) surgical approaches are presented to help organize the surgeons approach to these challenging patients. Each major subsite of the oral cavity (lip, cheek, tongue, palate, floor of mouth, mandible, etc.) is addressed through an individual and comprehensive chapter to provide the specific anatomical, physiological, and functional issues followed by a discussion of reconstructive options from simple to complex with the advantages and disadvantages of each reviewed. An effort is made to provide insight into the key factors that influence decision making by the surgeon as well as technical "tricks of the trade" to allow for maximal success and the avoidance of pitfalls.

We intend that this text will serve as a compilation of the current collective knowledge of how to manage defects of the oral cavity to provide the most functional and aesthetic results possible. We hope this will prove useful to the reconstructive neophyte and the experienced surgeon, as they face these most challenging of defects, to help provide individual patients with the best possible outcome.

Special thanks to LifeCell Corporation and Synthes Maxillofacial for the support to develop and publish this text.

Terry A. Day
Douglas A. Girod

Acknowledgment

The authors would like to thank the LifeCell Corporation, Branchburg, New Jersey and Synthes CMF, Paoli, Pennsylvania for the support of the original artwork found in this text.

Special thanks go to: Ann Durgun for administrative expertise and always being there! Dr. Jennifer Schnellman for professional scientific and editorial review. Anthony Pazos for wonderful and insightful artwork.

Contents

Foreword . . . . *v*
Preface . . . . *vii*
Acknowledgment . . . . *ix*
Contributors . . . . *xvii*

SECTION I: PRE-TREATMENT EVALUATION

1. Principles and History of Oral Cavity Reconstruction ***1***
Carsten E. Palme and Patrick J. Gullane
Introduction 1
Evaluation and Planning 2
Reconstructive Options 3
Conclusion 7
References 7

2. Anatomy of the Oral Cavity and Related Structures ***11***
Jeffrey H. Spiegel and Daniel G. Deschler
Introduction 11
Importance of Structure and Function 11
Conclusion 22
References 22

3. Functional Aspects and Physiology of the Oral Cavity ***23***
Gregory K. Hartig
Introduction 23
Embryology 23
Oral Competence 25
Salivation 27
Mastication 28
Bolus Formation and Propulsion 32
Taste 35
Conclusion 36
References 36

4. Pathology of Neoplastic Diseases of the Oral Cavity *39*
Mary Richardson
Introduction 39
Oral Squamous Malignancy by Anatomic Site 40
Oral Lichen Planus (OLP) 52
Osteoradionecrosis 52
Melanoma 52
Sarcoma 53
Tissue Procurement 54
Conclusion 54
References 54

5. Benign Lesions and Tumors of the Oral Cavity *59*
Charles L. Dunlap
Introduction 59
References 74

6. Planning and Diagnostic Evaluation in Oral Cavity Reconstruction *79*
Terance T. Tsue, David J. Kriet, Derrick I. Wallace, and Douglas A. Girod
Introduction 79
Evaluation and Planning 80
Reconstructive Options 87
Conclusion 91
References 91

SECTION II: TECHNICAL CONSIDERATIONS

7. Surgical Approaches to the Oral Cavity *95*
J. David Osguthorpe and Judith M. Skoner
Introduction 95
Evaluation and Planning 98
Reconstructive Options 102
Conclusion 116
References 117

8. Lip Reconstruction *119*
Gregory Renner
Introduction 119
Pertinent Anatomy 119
Evaluation and Planning 122
Reconstructive Options 124
Lip Repair Techniques 129
Simple Lip Advancement Flaps 132

Summary 153
References 153

9. **Reconstruction of the Buccal Mucosa and Salivary Ducts** *157*
Timothy M. McCulloch and D. Gregory Farwell
Introduction 157
Evaluation and Planning 158
Reconstructive Options 159
Summary 173
References 173

10. **Ventral Tongue and Floor of Mouth** *177*
Brian B. Burkey and C. W. David Chang
Introduction 177
Evaluation and Planning 177
Reconstructive Options 178
Conclusion 198
Problem-Based Discussion 199
References 200

11. **Reconstruction of Partial Glossectomy Defects** *205*
Judith M. Skoner, Joshua Hornig, and Terry A. Day
Introduction 205
Reconstructive Options 206
References 219

12. **Reconstruction of the Base of Tongue and Total Glossectomy Defects** *223*
Mark K. Wax and Dana S. Smith
Introduction 223
Evaluation and Planning 225
Reconstructive Options 227
Conclusion 249
References 250

13. **Hard Palate Reconstruction** *253*
J. Trad Wadsworth and Neal Futran
Introduction 253
Evaluation and Planning 253
Reconstructive Options 254
Decision Making Tips 263
Preoperative Considerations 269
Special Surgical Requirements 269
Conclusion 270
References 270

14. Reconstruction of the Soft Palate and Velopharyngeal Complex .. *273*
Craig W. Senders
Introduction 273
Evaluation and Planning 274
Reconstructive Options 275
Conclusion 281
References 281

15. Cleft Lip and Palate *283*
Jonathan M. Sykes and Travis T. Tollefson
Introduction 283
Evaluation and Planning 286
Reconstructive Options 292
Conclusion 305
References 305

16. Dental and Prosthetic Reconstruction of the Oral Cavity *307*
Betsy K. Davis and Eleni Roumanas
Introduction 307
Evaluation and Planning 308
Reconstruction Options 309
Conclusion 325
References 325

17. Mandibular Reconstruction *327*
Deepak Gurushanthaiah and Jeffrey R. Haller
Introduction 327
Evaluation and Planning 327
Reconstructive Options 328
Location of Mandibular Defects 337
Conclusion 343
References 344

18. Composite Defects of the Oromandibular Complex *347*
Douglas A. Girod and Terance T. Tsue
Introduction 347
Relevant Anatomy 348
Evaluation and Planning 348
Reconstructive Options for the Oromandibular Complex 350
Multiple Flaps for the Reconstruction of Oromandibular Defects 371
Implants and Biomaterials 373
Decision-Making Tips 376
References 378

19. Secondary Oral Cavity Reconstruction *383*
Theodoros N. Teknos, Douglas B. Chepeha, and Steven J. Wang
Introduction 383
Evaluation and Planning 383
Reconstructive Options 384
Decision-Making Tips 388
Conclusion 389
References 389

SECTION III: POST-RECONSTRUCTIVE ISSUES

20. Speech and Swallowing Rehabilitation *391*
Bonnie Martin-Harris and Julie Blair
Introduction 391
Vocal Subsystems 391
Swallowing 393
Evaluation Methods and Observations 396
Voice, Resonance, and Speech Disorders 399
Swallowing Disorders 401
Swallowing Treatment Strategies 403
Summary 409
Appendix A 411
References 415

21. Outcomes Research in Oral Cavity Reconstruction *421*
Michael G. Stewart
Introduction 421
Global QOL Instruments 423
Head and Neck Instruments 423
Functional Status After Reconstruction 425
QOL After Reconstruction 426
Cost-Effectiveness Issues 426
Summary 428
References 428

22. New Horizons in Oral Cavity Reconstruction *431*
Ahmed S. Ismail, Peter D. Costantino, David H. Hiltzik, Jason Moche, and Craig D. Friedman
Introduction 431
Distraction Osteogenesis 432
Bone Growth Factors 436
Tissue Engineered Oral Mucosal Lining 440
Conclusion 443
References 443

Index 449

Contributors

Julie Blair MUSC Evelyn Trammell Institute for Voice and Swallowing, Medical University of South Carolina, Charleston, South Carolina, U.S.A.

Brian B. Burkey Department of Otolaryngology—Head and Neck Surgery, Vanderbilt University, Nashville, Tennessee, U.S.A.

C. W. David Chang Department of Otolaryngology, University of Missouri, Columbia, Missouri, U.S.A.

Douglas B. Chepeha Department of Otolaryngology—Head and Neck Surgery, University of Michigan, Ann Arbor, Michigan, U.S.A.

Peter D. Costantino Department of Otolaryngology—Head and Neck Surgery, St. Luke's—Roosevelt Hospital Centers, New York, New York, U.S.A.

Betsy K. Davis Department of Oral and Maxillofacial Surgery, Medical University of South Carolina, Charleston, South Carolina, U.S.A.

Terry A. Day Department of Otolaryngology—Head and Neck Surgery, Medical University of South Carolina, Charleston, South Carolina, U.S.A.

Daniel G. Deschler Department of Otolaryngology—Head and Neck Surgery, Massachusetts Eye and Ear Infirmary, Harvard Medical School, Boston, Massachusetts, U.S.A.

Charles L. Dunlap Department of Oral and Maxillofacial Pathology and Radiology, School of Dentistry, University of Missouri—Kansas City, Kansas City, Missouri, U.S.A.

D. Gregory Farwell Otolaryngology—Head and Neck Surgery, Harborview Medical Center, University of Washington, Seattle, Washington, U.S.A.

Craig D. Friedman Facial Plastic and Reconstructive Surgery, New Haven Hospital, New Haven, Connecticut and Biomerix, Inc., New York, New York, U.S.A.

Neal Futran Department of Otolaryngology—Head and Neck Surgery, University of Washington, Seattle, Washington, U.S.A.

Douglas A. Girod Department of Otolaryngology—Head and Neck Surgery, University of Kansas School of Medicine, Kansas City, Kansas, U.S.A.

Patrick J. Gullane University Health Network, Wharton Chair in Head and Neck Surgery, Princess Margaret Hospital, Department of Otolaryngology, University of Toronto, Toronto, Ontario, Canada

Deepak Gurushanthaiah Department of Head and Neck Surgery, Oakland Medical Center, Oakland, California, U.S.A.

Jeffrey R. Haller Rocky Mountain Allergy Center, Missoula, Montana, U.S.A.

Gregory K. Hartig Department of Otolaryngology, University of Wisconsin—Madison, Madison, Wisconsin, U.S.A.

David H. Hiltzik Department of Otolaryngology—Head and Neck Surgery, Columbia University, New York, New York, U.S.A.

Joshua Hornig Department of Otolaryngology—Head and Neck Surgery, Medical University of South Carolina, Charleston, South Carolina, U.S.A.

Ahmed S. Ismail Department of Otolaryngology—Head and Neck Surgery, St. Luke's—Roosevelt Hospital Centers, New York, New York, U.S.A.

David J. Kriet Department of Otolaryngology—Head and Neck Surgery, University of Kansas School of Medicine, Kansas City, Kansas, U.S.A.

Bonnie Martin-Harris MUSC Evelyn Trammell Institute for Voice and Swallowing, Charleston, South Carolina, U.S.A.

Timothy M. McCulloch Otolaryngology—Head and Neck Surgery, Harborview Medical Center, University of Washington, Seattle, Washington, U.S.A.

Jason Moche Department of Otorhinolaryngology, University of Maryland, Baltimore, Maryland, U.S.A.

J. David Osguthorpe Department of Otolaryngology—Head and Neck Surgery, Medical University of South Carolina, Charleston, South Carolina, U.S.A.

Carsten E. Palme Oncologic Head and Neck Surgery, University of Toronto, Toronto, Ontario, Canada

Gregory Renner Department of Otolaryngology—Head and Neck Surgery, University of Missouri School of Medicine, Columbia, Missouri, U.S.A.

Mary Richardson Department of Pathology, Medical University of South Carolina, Charleston, South Carolina, U.S.A.

Eleni Roumanas Department of Biomaterials, Advanced Prosthodontics, and Hospital Dentistry, UCLA School of Dentistry, Los Angeles, California, U.S.A.

Craig W. Senders Department of Otolaryngology, University of California—Davis Medical Center, Sacramento, California, U.S.A.

Judith M. Skoner Department of Otolaryngology—Head and Neck Surgery, Medical University of South Carolina, Charleston, South Carolina, U.S.A.

Dana S. Smith Department of Otolaryngology—Head and Neck Surgery, Oregon Health and Science University, Portland, Oregon, U.S.A.

Jeffrey H. Spiegel Richard C. Webster Division of Facial Plastic and Reconstructive Surgery, Department of Otolaryngology—Head and Neck Surgery, Boston University School of Medicine, Boston, Massachusetts, U.S.A.

Michael G. Stewart Department of Otorhinolaryngology, Weill Medical College of Cornell University, New York, New York, U.S.A.

Jonathan M. Sykes Facial Plastic and Reconstructive Surgery, University of California—Davis Medical Center, Sacramento, California, U.S.A.

Theodoros N. Teknos Department of Otolaryngology—Head and Neck Surgery, University of Michigan, Ann Arbor, Michigan, U.S.A.

Travis T. Tollefson Facial Plastic and Reconstructive Surgery, Department of Otolaryngology—Head and Neck Surgery, University of California—Davis Medical Center, Sacramento, California, U.S.A.

Terance T. Tsue Medical Research Service, Veterans Affairs Medical Center, Kansas City, Missouri, and Department of Otolaryngology—Head and Neck Surgery, University of Kansas School of Medicine, Kansas City, Kansas, U.S.A.

J. Trad Wadsworth Eastern Virginia Medical School, Department of Otolaryngology—Head and Neck Surgery, Norfolk, Virginia, U.S.A.

Derrick I. Wallace Department of Otolaryngology—Head and Neck Surgery, University of Kansas School of Medicine, Kansas City, Kansas, U.S.A.

Steven J. Wang Department of Otolaryngology—Head and Neck Surgery, University of Michigan, Ann Arbor, Michigan, U.S.A.

Mark K. Wax Department of Otolaryngology—Head and Neck Surgery, Oregon Health and Science University, Portland, Oregon, U.S.A.

1
Principles and History of Oral Cavity Reconstruction

Carsten E. Palme
Oncologic Head and Neck Surgery, University of Toronto, Toronto, Ontario, Canada

Patrick J. Gullane
University Health Network, Wharton Chair in Head and Neck Surgery, Princess Margaret Hospital, and Department of Otolaryngology, University of Toronto, Toronto, Ontario, Canada

INTRODUCTION

Oral cavity cancer is an uncommon malignancy with a significant impact on both patients and health care resources. The current standard of treatment includes surgery and adjuvant external beam radiotherapy. Advances have been made with improved methods of reconstruction and rehabilitation that have significantly impacted on disease-specific outcome and quality of life.

A multidisciplinary approach in the treatment of oral cavity cancer is vital to achieve the best results. It provides close interaction between the head and neck oncologist and other members of the team. This is especially important for both ablation and reconstruction, as a careful balance needs to be established between tumor resection and quality reconstruction.

Tumors of the upper aerodigestive tract can be difficult to treat given the complex nature of the oral cavity. Great advances have occurred in both patient selection and tumor evaluation where radiology has become standard of care and includes computed tomography (CT) scans, magnetic resonance imaging (MRI), and positron emission tomography (PET) scanning. In addition, better medical management, improved anaesthetic techniques and close post-operative monitoring have allowed patients to undergo complex procedures with limited morbidity.

The goals of successful reconstruction are to recreate normal oral function, provide a satisfactory cosmetic result and permit prompt and careful follow up. This can be challenging as oral cavity tumors can extent to involve a number of critical sites (i.e., mandible, paranasal sinuses, orbit and skull base) and cause significant functional disabilities in terms of airway, speech, swallowing, and/or mastication.

A better understanding of normal oral function has resulted in the reconstruction of "like with like." Advances in surgical technique, improved knowledge in vascular anatomy and the development of more compatible biomaterials have allowed surgeons to perform the most complex of reconstructive techniques. A menu of reconstructive options includes free grafts, local tissue rearrangement, pedicled flaps, and vascularized free tissue transfer. This permits the successful transfer of skin, muscle, and/or bone to an otherwise hostile environment.

Successful rehabilitation would not be complete without the support of a variety of ancillary medical services including speech pathology, dietitians, and nursing staff. In addition, advances in the development of oral prostheses and dental implants have resulted in state-of-the-art and timely rehabilitation in patients with oral malignancies.

EVALUATION AND PLANNING

Evaluation of patient risk, tumor, and donor site factors are important prior to planning repair of the oral cavity defect. Patient factors include the presence of comorbidites such as diabetes, liver disease, chronic airway limitation, peripheral vascular disease, and a second malignancy. In addition, patient psychology plays a significant role and therefore may benefit from the assistance of a psychiatrist knowledgeable of the special needs of head and neck cancer patients. The subsequent selection of reconstructive options relies on a risk–benefit analysis that should always be considerate of the patient. Preoperative optimization of any intercurrent organic or functional disorder is vital prior to embarking on a surgical plan of management that requires prolonged anesthesia, lengthy hospitalization, and an extended period of rehabilitation.

Tumor factors should include knowledge of previous treatment, type of histology, primary site, size, and presence of distant disease. Previous external beam radiotherapy affects the microvasculature of the surrounding tissues that may result in significant problems such as soft tissue breakdown, fistula formation, osseous malunion, and carotid artery exposure. Repair generally requires the use of distant and vascularized tissue to achieve a successful outcome.

Squamous cell carcinoma (SCC) is the most common malignancy of the oral cavity but minor salivary gland tumors, primary bone tumors, and tumors of dental origin also occur with generous margins of > 1 cm required to achieve disease control.

The primary site of tumor within the oral cavity clearly influences the type of repair selected. Defects of the mobile tongue are best repaired with thin, soft, pliable, and sensate tissue whereas tumors originating from the inferior alveolar margin will likely require both bone and/or soft tissue. Palatal lesions are usually treated with simple excision and a dental prosthesis while large through-and-through defects will necessitate multiple reconstructive flaps.

Donor site factors are paramount in the selection of the tissue type used and can be divided into those specific to the patient and those vital to the reconstructive surgeon. Choice of donor tissue should result in minimal morbidity to the patient in terms of both function and form and be compatible with the needs of the defect. Qualities of donor tissue that are important include pliability, size of skin paddle, tissue volume, nature of the vascular pedicle, and the potential for both sensation and color match. Donor tissue should be relatively easy to harvest and ideally should permit a two-team approach to reduce operative time. Donor site factors that are contraindications to the successful harvest of tissue include prior injury or surgery (e.g., fractures, soft tissue trauma, peripheral vascular surgery), previous irradiation, recent intravenous cannulation (e.g., radial forearm free flap), and inadequate collateral circulation (e.g., peripheral vascular disease or dominant radial artery).

A thorough physical examination with appropriate imaging and examination under anesthesia in selected cases permits a comprehensive evaluation of the extent of the primary tumor and the type of reconstruction required. Magnetic resonance imaging provides superior soft tissue delineation of tumors especially within the tongue whereas tumors arising from or adjacent to bony structures are more accurately assessed using a CT scan. In addition, occlusal views or a dentascan may be helpful where minimal cortical bone erosion of the mandible is suspected. However, a combination of physical examination coupled with appropriate imaging as described improves both the sensitivity and specificity of tumor evaluation.

RECONSTRUCTIVE OPTIONS

Non-vascularized Grafts

The extensive vascularity of the upper aerodigestive tract has permitted the successful use of a number of free, non-vascularized grafts in the repair of oral cavity defects. Historically these have included skin, mucosa, and/or bone. Many authors have reported the successful use and good functional outcome of split thickness skin grafts following ablation of oral cavity tumors (1,2). Advantages include tissue availability, ease of harvest, and minimal donor site morbidity. In addition, techniques of skin harvesting have evolved from using a simple scalpel blade to a variety of commercially available powered dermatomes. However, prior history of radiation to either the donor or recipient site are contraindications to the use of split thickness skin. Despite these limitations, many authors continue to advocate their application for the repair of moderate- to large-sized defects following tumor ablation in the oral cavity (3).

Ollier (4) is credited with the first published paper in the French journal of physiology in 1860 detailing his experience with freebone graft and bone regeneration in lower animals and man. In 1892, the German surgeon Bardenheuer reported the reconstruction of both the bony and soft tissue defect of the lower jaw using a composite flap of skin, periosteum, and bone from the forehead (5). In 1949, Blocker and Stout (6) successfully transferred iliac bone for reconstruction of large mandibular defects. During the ensuing years, numerous reconstructive options were employed and these included the clavicle, sternum, radius, fibula, scapula, and metartarsal bone (7). Historically, all of these grafts had been used as either solid or particulate free bone grafts. Their successful outcome depended on the quality of the host environment and the type of soft tissue cover. In 1918, Blair (8) proposed the sterilization and reimplantion of autogenous mandible. A contemporary application of this technique was proposed in 1981 by Hamaker who reported the use of free autogenous irradiated mandible in seven cases (9). While initially this form of reconstruction was popular, the long-term poor results from a contaminated bed led surgeons to abandon this approach.

Converse and Campbell in 1954 were one of the first to use free particulate bone marrow and block grafts for the reconstruction of the mandible with varying results (10). Boyne (11) in 1969 employed vitalium metallic crib to support particulate iliac bone graft for the reconstruction of the non-irradiated mandible in patients with predominantly benign osseous neoplasms. He reported a successful outcome in excess of 80%. However in 1979, Adamo and Szal demonstrated an unsatisfactory outcome in 50% of cases and an 80% complication rate when employed in irradiated patients (12).

Local Tissue Rearrangement

Local flaps with either a random blood supply or a distinct axial vascular pedicle have been commonly used for the reconstruction of the oral cavity. A wide variety of options exist that date back to 600 B.C. when Indian surgeons first described this technique in the repair of nasal defects. Since then many different flaps have been used with varying success (13).

Malgaigne was the first to describe the successful use of the nasolabial flap in 1834 for repairing nasal defects. However, Rosenthal (1916), Esser (1918), and Thiersch (1968) expanded its usefulness for the repair of anterior or lateral oral cavity defects and remains a viable alternate option in select cases to date (13).

The palatal rotation flap as described by Gullane and Arena has been used to resurface defects involving the ipsilateral tonsil, retromolar trigone, and buccal mucosa (14). It is a simple local option, however, limited by pedicle length and contraindicated in the irradiated patient.

Klopp and Schurter (15) in 1956 proposed the tongue flap for the reconstruction of posterior oral cavity defects. It can be either based on an anterior or posterior pedicle. In 1969, Chambers and Jacques (16) popularized the use of this flap and DeSanto and Yarington (17) in 1983 reiterated the need for the contemporary head and neck surgeon to be aware of this option when treating oral cavity tumors.

A further contemporary option includes the buccinator musculomucosal flap as described by Bozola et al. (18) in 1989 and modified by Carstens et al. (19) in 1991. Its application and successful outcome makes this a reasonable local alternative in select patients with anterior or lateral oral cavity defects.

Over the past many years, lip reconstruction has significantly challenged many reconstructive surgeons. In general, defects less then one-third of the lip can be closed primarily. However, larger defects require local tissue transfer to provide an acceptable functional and cosmetic result. In 1837, Sabattini first proposed the concept of borrowing composite lip from the opposite side. Abbe in 1898 described this flap in detail, and therefore his name became associated with this technique. Similarly Stein's technique of lip reconstruction, as first described in 1848 became known as the Estlander flap in 1865 (13). In 1920, Gillies (20) described the rotation of adjacent residual lip around the commissure to repair moderate defects of the lower lip. Karapandzic (21) in 1974 recognized the need to maintain innervation when he proposed his modification of Gillies technique. Many local flaps have since been proposed to deal with total lip loss and these include the Bernard bilateral cheek advancement flap and Webster modification, which helped to improve both function and cosmesis (22,23).

Regional Flap Transfer

The use of adjuvant radiotherapy in the management of advanced oral cavity neoplasms has necessitated the need for distant, well-vascularised tissue for the reliable repair of the post-surgical defect. The evolution of pedicled regional flaps has fulfilled this reconstructive goal, the successful outcome of which has been further enhanced with modern advances in anesthesia, peri-operative care, and surgical techniques.

In 1791, Chopart is credited with the first description of using pedicled neck skin to repair a lip defect. Gersuny in 1887 expanded the usefulness of this approach in the reconstruction of oral cavity defects. Further developments of these techniques include the anterior and lateral apron flap and the Mutter flap (13). In 1968, Bakamjian (24) described the deltopectoral fasciocutaneous pedicled flap, which remained the "work horse" in head and neck reconstruction until the mid 1970s with the advent of free tissue transfer and pedicled musculocutaneous flaps. During that same era, the forehead flap as described by McGregor in 1969 was a popular alternative for primary reconstruction of the oral cavity (25). It provided primary repair for a number of subsites within the oral cavity with reliable blood supply but its cosmetic deformation was a significant contraindication. A more contemporary reconstructive option is the pedicled temporoparietal fascial flap, which can be employed in a small subset of patients with oral cavity neoplasms (26).

In 1896, Tansini (27) was the first to describe the use of a pedicled myocutaneous flap to repair a surgical defect. He employed the latissimus dorsi muscle with overlying skin for the reconstruction of a mastectomy defect. Owens (28) in 1955 first described this approach using the sternocleidomastoid myocutaneous flap for reconstruction in the head and neck region. This technique gained wide popularity in 1979 when Ariyan first described the pectoralis major myocutaneous flap in the reconstruction of the oral cavity (29). It subsequently became the work horse in head and neck reconstruction replacing the deltopectoral flap, and continues to be a viable alternative to date. Other pedicled musculocutaneous options include the sternocleidomastoid, the trapezius, the latissimus dorsi, and the temporalis muscle (30). Further variations of immediate mandibular reconstruction with regional osteomusculocutaneous flaps comprising the pectoralis major muscle, overlying skin, and a segment of the underlying 5th rib provided acceptable short-term results but few reports of reliable long-term outcome exist (31). Similar techniques using the sternocleidomastoid with the attached clavicle, the trapezius with the scapular wing and the temporalis with the outer cortical table have been described with successful outcomes varying from 30% to 80% in primarily non-irradiated beds (32). The unreliability and the many unacceptable donor site defects have made this method unattractive in primary reconstruction of the mandible after tumor ablation.

Distant Tissue Transfer

The advent of microvascular surgical techniques, knowledge of vascular territories, and improved systems of magnification have permitted the successful distant transfer and restoration of extensive defects in both irradiated and non-irradiated beds using vascularized skin, muscle and/or bone.

Harii et al. in 1976 and Panje et al. in 1976 were the first to employ free vascularized tissue transfer in the reconstruction of head and neck defects (33,34). However, it was not until the description of the radial forearm flap by Yang et al. (35) in 1981, that this technique gained widespread popularity and acceptance in soft tissue repair of the oral cavity. Factors such as ease of harvest, a long vascular pedicle, large skin paddle, pliability, potential for sensitivity, and low failure rates have supported the widespread use of this flap. Other soft tissue donor sites include the dorsalis pedis, the lateral arm, the scapular, rectus abdominus, latissimus dorsi, and groin flaps (36). More recently the recognition and description of perforator flaps such as the DIEP flap (i.e., deep inferior epigastric perforator) have helped to reduce tissue bulk and minimized donor site complications (37). A contemporary alternative is the anterolateral thigh flap, which is reliable, easy to harvest, has minimal donor site morbidity and allows for a two-team approach (38).

The pioneering experimental work by Ostrup and Frederickson (39) in 1975, in which they successfully demonstrated the ability to transfer free, vascularized rib graft into mandibular defects in an animal model, provided the background for the development of a number of bony reconstructive options for the management of oral cavity malignancies. Subsequently, a variety of vascularized free osseous flaps have included metatarsus, rib, radius, iliac crest, scapula, and fibula (40–45). The most popular contemporary options include both the fibula and the scapular osseocutaneous free flaps, which provide timely and efficient reconstruction of the entire spectrum of mandibular defects. One of the major advantages of osteocutaneous tissue is that the grafted site provides a bed in which the final stage of oral rehabilitation can be successfully completed using osseointegrated dental implant pegs.

Implants and Biomaterials

A number of synthetic biomaterials are available that help in the reconstruction of head and neck defects. These include mandibular reconstruction plates, maxillary prostheses, and dental implants. The ideal biomaterial should be inert, malleable, resilient, provide stablility over time, be cost effective, and easy to use.

Historically, a wide variety of materials have been used to reconstruct and alter the shape and function of the upper aerodigestive tract. These include a variety of metals, ivory, wax, and paraffin. Some of these were injected subcutaneously and moulded before solidification took place. The resultant significant foreign body reaction caused grotesque disfigurement. The early experience of most surgeons with alloplastic implants including steel, aluminum, brass, and magnesium were disappointing. They irritated the body tissues, produced necrosis and had to be discarded. The search for an ideal inert biomaterial resulted in numerous scientific evaluations of various combinations of metals. The earliest application of metals for mandibular reconstruction included the use of stainless steel wires by Scudder in 1912 (46). However, these resulted in loosening, migration, exposure, and malunion of the bony segments. Subsequently significant advances were made in 1936 when Venable and Stuck discovered vitallium (i.e., an alloy of cobalt, chromium, and molybdenum) (47). This was the most ideal alloplast available to date and was successfully used in reconstruction of the mandible by Winter et al. in 1945, Freeman in 1948, and Conley in 1951 (48–50). A major disadvantage of vitallium was its low malleability and significant failure rates in irradiated patients. In attempts to overcome the technical problems associated with this alloy, surgeons turned their attention to stainless steel devices using mesh trays and, subsequently, in the mid 1970s to a three-dimensional reconstruction plate (3-DBRP). In the early part of 1980, titanium began to replace stainless steel because of its superior malleability and inertness. Modifications of the titanium reconstruction system have resulted in a thinner and more pliable plate with improved screw design and reduced failure rates. Finally, the compatibility of stainless steel and titanium with either pre- or post-operative radiotherapy was confirmed in 1991 with the recognition of limited dose uptake, minimal effect on adjacent bone, and soft tissue with the use of parallel apposed fields (7).

The first use of prosthetics as cited by Conley (50) dates back to 1565 when Petronius devised a gold plate for the repair of a cleft palate defect. Since then the emergence of synthetic polymers has permitted the development of a wide range of oral prosthetics, which attempt to recreate normal oral anatomy, separate the sinonasal and oral cavity, and provide both form and function. This has resulted in prompt rehabilitation with an improvement in the overall quality of life in patients with oral cavity malignancies.

CONCLUSION

The past 50 years have seen a significant renaissance in surgical techniques in the management of oral cavity reconstruction. The first phase in reconstruction used local flaps with non-vascularized free grafts. The resultant functional and cosmetic outcome was often poor with an associated significant mortality due to tissue necrosis, flap failure, and severe nutritional depletion. The classic "Andy Gump" deformity reminds us of the limitations in reconstruction during this period.

The second phase commenced with the development of the pedicled myocutaneous and free tissue transfer. This period resulted in a significant reduction in mortality and improved quality of life in this patient population.

The third phase resulted in neural reinnervation of free tissue transfer and state-of-the-art oral rehabilitation with osseointegrated dental implants and prosthetics.

These reconstructive innovations have permitted the successful and reliable use of combined therapy with either pre- or post-operative chemoradiotherapy in an attempt to improve both survival and quality of life in patients with oral cavity malignancies.

REFERENCES

1. Helsper JT, Fister HW. Use of skin grafts in the mouth in the management of oral cancer. Am J Surg 1967; 114(4):596–600.
2. Myers EN. Reconstruction of the oral cavity. Otolaryngol Clin North Am 1972; 5(3):413–433.
3. Petruzzelli GJ, Johnson JT. Skin grafts. Otolaryngol Clin North Am 1994; 27(1):25–37.
4. Ollier L. Recherches Experimentales sur les Greffes Oseuses. J Physiol L'Homme Par 1860; 3:88–108.
5. Bardenheuer D. Ueber Unterkiefer und Oberkiefer Resektion. Arch Klin Chir 1892; 4:153–156.
6. Blocker TG, Stout RA. Mandibular reconstruction in World War II. Plast Reconstr Surg 1949; 4:153–156.
7. Gullane PJ. Primary mandibular reconstruction: analysis of 64 cases and evaluation of interface radiation dosimetry on bridging plates. Laryngoscope 1991; 101(6):S1–S24.
8. Blair VP. Surgery and Diseases of the Mouth and Jaws. St. Louis: CV Mosby, 1918.
9. Hamaker RC. Irradiated autogenous mandibular grafts in primary reconstruction. Laryngoscope 1981; 7:1031–1051.
10. Converse JM, Campbell RM. Bone grafting in surgery of the face. Surg Clin North Am 1954; 34:375–401.
11. Boyne PJ. Restoration of osseous defects in maxillofacial casualties. J Am Dent Assoc 1969; 78:767–776.
12. Adamo A, Szal RL. Timing, results and complications of mandibular reconstructive surgery: report of 32 cases. J Oral Surg 1979; 37:755–763.
13. Yarington CT. The evolution of reconstructive facial surgery. Otolaryngol Clin North Am 1983; 16(2):305–308.
14. Gullane PJ, Arena S. Palatal island flap for reconstruction of oral defects. Arch Otolaryngol 1977; 103(10):598–599.
15. Klopp CT, Schurter M. The surgical treatment of cancer of the soft palate and tonsil. Cancer 1956; 9:1239–1243.

16. Chambers RG, Jacques DA, Mahoney WD. Tongue flaps for intraoral reconstruction. Am J Surg 1969; 118:783–786.
17. DeSanto LW, Yarington CT Jr. Tongue flaps: repair of oral and pharyngeal defects after resection for cancer. Otolaryngol Clin North Am 1983; 16(2):343–351.
18. Bozola AR, Gasques JA, Carriquiry CE, Cardosos de Oliveira M. The buccinator musculomucosal flap: anatomic study and clinical application. Plast Reconstr Surg 1989; 84:250.
19. Carstens MH, Stofman GM, Hurwitz DJ, Futrell JW, Patterson GT, Sotereanos GC. The buccinator myomucosal island pedicle flap: anatomic study and case report. Plast Reconstr Surg 1991; 88:39.
20. Gillies HD. Plastic surgery of the face, London, 1920, Frowde, Hodder & Stoughton: Oxford University Press, 1920.
21. Karapandzic M. Reconstruction of lip defects by local arterial flaps. Br J Plast Surg 1974; 27(1):93–97.
22. Bernard C. Cancer de la levre inferieure; restauration a l aide de deux lambeaux lateraux quadrilataires, guerison. Bull Mem Soc Chir Paris 1853.
23. Patterson HC, Anonsen C, Weymuller EA, Webster RC. The cheek-neck rotation flap for closure of temporozygomatic-cheek wounds. Arch Otolaryngol 1984; 110:388–393.
24. Bakamjian VY. Total reconstruction of pharynx with medially based deltopectoral skin flap. North Y State J Med 1968; 68(21):2771–2778.
25. McGregor IA. The temporal flap in intraoral reconstruction. In: Gaisford JC, ed. Symposium on Cancer of the Head and Neck. St. Louis: The CV Mosby Co., 1969:72–88.
26. Cheney ML, Varvares MA, Nadol JB Jr. The temporoparietal fascial flap in head and neck reconstruction. Arch Otolaryngol Head Neck Surg 1993; 119(6):618–623.
27. Tansini I. Nouvoprocesso per l'amputazione della mammaella per cancro. Riforma Med 1896; 12:3–5.
28. Owens NA. A compound neck pedicle designed for the repair of massive facial defects: formation, development and application. Plast Reconstr Surg 1955; 15:369–374.
29. Ariyan S. The pectoralis major myocutaneous flap. A versatile flap for reconstruction in the head and neck. Plast Reconstr Surg 1979; 63(1):73–81.
30. Shindo ML, Sullivan MJ. Muscular and myocutaneous pedicled flaps. Otolaryngol Clin North Am 1994; 27(1):161–172.
31. Panje W, Cutting C. Trapezius osteomyocutaneous island flap for reconstruction of the anterior floor of the mouth and the mandible. Head Neck Surg 1980; 3(1):66–71.
32. Cuono CB, Ariyan S. Immediate reconstruction of a composite mandibular defect with a regional osteomusculocutaneous flap. Plast Reconstr Surg 1980; 65(4):477–484.
33. Harii K, Ohmori K, Sekiguchi J. The free musculocutaneous flap. Plast Reconstr Surg 1976; 57(3):294–303.
34. Panje WR, Bardach J, Krause CJ. Reconstruction of the oral cavity with a free flap. Plast Reconstr Surg 1976; 58(4):415–418.
35. Yang GF, Chen PJ, Gao YZ, Liu XY, Li J, Jiang SX, He SP. Forearm free skin flap transplantation: a report of 56 cases. 1981. Br J Plast Surg 1997; 50(3):162–165.
36. Shindo ML, Sullivan MJ. Soft-tissue microvascular free flaps. Otolaryngol Clin North Am 1994; 27(1):173–194.
37. Koshima I, Handa T, Satoh Y, Akisada K, Orita Y, Yamamoto H. Free rectus abdominis muscle perforating artery flaps for reconstruction of the head and neck defects. Nippon Jibiinkoka Gakkai Kaiho 1995; 98(1):1–7.
38. Song YG, Chen GZ, Song YL. The free thigh flap: a new free flap concept based on septocutaneous artery. Br J Plast Surg 1984; 37:149.
39. Ostrup LT, Fredrickson JM. Reconstruction of mandibular defects after radiation, using a free, living bone graft transferred by microvascular anastomose. An experimental study. Plast Reconstr Surg 1975; 55(5):563–572.
40. MacLeod AM, Robinson DW. Reconstruction of defects involving the mandible and floor of mouth by free osteo-cutaneous flaps derived from the foot. Br J Plast Surg 1982; 35(3):239–246.

41. Serafin D, Villarreal-Rios A, Georgiade NG. A rib-containing free flap to reconstruct mandibular defects. Br J Plast Surg 1977; 30(4):263–266.
42. Soutar DS, McGregor IA. The radial forearm flap in intraoral reconstruction: the experience of 60 consecutive cases. Plast Reconstr Surg 1986; 78(1):1–8.
43. Taylor GI, Townsend P, Corlette RJ. Superiority of the deep circumflex iliac vessels as the supply for the free groin flap. Plast Reconstr Surg 1984; 104:238–242.
44. Gilbert A, Teot L. The free scapular flap. Plast Reconstr Surg 1982; 69(4):601–604.
45. Hidalgo DA. Fibula free flap: a new method of mandible reconstruction. Plast Reconstr Surg 1989; 84(1):71–79.
46. Scudder CL. Tumors of the Jaws. Philadelphia: Saunders and Co., 1912:325–339.
47. Venable CS, Stuck WG. The effects of bone of the presence of metals based on electrolysis: an experimental study. Ann Surg 1937; 105:917–929.
48. Winter L, Lifton JC, McQuillan AS. Embedment of a vitallium mandibular prosthesis as an integral part of the operation for removal of an adamantinoma. Am J Surg 1945; 69:318–324.
49. Freeman BS. The use of vitallium plates to maintain function following resection of the mandible. Plast Reconstr Surg 1948; 3:73–79.
50. Conley JJ. The use of vitallium prostheses and implants in the reconstruction of the mandibular arch. Plast Reconstr Surg 1951; 8:150–162.

2

Anatomy of the Oral Cavity and Related Structures

Jeffrey H. Spiegel
Richard C. Webster Division of Facial Plastic and Reconstructive Surgery, Department of Otolaryngology—Head and Neck Surgery, Boston University School of Medicine, Boston, Massachusetts, U.S.A.

Daniel G. Deschler
Department of Otolaryngology—Head and Neck Surgery, Massachusetts Eye and Ear Infirmary, Harvard Medical School, Boston, Massachusetts, U.S.A.

INTRODUCTION

The oral cavity comprises the area within the confines of the vermilion border of the lips, the floor-of-mouth mucosa, the buccal mucosa of the cheeks, and a plane passing through the junction of the hard and soft palates to the circumvallate papillae of the tongue. The space is divided into several distinct areas including the lip, buccal mucosa, alveolar ridges (maxillary and mandibular), floor of mouth, retromolar trigone, hard palate, and oral tongue. Many structures are intimately related to the oral cavity, including the immediately related teeth, mandible, palatine tonsils, and soft palate, and the more distantly related (but equally important) muscles of mastication, oral pharynx, and neck. The oral cavity is not synonymous with the mouth. Anteriorly, the vestibule represents the space between the lips and the gingiva and teeth. The mouth is that space bounded by the lingual surface of the teeth and alveolar ridges, the hard and soft palates, the entire tongue and floor of mouth, and extends back to enter the oropharynx at the tonsillar pillars.

IMPORTANCE OF STRUCTURE AND FUNCTION

An ideal reconstruction of the oral cavity is one that very closely resembles the original structures in both form and function. To approach this ideal, the interactions between structures both within and beyond the oral cavity must be considered (Fig. 1). Furthermore, advanced reconstructive techniques typically require utilizing or transversing structures adjacent to the oral cavity. Thus, a detailed understanding of both the structures within the oral cavity, and those related to it, is necessary to achieve the best reconstructive results.

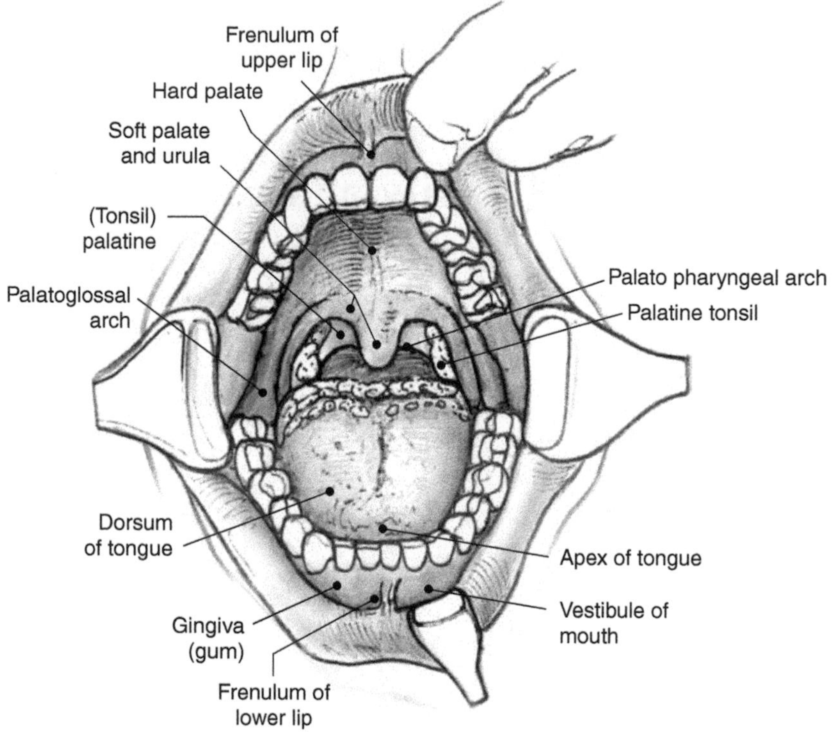

Figure 1 Anterior and intra-oral view of the oral cavity.

Lips

The lips function as a sphincter, controlling ingress to and egress from the oral cavity. The full anatomic extent of the upper lip reaches superiorly to the base of the nose, and superolaterally to the deepest part of the nasolabial fold. The lower lip extends inferiorly to the labiomental groove. With relation to the oral cavity, however, the lip begins as the vermilion border and includes only those areas that are red in color. This red color is the result of blood being seen through a translucent mucous membrane, rather than from inherent red pigmentation. This is easily demonstrated by blanching the lip with pressure.

The upper lip skin contains a central groove, the philtrum, the lateral ridges of which end inferiorly at the labial tubercles of the upper lip. These tubercles contribute to the desirable cupid's bow shape to the upper lip. Displacement or effacement of the philtrum is quickly noticed; thus, this area represents an important region during lip reconstruction.

Beneath the lip skin is a layer of subcutaneous tissue with many muscles, nerves, and vessels (Fig. 2). This subcutaneous tissue lies just superficial to the orbicularis oris. The orbicularis oris provides the muscle tone and motion necessary for a competent oral sphincter. In addition to intrinsic muscle fibers, which run both circumferentially and obliquely from skin to mucosal membrane, the orbicularis is made of muscle fibers contiguous with the mentalis and buccinator muscles, as well as of fibers from the zygomaticus major, levator labii superioris, and depressor labii inferion. The contributions from the buccinator connect to muscle fibers extending from the commissures towards the maxillary or mandible alveolar ridges. These fibers form two commissures

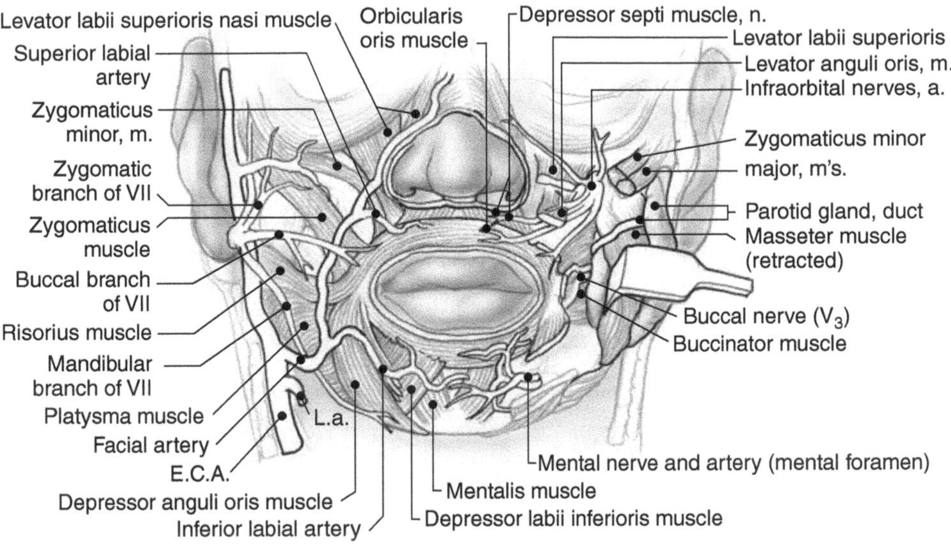

Figure 2 Frontal view of deep structures of the soft tissues of the face and lips.

towards the maxillary or mandibular alveolar ridges. These fibers form two muscles, the incisivus labii superioris and inferioris. Buccal branches of the facial nerve innervate the orbicularis oris. The mentalis muscle, inferior to the orbicularis, receives innervation from the marginal mandibular branch of the facial nerve. Deficiency of mentalis function can be very noticeable in affecting lip position and function.

Blood supply to the lip is from the superior and inferior labial arteries that branch from the facial arteries, which run along the margin of the orbicularis oris deep to the vermilion of the lip. Deep to the orbicularis oris are numerous labial salivary glands, each with a small duct penetrating the mucosal membrane. The mucosal membrane forms a superior and inferior midline fold connecting to the alveolar gingiva, forming the superior and inferior labial frenulum.

Sensory supply to the lip arises from branches of the fifth cranial nerve. The infraoribtal nerves extend to the upper lip, and the mental nerve provides sensation to the lower lip. Lymphatic drainage is to the submental and submandibular lymph nodes, and can often be bilateral.

Buccal Mucosa and Cheek

The main structural component of the cheek is provided by the buccinator muscle. This muscle arises from the alveoli of the maxilla and mandible, as well as from the pterygomandibular raphe. This ligamentous raphe separates the superior constrictor muscle from the buccinator, and extends from the hamulus of the pterygoid to the mylohyoid line of the mandible. Anteriorly, the buccinator muscle extends to contribute to the orbicularis oris. Lateral to the buccinator is the buccal fat pad, which extends between the masseter and temporalis muscles. The buccinator muscle is pierced by the parotid duct that enters the oral cavity through the buccal mucosa across from the second maxillary molar. The buccinator muscle is continuous embryologically with the superior pharyngeal constrictor muscles. It is readily apparent that the external cheek skin covering, buccinator muscle, and buccal mucosa are

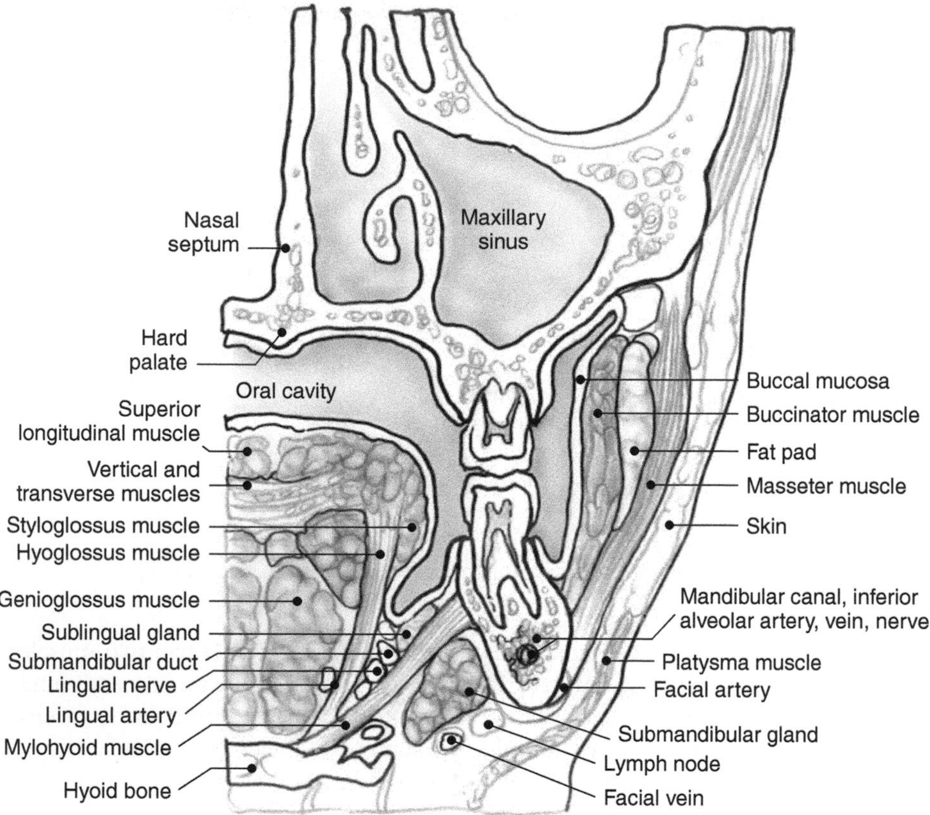

Figure 3 A coronal image through the cheek showing the mucosa, muscle, fat pad, masseter, and a cross-section of the tongue and floor of mouth.

intimately related anatomically and functionally (Fig. 3). Buccal salivary glands are present in the submucosa, but are smaller than those in the lip.

Alveolar Ridges

The alveolar ridges represent bony extensions from the maxilla, superiorly, and mandible, inferiorly (Fig. 4). The teeth are present in alveolar sockets, and within these two ridges is a vascular mucosal membrane which is firmly attached by fibrous connective tissue. This mucosal membrane extends to be contiguous with the mucosa of the lips and buccal membranes, and also with the floor of mouth on the lingual side of the alveolar ridge, inferiorly, and with the hard palate, superiorly. Within the tooth sockets, the mucosa becomes contiguous with the periosteum.

Retromolar Trigone

The retromolar trigone (retromolar gingiva) is the term given to the tightly attached mucosa overlying the mandible from posterior to the first molar, along the ramus to the apex (Fig. 4). Tumors, such as those of the base of tongue or tonsillar fossa, onto the retromolar trigone must be carefully assessed for bone involvement as there is minimal tissue between the overlying mucosa and periosteum of the mandible.

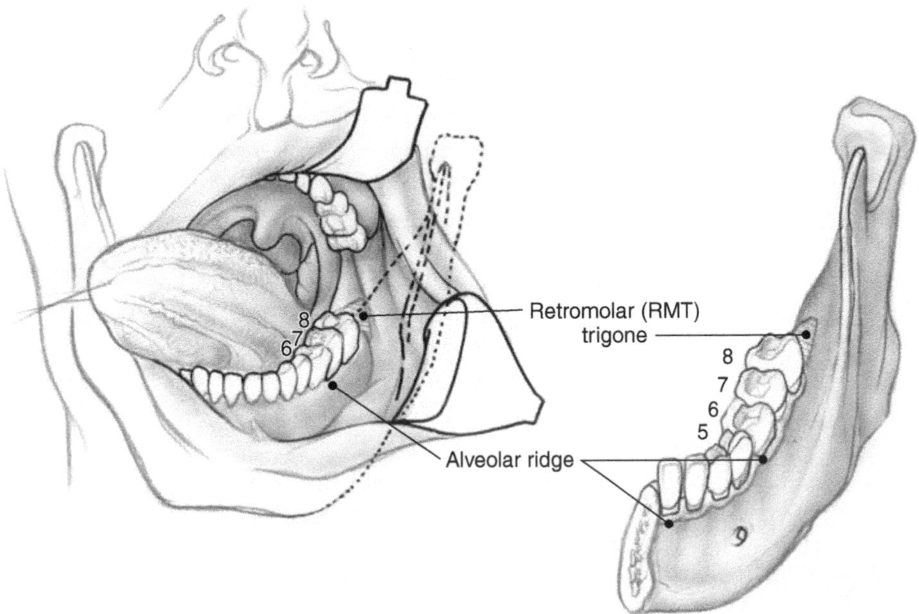

Figure 4 Transoral view of the alveolar ridge, retromolar region, and mandible of the left side of the oral cavity.

Floor of Mouth

The floor of the mouth is a mucosal covered space that extends from the lingual surface of the mandibular alveolar ridge to the ventral surface of the tongue. Posteriorly, it extends to the base of the anterior tonsillar pillar. The left and right sides meet at the lingual frenulum along the anterior midline.

The underlying geniohyoid and mylohyoid muscles provide support for the floor of mouth. The mylohyoid muscle arises along the mylohyoid line of the mandible and inserts posteriorly into the hyoid and elsewhere into a median raphe. The geniohyoid is a paired midline muscle just superior to the mylohyoid. It originates along the posterior aspect of the symphysis at the mental spine and inserts on the hyoid. The floor of mouth is pierced anteriorly on either side of the lingual frenulum by the end of the submandibular duct forming the sublingual caruncle. Laterally, an elevation in the floor of mouth known as the sublingual fold represents the area of the underlying sublingual glands within the paralingual space (Fig. 5).

Also within the paralingual space courses the lingual nerve. This nerve arises from the mandibular division of the trigeminal nerve and courses across the submandibular duct to spiral around the duct from lateral to medial and then upward into the tongue (Fig. 6A). More medially, the hypoglossal nerve, cranial nerve XII, lies inferior (superficial) to the mylohyoid muscle before crossing the muscle into the tongue to supply motor innervation the intrinsic and extrinsic tongue musculature (Fig. 6B).

Hard Palate

The hard palate comprises the arched area extending from the inner portion of the superior alveolar ridge to the posterior edge of the palatine bone (Fig. 7). The bony

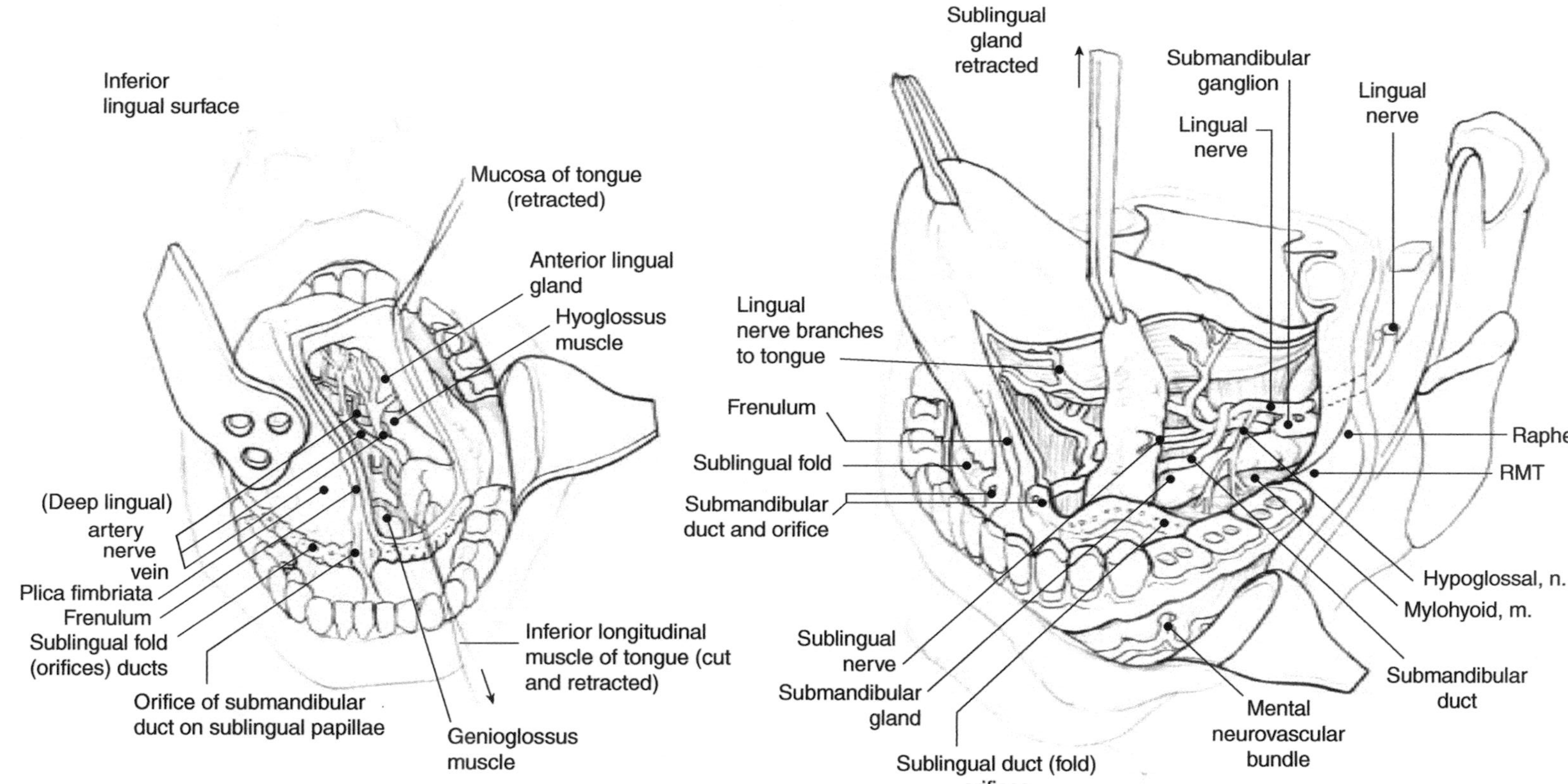

Figure 5 Intra-oral view of the neurovascular structures of the tongue and floor of mouth with surface and deep anatomic details.

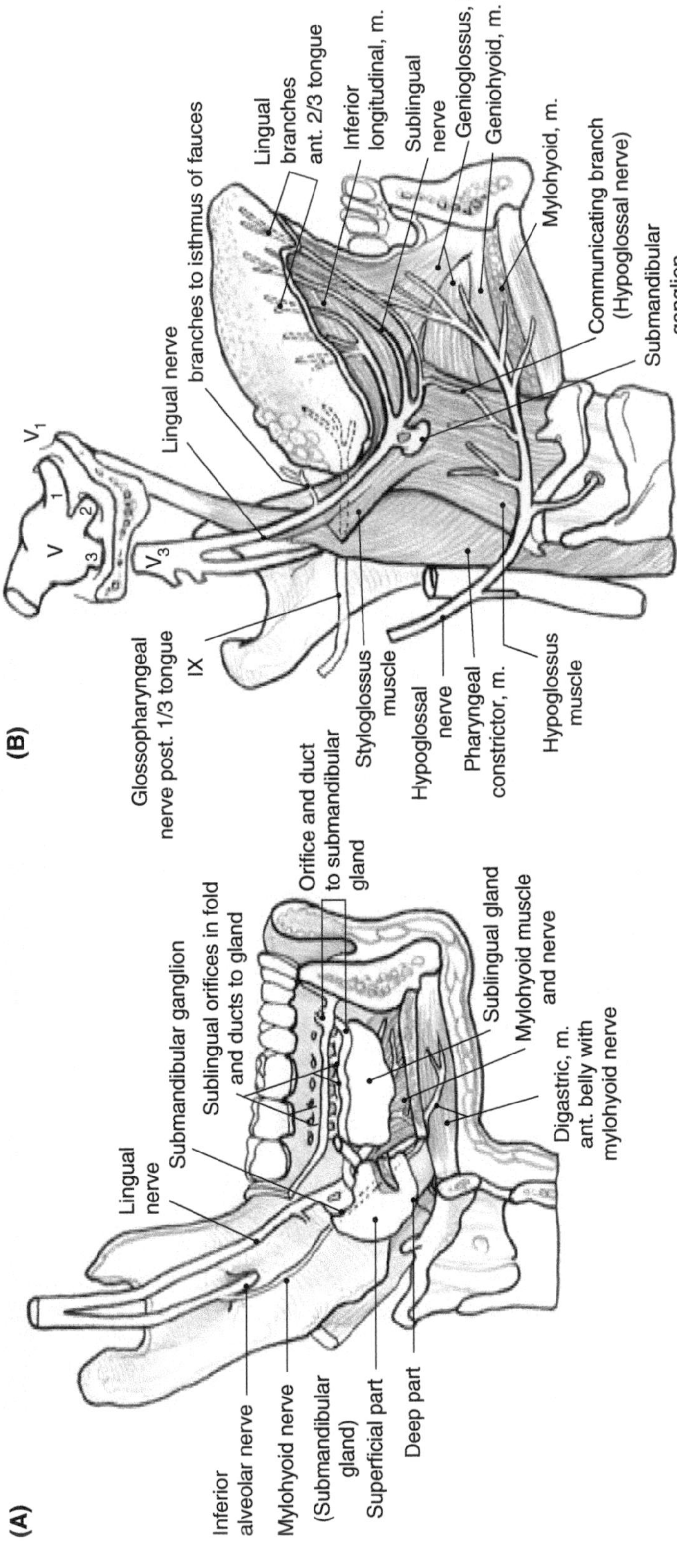

Figure 6 (A) View from right to left of the left interior oral cavity revealing detailed anatomy of salivary gland structures and neurovascular and muscular attachments. (B) View from right to left of interior right oral cavity revealing detailed neuromuscular anatomy of the tongue and floor of mouth.

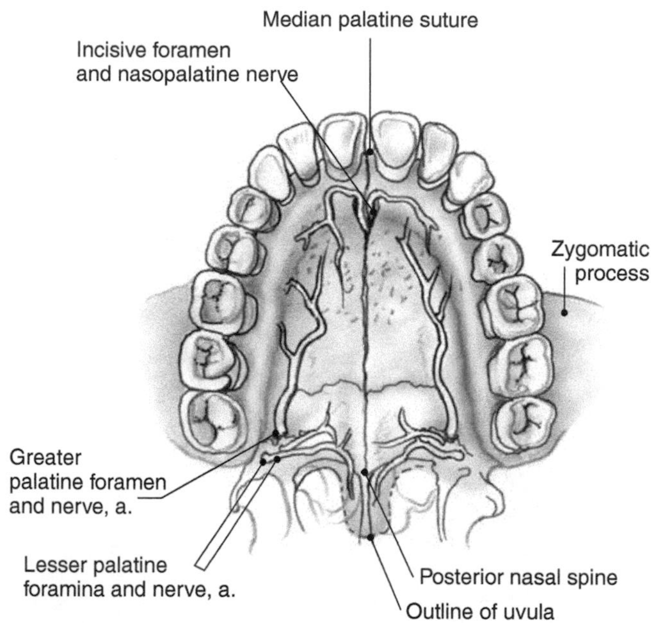

Figure 7 View of the hard palate and anterior soft palate deep structures looking from inferior to superior.

structure of the hard palate consists of the horizontal portions of the palatine bones and the palatine processes of the maxillae. These paired midline bones completely separate the oral cavity from the nasal cavity superiorly.

The bony structure is covered with periosteum tightly adherent to the overlying mucosa. Minor salivary glands, towards the posterior aspect of the hard palate, drain directly through the overlying mucosa into the oral cavity. Along the midline of the hard palate is the raised palatine raphe ridge, which ends anteriorly at the incisive papilla through which opens the incisive canal. This canal transmits sensory branches of the nasopalatine nerve to the anterior third of the hard palate. The posterior two-thirds of the hard palate receive sensory innervation through left and right greater palatine nerves, which penetrate the bony palate through left and right greater palatine foramina. These foramina lie along the lateral aspect of each of the horizontal parts of the palatine bones. The greater palatine branch of the maxillary artery also goes through the greater palatine foramen, traveling anteriorly on either side of the palate to meet branches of the sphenopalatine artery coming through the incisive canal. Lymphatic drainage is lateral to the tonsils towards the deep cervical nodes.

Although strictly part of the oral pharynx, the soft palate begins directly posterior to the hard palate at the posterior aspect of the horizontal palatine bones. The soft palate is a fold of mucous membranes containing muscle fibers, glands, nerves, and vessels. Laterally, the soft palate extends into the anterior (palatoglossal fold) and posterior (palatopharyngeal fold) tonsillar pillars. Between these, on either side, sits the palatine tonsil. A midline extension of the soft palate, the uvula, contains the musculus uvulae, which arises off of the palatine bones and soft palate aponeurosis. Many muscles contribute to the soft palate, including the levator veli palatini, tensor veli palatini, palatoglossus, palatopharyngeus, and musculus uvulae.

The tensor veli palatini is innervated by the mandibular branch of the trigerninal nerve, while these other muscles receive branches from the vagus through the pharyngeal plexus.

Oral Tongue

The oral tongue is that area of the tongue anterior to the circumvallate papillae extending to the floor of mouth mucosa and is generally considered to represent the anterior two-thirds of the entire tongue. Separating the tongue into an anterior two-thirds and posterior one-third is legitimate as the two areas have different innervation, structure, and embryonic development. The division is the sulcus terminalis whose apex ends in the median foramen cecum. Anterior to the sulcus are 8–12 circumvallate papillae, each 1–2 mm wide and each with its own circumferential sulcus containing numerous taste buds.

The tongue is suspended by three bilateral attachments. On each side, there are connections to the mandible, hyoid bone, and styloid process. The tongue is also connected to the palate through the anterior tonsillar pillars, or palatoglossal arches. The midline of the tongue is incompletely divided by an areolar lingual septum that makes a relatively surgically bloodless plane of dissection. This midline septum is visible as a median sulcus along the dorsum of the tongue. Overall, the oral tongue is considered to have four parts: tip (or apex), lateral aspects, dorsum, and undersurface or ventral aspect.

The mucous membrane of the tongue has a rough surface that is distinct from the smooth surface of the floor of mouth or buccal mucosa. This roughness is a result of numerous papillae including fungiform papillae (present on the side and tip) and filiform papillae (prominent along the dorsum).

Tongue musculature is divided into intrinsic and extrinsic groups. The extrinsic groups include the genioglossus, styloglossus, and hyoglossus (Fig. 3). These serve to connect the tongue and move it relative to the three main bony attachments. The genioglossus arises from the mental spine of the symphysis before fanning along the inferior aspect of the tongue from the tip down to the hyoid. The styloglossus travels from the styloid process and stylomandibular ligament to lie predominantly superficially along the lateral aspects of the tongue extending to the tip. Some fibers travel through the hyoglossus towards the deep tongue. The hyoglossus arises from the hyoid bone and ascend into the tongue to run transversely, obliquely, and longitudinally.

Intrinsic tongue muscles lack origins or insertions outside of the body of the tongue. Their names are descriptive of their overall position and include the superior longitudinal muscles, inferior longitudinal muscles, transverse lingual muscles, and verticalis muscle.

Blood supply to the oral tongue is via the lingual artery, branching from the external carotid. Several branches that include the hyoid, dorsal lingual, deep lingual, and sublingual extend from the main lingual artery. Venous drainage is via the lingual veins, which meet the dorsal lingual veins to join the internal jugular. However, the vena comitans nervi hypoglossi travelling with the hypoglossal nerve is often larger than the lingual veins and drains into the facial vein.

Lingual lymphatics are rich and divided into four primary groups. The apical channels drain to the superior deep cervical chain, and specifically to the juguloomohyoid nodes, via the submental and submandibular nodes. Marginal channels drain around the sublingual gland to the submandibular nodes and superior deep cervical nodes near the digastric. Basal channels drain the posterior tongue into the jugulodigastric nodes, and the central channels drain between the genioglossus muscles to the superior deep cervical nodes. Median areas may drain bilaterally or contralaterally.

Muscular innervation is via the hypoglossal nerve. Taste sensation includes contributions from the seventh (chorda tympani), ninth (glossopharyngeal), and tenth (superior laryngeal) cranial nerves. General sensation is via the lingual nerve, branching from the trigeminal for the oral tongue, and via the ninth and tenth cranial nerves for the pharyngeal tongue (Fig. 6B).

Mandible

Although not specifically part of the oral cavity, the mandible contributes to the alveolar rides and retromolar trigone. The mandible is clinically divided into several regions including the condyle, condylar neck, coronoid process, ramus, angle, body, and symphysis (Fig. 8). Anteriorly, a protrusion along the lower border of the symphysis forms the mental protuberance. The mental foramen, which transmits the mental nerve, is located on the right and left along the midportion of the mandible at the point of the second bicuspid tooth. In the mandible of the elderly edentulous patient, resorption of alveolar bone places the mental foramen in a relatively more superior location. An oblique line is palpable running inferior to the foramen to the ramus. This line can be of significance when using miniplates to reconstruct mandible fractures.

The mental spines are along the lingual surface of the mandible at the symphysis and provide attachment for the genioglossus muscles. The geniohyoid arises from a ridge just below this, and the mylohyoid along the inferior surface.

The ramus arises from the angle (an area of relatively thin bone) in a more vertical plane (approximately 110–120°). It provides attachments for the masseter along its lateral surface and for the medial pterygoid muscle on the medial surface. Also on the medial surface, the mandibular foramen allows for passage of the inferior alveolar nerve (off the third branch of the trigeminal nerve) and several blood vessels to enter the mandibular canal for travel towards the mental foramen. Several branches from the canal extend to each tooth socket.

The condylar neck is superior to the ramus and provides an insertion for the lateral pterygoid muscle. The condyle itself interfaces with the temporal bone at the temporomandibular joint. Anterior to the neck is a notch through which the masseter receives its neurovascular supply, and anterior to the notch is the coronoid process onto which the temporalis muscle inserts both laterally and medially.

Function

The oral cavity performs several critical functions. It has several specific roles in eating and processing of the food bolus. Beginning at the lips, proper sphincter function is necessary for delivery of food to the mouth and its containment during mastication. The tongue assists in mastication, along with the cheeks, by keeping food in the proper position to be chewed, and then helps deliver the bolus into the oral pharynx. Salivary glands, which drain into the oral cavity, contribute to formation of the food bolus, provide initial contact with digestive enzymes, as well as form a protective layer for the oral cavity mucosa and teeth.

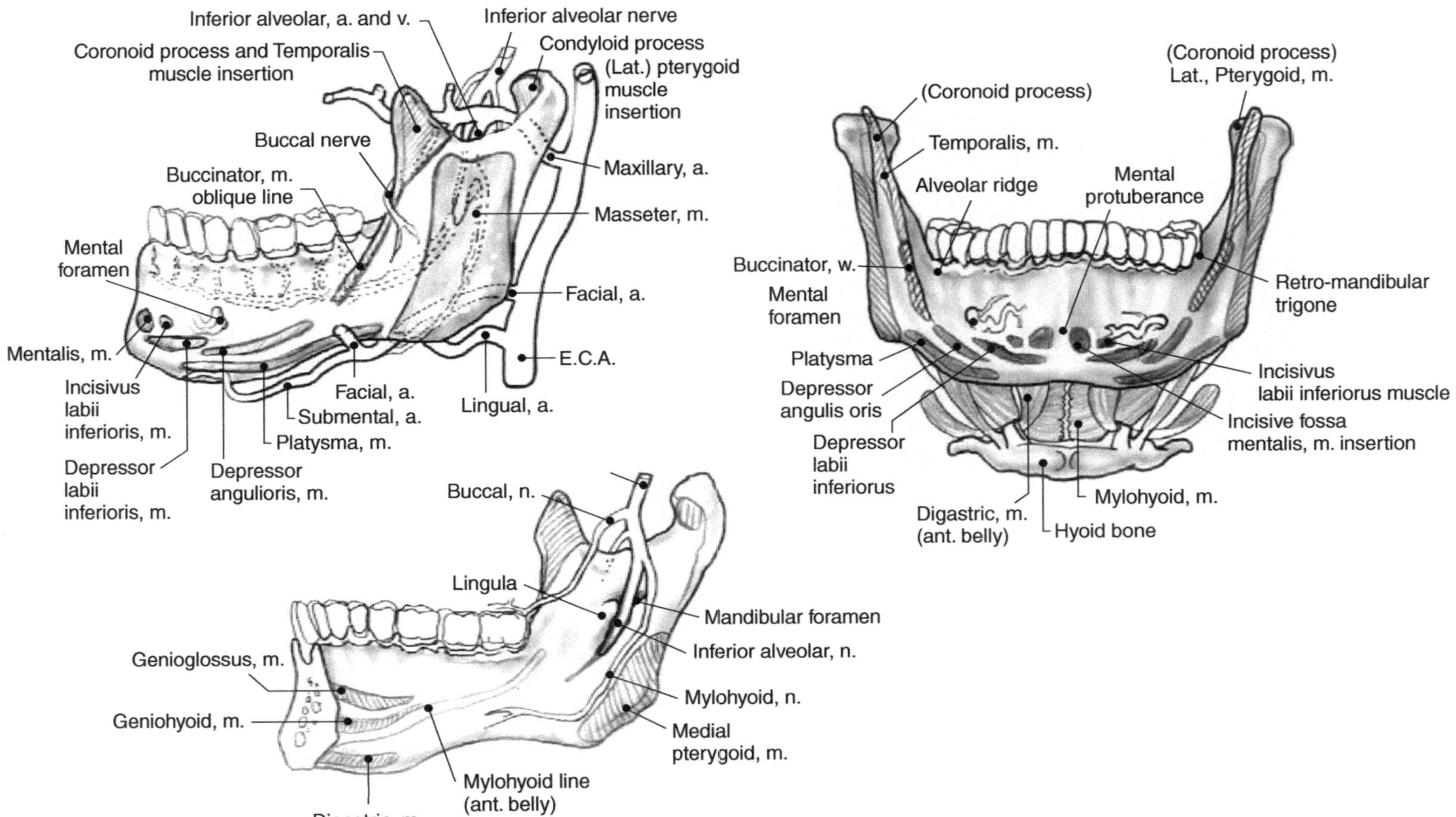

Figure 8 Detailed bony and neuromuscular anatomy of the mandible.

The lips contribute to facial expression. Smiling, frowning, surprise, anger, and other emotions can all be quickly communicated through changing lip position. Inability to move the lips can significantly impact non-verbal communication.

Enunciation and speech are additional critical functions of the oral cavity. Although the larynx generates much of the sound of speech, these tones are shaped into words through the combined actions of oral cavity components. For example, interactions among the tongue, teeth, and lips help escaping air form fricative versus plosive consonant sounds. Similarly, cheek and mandible position affect vowel formation.

The hard and soft palates function to separate the nasal cavity and nasal pharynx from the oral cavity and oral pharynx below. Malfunction or absence of parts of the palate can result in hypernasal speech and regurgitation of the food bolus into the nasal cavity or nasal pharynx. Children with cleft palates suffer difficulties with both speech and eating.

CONCLUSION

The oral cavity represents a complex anatomic area. Malfunction or absence of any one area can lead to significant functional problems. For example, subtle lip weakness or malposition can result in a speech impediment and loss of oral sphincter competence. Resection of part of the palate can result in velopalatal insufficiency or oronasal fistula with resulting hypernasal speech and dysphagia. The important functions of each small area of the oral cavity make reconstruction of this region particularly challenging as many ablative and traumatic defects of the oral cavity may involve several subsets of the anatomic area. Because a composite resection of the oral cavity can involve removal of part of the soft palate, buccal mucosa, retromolar trigone, floor of mouth, and tongue, a detailed knowledge of oral cavity anatomy is required for good judgment during resection, and it can guide the surgeon in providing maximal restoration of function.

REFERENCES

1. Clemente CD. Anatomy. Baltimore: Urban & Schwartzenberg, 1981.
2. Netter FH. Atlas of Human Anatomy. New Jersey: Novartis Medical Education, 1997.
3. Sessions DG, Cummings CW, Weymuller EA Jr, Makielski KH, Wood P. Atlas of Access and Reconstruction in Head & Neck Surgery. New York: Mosby Year Book, 1992.
4. Woodburne RT. Essentials of Human Anatomy. New York: Oxford University Press, 1978.

3
Functional Aspects and Physiology of the Oral Cavity

Gregory K. Hartig
Department of Otolaryngology, University of Wisconsin—Madison, Madison, Wisconsin, U.S.A.

INTRODUCTION

Wide excision remains the usual method for management of oral cavity carcinomas. With more advanced lesions, these resections often involve sacrifice of multiple subunits of the oral cavity. The resultant defect is rightfully of secondary concern in this ablative effort; however, our subsequent reconstructive efforts must then attempt to restore the form and function that has been lost. This effort requires an understanding of the normal physiology and function of the oral cavity and an understanding of which oral functions are most affected by which type of resection. Furthermore, we must understand the plasticity of these various functions and the potential for their recovery. Additionally, we must appreciate the effect of loss of these functions on a patient's overall quality of life. To this end, this chapter provides a brief review of the embryology of the oral cavity followed by a discussion of normal oral cavity functions, then, a discussion of abnormal functions imposed by resection, and finally, the aspects of our reconstructive efforts, which relate directly to preservation and restoration of these functions.

EMBRYOLOGY

The embryologic origins of the various tissues composing the oral cavity can be traced back to the mesoderm of the paraxial and lateral plates, the ectodermal placodes, and neural crest tissue (1). However, the most straightforward organization of these derivatives is to consider their origins from the pharyngeal arches, which form in the fourth and fifth weeks of gestation. Each arch contains all three germ cell layers and gives rise to a major arterial derivative, a bone or cartilaginous derivative, a cranial nerve, and the musculature associated with that cranial nerve (2). Although the arches are separated by clefts externally and pouches internally, the pouches and clefts never communicate, as in the branchia of lower animals (2,3).

The first pharyngeal arch consists of a dorsal maxillary process and a ventral mandibular process. The Meckel's cartilage of the first arch gives rise to the bone of the palate (maxilla and premaxilla) and the mandible. In addition, the first arch also forms the zygoma, part of the temporal bone, and the incus and malleus. The first arch also gives rise to the trigeminal nerve, which in turn supplies the muscles of mastication (medial and lateral pterygoid, temporalis, masseter, anterior belly of the digastric, mylohyoid, and tensor veli palatini) (2,3).

The second arch cartilage (Reichert's cartilage) gives rise to the upper part of the hyoid body, the lesser horns of the hyoid, the styloid process, and the stapes. The facial nerve arises from the second pharyngeal arch and supplies the muscles of facial expression, the posterior belly of the digastric muscle, the stylohyoid muscle and ligament, and the stapedeus and auricular musculature (2,3).

The third pharyngeal arch cartilage gives rise to the lower portion of the hyoid body and its greater horns. Its cranial nerve is the glossopharyngeal, which innervates the stylopharyngeous muscle. The fourth pharyngeal arch is associated with the superior laryngeal branch of the vagus, which supplies the levator veli palatini as well as the cricothyroid muscle (1,2). Because they are in close proximity to the oral cavity, the first pharyngeal pouch gives rise to the Eustachian tube and middle ear cavity, and the second pharyngeal pouch to the palatine tonsils.

The tongue begins to develop at four weeks gestation as a single medial tongue bud (tuberculum impar) and two laterally positioned tongue buds, all of which arise from the first pharyngeal arch. The two lateral tongue buds overgrow the medial tongue bud and fuse at the midline, forming the anterior two-thirds of the tongue. Posteriorly, the copula is formed from fusion of ventromedial aspects of the second pharyngeal arches. The hypobranchial eminence, formed from the ventromedial aspects of the third and fourth pharyngeal arches, eventually overgrows the copula and develops into the posterior third of the tongue. The anterior and posterior aspects of the tongue fuse at the terminal sulcus. The tongue musculature develops from myocytes derived from the occipital myotomes and is innervated by the hypoglossal nerve (2,3).

The facial prominences also begin to develop during the fourth week of gestation. Paired maxillary prominences develop lateral to the stomodeum (primordial mouth), paired mandibular prominences caudal to it, and the frontonasal prominence rostral to it. The mandibular prominences fuse across the midline forming the lower jaw, lower lip, and lower cheeks. Nasal placodes develop on the inferior border of the frontonasal prominence. These invaginate, producing nasal pits and medial and lateral nasal prominences. The maxillary prominences grow medially causing the lateral and medial nasal prominences to fuse with each other and the maxillary prominences, thus forming the upper cheeks and maxilla. The fused maxillary prominences form the intermaxillary segment, which gives rise to the philtrum of the upper lip, four incisors, premaxillary aspect of the maxilla, and the primary palate. Outgrowths from the maxillary prominences, known as palatine shelves, migrate into a horizontal position and fuse at the midline to produce the secondary palate. The secondary palate fuses anteriorly with the primary palate, separated by the incisive fossa. Bone develops in the primary palate and then migrates posteriorly to the anterior portion of the secondary palate (1,2).

The salivary glands develop between the sixth and twelfth weeks of gestation. The parotid glands arise first, in the sixth week of development, as invaginations of the ectodermal epithelium at the angles of the stomodeum. They migrate posteriorly to the ascending rami of the mandible. During this migration, the facial nerves migrate anteriorly. The submandibular glands develop late in the sixth week of gestation from the endoderm in the floor of the stomodeum. Then the sublingual glands develop in the eighth week from endodermal buds in the paralingual sulcus. The minor salivary glands develop last, in the twelfth week of gestation (1,3).

ORAL COMPETENCE

Normal

The primary function of the lips and the corresponding musculature is to provide oral competence. The basic structure of the lips appears simple with a musculature core covered with skin on its outer surface and mucosa on its inner surface. However, the sensory and motor functions of the lips are complex (Fig. 2, chap. 1). The primary muscle involved is the orbicularis oris, which is composed of four independent quadrants, each separated into a pars peripheralis and a pars marginalis (4). From a functional standpoint, it is more straightforward to consider the obicularis oris muscle a solid ring of muscle divided into a deep and superficial component. The deep component provides the lips with sphincteric action, which includes a unique association between the obicularis fibers of the upper and lower lips where the upper lip fibers split and the lower lip fibers pass through the split. Upon contraction, this forms a seal at the angles of the mouth (5). Contraction of the deep muscle fibers of the orbicularis oris allows the lips to form a seal around eating utensils in order to bring food into the mouth, prevent food from exiting the oral cavity anteriorly, and prevent drooling (6). The orbicularis oris receives motor innervation via the buccal and marginal mandibular divisions of the facial nerve (4).

The superficial muscle fibers of the orbicularis oris function in the finer movements of the lips, as do many muscles of facial expression (4). The incisivus superioris and inferioris are considered to be accessory muscles to the orbicularis oris, serving to press the upper lip against the teeth. The levator anguli oris raises the corners of the mouth; the depressor anguli oris moves the corners of the mouth down and laterally; the risorius retracts the angle of the mouth laterally. The zygomaticus major brings the angle of the mouth superiorly and laterally. Collectively, these muscles (orbicularis oris, incisvus superioris and inferioris, levator anguli oris, depressor anguli oris, risorius, and zygomaticus major), along with the buccinator, converge at the angle of the mouth, forming the modiolus. Another group of muscles (levator labii superioris, levator labii superioris alaeque nasi, and zygomaticus minor) enters the upper lip. The levator labii superioris is the main elevator of the lip but also causes slight eversion of the upper lip. The levator labii superioris alaeque nasi dilates the nostril and elevates and everts the upper lip, whereas the zygomaticus minor elevates and curls the upper lip. Finally, the muscle group comprised of the depressor labii inferioris, mentalis, and platysma enters the lower lip. The depressor labii inferioris depresses and pulls the lower lip slightly laterally. The mentalis maintains the position of the lower lip and chin while at rest, but upon contraction protrudes and elevates the lower lip. Most of the muscles in the lips are paired, with the exception of the mentalis muscle of the lower lip, which provides the lower lip with greater speed and force than the upper lip (5). Although the lips often act simultaneously, they can be activated separately, as proven by phonation of sounds such as "f" (4). The platysma assists in opening the mouth and may play a role in depression and lateral movement of the mouth (4,5). Sensory innervation of the upper lip is provided by the infraorbital nerve (V2), whereas lower lip sensation is supplied by the mental nerve (terminal component of inferior alveolar branch of V3) (5).

Abnormal

Difficulties in oral competence can take several forms. Loss of sensory input can result in loss of competence even with an intact muscular sphincter. For example, Sandstedt and Sorensen sent out a questionnaire to individuals who had suffered trigeminal nerve damage (6,7). Of the 226 individuals who responded, greater than 70% had sensory disturbances. Of those with sensory deficits in the lower lip, 54% had issues of insecurity; 56% had decreased oral competence, manifested by drooling; 50% complained of biting their lip.

Sacrifice of the mental nerve (lower lip) or inferior alveolar nerve (upper lip) might occur with resection of soft tissue alone or with resection of the mandible or maxilla, respectively. Loss of upper lip sensation alone does not result in oral incompetence. Mental nerve loss, however, is more problematic and with nerve grafting, some of this lost sensation can be recovered. When a lateral or anterior segmental resection has been performed for carcinoma of the mandible, the proximal and distal inferior alveolar nerve stumps are typically sampled using frozen section to rule out perineural tumor involvement. Assuming a clear margin, the remaining proximal nerve stump within the mandible is in a poor position for grafting, especially if an osseous flap is being used for reconstruction. However, the remaining nerve can usually be pulled out of the mandible with gentle traction and brought through the inferior alveolar canal. This provides a more easily approached proximal nerve stump for placement of an interposition cable nerve graft to re-establish connection between this proximal inferior alveolar nerve stump and the distal mental nerve stump.

Loss of muscular control of the oral sphincter can occur with loss of the lower division of the facial nerve or with loss of the soft tissues including the obicularis muscle of the lower lip. The marginal mandibular and buccal branches supply the obicularis oris and the additional musculature of the lower lip. Loss of the marginal mandibular nerve is a more likely event than loss of the buccal branches. With loss of the marginal mandibular nerve, one loses function of the depressor musculature of the lower lip, resulting in elevation of the ipsilateral lower lip and consequent asymmetry of the smile. Loss of the marginal mandibular nerve alone typically does not result in significant loss of oral competence; however, when coupled with mental nerve loss, significant incompetence often occurs. Such losses of oral competence can be addressed with re-innervation or suspension in the form of passive or active sling procedures.

When the oral sphincter is impaired by significant resection, again, typically involving the lower lip, re-establishment of the oral sphincter is most successful when innervated lip tissues can be utilized. In general, lip-switch procedures and use of local- or distant-tissue transfers for lip reconstruction will produce an asensate lower lip segment, which can result in incompetence due to loss of sensory and motor function. However, there is some initial return of sensory function along with partial motor function (8). As expected, this is less important with upper lip reconstruction. In contrast, advancement of lip tissues with an intact neurovascular pedicle, like the Karapanzic flap, is preferred because sensory and motor functions are preserved (9).

Another issue affecting oral competence is that of lip height. When malignancies of the anterior mandibular arch involve the mucosa and soft tissue of the lower lip, our reconstructive efforts must allow the re-establishment of lower lip height. The physician should consider the potential for contracture to reduce the reconstructed lip height. Given the thickness of the cutaneous component of the flap relative to normal lip thickness, persons undergoing osteocutaneous free-flap reconstruction of this area will often have what appears to be excessive bulk of the lower lip early in their recovery. Adequate wound maturation should be allowed prior to debulking, because efforts to thin this tissue or to prepare the site for dental implants can result in further wound contracture and loss of lip height.

SALIVATION

Normal

The role of saliva is to moisten and protect oral and pharyngeal mucosa, lubricate, transmit taste information, buffer chemicals, initiate carbohydrate digestion, act as an antimicrobial agent, prevent dental caries, and participate in enamel formation (10,11). The oral cavity houses three major paired salivary glands [parotid, submandibular (submaxillary), and sublingual] and hundreds of minor salivary glands. The minor salivary glands are primarily located in the buccal, labial, palatal, and lingual regions, but are also found at the superior pole of the tonsils, tonsillar pillars, and base of the tongue (10). Together, the major and minor salivary glands produce 1000–1500 mL of saliva per day, equivalent to an average salivary flow rate of 1 mL/min, depending on salivary gland stimulation (12). Each gland at rest secretes at a rate of 0.001–0.2 mL/min, and secretion increases to 0.18–1.7 mL/min when the glands are stimulated (10). The gland distribution of salivary production also depends on whether a stimulus is present: the parotid gland produces approximately two-thirds of the total saliva when stimulated, but, under resting conditions, is responsible for only 26% of total production (13,14). At rest, the submandibular and sublingual glands produce 69% and 5% of total saliva, respectively (14). Minor salivary gland output varies little with stimulation and accounts for less than 10% of total overall salivary production (15). The parotid gland consists mainly of serous acinar cells that produce watery saliva, whereas the sublingual gland has mainly mucous acinar cells that produce viscous saliva. The submandibular glands have both mucous and serous acinar cells and produce saliva of intermediate viscosity (10).

Once saliva is produced, it travels by ducts to enter the oral cavity. Stensen's duct exits the parotid gland from its anterior border, travels anterior to the masseter muscle and through the buccinator muscle to enter the oral cavity through a papilla opposite the second upper molar. The Wharton's duct orifice exits from the medial surface of the submandibular gland and opens to the oral cavity lateral to the lingual frenulum. Saliva from the sublingual glands travels through multiple (usually 10) separate ducts, collectively referred to as Ducts of Rivinus, which open into the sublingual fold or plica of the mouth floor. Occasionally, a number of these ducts converge to form a Bartholin's duct, which empties into Wharton's duct (10).

Both sympathetic and parasympathetic nerve stimulation cause salivary secretion. Sympathetic nerve fibers from the superior cervical ganglion enter the glands with the arterial supply (external carotid artery to the parotid gland, facial artery to submandibular gland, and lingual artery to sublingual gland). Such stimulation produces a small volume of viscous saliva, which ceases after prolonged stimulation. Parasympathetic nerve stimulation is provided through cranial nerves 7 and 9. Preganglionic parasympathetic fibers from the glossopharyngeal nerve reach the otic ganglion via the lesser superficial petrosal nerve, and the postganglionic fibers continue to the parotid gland via the auriculotemporal nerve (branch of V3). Preganglionic fibers in the chorda tympani travel with the lingual nerve to the submandibular ganglion (Fig. 6, chap. 1). Postganglionic fibers then cause stimulation of the submandibular gland. Some of these postganglionic fibers travel in the lingual nerve to the sublingual glands. Parasympathetic stimulation produces a large volume of watery saliva that is secreted throughout the entire time of stimulation (11).

The composition of saliva varies according to a number of factors including rate of secretion, stimulus duration, dominant gland involved, time of day, and season of the year (17). The average pH of saliva is between 6.2 and 7.4, consisting chiefly of water (99.5%) and organic and inorganic solvents (0.5%). Saliva also contains sodium (10 mEq/L) potassium (26 mEq/L) chlorine (10 mEq/L), and bicarbonate (30 mEq/L) (16). Saliva also contains proteins, calcium, magnesium, and phosphate (17,18). With a slight increase in salivary flow rate, sodium and bicarbonate concentration and pH increase while potassium, calcium, phosphate, chloride, and protein content decrease. When flow rate is greatly increased, concentrations of sodium, calcium, chloride, bicarbonate, protein, and pH increase. At the highest flow rate, phosphate concentration decreases and potassium concentration remains unchanged. An increased duration of stimulation is known to increase protein, calcium, and bicarbonate concentrations and pH while chloride concentration decreases (17).

Abnormal

Although, resection of major salivary glands does negatively impact overall saliva production, in most patients, there will be few complaints of xerostomia with resection alone. In contrast, those who have undergone either primary or post-operative radiotherapy to the oral cavity will usually complain of some degree of xerostomia. Often patients find that xerostomia is their most problematic long-term side effect of treatment. Although, salivary substitutes and parasympathetic agonists help somewhat, most patients opt for keeping their oral cavity moist with regular and frequent small sips of water. Without this regular moistening of the oral cavity, speech becomes distorted by adherence of oral mucous membranes to one another. Ease of mastication is obviously dependent on the water content of the foodstuff in question, and as expected, increased water intake is required for drier foods. These difficulties with xerostomia are further exacerbated by the presence of cutaneous surfaces within the oral cavity. The keratin produced by the skin has poorer clearance in patients with xerostomia.

MASTICATION

Normal

Mastication involves coordination of complex movements of the mandible, tongue, and teeth. The muscles of mastication (masseter, temporalis, and medial and lateral pterygoids) control the movements of the mandible. The masseter elevates and protrudes the mandible while the temporalis elevates it further (19). When unilaterally contracted, the medial and lateral pterygoids move the mandible laterally, but bilateral contraction causes the medial pterygoids to elevate the mandible while the lateral pterygoids cause depression and protrusion (17). Motor innervation of these muscles is provided by the mandibular division of the trigeminal nerve (V3). The paired mylohyoid and digastric muscles also have a role in mandibular motion, as both contribute to depression of the mandible (5). Motor innervation of the mylohyoid and anterior belly of the digastric is provided by the mylohyoid nerve, a branch of the inferior alveolar nerve (5). The posterior belly of the digastric is innervated by the facial nerve (5). The first phase of jaw closure is caused by elastic recoil of the stretched jaw-closing muscles in coordination with relaxation of jaw-opening muscles. Jaw closure then continues with the medial pterygoids, followed by the anterior temporalis and then the posterior temporalis and masseter muscles (18). Jaw opening is initiated by the mylohyoid and continues with the digastric and lateral pterygoid muscles (18). The masseter muscles also contribute to jaw opening as they relax and are stretched under the weight of the mandible. Rotational movement of the mandible is produced by the pterygoids (18). During opening and closing of the jaw, the muscles are in an isotonic state, but during occlusion or when crushing a bolus, the muscles are in an isometric state (18).

The tongue musculature consists of both intrinsic and extrinsic muscles. The intrinsic muscles (superior longitudinal, inferior longitudinal, vertical, and transverse) have no bony connections and serve to alter the form of the tongue and receive their motor innervation via the hypoglossal nerve. The extrinsic muscles (genioglossus, hyoglossus, styloglossus, and palatoglossus) cause movement of the tongue relative to other oral cavity structures. The extrinsic muscles also receive motor innervation via the hypoglossal nerve except for the palatoglossus, which is innervated via the pharyngeal plexus (18).

The palate is controlled by numerous muscles which receive motor innervation from the pharyngeal plexus (18). The palatoglossus raises the tongue, and the palatopharyngeous elevates the larynx and pharynx, all of which narrow the oropharyngeal opening. The musculus uvulae alters the uvula, and the levator veli palatini elevates the soft palate to bring it in contact with the posterior pharyngeal wall. The tensor veli palatini moves the soft palate laterally, producing rigidity.

The average adult mouth houses 32 permanent teeth, obviously varying greatly among individuals. Each quadrant of the jaw typically contains two incisors (maxillary larger than mandibular), one canine, two premolars, and three molars (decreasing in size distally). An individual tooth is comprised of a crown, coated with a 1.5 mm layer of enamel, and a root, covered with cement and separated by the cervical margin. The body of the tooth is made of dentine and contains a pulp cavity at its core. The root is surrounded by alveolar bone, which undergoes resorption when teeth are lost, and a 0.2-mm thick periodontal ligament separates the two structures. Gingiva surrounds the tooth, periodontal ligament, and bone near the cervical margin (5).

During central occlusion, teeth achieve maximum contact. In this position, the mandibular canines and post-canines are slightly in front of their maxillary counterparts. The mandibular incisors make contact with the lingual aspect of their maxillary counterparts during mastication (5). Mastication is neither completely voluntary or involuntary: masticatory movements can be voluntarily initiated, but these motions continue without further voluntary input. This involuntary activity is thought to be mediated by the chewing reflex as shown by Sherrington in his work with decerebrate animals (19). In this study, with downward forces on the jaw, possibly due to gravity or food, the stretching of muscles activates muscle spindle receptors, which in turn lead to contraction of the jaw-closing musculature. As the jaw closes, food in the oral cavity comes in contact with the teeth, gingiva, or hard palate, inhibiting further contraction of these jaw-closing muscles and stimulating contraction of jaw-opening muscles. As this cycle continues, the stimuli grow weaker, decreasing inhibition of the jaw-closing musculature. A chewing cycle lasts approximately two-thirds of a second and the bolus is in contact with the teeth for

20% of this time (20). This reflex is unilateral, reacting only to the side of the mouth containing the food bolus (19).

The rate of chewing is quite variable but is thought to have an average rate of 1–2 strokes/sec. The time necessary for mouth opening is not significantly different than that for mouth closing: the mouth opens at a rate of about 7–8 cm/sec, with a rotary downward movement toward the side with the bolus, and when closing, the mandible returns to the position of central occlusion at a rate of over 10 cm/sec. Chewing generally takes place bilaterally for the first 3–4 strokes, after which the food bolus is moved to a preferred side (19).

We are capable of producing chewing forces much greater than those needed for a normal human diet. In 1948, Howell and Manly measured the maximal force between incisors to be 130–240 N and that between molars to be 22–881 N in tested subjects ($n=4$) (21). A more recent study has shown the mean maximal bite force of the molar and premolar area to be 738 N $\pm$ 209 N whereas investigators in a similar study reported that the mean maximal bite force of the molar area is 847 N in men and 597 N in women (22,23). However, these maximal forces are 25–30% less in individuals with full dentures (18). The actual force used during mastication varies according to the properties of the food, with harder foods necessitating higher pressures (20).

Chewing efficiency is dependent on a number of factors including dental occlusion, producible force, number and position of teeth, strength of teeth, and their periodontal structure, function of musculature involved in mastication, and time given to chew. Molars are important to chewing efficiency because the first and second molar can provide up to 70% of the chewing surface area. Some individuals have decreased efficiency secondary to limited chewing tolerance due to factors such as pain.

It has also been shown that chewing efficiency is best in individuals with normal teeth and better in those with partials than complete dentures. Duration of mastication is prolonged in patients with partials compared to complete dentures, but this is thought to be due to the increased periodontal proprioception in this group (24). Also, persons with partial dentures tend to seek regular dental follow-up because they have a high desire to retain their remaining natural teeth. In contrast, patients with complete dentures tend to neglect dental follow-up. The mandibular alveolus undergoes a slow but progressive resorption in the edentulous patient, and as this resorption becomes more dramatic over time, the ability to use a tissue-borne denture is eventually lost because the alveolar ridge necessary for stabilization is progressively shallower.

Abnormal

Discussion of abnormal mastication will be limited to impairments in the movement of the mandible. Although resections of the tongue can negatively effect mastication, these will be discussed as impairments in bolus formation and propulsion in a later section of this chapter.

Resection of the lateral oral cavity soft tissues is often performed with preservation of the ipsilateral mandible. In this setting, scar contracture can result in significant limitation in temporomandibular joint (TMJ) range of motion with resultant trismus. This is particularly true with larger resections of the buccal soft tissues and muscles of mastication.

The amount of scar contracture that forms is governed by multiple issues, including the volume of resection, the amount and location of pterygoid or masseter muscle loss, the addition of post-operative radiotherapy, and the type of reconstruction employed. For example, one would expect the maximal amount of contracture with healing by secondary intent, some improvement with a split-thickness skin graft, more with a full-thickness graft and the best result with vascularized tissue such as a radial forearm, free-tissue transfer. Heavier and thicker flaps will produce excessive bulk, which can prevent adequate mastication by placing soft tissue between the occlusal surfaces of the mandibular and maxillary alveolus. Often, even with a well-planned and ultimately successful reconstruction, the temporary swelling associated with the inflammatory phase of healing will produce this difficulty with mastication.

Although, replacement with a vascularized flap is helpful, a second important component of minimizing trismus is the use of aggressive post-operative physical therapy. This therapy should be initiated early to counteract the contraction that occurs during maturation of the wound.

Most difficulties with mastication are the result of segmental resections of the mandible. Resection of the lateral mandible creates an unbalanced set of forces in the pterygoid and masseter muscles. The pterygoids are greater in bulk and stronger than the masseters and will therefore overpower the masseter and pull the remaining intact mandible inwardly or medially. Some physicians think that this medial displacement lessens the cosmetic deformity produced by resection of the hemimandible (25). This jaw shift produces a cross-bite malocclusion. However, with guide training, the patient can be taught to correct much of this malocclusion (25). With a lateral mandibular defect, most dentulous patients will resume chewing and often have surprisingly little deterioration in their diet when compared to their preoperative diet status. In edentulous patients, the loss of masticatory ability with lateral resection is also surprisingly minor. Even so, these unbalanced movements produce an abnormal set of forces on the TMJ. In younger patients with anticipated longevity, TMJ arthritis is more likely.

Reconstruction of the lateral mandible with an osteocutaneous free flap or with a soft-tissue flap and plate will maintain the original size and contour of the oral cavity. Heavier bone flaps such as the iliac crest or fibula will also allow for implant-borne dental restoration. However, in most cases these osteocutaneous flaps also bring in a cutaneous soft tissue component, which remains largely asensate and adynamic. In some cases, this cutaneous component becomes problematic with bolus formation or food retention in this portion of the oral cavity. This is most likely to occur in areas with a natural concavity, which might harbor foodstuffs, such as the floor of mouth (FOM) and labial/buccal sulcus. In contrast, in the non-reconstructed patient, the oral cavity can often be closed primarily. The size of the oral cavity can then be significantly decreased, because the mandibular arch no longer restricts it. This avoids the previously mentioned difficulties that can be encountered with asensate skin in the oral cavity. Also, with these primary closures, the slope of the closure tends to slant toward the unresected side, which helps keep food on the "normal" side of the mouth. Typically, in patients with a higher performance status, the advantages of reconstruction of the lateral mandible will outweigh these negatives. A comparison of pectoralis major or radial forearm flap plus plate reconstructions demonstrated a slight reduction in plate extrusion with the free forearm group. Also, no real difference in oral deglutition or facial contour was seen when these soft-tissue-plus-plate options were compared with osteocutaneous free-flap reconstruction of the lateral mandible (26). However, only the latter reconstruction allows for consideration of implants.

Loss of the anterior mandibular arch produces profound impairment in mastication and all other oral functions. Even those who are less inclined toward free-tissue transfer will agree that osteocutaneous free flaps are the best reconstruction option for these defects. However, even with bony free-flap reconstruction, aberrations in mastication can occur. For example, loss of the anterior musculature of the mandible (mylohyoid and digastric muscles) results in impairment in jaw opening. In addition, loss of this portion of the mandible results in loss of hyoid suspension with consequent downward displacement of the larynx and resultant propensity for aspiration. As a result, hyoid suspension is helpful with anterior mandibular reconstruction.

BOLUS FORMATION AND PROPULSION

Normal

During oral preparation, the stage in which pleasure for food and eating is experienced, food is manipulated to a texture that is appropriate for swallowing (27). The incisors are used for vertical movements such as biting, during which the lips and anterior portion of the tongue manipulate the food (18,21). The anterior third of the tongue is responsible for the manipulation of food such as taking the food off a utensil, lapping, or licking, etc. (28). The molars use lateral and vertical movements to crush and grind food (18), whereas the cheek and the body of the tongue manipulate food into the correct position (29). The middle third of the tongue is used to maintain appropriate placement of food during mastication. This portion of the tongue moves the food into the lateral food channels positioned over the sides of the tongue and between the teeth (28). The tongue is also used to crush food against the hard palate (17), manipulating food into particles that are only a few cubic millimetre in volume (20). Facial tone from contraction of the buccal musculature prevents food from entering anterior and lateral sulci, between the lips or buccal mucosa and the mandible, thus keeping the food in the medial oral cavity (27). During this phase, the palatoglossus muscle descends the soft palate to prevent food from prematurely entering the oropharynx as well as to increase the width of the nasal airway (27,30).

After the oral preparatory stage of the swallow just described, the next stage of swallowing is known as the oral phase, which takes approximately 0.7–1.2 seconds (31). This stage is voluntary and causes the food bolus to move from the oral cavity to the oropharynx. Once a bolus is formed, it can be held between the dorsal surface of the tongue and the hard palate or between the tongue and the floor of the mouth (27). If the bolus is in the latter position, the tongue must maneuver the bolus to its dorsal surface prior to bolus propulsion (27). The intrinsic muscles of the tongue move the bolus to the dorsal surface of the tongue, which is referred to as the preparatory position (18). The elevating movement of the anterior and lateral portions of the tongue is also used to separate the 5–15 cm^3 portion of the bolus that is an acceptable texture to be swallowed from other oral cavity contents (20,29). If a smaller volume of only several cubic centimetre is swallowed, the oral cavity does not close around this small volume as it does with a larger bolus. Instead, assuming an anterior seal (i.e., competent oral sphincter) there is significant admixture with air such that, for small bolus sizes, there is significant aerophagia (31).

Two distinct but not mutually exclusive theories are thought to explain the neural control of the oral and pharyngeal stages of swallowing. The first, the reflex chain hypothesis, suggests that the act of swallowing is a chain of reflexes in which one action (movement of the bolus) stimulates the next. The second hypothesis, the central pattern generator hypothesis, states that deglutition is controlled by the medullary swallowing center (32). Thus, once swallowing is initiated, the process continues independent of sensory feedback (32).

After the bolus is formed, it is necessary to move it from the oral cavity to the oropharynx, which is known as bolus propulsion. The mandible is kept in a closed position to stabilize the tongue musculature (32). The posterior third of the tongue plays a major role in bolus propulsion, especially when the bolus volume is large (28,31). The posterior third of the tongue acts like a wedge once food has entered the oropharynx by opposing the soft palate and pharyngeal constrictors, which, in turn, pushes the bolus downward. With smaller bolus volumes, the pharyngeal constrictors play a larger role in this propulsion, because a bolus of this size can simply be spilled into the oropharynx (29,31). The anterior tip of the tongue comes in contact with the hard palate and the lateral aspects of the tongue contact the alveolar ridge or the pharyngeal wall, which provides the pressure necessary to propel the bolus into the pharynx (30). The central groove of the tongue then undergoes centripetal (contraction of the genioglossus muscle and vertical and transverse intrinsic muscles of the tongue) and centrifugal motion, causing a wave-like or rolling movement, which acts to transport the bolus (31). The mylohyoid elevates the floor of the mouth (16). The soft palate is then elevated by musculus uvulae, levator veli palatini, and tensor veli palatini to close off the nasopharynx, thereby preventing the generated pressure from dissipating through the nasopharynx and preventing the bolus from being refluxed into the nasopharynx (18). When the bolus reaches the facial arches, sensory receptors are triggered and the pharyngeal swallow reflex is initiated (27). Pharyngeal pressure generators activate when the pharyngeal swallow is initiated (30). In general, that part of a food bolus which falls behind the glossopalatal junction will be swallowed, where as that component anterior to this junction remains in the oral cavity (31).

The frequency of deglutition varies among individuals and also according to the activity being performed. An average value for number of swallows/hr was determined to be 24, which is equivalent to about 585 swallows/day (5). This frequency of swallowing increases 7- to 12-fold during the act of eating (33). When an individual is asleep, the rate of swallowing decreases to an average of 5.8–7.5 swallows/hr, and this activity chiefly occurs during the processes of falling asleep or waking or during periods associated with movement arousals (32,34).

Abnormal

Abnormalities in bolus formation and propulsion can occur with disease processes or anatomical changes created by surgical manipulation that promote food retention, result in loss of bolus manipulation and propulsion, and/or result in bolus escape.

The creation of asensate concavities or pockets within the oral cavity produces problems with food retention for different reasons depending on the reconstruction options. For example, the pectoralis major flap has excess weight and bulk, which can pull the oral soft tissues downward. The lighter platysma flap has a pedicle, which is shorter along its medial skin edge than along the lateral edge; therefore, when a platysma flap is brought into the FOM, the medial edge between the ventral tongue and the platysma skin will pull downward, creating a "pedicle pull." This problem can be avoided with the similar but better vascularized submental island skin flap or other free-tissue transfer options such as the radial forearm or lateral arm flap for FOM and tongue reconstruction. However, when using the radial forearm flap, it is easy to place too much tissue in the FOM, so limiting the flap size to the size of the resected area provides enough soft tissue to avoid limitation in tongue mobility, but avoids excess tissue that would result in bolus retention and stasis.

Another problem associated with reconstruction is re-establishing sensory input through re-innervation, which may improve overall function but does not fully restore normal function. Logemann and Bytell (35) found that patients with anterior FOM resection had significant problems with anterior stasis of the bolus with consequent oral incompetence and drooling.

Generally, most problems arising from reconstruction efforts can be eliminated via smaller revision procedures. Pedicles can be divided when adequate neovascularization has occurred, flaps can be debulked, and areas of cutaneous surface redundancy can be eliminated. When problems of food retention do occur despite the best efforts, patients can work with a swallowing therapist to develop strategies to clear the material during the act of eating. Also, with more fastidious oral care, problems with halitosis can be avoided.

Problems of bolus formation relate primarily to loss of anterior tongue function. As described above, the intrinsic musculature allows the shape of the tongue to be altered while the extrinsic musculature moves the tongue relative to the remainder of the oral cavity. In persons undergoing anterior tongue resection, reconstruction should focus on maintaining the sensory and motor function of the remaining anterior tongue. Often when less than half of the anterior tongue is involved, and the resection does not extend into the FOM, primary closure is the best method.

Although the patient will have less tongue bulk, the remaining tongue will be fully sensate and retain good mobility. In contrast, when FOM and alveolar subunits are also involved, reconstruction with skin grafts or vascularized flaps is required to retain tongue mobility; although, even this point is open to debate. A prospective analysis of speech and swallowing was conducted in patients ($n = 284$) who were divided into three groups based on the method of oral cavity and oropharyngeal resection (primary closure, myocutaneous flap, and free-tissue transfer). The study results suggested that, contrary to popular belief, primary closure resulted in equal or better function than the use of flap reconstruction in patients with a comparable locus of resection and percentage of oral tongue and tongue base resection (36). In general, patients often compensate better than expected with oral tongue reconstruction. It is important to emphasize the significant improvements that occur over time in those discouraged by initially poor speech and bolus formation/propulsion performance. This concept was demonstrated in a simple study by McFarland and colleagues, in which significant adaptive improvements were made in a very short interval (15 minutes) after patients received a palatal obturator (37).

In patients who have undergone near total or total glossectomy, the problems are somewhat different. Logemann and Bytell (35) found that oral transit time increased as the amount of resected lingual tissue increased. This finding was reinforced by studies that examined compensatory features of patients who have undergone near total or total glossectomy. Specifically, Kothary and Desouza clarified functional compensatory swallowing mechanisms in patients ($n = 25$) with total glossectomy. Because the patients lack a tongue for bolus propulsion, the food was passed by quickly tilting the head posteriorly, which placed the food in the oropharynx to initiate the pharyngeal phase of the swallow (38). A liquid or pureed diet is often most appropriate for total glossectomy patients in as much as the absence of tongue movement makes bolus formation and propulsion very difficult.

Restoration of form and bulk in patients who have undergone total glossectomy can greatly improve swallowing function. If the reconstructed oral mound (residual tongue or flap tissues) can make contact with the palate, the food bolus can be pushed posteriorly rather than simply using the head tilt maneuver previously described. The importance of apposition of the residual or reconstructed tongue with the palate was also proved by Robbins et al., who found improvements in speech with a palatal augmentation prosthesis that allowed improved contact of the oral mound with the palate and thus allowed improvement in articulation, voice speed, and intelligibility (39).

With regard to extent of resection and its relation to risk of aspiration, persons with good pulmonary reserve who undergo total glossectomy with resection of both hypoglossal nerves can be taught to swallow safely if their palatal and supraglottic sensation is preserved. Similarly, those who undergo resection of the entire tongue base and the epiglottis can be taught to swallow safely. In contrast, those who undergo total or near total glossectomy and also require epiglottic resection or resection of lateral oropharyngeal/palatal soft tissues will have significant aspiration difficulties. Similarly, those patients who undergo resection of the entire tongue base in conjunction with the entire supraglottic larynx will also perform poorly. Thus, the surgeon must determine when evidence suggests post-surgical swallowing failure, and he/she must attempt to prevent or manage the problem.

When deciding which patients will tolerate total glossectomy, the criterion for open supraglottic laryngectomy can be considered. First, the patient should have pulmonary function indices of at least 70% of predicted values. Next, the patient should understand that longer recovery time is required, that swallowing retraining may be necessary and is highly likely, and that a perioperative gastrostomy tube is generally necessary. The patient's age should also be considered. In general, younger patients do relatively well and those over the age of 70 do more poorly, even when preoperative functional status indicators look favorable.

Use of laryngeal suspension may also be beneficial. When near-total or total glossectomy is performed, the suprahyoid musculature has been divided and therefore the larynx descends inferiorly. Suspending the hyoid from the anterior mandible brings the larynx anteriorly and superiorly. In Weber et al.'s review of total and near-total glossectomy patients, none of the patients who had undergone laryngeal suspension had persistent aspiration, whereas 20% of those who did not undergo larygneal suspension had serious problems with aspiration (40).

TASTE

Normal

Taste buds are the receptors for the sensation of taste. These taste receptors are mainly located on the tongue, but can also be found on the palate, epiglottis, larynx, pharynx, uvula, proximal third of the esophagus, lips, and cheeks. On the tongue, taste buds are contained in three of the four varieties of papillae, which include fungiform, circumvillate, and foliate papillae; filiform papillae do not contain taste buds. Fungiform papillae are located on the anterior two-thirds of the tongue and each house 1–18 taste buds. The circumvillate papillae form a "V" on the posterior aspect of the tongue, just anterior to the sulcus terminalis. Foliate papillae can be found on the lateral aspect of the tongue, just anterior to the circumvillate papillae (41). Taste receptors undergo atrophic changes with age, generally beginning after the age of 45 (18).

Three cranial nerves are involved in the sensation of taste. The anterior two-thirds of the tongue (fungiform papillae, anterior foliate papillae) and the soft palate are innervated by the chorda tympani (branch of the facial nerve), which travels in the lingual nerve sheath. The posterior third of the tongue (circumvillate papillae and posterior foliate papillae) is innervated by the glossopharyngeal nerve. The vagus nerve innervates the tongue base, pharynx, larynx, uvula, and epiglottis. The tongue has four basic taste dimensions, each of which is sensed best at a specific location on the tongue. Sweet, bitter, sour, and salty tastes are discriminated at the tip, base, middle and lateral, and tip of the tongue, respectively (18).

Abnormal

The sense of smell and taste together are responsible for conveying the appeal of food. Loss or distortions in olfaction or the sense of taste will have negative impacts on quality of life and even on overall health. Persons who have an adequate swallowing mechanism but significant hypoguesia or dysguesia may become nutritionally depleted and even cachectic due to the loss of interest in food.

Abnormalities in taste occur in persons who have undergone operations that result in loss of olfaction such as anterior craniofacial resection and laryngectomy. Surprisingly, unless an individual has had a total glossectomy, most persons do not complain of hypoguesia or dysguesia as a result of surgical resection of the tongue alone. In contrast, those who have also undergone radiotherapy to the oral cavity have significant difficulties with loss of taste or more commonly, impairments of taste.

CONCLUSION

In conclusion, the normal physiologic functions of the oral cavity are almost always affected in some way by the treatment of oral cavity carcinomas. Given the heterogeneity of these lesions, and the variable health of the patents affected, consistently accurate predictions of impairment can be difficult. However, with thorough pre-treatment counseling, thoughtful use of reconstructive options, and early and continued post-treatment rehabilitation, we can minimize the functional morbidities experienced by our patients.

ACKNOWLEDGMENT

The author would like to thank Dr. Susan Martinelli for her assistance and research in preparation of this chapter.

REFERENCES

1. Moore K, Persaud T, Moore K, Persaud T. The Pharyngeal (Branchial) Apparatus, Before We Are Born. Philadelphia: Saunders, 1998:197–239.
2. Sadler T. Head and neck. In: Sadler T, ed. Langman's Medical Embryology. Baltimore: Williams & Wilkins, 1995:312–346.
3. Moore K, Persaud T. The Pharyngeal (Branchial) Apparatus, Before We Are Born. Philadelphia: Saunders, 1998:197–239.

4. Calhoun K. Lip anatomy and function. In: Stiernberg C, ed. Surgery of the Lip. New York: Thieme Medical Publishers, Inc., 1992:1–10.
5. Williams PL, et al. Gray's Anatomy. New York: Churchill Livingston, 1995.
6. Dao TT, Mellor A. Sensory disturbances associated with implant surgery. Int J Prosthodont 1998; 11:462–469.
7. Sandstedt P, Sorensen S. Neurosensory disturbances of the trigeminal nerve: a long-term follow-up of traumatic injuries. J Oral Maxillofac Surg 1995; 53:498–505.
8. Renner GJ, Zitsch RP III. Reconstruction of the lip. Otolaryngol Clin N Am 1990; 23:975–990.
9. Hamilton MM, Branham GH. Concepts in lip reconstruction. Otolaryngol Clin N Am 1997; 30:593–606.
10. Kontis T, Johns M. Anatomy and physiology of the salivary glands. In: Healy G, et al., eds. Head & Neck Surgery-Otolaryngology. Philadelphia: Lippincott Williams & Wilkins, 2001:429–451.
11. Shemen L. Salivary glands: benign and malignant disease. In: Lee K, ed. Essential Otolaryngology Head & Neck Surgery. New Jersey: Appleton & Lange, 1995:505–533.
12. Nachlas N, Johns M. Physiology of the salivary glands. In: Meyerhoff WL, ed. Otolaryngology. Philadelphia: WB Saunders, 1991:391–405.
13. Enfors B. The parotid and submandibular secretion in man. Acta Otol Laryngol 1962; 172:1–67.
14. Schneyer L, Levin L. Rate of secretion by individual salivary gland pairs of man under conditions of reduced expoenous stimulations. J Appl Physiol 1955; 7:508–512.
15. Dawes C, Wood CM. The contribution of oral minor mucous gland secretions to the volume of whole saliva in man. Arch Oral Biol 1973; 18:337–342.
16. Jones K. The oral cavity, oropharynx, and hypopharynx. In: Lee K, ed. Essential Otolaryngology: Head & Neck Surgery. New Jersey: Appleton & Lange, 1995:461–479.
17. O'Rourke J. Oral Physiology. St. Louis: Mosby, 1951.
18. Hanson K. Physiology. In: Schuller D, ed. Otolaryngology: Head and Neck Surgery. St. Louis: Mosby, 1986:1103–1116.
19. Sherrington C. Reflexes elicitable in the cat from pinna vibrissae and jaws. J Physiol 1917:404–431.
20. Davenport H. Chewing and swallowing. In: Davenport H, ed. Physiology of the Digestive Tract. Chicago: Year Book, 1982:35–51.
21. Howell A, Manly R. An electronic strain gauge for measuring oral forces. J Dental Res 1948; 27:705–712.
22. Braun S, Bantleon HP, Hnat WP, Freudenthaler JW, Marcotte MR, Johnson BE. A study of bite force, part 1: relationship to various physical characteristics. Angle Orthod 1995; 65:367–372.
23. Waltimo A, Kononen M. A novel bite force recorder and maximal isometric bite force values for healthy young adults. Scand J Dent Res 1993; 101:171–175.
24. Rissin L, House JE, Manly RS, Kapur KK. Clinical comparison of masticatory performance and electromyographic activity of patients with complete dentures, overdentures, and natural teeth. J Prosthet Dent 1978; 39:508–511.
25. Marchetta FC. Function and appearance following surgery for intraoral cancer. Clin Plast Surg 1976; 3:471–479.
26. Shpitzer T, Gullane PJ, Neligan PC, Irish JC, Freeman JE, Van den Brekel M, Gur E. The free vascularized flap and the flap plate options: comparative results of reconstruction of lateral mandibular defects. Laryngoscope 2000; 110:2056–2060.
27. Logemann JA. Effects of aging on the swallowing mechanism. Otolaryngol Clin N Am 1990; 23:1045–1056.
28. Lund W. Some thoughts on swallowing—normal abnormal and bizarre. J R Soc Med 1910; 83:138–142, 132.
29. Bosma J. Physiology of the mouth pharynx and esophagus. In: Meyerhoff W, ed. Otolaryngology. Philadelphia: WB Saunders, 1991:361–389.

30. Logemann J. Upper digestive tract anatomy and physiology. In: Tardy M, ed. Head & Neck Surgery–Otolaryngology. Philadelphia: Lippincott-Raven, 1998:571–578.
31. Kahrilas PJ, Lin S, Logemann JA, Ergun GA, Facchini F. Deglutitive tongue action: volume accommodation and bolus propulsion. Gastroenterology 1993; 104:152–162.
32. Dodds W. The physiology of swallowing. Dysphagia 1989:171–178.
33. Lear C, Flanagan J Jr, Moorrees C. The frequency of deglutition in man. Arch Oral Biol 1965; 10:83–99.
34. Lichter I, Muir RC. The pattern of swallowing during sleep. Electroencephalogr Clin Neurophysiol 1975; 38:427–432.
35. Logemann JA, Bytell DE. Swallowing disorders in three types of head and neck surgical patients. Cancer 1979; 44:1095–1105.
36. Reece GP, Kroll SS, Miller MJ, Evans GR, Chang DW, Langstein HN, Robb GL, Wang B, Goepfert H. Functional results after oropharyngeal reconstruction: a different perspective. Arch Otolaryngol Head Neck Surg 1999; 125:474–477.
37. McFarland D, Baum S, Chabot C. Speech compensation to structural modifications of the oral cavity. J Acoust Soc Am 1996; 100(2 Pt 1):1093–1104.
38. Kothary P, Desouza L. Bombay Hosp J 1973; 15:58–60.
39. Robbins KT, Bowman JB, Jacob RF. Postglossectomy deglutitory and articulatory rehabilitation with palatal augmentation prostheses. Arch Otolaryngol Head Neck Surg 1987; 113:1214–1218.
40. Weber RS, Ohlms L, Bowman J, Jacob R, Goepfert H. Functional results after total or near total glossectomy with laryngeal preservation. Arch Otolaryngol Head Neck Surg 1991; 117:512–515.
41. Schiffman SS, Gatlin CA. Clinical physiology of taste and smell. Annu Rev Nutr 1993; 13:405–436.

4

Pathology of Neoplastic Diseases of the Oral Cavity

Mary Richardson
Department of Pathology, Medical University of South Carolina, Charleston, South Carolina, U.S.A.

INTRODUCTION

Throughout the world, the incidence of oral cavity cancer varies widely. Malignancies within the confines of the oral cavity represent approximately 30% of all head and neck cancers, and 95% of these malignancies are squamous cell carcinoma (1). Globally, a variety of local customs, a myriad of tobacco uses, and chronic alcohol consumption increase the risk for oral cancer (2).

Within the United States, oral and pharyngeal cancer represents about 3% of all cancers (3), and roughly 30,000 new cases are diagnosed annually (4), accounting for approximately 4000 deaths per year. Oral and pharyngeal cancers have one of the lowest five-year survival rates (53%) which unfortunately have remained constant for the last three decades (5), likely due to the fact that most oral cancer patients present with advanced stage disease (T3, T4): 40% have regional disease, and 10% have distant metastasis (6).

Ninety percent of oral cancers occur in males older than 45 years of age. In the last several decades; however, the ratio of male to female cancer cases has decreased from 6:1 in 1950 to 2:1 in 1987 until the present (7,8). This change may reflect greater numbers of aging females and an increased use of tobacco products and alcohol among women.

As noted above, approximately 75% of oral cancers are associated with two important risk factors, alcohol ingestion and use of tobacco in any form (9). When alcohol and tobacco are used in combination, the deleterious effects are synergistic (3,10). Data suggest additional risk factors for oral cancers, such as smoking of marijuana (11), presence of the human papilloma virus (12), and malnutrition (13).

Epidemiologic studies have shown not only an increased risk for oral cancer in populations with increased consumption of alcohol and tobacco products but also a risk for a second primary tumor in patients previously cured of a first head and neck primary (9). Within the confines of the oral cavity, cancer patients with primary tumors located in the floor of mouth (FOM), retromolar area, or lower alveolar process have the greatest risk for a second primary squamous cell carcinoma (14).

Research continues in pursuit of meaningful screening tests to identify and monitor patients at risk for this form of carcinoma. Although, oncology surgeons have improved multi-modality treatment options and reconstructive surgery to increase patients' quality of life and function, screening tests lag behind these advances. Each oral cavity area presents its own challenge to obtaining the optimal resection of cancer, restoration, and maintenance of function and continued assessment for new or recurrent disease.

ORAL SQUAMOUS MALIGNANCY BY ANATOMIC SITE

Anatomic Sites

The parameters of oral cavity as defined by the American Joint Committee on Cancer (15) include the region extending from the circumferential mucocutaneous border of the lips to the junction of the hard and soft palate superiorly and inferiorly to the line of the circumvallate papillae of the tongue (15). The oral cavity is divided into seven areas: the lips, buccal mucosa, upper and lower alveolar ridges, retromolar gingiva (retromolar trigone), FOM, hard palate, and anterior two-thirds of the tongue (oral or mobile). These designated areas allow for assessment and comparison of varied treatment modalities and prognosis. The frequency of oral cancer in these various areas, in descending order, are: lip, oral tongue, FOM, gingival, retromolar trigone, buccal mucosa, and palate. The various areas are considered separately in this chapter.

A number of significant groups of lymph nodes serve as the primary echelon nodes for the oral cavity. Submental lymph nodes are framed in the submental triangle by the anterior bellies of the digastric muscles and the hyoid bone. Submandibular lymph nodes are positioned around the submandibular gland in proximity to the lower jaw and facial artery. The upper deep jugular nodes are found along the upper internal jugular vein between the posterior bellies of the digastric muscles and the omohyoid muscles. Two lymph nodes, which frequently herald cancer in the oral cavity, are contained in the upper deep jugular nodes: the uppermost node is the jugular digastric (tonsillar node), and the middle node is the jugular carotid (principle node of the tongue). Lymph nodes less frequently receiving primary lymphatic drainage from the oral cavity are the lateral retropharyngeal and preparotid lymph nodes. Regional metastatic squamous cell carcinoma of the oral cavity frequently proceeds in an orderly fashion from nodes in the upper levels of the neck toward nodes in the lower aspects of the neck with rare exceptions (16,17). Metastatic deposits from the lips, anterior FOM, adjacent gingival, and buccal mucosa tend to present in submandibular nodes. Malignancies located posteriorly in the oral cavity frequently metastasize to the upper deep jugular nodes first and as disease advances to the middle and lower deep jugular nodes. A single metastatic deposit in the lower posterior cervical nodes from the oral cavity from carcinoma is unlikely. There are, however, lymphatic channels that directly connect the oral cavity with lower jugular nodes, which provides an anatomic justification for a lower jugular lymphadenectomy (18).

Lips

The lips are composed of the vermillion or that portion of the lip mucosa that extends from the anterior cutaneous border to the posterior contact area with the opposing lip. The obicularis oris muscle is a subjacent sphincter muscle surrounding the mouth that maintains oral competence. The loosely attached mucous membrane of the oral cavity contains numerous minor salivary glands and is attached to the deep surface of the obicularis oris. In the subjacent connective tissue of the vermilion border, lymphatic channels of the lip begin as a fan of delicate capillaries that merge to form larger connecting vessels. Lymphatics from the upper lip and commissure drain to the ipsilateral preauricular, infraparotid, submandibular, and submental lymph nodes (19). The lymphatics of the lower lip proceed to the submental and submandibular lymph nodes. During embryonic development, the mandibular process fuses in the midline; therefore numerous anastomoses cross the midline allowing drainage to occur bilaterally. Of note, the lower lip lymphatic channels enter the mental foramen of the mandible in approximately 22% of patients (19).

Lip carcinoma is the most common malignant tumor of the oral cavity representing about one-third of these cancers (20). The incidence is approximately 1.8 per 100,000 (20,21). Roughly 90% of the lip carcinomas are squamous cell carcinoma (21). Prolonged exposure to sunlight and having a fair complexion predispose a person to lip carcinoma. Lip cancer is seen most commonly in white male smokers. The majority of lip carcinoma originates near the midline of the exposed vermilion of the lower lip (90%). The oral commissure is the site of origin for 1–6% of lip carcinomas (21,22). Lip cancer is commonly seen in association with primary skin malignancies (21). Often, adjacent to a lip carcinoma, the histologic effects of sun exposure are seen: hyperkeratosis and solar cheilitis (21,23,24). These findings have been reported in association with squamous cell carcinoma of the lip in 46% of patients (23).

Clinically, lip carcinoma presents with a crust on the lip that may bleed upon removal or as a non-healing "blister" which is present for several months. On physical examination, an ulcerated area with surrounding induration is found. The diagnosis is established by an incisional biopsy, which should include part of the deep and lateral margin of the tumor. The deep and lateral margin allows the pathologist to determine the presence of invasive tumor, the pattern of invasion and search for the presence of perineural and lymphovascular invasion. These findings are valuable in the planning of treatment options, evaluating the need for intra-operative frozen section and prognosis.

Due to its prominent location, lip carcinoma can be detected early and is one of the most curable malignancies of the head and neck. Important prognosticators for lip cancer include: size of the tumor, tumor thickness, perineural invasion, and lymph node status (22,24–26). The overall determinate five-year survival rate is 89% (21,23). If left untreated, lip carcinoma will progress to involve skin of the mentum and alveolar mucosa. The mandibular bone may become involved either by direct extension or via lymphovascular or perineural invasion (mental nerve). The perineural invasion may be detected radiographically by unilateral widening of the mental foramen or noted clinically as sensory disturbances (27). Primary lip lesions less than 2 cm have an excellent prognosis with a five-year survival of 90%. Lesions larger than 3 cm, however, have a determinate five-year survival of 64%, and with involvement of the mandible; the five-year survival is less than 50% (21,22). Lip carcinoma recurrences generally increase as the size of the primary tumor increases. The incidence of recurrence is approximately 40% in tumors that are greater than 3 cm in size (22). Those patients with tumors greater than 6 cm have the highest incidence of bilateral lymph node metastasis, and thus have the poorest prognosis (21,26).

Aggressiveness of carcinomas located at the oral commissure is often debated. Generally tumors at this site tend to be larger, therefore increasing the probability of poor prognostic factors such as metastasis, lymphovascular, and perineural invasion.

Investigators who conducted a study involving 46 patients with squamous cell carcinoma at the commissure concluded that the involvement of oral commissure was no more aggressive, but rather, tumors at this location frequently were inadequately resected due to reconstructive considerations (28).

Buccal Mucosa

The buccal mucosa extends from the intra-oral surface of the lips in a superior direction to the attachment of mucosa to the maxilla, posteriorly to the mandibular raphae, and inferiorly to the mandibular alveolar ridges. The buccal mucosa is supported by a thin, delicate, loose connective tissue. The buccinator muscle is immediately subjacent to the connective tissue and perforated by the parotid duct.

Although uncommon, squamous cell carcinoma of the buccal mucosa is an aggressive neoplasm of the oral cavity. The reported frequency of squamous cell carcinoma at this site ranges anywhere from 2% to 10% (29,30). The greatest risk factors associated with carcinoma of this site and elsewhere in the oral cavity are smoking and alcohol. In countries such as Asia or India where chewing beetle nut is a common practice, squamous cell carcinomas of the buccal mucosa may constitute approximately 44% of all oral cavity squamous cell carcinomas (31).

Squamous cell carcinoma in the buccal mucosa occurs most often in the sixth and seventh decades of life with the majority of cases being in male patients greater than 40 years of age. The male-to-female ratio ranges from 2:1 to 9:1 in most series (32). In the southeastern and southwestern United States, however, carcinoma of the buccal mucosa is frequently seen in elderly females and attributed to the use of chewing tobacco or snuff (33,34). On the mucosa adjacent to the carcinoma, frequently erythroplasia or leukoplakia can be found (1,2). Invasive carcinoma will generally have one of three clinical growth patterns: exophytic, ulcerative/infiltrative, or a verrucous form. On histologic evaluation, the tumor frequently will have marked infiltration of the lamina propria with deep invasion into musculature may be present (1). The location of the most of these cancers is along or inferior to the plane of occlusion at the middle or posterior aspect of the buccal mucosa (32). Tumors at this site in the early stages are usually completely asymptomatic. As the carcinoma continues to grow, eventually it will become enlarged, traumatized and frequently infected. The tumor can infiltrate the cheek and invade the vicinity of the pterygoid and temporalis muscles, causing trismus. T1 and T2 carcinomas are usually amenable to either surgery or radiation therapy as a single modality (31). Larger tumors (T3, T4) may require excision with cheek flap replacement. Proximity of these lesions to the mandible may require resection of a portion of the mandible. Regardless of the treatment, local recurrences (30–80%) are common (30). Even patients with T1 and T2 tumors that are resected with negative margins (equal to or greater than 5 mm) have 40% local recurrence in some studies (30). Others have shown that combining the T-size of the lesion with tumor thickness (6 mm) has been useful in predicting outcomes (35). The five-year survival for patients of T1 or T2 with less than 6-mm tumor thickness was 98% whereas the corresponding values for T1 or T2 and T3 or T4 that were greater than 6-mm tumor thickness were 65% and 40%, respectively (35). Prognosis is determined by three major factors: the presence/absence of lymph node metastasis, the position of the lesion within the buccal mucosa, and tumor thickness (30,32,35). Generally, the more posterior the lesion is located the poorer the prognosis due to a tendency to invade adjacent structures such as the maxilla, mandible, tonsillar pillars, and soft palate.

Gingiva and Alveolar Mucosa

The soft tissue that interdigitates between and around the teeth is the free and attached gingiva. Free gingiva forms a collar around the tooth that extends from the gingival margin to the base of the gingival sulcus. The attached gingiva is pink with a stippled surface and, unlike the free gingiva, is tightly bound to the underlying periosteum. The attached gingiva extends from the base of the sulcus to the mucogingival junction, which appears as a scalloped line. The alveolar mucosa is red, smooth, and mobile. The alveolar mucosa covers the edentulous arches in the maxilla and mandible.

Gingival cancer is insidious and frequently masquerades for extended periods of time as a benign inflammatory process such as periodontal disease (36). A number of risk factors have been identified, and include use of tobacco products, alcohol consumption, and probably poor oral hygiene (36). Carcinoma of the gingiva within the United States represents about 4–16% of all oral cancers (37,38). If carcinoma of the lips is excluded, carcinoma of the gingiva is the third most common intra-oral malignancy. This is a disease primarily of the elderly, most often affects the mandibular region over the maxilla and men more frequently than women. Due to the close proximity to the underlying bone, there is usually invasion of the bone early in the course of the disease. Clinical evidence of osseous invasion has been reported to be between 30% and 56% of patients (39). The incidence of osseous invasion appears to be dependent on the proximity of the tumor to adjacent bone and not to the stage of the disease (39). If the tumor reaches the mandibular canal within the mandible, then invasion of the inferior alveolar nerve may result in pain or paraesthesia and possible extension to the skull base (40). There is a particular propensity for nerve involvement in edentulous arches (41).

Two types of bone involvement by tumor have been described: an erosive pattern and a diffuse infiltrative pattern (42). The erosive pattern is a tumor with a pushing border at the bony interface and shows a pattern of resorption at the bony borders of the advancing tumor. In this type of pushing border, there are usually no remnants of bone entrapped within the neoplasm and cancellous spaces are separated from the tumor by a continuous layer of newly formed bone and fibrous tissue. In contrast, the diffuse infiltrative type growth pattern may progress insidiously through the cancellous bone and around neural structures (42). The infiltrative pattern is composed of nests, strands, and cords of tumor cells, which have a tentacular spread along the tumor front (Fig. 1).

Surgery is the preferred treatment for gingival carcinoma and the extent of the surgical procedure is usually determined by the degree and nature of any bony involvement. Those tumors having the erosive pattern of bony involvement may be amenable to conservative procedures. Tumors, however, exhibiting the diffuse infiltrative pattern may require segmental resection of the mandible (42,43).

The erosive pattern of bone invasion has been hypothesized to extend in a more predictable manner than the infiltrative pattern. This non-expansive growth pattern can lead to underestimating the tumor size. The separation of these two distinct histological growth patterns has called into question the previously held assumption that mandibular bone invasion universally was a poor prognosticator (42). A recent study evaluated the significance of these two growth patterns and concluded that infiltrative lesions were more likely to result in death with disease or recurrent disease (43). The three-year disease-free survival for the infiltrative pattern and erosive growth pattern was 30% and 73%, respectively. The tumors' with the infiltrative growth pattern in bone more often had primary, regional, and distant recurrence,

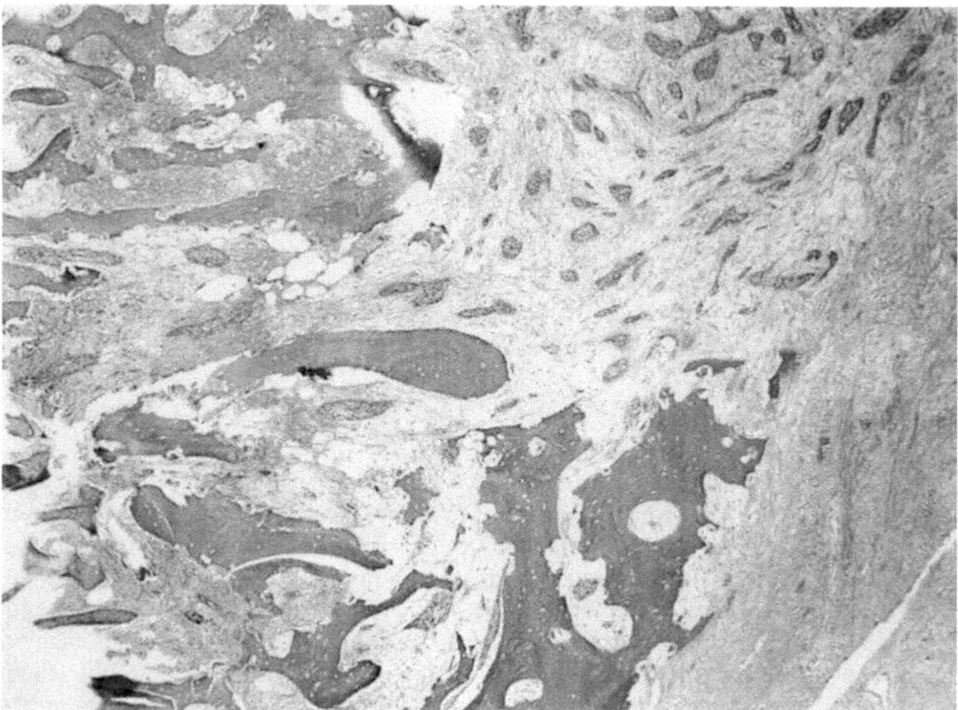

Figure 1 Tentacular strands of invasive squamous cell carcinoma can be seen infiltrating cortical bone.

and positive surgical margins (soft tissue and bony). Unfortunately, intra-operative and preoperative determination of invasion pattern remains problematic. Intra-operative assessment of bone by frozen section is difficult due to the inherent problems in performing frozen sections on bone. Touch prep of curetted soft bone marrow can be useful for intra-operative evaluation for presence of tumor; however, the histology growth pattern cannot be determined via cytologic touch preparation. Knowledge of the growth pattern intra-operatively may alter the surgical parameters. Post-operative pathologic assessment of the pattern of bony invasion is easily made and provides important reconstructive and prognostic information (43).

Retromolar Trigone

The retromolar trigone is a triangular shaped area of attached gingiva overlying the ascending ramus of the mandible. The base of the triangle is from the distal surface of the last molar and the apex terminates superiorly at the maxillary tuberosity. The lateral aspect of this area is continuous with the buccal mucosa and the medial aspect abuts the anterior tonsillar pillars. The mucosa is adherent to the bone. The inferior alveolar nerve and lingual nerves lie just inferior and medial to the mid-point to the retromolar trigone. Tumors involving the retromolar area may penetrate deep into the parapharyngeal soft tissues and extend along the lingual and inferior alveolar nerves ultimately gaining access to the skull base (36,44).

Squamous cell carcinomas of the retromolar trigone occur chiefly in men between 55 years and 70 years of age. Common presenting symptoms are sore throat, otalgia, and trismus. At the time of diagnosis, the majority of tumors are smaller than

4 cm with 27–60% presenting with positive cervical lymph nodes, particularly the submandibular and jugular digastric lymph nodes (36,44–50). Although, the retromolar area is firmly adhered to bone, it has been reported that 14% actually show histologic invasion of the mandible (44). See discussion of bone invasion in alveolar ridge section. T1 and T2 lesions of this area can be affectively treated with radiation or surgery.

Floor of Mouth

The FOM is a crescent-shaped region of mucosa extending from the lingual aspect of the lower alveolar ridge to the interface with ventral surface of the anterior two-thirds of the oral tongue. Posteriorly, the FOM proceeds to the anterior tonsillar pillar, and in the anterior the frenulum of the tongue divides the space into two sides. A sublingual caruncle is on either side of the frenulum anteriorly designating the orifices of the submandibular gland duct (Wharton's duct). Orifices appear as rounded ridges of the mucosa known as the sublingual fold, which overlies the upper border of the sublingual salivary glands. Paired mylohyoid muscles, which act as a muscular diaphragm for the anterior portion of the FOM. The hyoglossus muscle supports the extreme posterior portion of the FOM. The lymphatic vessels of the FOM come from an extensive submucosal plexus. These lymphatic channels drain into ipsilateral and contralateral lymph nodes. Malignancies of the FOM frequently have bilateral metastases.

Squamous cell carcinomas of the FOM are commonly located in the anterior portion near the midline. Carcinomas at this site easily spread to such contiguous structures, such as the alveolar ridge or the ventral aspect of the tongue, or track along the submandibular gland duct. Squamous cell carcinoma of the FOM represents approximately 15–20% of all malignant lesions of the oral cavity. If carcinoma of the lips is excluded from the oral cavity, FOM carcinoma is the second most common malignancy only being surpassed by carcinoma of the tongue. Men are affected two to three times as often as women are with this carcinoma. Carcinoma of the FOM in women frequently presents a decade earlier than in men (51), but increased incidence of FOM cancers in women and the margin between the men and women is narrowing (51).

Although any area within the FOM can be affected by carcinoma, the most frequent site of occurrence is the anterior aspect adjacent to the lingual frenulum. Approximately 70% of all FOM tumors occur in this location. The middle third and posterior third of the FOM are roughly split for the remaining 30% (52). The typical initial clinical presentation of FOM carcinoma is that of a non-healing ulcer with or without xerostomia. As neoplasms developing in the anterior FOM advance, they frequently will involve the midline and the papilla of Wharton's duct of the submandibular gland. This involvement of Wharton's duct can lead to subsequent obstruction of the salivary gland with ensuing sialadenitis or xerostomia (53). The mucosal borders of these tumors may contain clinically notable leukoplakia or erythroplakia. The deceiving benign appearance and lack of symptoms in these patients may cause early lesions often to be dismissed or misdiagnosed as some inflammatory process. Due to this delay in detection, most lesions in this area at time of diagnosis are greater than 2 cm before the nature of the lesion has been established (53).

Invasion of the mandible at this site has been reported in approximately 15–29% of the patients at the time of diagnosis (39). As with carcinoma of the alveolar ridge and retromolar trigone, proximity to the bone seems to determine this event rather than the size of the carcinoma (42,53).

Several studies have been undertaken to determine predictive tumor features for the likelihood of metastasis to lymph nodes. It appears that tumor stage,

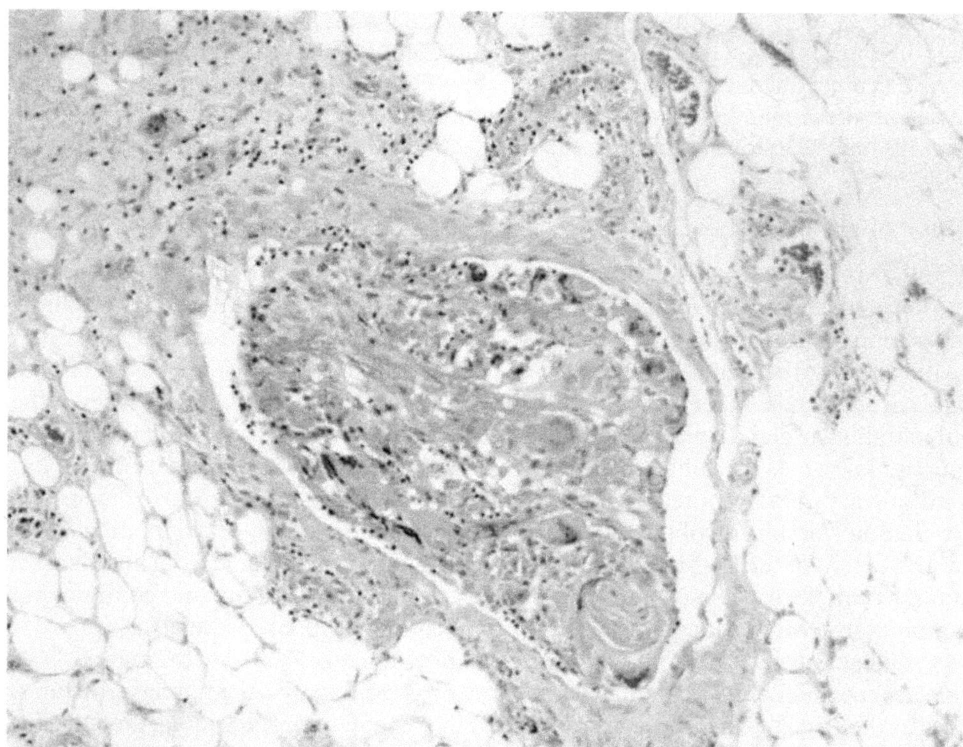

Figure 2 Tumor embolus is seen distending a small lymphovascular structure.

perineural invasion, and intralymphatic tumor emboli (Fig. 2) are often associated with the development of metastasis within the neck. The T-stage, however, in other studies proved to be of little prognostic significance (41,54). Another developing prognostic parameter under investigation is tumor thickness. Some studies have shown that the tumor thicknesses of less than 3 mm correlate with increased survival (55–58). Elective neck dissection for a clinically negative neck for early disease (T1 or T2 lesion) within the FOM is still controversial (59). The growth pattern of T1 and T2 lesions has been analyzed and may be a useful predictor in superficial or micro-invasion of the submucosa. The majority of T1 tumors and some T2 tumors tend to grow in a horizontal manner rather than deeply invading the submucosal tissues. If tumors are confined to this horizontal spread without invasion into the submucosa gaining access to larger lymphatic trunks, then tumor dissemination to the cervical lymph nodes is less likely (58). In a recent study of FOM cancers, just looking at tumor size, the incidence of occult metastatic disease was 21% for T1 lesions (59). The importance of "negative" surgical margins (0.5 cm from dysplasia or invasive tumor) has been evaluated several times and the local recurrences have been reported to be 3–32% (60,61).

Tongue

The tongue is divided into two portions, the anterior two-thirds (oral and mobile tongue) that lies within the oral cavity and the posterior one-third (base of tongue), which is within the confines of the oropharynx. The anterior portion of the tongue, which is in the oral cavity, is arbitrarily divided into four areas: tip, lateral borders, dorsum, and ventral surface (underside adjacent to FOM). Squamous cell carcinoma of the tongue represents approximately 50% of all intra-oral carcinomas. Roughly two-thirds of these carcinomas are located on the mobile aspect of the tongue. The most common site of occurrence for squamous cell carcinoma on the mobile tongue is the lateral border. These lateral border tumors may extend onto the FOM (36). Clinically, squamous cell carcinoma of the tongue most often grows as an ulcerating lesion and can be deeply invasive. The frequency of metastatic disease from carcinoma of the oral tongue is highest for all intra-oral squamous cell carcinoma: 20–40% for T1 lesions; 40% for T2 lesions; 75% for T3 lesions (36).

Squamous cell carcinoma of the mobile tongue can penetrate deeply between the multi-directional tongue muscle fibers and often "skip" to apparently uninvolved areas. The median raphe of the tongue conveys no special resistance to tumor invasion to the contralateral side. The incidence of contralateral or bilateral lymph node metastasis in patients with carcinomas of the tongue is high. Perineural invasion is a frequent finding in these tumors (62). Squamous cell carcinoma of the tongue invades adjacent structures such as the FOM, gingiva, mandible, or base of tongue in roughly 25% of cases (63).

Squamous cell carcinoma of the anterior two-thirds of the tongue tends to be histologically well to moderately differentiated tumors. Perineural invasion can be demonstrated in roughly 30% of the cases and is an ominous sign. Approximately 76% of patients with perineural invasion develop positive cervical lymph nodes (Fig. 3) (62,64).

Nodal metastasis is considered to be one of the most common sites of recurrence and treatment failure in tongue carcinoma (65). The predictive value of tumor diameter and T-staging in differentiating the patients with high risk and low risk of nodal metastasis, local recurrence, and survival has been challenged. Recent studies suggest that tumor thickness is a better predictor than T-stage (64) while others have found only perineural invasion to be a significant predictor of patient progression and outcome (66). In one study, tumor-size parameters were evaluated with the use of 3-mm and 9-mm depth of invasion as a division. Tumors up to 3 mm had 10% nodal metastasis, 0% local recurrence, and 100% five-year actual disease-free survival (64). In lesions with tumor thickness more than 3 mm and up to 9 mm, 50% nodal metastasis, 11% local recurrence, and 77% five-year actual disease-free survival was noted; tumors of greater than 9 mm had 65% nodal metastasis, 26% local recurrence, and 60% five-year actual survival (64). Although tumor thickness is currently not a component to the T-stage in the AJCC and UIC TNM staging manuals, as the literature evolves, these parameters may become widely endorsed for evaluation of neck dissections.

A recent epidemiologic observation regarding squamous cell carcinoma of the tongue suggests an increase in occurrence of tumors in patients under the age of 40: squamous cell carcinomas of the tongue increased in patients under the age of 40 from 4% in 1971 to 18% in 1993 (67). More studies are needed to validate this finding.

Palate

The palate is divided anatomically into the hard palate, which lies within the oral cavity, and the soft palate, which lies within the oropharynx. The mucosa of the hard palate is located between the horseshoe-shaped maxillary alveolar ridges anteriorly and is attached posteriorly to the ridge of the palatine bone. The mucosa is firmly attached to the periosteum of the underlying bone. The submucosa of the palate

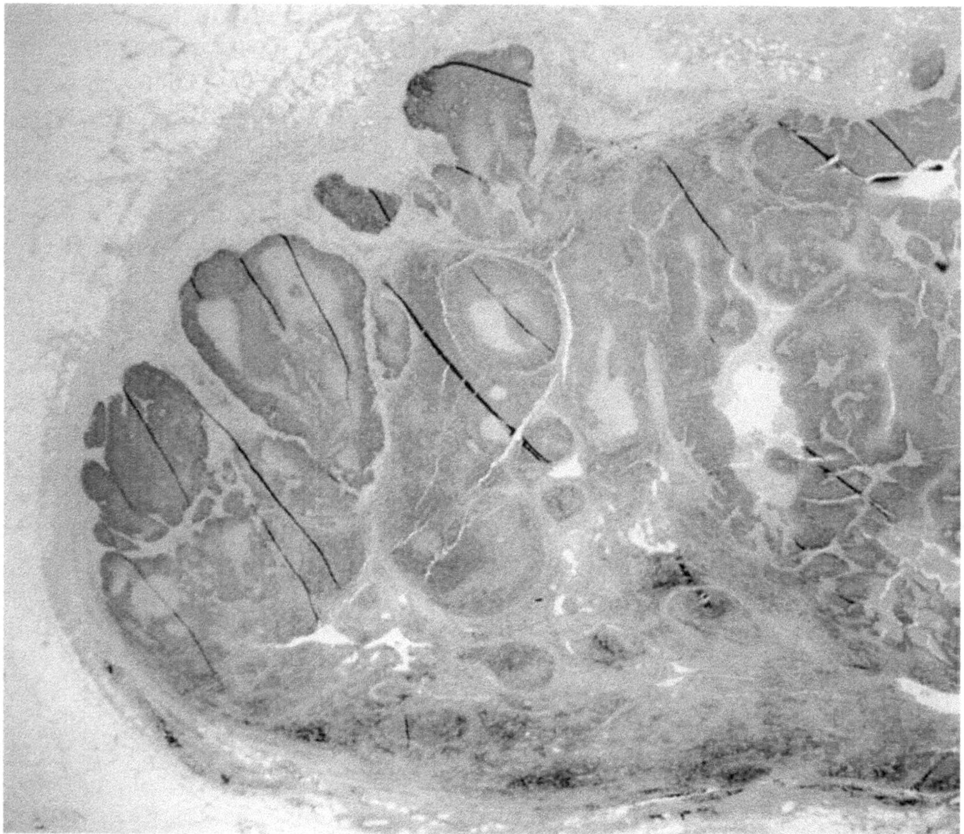

Figure 3 A lymph node is almost entirely replaced by metastatic squamous cell carcinoma. Along the capsular surface of the lymph node an area of extracapsular extension is identified. This finding is a useful prognostic finding.

contains more minor salivary glands than any other location within the oral cavity. It is not surprising that this location is particularly prone to salivary gland neoplasms.

In the United States, the hard palate is the rarest site of intra-oral squamous cell carcinoma. The initial lesion usually presents as leukoplakia in about 25% of the cases (68). Half the tumors will be localized to the palate at diagnosis, a third will have extended to adjacent structures, and 15–25% will have metastasized to regional lymph nodes (5% are bilateral) (68).

Although squamous cell carcinoma of the palate is extremely rare in the United States, other types of neoplasms are more frequent at this site. The palate is the most common site for salivary gland malignancies within the oral cavity (69).

The proximity of the greater palatine nerve to a palatal malignancy is noteworthy. Perineural invasion allows tumors to spread in a longitudinal as well as a radial fashion through the planes of least resistance (58). The presence of perineural invasion should alert the surgeon and the pathologist to an increased likelihood of perineural extension beyond the confines of the resection margins and extension to the skull base (Fig. 4). This tendency for extension along the nerves is of great significance when planning the treatment of certain tumors (e.g., adenoid cystic carcinoma of salivary gland origin, mucosal, and cutaneous squamous cell carcinomas).

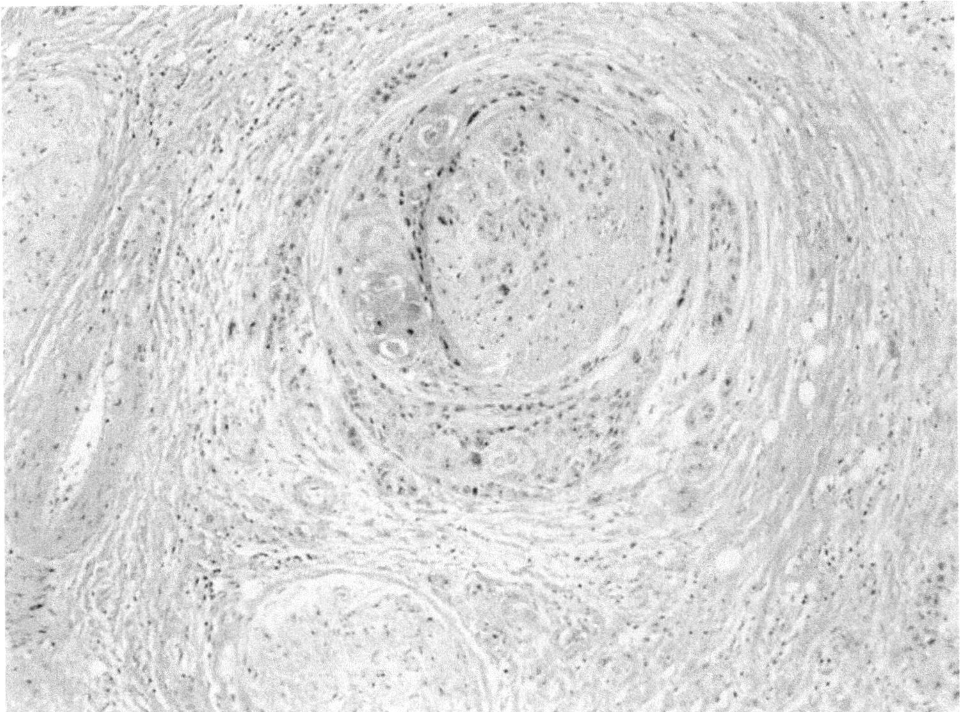

Figure 4 Both perineural and intraneural invasion are present in this nerve.

Salivary Gland

Salivary glands are divided into two groups, major salivary glands (paired); parotid, submandibular, and sublingual, and minor salivary glands of which approximately 300–600 are dispersed within the submucosa of the upper aerodigestive tract. Within the confines of the oral cavity, the major salivary gland group is represented by the submandibular glands and the sublingual glands. Both glands are found in the superficial and deep soft tissue of the FOM. The minor salivary glands are widely distributed throughout the oral cavity but are in greatest concentration within the submucosa of the palate. Anatomically, a major difference between the major salivary glands and minor salivary glands is encapsulation. The major salivary glands have a capsule surrounding them thus defining the borders of the gland. The sublingual gland is the only major gland that may have an incomplete capsule. In contrast, the minor salivary glands are dispersed freely within the submucosa devoid of capsules.

Malignancies of the minor salivary gland represent approximately 10% of all oral cavity cancers and between 10% and 23% of all salivary gland cancers (69). These tumors, due to the diversity of anatomic site and histology, have an unpredictable course and a long natural history. The most common histologic type of tumor in the oral cavity in most series is adenoid cystic carcinoma followed by polymorphous low-grade adenocarcinoma and mucoepidermoid carcinoma (MEC) (70).

Pleomorphic adenomas (PA) represent 50–75% of all salivary gland tumors (71). Intra-orally, the most common sites for PA to occur are the hard palate, lips, and buccal mucosa. Both mesenchyme-like and epithelial elements histologically characterize these tumors. PA of the submandibular and sublingual glands are treated by total glandectomy. When these tumors occur in the minor glands they are excised with the rim of normal tissue (72). Malignant transformation can occur in longstanding PA. In one series of carcinoma expleomorphic adenoma, 18% occurred in minor salivary glands (73). Diagnosis requires the presence or a remnant of pleomorphic adenoma to be in association with the carcinoma. The extension beyond the capsule has prognostic significance. If confined by the capsular tissue, the carcinoma is called encapsulated, carcinoma in situ or non-invasive carcinoma expleomorphic adenoma (74), and behavior of these lesions is characterized by local recurrence similar to PA.

MEC is the most common salivary gland malignancy. Within the minor salivary gland sites, MEC is most frequent in the palate followed by the buccal mucosa and lips. In the major glands, this tumor presents as a solitary, painless mass frequently associated with obstruction. In the minor glands, the clinical appearance is variable but frequently appears as a blue semi-translucent fluctuant swelling. Symptoms of parathesia, pain, and dysphasia are more often associated with minor gland lesions (75). The tumor is histologically composed of three cells types, mucin-filled globet cells, squamous cells, and intermediate cells. A variety of histologic grading systems exist (71,74). The histologic grade of MEC of the submandibular gland, however, has not correlated well with biologic behavior

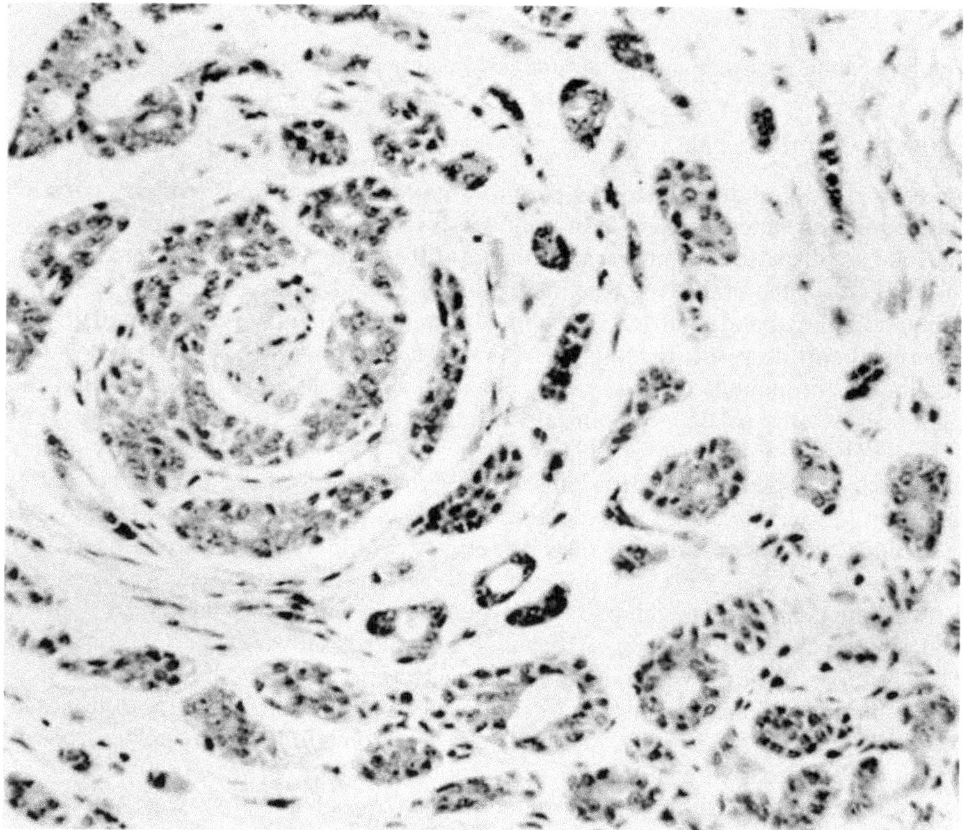

Figure 5 Adenoid cystic carcinoma has a distinctive biphasic cellular pattern with a marked propensity for perineural invasion (*upper left*).

(71,76). Generally clinical stage, histologic grade and adequacy of treatment influence the prognosis.

Adenoid cystic carcinoma (ACC) represents about 8% of carcinoma of all salivary glands. Just under half of the intra-oral ACC occur in the palate. The tumor is composed of two cell types: basaloid myoepithelial cells and intercalated duct-type cells. Tubular, cribriform, and solid architectural growth patterns are recognized. Cribriform growth, with tissue spaces filled with glycoaminoglycans and basal lamina, and extensive perineural invasion are characteristic of this tumor (Fig. 5). The tumor may be circumscribed but frequently frozen section examination of radiating nerve segments will demonstrate the tumor extending beyond the visible borders. Tumors having greater than 30% of the solid growth pattern have a more aggressive clinical course. The solid growth pattern, however, is more often seen in tumors with a high T-stage (77–81). The natural history of this tumor is a long relentless course characterized by late (20 years) recurrences (81).

Polymorphous low-grade adenocarcinoma occurs almost exclusively in the minor salivary glands. In the minor salivary glands, this entity represents 20–25% of all malignant minor salivary gland tumors (71). The tumors are usually circumscribed. There is focal infiltration of the adjacent tissue and notable neurotropism (Fig. 6). This tumor type has a 17% recurrence rate, and about 9% rate of metastases to regional lymph nodes (82). Wide surgical excision for tumor-free margins and long-term follow-up are recommended (71). The vast majority of patients do extremely well following complete excision.

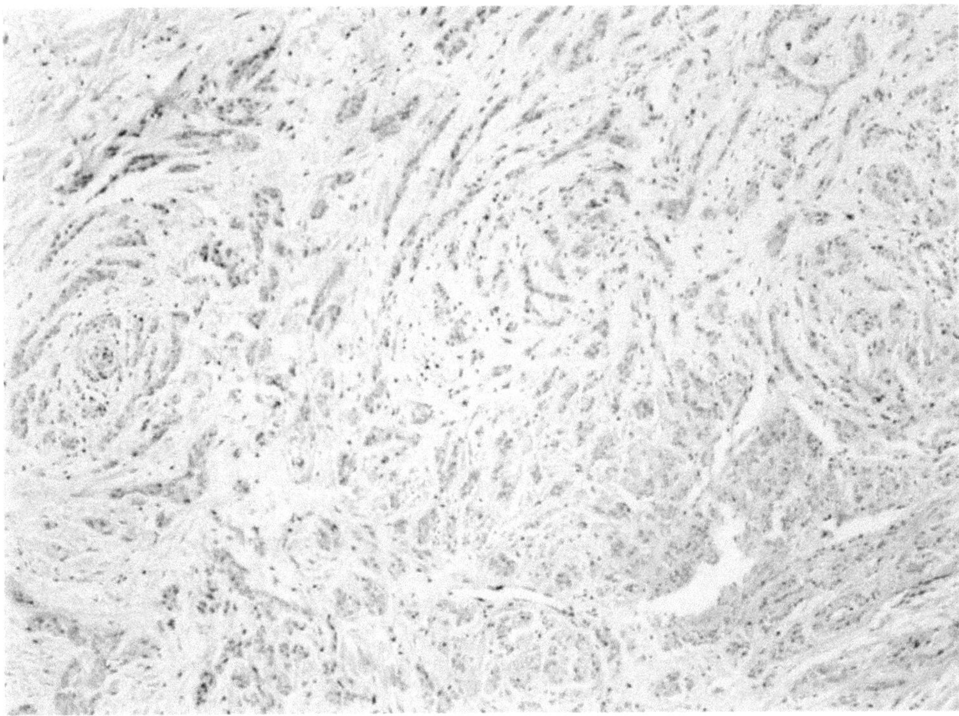

Figure 6 Polymorphous low-grade adenocarcinoma has a "targetoid" growth pattern with focal neurotopism identified.

ORAL LICHEN PLANUS (OLP)

Lichen planus is a mucocutaneous inflammatory disease. OLP is clinically different from the dermal counterpart but has similar histopathology. The mechanism of the disease is thought to involve a cell-mediated immune response induce by an antigenic change in the mucosa. A variety of antigens have been proposed which include drugs, viral and bacterial infections, and amalgam restorations. The majority of patients are middle-aged with a slight female predominance (60%). A number of clinical variants have been described (erosive, atrophic, and hypertrophic) and exist with a notable amount of overlap.

A number of reports of malignant transformation of OLP exist (83). Malignant transformation of OLP is still controversial and the reported rates of malignant transformation range from 0% to 5.6% (83–85). A lack of consensus as to the exact criteria used in the clinical and histopathologic diagnosis of OLP has confounded the matter. The diagnosis of OLP may be complicated by some overlap with other entities such as chronic discoid lupus erythematous and leukoplakia. Aggressive use of steroids for treatment of OLP has been proposed as a possible reason why OLP patients may be vulnerable to malignant transformation (86). Clinicians should have a high index of suspicion of patients with OLP developing an oral malignancy. The clinical variants most often associated with the transformation are the erosive and atrophic forms. In one study based on the outcome of 832 patients, investigators found a transformation rate of 0.8% and recommended a follow-up of at least six years for patients with OLP (83).

OSTEORADIONECROSIS

Osteoradionecrosis is one of the most serious and dreaded complications of irradiation therapy for head and neck tumors. The reported frequency ranges from 1% to 35% (87). Osteoradionecrosis was traditionally thought to represent a form of osteomyelitis; however, the concept has been redefined and is no longer a primary infection of bone but rather a radiation-induced vascular defect. There is a sequence that is described within this defect that entails a hypocellular hypoxic tissue and finally a non-healing wound that may or may not become secondarily infected.

Pathologically, osteoradionecrosis consists of six basic processes, which include hyperemia, inflammation, thrombosis, cell loss, hypovascularity, and fibrosis (87). This loss of blood vessels leads to devitalized tissue, which usually appears six months after the irradiation (88).

Within the oral cavity, the mandible is far more susceptible to osteoradionecrosis than the maxilla. Consequently, this difference is believed to be due to the small blood supply to the mandible and the predominance of compact bone in the composition of the mandible (89). The onset of osteoradionecrosis is related to the dose of irradiation, the dental status of the patient, and the anatomic site of the tumor. The risk for osteoradionecrosis increases with the dosage is more likely to occur in dentulous rather than edentulous patients and is usually found in patients with a poor oral hygiene (89).

MELANOMA

Mucosal melanomas fortunately are rare. Mucosal melanomas of the oral cavity and head and neck areas have not been as well characterized as their cutaneous counterparts (90). Certainly, the paucity in melanoma in mucosal surfaces, accounts for less than 1% of all cases of melanomas, contributes to this lack of understanding. Mucosal melanomas as a rule tend to present at a higher stage and are more aggressive than cutaneous melanomas. With oral melanomas, the incidence is very low, in the order of 1.2 cases/10 million per year. Overall, the most common sites for mucosal melanomas are head and neck (55%), followed by the anal/rectal region (24%), female genital tract (18%), and urinary tract (3%) (90). In the literature, about one-half of all melanomas that occur within the oral/nasal region are located in the oral cavity (48%) (90). The survival rate for mucosal melanomas is much less than that of cutaneous melanomas, likely due to a more prominent vertical growth phase in mucosal melanomas, higher stage of discovery, and the inability of surgeons to adequately resect lesions for negative surgical margins. A recent report suggested hopeful prognostic indicators: clinical stage of presentation, tumor thickness greater than 5 mm, vascular invasion on histologic slides, and development of distant failures are the only independent predictors for mucosal malignant melanomas (91).

SARCOMA

Sarcomas of the head and neck are also rare. Most commonly encountered sarcomas are those involving the mandible and maxilla as an osteosarcoma. Also seen within the oral cavity are lymphomas. Other tissue sarcomas seen in children and young adults are rhabdomyosarcoma.

Rhabdomyosarcoma is the most common sarcoma in children. Overall, rhabdomyosarcoma accounts for 8–20% of sarcomas in patients of all ages (92). Distribution of the tumor type depends on anatomic region; however, in children head and neck sarcomas account for 30–50% of these cases (92). There are four histologic subtypes of rhabdomyosarcoma: embryonal, alveolar, pleomorphic, and botryoid.

Cytogenetic typing and histologic subtyping has prognostic significance in rhabdomyosarcoma. Due to the histologic subtypes having significant impact on prognosis, tumor procurement for cytogenetic analysis and molecular investigation are paramount in patient treatment (93). Tissue biopsy for purposes of standard histologic examination should be submitted as well as fresh tissue for the purposes of ancillary molecular studies (see intra-operative consultation). Radical surgery for head and neck rhabdomyosarcoma has been largely replaced by the use of irradiation and chemotherapy. Surgical intervention has been used to excise small accessible tumors, reduce tumor bulk followed by other Multi-modality treatments or as a post-therapy resection (92).

Osteosarcomas of the head and neck are relatively infrequent. In a rather large study of osteosarcoma, approximately 6.5% of the cases involved skull, mandible, maxilla, facial bones, or cervical vertebrae (92). In the United States, osteosarcoma of head and neck accounts for approximately 6–13% of all osteosarcomas (94). Osteosarcoma of the long bones occurs most commonly in the second decade of life. In contrast, head and neck osteosarcomas typically occur in the third and fourth decades of life with equal gender distribution (95). Head and neck osteosarcomas are more problematic from a surgical standpoint due the anatomic constraints of obtaining negative surgical margins. Within the oral cavity, osteosarcoma of the mandible is a more favorable surgical site while the maxillary antrum is the most difficult site to manage surgically (94). Review of multi-modality studies has been addressed elsewhere (94).

TISSUE PROCUREMENT

Procuring viable tumor for molecular studies may be necessary for diagnostic, therapeutic and prognostic purposes. This is most often required when the neoplasm is a sarcoma. Whether submitting tissue for evaluation of a possible lymphoma or soft tissue sarcoma, the tissue should be sent fresh, without formalin, for an intra-operative consultation to determine if the specimen is adequate (enough viable tumor is present to complete the studies). Surgical closure should occur after the adequacy of the tissue has been assessed and reported to the surgeon. The pathologist can then divide the tumor into the necessary quantities and place it in the appropriate media.

CONCLUSION

Due to the complex anatomy, evaluation of resection margins from oral cavity cancer specimens is difficult and not amenable to a single, simple set of guidelines. Proper orientation of the specimen requires accurate and exact communication between the surgeon and pathologist. This level of communication is particularly necessary when performing intra-operative frozen sections.

One of the chief indicators of completeness of surgical excision is the margin of uninvolved tissue surrounding the extirpated neoplasm. To facilitate optimal excision, intra-operative evaluation is frequently used to guide margins of resection. Mucosal surgical margins should be received oriented as to which side is the true surgical margin. This orientation facilitates cutting the frozen section from the appropriate surface, and therefore in the correct direction (cutting the sections toward the true margin and not toward the tumor size). The surgeon, by placing strategic sutures on the specimen and rendering a simple illustration key to the placement of the sutures, can facilitate this type of coordination.

Recent studies found that in resection specimens of squamous cell carcinoma in the head and neck the presence of lesional tissue (severe dysplasia, carcinoma in situ, or invasive carcinoma) within 5 mm of the resection margin puts a patient at equal risk for local recurrence (96). If a 5-mm negative surgical margin is to be obtained and the surgical margins are to be removed and submitted by the surgeon, it is necessary to designate for the pathologist which surface is the "true" surgical margin (96).

REFERENCES

1. Muir C, Weiland L. Upper aerodigestive tract cancers. Cancer 1995; 75:147–153.
2. Boyle P, Macfarlane GJ, Zheng T, Maisonneuve P, Evstifeeva T, Scully C. Recent advances in epidemiology of head and neck cancer. Curr Opin Oncol 1992; 4:471–477.
3. Vokes EE, Weichselbaum RR, Lippman SM, Hong WK. Head and neck cancer. N Engl J Med 1993; 328:184–194.
4. American Cancer Society. Cancer Facts and Figures. Atlanta: American Cancer Society, 1996.
5. Swango PA. Cancers of the oral cavity and pharynx in the United States: an epidemiologic overview. J Public Health Dent 1996; 56:309–318.
6. Taneja C, Allen H, Koness RJ, Radie-Keane K, Wanebo HJ. Changing patterns of failure of head and neck cancer. Arch Otolaryngol Head Neck Surg 2002; 128:324–327.

7. Ries L, Kosary C. SEER Cancer Statistics Review, 1973–1996. National Cancer Institute, 1999.
8. Horowitz AM, Goodman HS, Yellowitz JA, Nourjah PA. The need for health promotion in oral cancer prevention and early detection. J Public Health Dent 1996.
9. Wynder EL, Mushinski MH, Spivak JC. Tobacco and alcohol consumption in relation to the development of multiple primary cancers. Cancer 1977; 40:1872–1878.
10. Spitz MR. Epidemiology and risk factors for head and neck cancer. Semin Oncol 1994; 21:281–288.
11. Zhang ZF, Morgenstern H, Spitz MR, Tashkin DP, Yu GP, Marshall JR, Hsu TC, Schantz SP. Marijuana use and increased risk of squamous cell carcinoma of the head and neck. Cancer Epidemiol Biomarkers Prev 1999; 8:1071–1078.
12. Gillison ML, Koch WM, Shah KV. Human papillomavirus in head and neck squamous cell carcinoma: are some head and neck cancers a sexually transmitted disease? Curr Opin Oncol 1999; 11:191–199.
13. Horowitz AM, Nourjah P, Gift HC. U.S. adult knowledge of risk factors and signs of oral cancers: 1990. J Am Dent Assoc 1995; 126:39–45.
14. Jovanovic A, van der Tol IG, Kostense PJ, Schulten EA, de Vries N, Snow GB, van der Waal I. Second respiratory and upper digestive tract cancer following oral squamous cell carcinoma. Eur J Cancer B Oral Oncol 1994; 30B:225–229.
15. Greene F, Page D, Fleming I. American Joint Committee on Cancer. Berlin: Springer-Verlag, 2002.
16. Lindberg R. Distribution of cervical lymph node metastases from squamous cell carcinoma of the upper respiratory and digestive tracts. Cancer 1972; 29:1446–1449.
17. Mukherji SK, Armao D, Joshi VM. Cervical nodal metastases in squamous cell carcinoma of the head and neck: what to expect. Head Neck 2001; 23:995–1005.
18. Shah JP. Patterns of cervical lymph node metastasis from squamous carcinomas of the upper aerodigestive tract. Am J Surg 1990; 160:405–409.
19. Ward G, Hendrick J. Results of treatment of carcinoma of the lip. Surgery 1950; 27:321.
20. Wilson JS, Walker EP. Reconstruction of the lower lip. Head Neck Surg 1981; 4:29–44.
21. Baker SR. Risk factors in multiple carcinomas of the lip. Otolaryngol Head Neck Surg 1980; 88:248–251.
22. Zitsch RP III, Park CW, Renner GJ, Rea JL. Outcome analysis for lip carcinoma. Otolaryngol Head Neck Surg 1995; 113:589–596.
23. Baker SR, Krause CJ. Carcinoma of the lip. Laryngoscope 1980; 90:19–27.
24. Cruse CW, Radocha RF. Squamous cell carcinoma of the lip. Plast Reconstr Surg 1987; 80:787–791.
25. Frierson HF Jr, Cooper PH. Prognostic factors in squamous cell carcinoma of the lower lip. Hum Pathol 1986; 17:346–354.
26. McGregor GI, Davis NL, Hay JH. Impact of cervical lymph node metastases from squamous cell cancer of the lip. Am J Surg 1992; 163:469–471.
27. Bagatin M, Orihovac Z, Mohammed AM. Perineural invasion by carcinoma of the lower lip. J Craniomaxillofac Surg 1995; 23:155–159.
28. Teichgraeber JF, Larson DL. Some oncologic considerations in the treatment of lip cancer. Otolaryngol Head Neck Surg 1988; 98:589–592.
29. Bloom ND, Spiro RH. Carcinoma of the cheek mucosa. A retrospective analysis. Am J Surg 1980; 140:556–559.
30. Sieczka E, Datta R, Singh A, Loree T, Rigual N, Orner J, Hicks W Jr. Cancer of the buccal mucosa: are margins and T-stage accurate predictors of local control? Am J Otolaryngol 2001; 22:395–399.
31. Rao DN, Ganesh B, Rao RS, Desai PB. Risk assessment of tobacco, alcohol and diet in oral cancer–a case-control study. Int J Cancer 1994; 58:469–473.
32. Martin H, Pflueger O. Cancer of the cheek (buccal mucosa). Study of 99 cases with results of treatment at the end of five years. Arch Surg 1935; 30:731–747.

33. Brown R, Suh J, Scarborough J. Snuff Dippers intra-oral cancer: clinical characteristics and response to therapy. Cancer 1965; 18:2–13.
34. Rosenfeld L, Callaway J. Snuff Dipper's cancer. Am J Surg 1963; 106:840–844.
35. Urist MM, O'Brien CJ, Soong SJ, Visscher DW, Maddox WA. Squamous cell carcinoma of the buccal mucosa: analysis of prognostic factors. Am J Surg 1987; 154:411–414.
36. Slootweg PJ, Richardson M. Squamous cell carcinoma of the upper aerodigestive system. Philadelphia: WB Saunders, 2001.
37. Krolls SO, Hoffman S. Squamous cell carcinoma of the oral soft tissues: a statistical analysis of 14,253 cases by age, sex, and race of patients. J Am Dent Assoc 1976; 92: 571–574.
38. Martin H. Cancer of the Head and Neck. J Am Med Assoc 1948; 137:1306–1315, 1366–1376.
39. Gilbert S, Tzadik A, Leonard G. Mandibular involvement by oral squamous cell carcinoma. Laryngoscope 1986; 96:96–101.
40. McGregor AD, MacDonald DG. Patterns of spread of squamous cell carcinoma within the mandible. Head Neck 1989; 11:457–461.
41. McGregor AD, MacDonald DG. Routes of entry of squamous cell carcinoma to the mandible. Head Neck Surg 1988; 10:294–301.
42. Slootweg PJ, Muller H. Mandibular invasion by oral squamous cell carcinoma. J Craniomaxillofac Surg 1989; 17:69–74.
43. Wong RJ, Keel SB, Glynn RJ, Varvares MA. Histological pattern of mandibular invasion by oral squamous cell carcinoma. Laryngoscope 2000; 110:65–72.
44. Byers RM, Anderson B, Schwarz EA, Fields RS, Meoz R. Treatment of squamous carcinoma of the retromolar trigone. Am J Clin Oncol 1984; 7:647–652.
45. Lo K, Fletcher GH, Byers RM, Fields RS, Peters LJ, Oswald MJ. Results of irradiation in the squamous cell carcinomas of the anterior faucial pillar-retromolar trigone. Int J Radiat Oncol Biol Phys 1987; 13:969–974.
46. Kowalski LP, Hashimoto I, Magrin J. End results of 114 extended "commando" operations for retromolar trigone carcinoma. Am J Surg 1993; 166:374–379.
47. Fletcher GH, Lindberg RD. Squamous cell carcinomas of the tonsillar area and palatine arch. Am J Roentgenol Radium Ther Nucl Med 1966; 96:574–587.
48. Skolnik EM, Campbell JM, Meyers RM. Carcinoma of the buccal mucosa and retromolar area. Otolaryngol Clin North Am 1972; 5:327–331.
49. Shumrick DA, Quenelle DJ. Malignant disease of the tonsillar region, retromolar trigone, and buccal mucosa. Otolaryngol Clin N Am 1979; 12:115–124.
50. Brennan CT, Sessions DG, Spitznagel EL Jr, Harvey JE. Surgical pathology of cancer of the oral cavity and oropharynx. Laryngoscope 1991; 101:1175–1197.
51. Ballard BR, Suess GR, Pickren JW, Greene GW Jr, Shedd DP. Squamous-cell carcinoma of the floor of the mouth. Oral Surg Oral Med Oral Pathol 1978; 45:568–579.
52. Mashberg A. Diagnosis of early oral and oropharyngeal squamous carcinoma: obstacles and their amelioration. Oral Oncol 2000; 36:253–255.
53. Nason RW, Sako K, Beecroft WA, Razack MS, Bakamjian VY, Shedd DP. Surgical management of squamous cell carcinoma of the floor of the mouth. Am J Surg 1989; 158:292–296.
54. Woolgar JA, Scott J. Prediction of cervical lymph node metastasis in squamous cell carcinoma of the tongue/floor of mouth. Head Neck 1995; 17:463–472.
55. Spiro RH, Huvos AG, Wong GY, Spiro JD, Gnecco CA, Strong EW. Predictive value of tumor thickness in squamous carcinoma confined to the tongue and floor of the mouth. Am J Surg 1986; 152:345–350.
56. Shingaki S, Suzuki I, Nakajima T, Kawasaki T. Evaluation of histopathologic parameters in predicting cervical lymph node metastasis of oral and oropharyngeal carcinomas. Oral Surg Oral Med Oral Pathol 1988; 66:683–688.
57. Mohit-Tabatabai MA, Sobel HJ, Rush BF, Mashberg A. Relation of thickness of floor of mouth stage I and II cancers to regional metastasis. Am J Surg 1986; 152:351–353.

58. Brown B, Barnes L, Mazariegos J, Taylor F, Johnson J, Wagner RL. Prognostic factors in mobile tongue and floor of mouth carcinoma. Cancer 1989; 64:1195–1202.
59. Hicks WL Jr, Loree TR, Garcia RI, Maamoun S, Marshall D, Orner JB, Bakamjian VY, Shedd DP. Squamous cell carcinoma of the floor of mouth: a 20-year review. Head Neck 1997; 19:400–405.
60. van Es RJ, van Nieuw Amerongen N, Slootweg PJ, Egyedi P. Resection margin as a predictor of recurrence at the primary site for T1 and T2 oral cancers. Evaluation of histopathologic variables. Arch Otolaryngol Head Neck Surg 1996; 122:521–525.
61. Weijers M, Snow GB, Bezemer PD, van der Wal JE, van der Waal I. The clinical relevance of epithelial dysplasia in the surgical margins of tongue and floor of mouth squamous cell carcinoma: an analysis of 37 patients. J Oral Pathol Med 2002; 31: 11–15.
62. Carter RL, Tanner NS, Clifford P, Shaw HJ. Perineural spread in squamous cell carcinomas of the head and neck: a clinicopathological study. Clin Otolaryngol 1979; 4:271–281.
63. Spiro RH, Strong EW. Surgical treatment of cancer of the tongue. Surg Clin N Am 1974; 54:759–765.
64. Yuen AP, Lam KY, Wei WI, Ho CM, Chow TL, Yuen WF. A comparison of the prognostic significance of tumor diameter, length, width, thickness, area, volume, and clinicopathological features of oral tongue carcinoma. Am J Surg 2000; 180:139–143.
65. Asakage T, Yokose T, Mukai K, Tsugane S, Tsubono Y, Asai M, Ebihara S. Tumor thickness predicts cervical metastasis in patients with stage I/II carcinoma of the tongue. Cancer 1998; 82:1443–1448.
66. Morton RP, Ferguson CM, Lambie NK, Whitlock RM. Tumor thickness in early tongue cancer. Arch Otolaryngol Head Neck Surg 1994; 120:717–720.
67. Myers JN, Elkins T, Roberts D, Byers RM. Squamous cell carcinoma of the tongue in young adults: increasing incidence and factors that predict treatment outcomes. Otolaryngol Head Neck Surg 2000; 122:44–51.
68. Petruzzelli GJ, Myers EN. Malignant neoplasms of the hard palate and upper alveolar ridge. Oncology (Huntingt) 1994; 8:43–48; discussion 50, 53.
69. Anderson JN Jr, Beenken SW, Crowe R, Soong SJ, Peters G, Maddox WA, Urist MM. Prognostic factors in minor salivary gland cancer. Head Neck 1995; 17:480–486.
70. Vander Poorten VL, Balm AJ, Hilgers FJ, Tan IB, Keus RB, Hart AA. Stage as major long term outcome predictor in minor salivary gland carcinoma. Cancer 2000; 89: 1195–1204.
71. Ellis GL, Auclair PL. Tumors of the Salivary Glands, Atlas Pathology, Third Series, Fascicle 17. Washington DC: Armed Forced Institute of Pathology, 1996.
72. Chau MN, Radden BG. A clinical-pathological study of 53 intra-oral pleomorphic adenomas. Int J Oral Maxillofac Surg 1989; 18:158–162.
73. Gnepp DR. Malignant mixed tumors of the salivary glands: a review. Pathol Annu 1993; 28(Pt 1):279–328.
74. Brandwein M, Huvos AG, Dardick I, Thomas MJ, Theise ND. Noninvasive and minimally invasive carcinoma ex mixed tumor: a clinicopathologic and ploidy study of 12 patients with major salivary tumors of low (or no?) malignant potential. Oral Surg Oral Med Oral Pathol Oral Radiol Endod 1996; 81:655–664.
75. Auclair PL, Goode RK, Ellis GL. Mucoepidermoid carcinoma of intraoral salivary glands. Evaluation and application of grading criteria in 143 cases. Cancer 1992; 69:2021–2030.
76. Hanna DC, Clairmont AA. Submandibular gland tumors. Plast Reconstr Surg 1978; 61:198–203.
77. Xie X, Nordgard S, Halvorsen TB, Franzen G, Boysen M. Prognostic significance of nucleolar organizer regions in adenoid cystic carcinomas of the head and neck. Arch Otolaryngol Head Neck Surg 1997; 123:615–620.

78. Szanto PA, Luna MA, Tortoledo ME, White RA. Histologic grading of adenoid cystic carcinoma of the salivary glands. Cancer 1984; 54:1062–1069.
79. Hamper K, Lazar F, Dietel M, Caselitz J, Berger J, Arps H, Falkmer U, Auer G, Seifert G. Prognostic factors for adenoid cystic carcinoma of the head and neck: a retrospective evaluation of 96 cases. J Oral Pathol Med 1990; 19:101–107.
80. Batsakis JG, Luna MA, el-Naggar A. Histopathologic grading of salivary gland neoplasms: III. Adenoid cystic carcinomas. Ann Otol Rhinol Laryngol 1990; 99:1007–1009.
81. Spiro RH, Huvos AG. Stage means more than grade in adenoid cystic carcinoma. Am J Surg 1992; 164:623–628.
82. Evans HL, Batsakis JG. Polymorphous low-grade adenocarcinoma of minor salivary glands. A study of 14 cases of a distinctive neoplasm. Cancer 1984; 53:935–942.
83. Rajentheran R, McLean NR, Kelly CG, Reed MF, Nolan A. Malignant transformation of oral lichen planus. Eur J Surg Oncol 1999; 25:520–523.
84. Scully C, Beyli M, Ferreiro MC, Ficarra G, Gill Y, Griffiths M, Holmstrup P, Mutlu S, Porter S, Wray D. Update on oral lichen planus: etiopathogenesis and management. Crit Rev Oral Biol Med 1998; 9:86–122.
85. Holmstrup P. The controversy of a premalignant potential of oral lichen planus is over. Oral Surg Oral Med Oral Pathol 1992; 73:704–706.
86. Duffey DC, Eversole LR, Abemayor E. Oral lichen planus and its association with squamous cell carcinoma: an update on pathogenesis and treatment implications. Laryngoscope 1996; 106:357–362.
87. Marx RE. Osteoradionecrosis: a new concept of its pathophysiology. J Oral Maxillofac Surg 1983; 41:283–288.
88. Koka VN, Deo R, Lusinchi A, Roland J, Schwaab G. Osteoradionecrosis of the mandible: study of 104 cases treated by hemimandibulectomy. J Laryngol Otol 1990; 104:305–307.
89. Curi MM, Dib LL. Osteoradionecrosis of the jaws: a retrospective study of the background factors and treatment in 104 cases. J Oral Maxillofac Surg 1997; 55:540–544; discussion 545–546.
90. Hicks MJ, Flaitz CM. Oral mucosal melanoma: epidemiology and pathobiology. Oral Oncol 2000; 36:152–169.
91. Patel SG, Prasad ML, Escrig M, Singh B, Shaha AR, Kraus DH, Boyle JO, Huvos AG, Busam K, Shah JP. Primary mucosal malignant melanoma of the head and neck. Head Neck 2002; 24:247–257.
92. El-Mofty S, Kyriakos M. Soft tissue and bone lesions. In: Gnepp DR, ed. Diagnostic Surgical Pathology of the Head and Neck. Philadelphia: WB Saunders, 2001:505–604.
93. Hill DA, O'Sullivan MJ, Zhu X, Vollmer RT, Humphrey PA, Dehner LP, Pfeifer JD. Practical application of molecular genetic testing as an aid to the surgical pathologic diagnosis of sarcomas: a prospective study. Am J Surg Pathol 2002; 26:965–977.
94. Oda D, Bavisotto LM, Schmidt RA, McNutt M, Bruckner JD, Conrad EU III, Weymuller EA Jr. Head and neck osteosarcoma at the University of Washington. Head Neck 1997; 19:513–523.
95. Garrington GE, Scofield HH, Cornyn J, Hooker SP. Osteosarcoma of the jaws. Analysis of 56 cases. Cancer 1967; 20:377–391.
96. Batsakis JG. Surgical excision margins: a pathologist's perspective. Adv Anat Pathol 1999; 6:140–148.

5
Benign Lesions and Tumors of the Oral Cavity

Charles L. Dunlap
Department of Oral and Maxillofacial Pathology and Radiology, School of Dentistry, University of Missouri—Kansas City, Kansas City, Missouri, U.S.A.

INTRODUCTION

There is an ancient axiom that "all trouble comes from the mouth, but not all troubles leave." True to that axiom, numerous disfiguring developmental abnormalities, infections, and neoplasms take seed and remain in the oral and perioral tissues. Not only does the mouth have its own unique diseases, but also it often provides clues to wider problems. For example, failure of the immune system may initially be announced by oral candidiasis or hairy leukoplakia. Oral ulcers may signal inflammatory bowel disease before it is discovered in the bowel. The majority of substances that enter the body pass through the mouth, exposing the oral cavity to various elements such as cigarette smoke, which makes contact with oral tissues during inhalation and exhalation. Hematopoietic diseases such as leukemia, lymphoma, and myeloma and a host of venereal diseases are often initially evident in oral tissues. Thus, this chapter is devoted to benign, but not always harmless, lesions of this complicated structure.

Mucosa and Soft Tissue Traumatic Fibroma (Irritation Fibroma)

Nodules of hyperplastic fibrous connective tissue are among the most common of oral mucosal lesions. Their occurrence at sites that are easily bitten is circumstantial evidence that trauma is the causative factor. They are found mostly in adults and their duration is months to years with little change in size. The usual presentation is a broad-based, normal colored nodule, seldom larger than 1.5 cm. Patients are aware of the lesion but are asymptomatic unless the site has been recently irritated. Histologically the lesions consist of collagenous, acellular fibrous connective tissue covered by unremarkable squamous epithelium. The collagen fibers are coarse, interlacing, and brightly eosinophilic with few identifiable fibroblast nuclei. The term "collagenoma" would be an apt description for these lesions. Treatment is usually elective surgical excision. Tumors of minor salivary gland and soft tissue tumors such as neurofibroma may have a similar appearance and should be considered in the differential diagnosis.

Pyogenic Granuloma (Pregnancy Tumor, Lobular Capillary Hemangioma)

The exuberant proliferation of granulation tissue produces a sessile or polypoid mucosal mass, a pyogenic granuloma, which is found in people of all ages. The increased frequency with which it is encountered in pregnancy accounts for the term "pregnancy tumor," but the absence of estrogen and progesterone cell surface receptors leaves the relationship to pregnancy unexplained: the cause is unknown. Although pyogenic granulomas may occur on any skin or mucosal surface, the oral mucosal and especially the gingiva are among the most common sites. Clinically, pyogenic granulomas present as an easily bleeding, red mass that ranges in size from a few millimeters to several centimeters and lasts for weeks or months. In dentulous areas, the lesion may partially encircle or form a collar around a tooth. The tongue, lips, and buccal mucosa are other common sites. Microscopic examination reveals a unicentric or polylobate proliferation of granulation tissue. The vessel size ranges from capillary to small venules. Much of the surface is ulcerated and inflammation spreads into the underlying vascular connective tissue. The term "pyogenic granuloma" is misleading because pus is seldom encountered. The treatment is surgical excision, and the recurrence rate is unknown but is in the order of 10%. Pregnancy tumors may regress after parturition.

Peripheral Giant Cell Granuloma (Giant Cell Epulis)

The peripheral giant cell lesion is the gingival counterpart of the intrabony central giant cell granuloma. It is found almost exclusively in the mouth: two-thirds of all cases occurring in the mandibular gingiva, one-third in the maxillary gingiva. Peripheral giant cell lesions occur in both dentulous and edentulous alveolus. Approximately 8% occur in or adjacent to a recent dental extraction wound. It may be seen in children but occurs mainly in the midyears and is slightly more prevalent in females, although there is no increased incidence in pregnancy. The lesions range in size from millimeters to several centimeters. The red-to-purple color is accounted for by the percolation of blood through ill-defined, sinusoidal spaces and small areas of hemorrhage. The histomorphology is characterized by a proliferation of mononuclear cells with an overlay of multi-nucleated giant cells. Giant cells may be found within the lumen of thin-walled vascular channels. Foci of hemorrhage are found in almost 90% of cases and about 40% exhibit formation of osteoid and immature bone. Hemosiderin is plentiful and tends to concentrate at the superior pole of the lesion. The mononuclear cells and giant cells express vimentin, alpha 1-antichymotrypsin, and CD-68, suggesting a mononuclear macrophage lineage. Birbeck-granule-positive dendritic cells are found in 65% of cases, evidence of the presence of Langerhans histiocytes, although the significance of this presence is unknown. Treatment consists of surgical excision, with a recurrence rate of 10%. The clinician should confirm that the peripheral lesion is not a central lesion that has perforated the cortex, masquerading as a peripheral lesion. Peripheral giant cell epulis occurring as a manifestation of neurofibromatosis is rare.

Peripheral Ossifying Fibroma (Fibroid Epulis)

As the name implies, this lesion is a neoplasm but evidence suggests that peripheral ossifying fibroma originates as a reactive lesion, an inflammatory fibrous hyperplasia. These lesions are more common in the young and in females. They appear as a nodular mass and are not known to occur at sites other than the gingiva. The color is normal-to-red, and the size seldom exceeds 2.0 cm. Large lesions may cause the separation of teeth. The typical histologic finding is a proliferation of benign, cellular, fibrous connective tissue from which arise trabeculae of bone or droplets of acellular calcified matrix, putative cementum. The base of the lesion may harbor a florid infiltrate of plasma cells. Treatment is surgical excision and the recurrence rate is approximately 15%. Multiple recurrences are not uncommon.

Squamous Papilloma

Squamous papilloma is a hyperplastic proliferation of squamous epithelium and is a member of the family of mucocutaneous lesions that includes verrucous vulgaris and condyloma acuminatum. They are thought to be caused by the human papillomavirus (HPV), a large and growing family of viruses with more than 90 subtypes. No single member of this family is constantly associated with oral papillomas. HPV types 1, 2, 4, 6, 7, 11, 13, 16, 32, 57, 72, and 73 have been identified in oral papillomas and the virus is found in approximately 13% of specimens of normal oral mucosa. The ability to find the virus and identify the subtype may be related to the experience, skill, and tools of the clinician. The virus infects basal keratinocytes, and the portal of entry is created by a breach in the epithelial barrier. It is believed that the virus attaches to cell surface integrins and is internalized by endocytosis of the integrin-virus complex. Viral proteins E6 and E7 disable cellular proteins p53 and retinoblastoma (rb), respectively. Inactivation of these two important regulators of the cell cycle permits cells to pass through the Gl checkpoint unchallenged. Oral papillomas are commonly referred to as epithelial tumors but their behavior is that of a hyperplastic, not neoplastic lesion. Clinically they appear as exophytic, verrucous, or papillary lesions that are ordinarily a few millimeters in size. They lesions may be broad-based and sessile with a histomorphology is characterized by fronds of squamous epithelium, each with a core of edematous connective tissue. Increased numbers of mitoses are encountered but they are of normal morphology. Koilocytes are generally absent. The treatment is elective surgical removal and recurrences are rare. Oral squamous papillomas are associated with low-risk HPV and they do not undergo malignant transformation.

Mucocele

A breach in the duct of a minor salivary gland allows for the extravasation of saliva creating a mucocele. If the mucous escape is near or within the intraepithelial portion of the duct, the lesion appears as a small translucent vesicle, the superficial mucocele. Multiple superficial mucoceles should not confused with vesiculobullous diseases. More commonly, the breach occurs in the deeper portions of the duct resulting in a more deeply seated, broad-based mucosal swelling that may be blue-tinged. Those that occur in the floor of the mouth may grow to several centimeters in size, fill the floor of the mouth, and elevate the tongue. The resemblance to the abdomen of a frog (Rana frog) gives rise to the name, "ranula." Large ranulas may separate the fibers of the mylohyoid muscle and spread into the neck, referred to as plunging ranula. The lower lip is the most common location for mucoceles but any mucosa in which there are minor glands is a potential target. Sometimes forgotten are the glands of Blandin, located in the midline of the ventral tongue, the only site on the tongue where mucoceles are regularly encountered. Von Ebner's glands on the posterior dorsal tongue seem peculiarly immune. The typical presentation is a painless swelling of several weeks duration that has waxed and waned in size, a finding explained by cyclical episodes of secretion-resorption that alternately fill and empty the mucous lake. Microscopic examination reveals an intramucosal lake of extravasated salivary secretion walled off by a margin of cellular fibrous connective tissue from which is shed foamy histiocytes. The accumulation of histiocytes may be so dense that the lesion resembles a clear cell salivary tumor. Late lesions may be virtually obliterated by the ingrowth of granulation tissue. Mucoceles do not voluntary resolve and require surgical excision including the gland that feeds them. It is surprising that the procedure does not create new mucoceles. Large lesions in the floor of the mouth respond to marsupialization.

Granular Cell Tumor

Formerly referred to as granular cell myoblastoma and then as granular cell Schwannoma, this lesion is now referred to as granular cell tumor because of the certainty that it is not myoblastic and the continuing uncertainty of a Schwann cell parentage. It has been described in many viscera, soft tissues, and skin but in most series, the tongue is the most common site. It is found mostly in adults and ordinarily is solitary, but 10% are multiple. Multiple granular cell tumors have been linked to neurofibromatosis. Oral lesions appear as an intramucosal nodule that is painless, pale, and firm. Microscopic examination reveals sheets of tumor cells with abundant, eosinophilic granular cytoplasm and nuclei that show minimal pleomorphism. There is no capsule, and tumor cells extend into surrounding tissues including skeletal muscle where tumor cells may even appear within the sarcolemma. Similarly, nerve trunks may have a halo of tumor cells and they may appear within the nerve sheath. Ultrastructure images show the cytoplasm to be rich in lysosomes that account for the eosinophilic granules and the uptake of the McMannus' Periodic Acid Schiff's stain. Anti S-100 immunoperoxidase stain is positive, lending support to the Schwann cell lineage. Where tumor cells lie near squamous epithelium, it is not unusual to find florid pseudocarcinomatous hyperplasia. It may dominate the field and can easily be mistaken for superficially invasive squamous cell carcinoma. This lesion is treated by surgical excision; recurrences are infrequent. Congenital epulis of the newborn may resemble granular cell tumors histologically but the clinical presentation, negative response to S-100 stain, and the absence of pseudocarcinomatous hyperplasia are distinguishing features.

Cheilitis Granulomatosa (Miescher's Cheilitis)

There are few diseases that will cause chronic swelling of one or both lips other than cheilitis granulomatosa or Miescher's cheilitis. This form of cheilitis combined with fissured tongue and facial nerve paralysis constitutes the Melkersson–Rosenthal syndrome. Although labial swelling is the most common presentation, no orofacial tissue is immune. Facial skin, gingiva, buccal mucosa, tongue, and palate may be affected. The term orofacial granulomatosis recognizes the disparate forms of this condition. Females are more often affected than are males and the mean age of onset is 33 years. It is ushered in by cycles of unexplained edema and resolution that ultimately lead to swelling without remission. Examination of biopsy material reveals non-caseating, epithelioid granulomas devoid of foreign material and organisms. Granulomas may be few in number and multiple sections may be required to find them. In some instances, edema and a subtle lymphocytic infiltrate are the sole finding. It has been claimed that Miescher's cheilitis is an oligosymptomatic form of sarcoidosis and there are published accounts linking it to Crohn's disease. Though infrequently found, these conditions should be considered in the differential diagnosis. Intralesional injection of steroid suspension is standard treatment, and more than one round may be required. The literature contains reports of success with clofazimine and ciproheptadine. The role of cheiloplasty is controversial and probably should be reserved for debulking of advanced disease.

Epulis Fissuratum

Epulis fissuratum is an inflammatory fibrous hyperplasia of oral mucosa caused by frictional irritation due to a denture. The lesion usually occurs in the labial vestibule and appears as folds of redundant mucosa separated by a fissure. The depth of the fissure may be ulcerated. Biopsy reveals hyperplasia of moderately cellular fibrous connective tissue covered by squamous epithelium that ranges from atrophic to hyperplastic with focal ulceration. The inflammatory infiltrate is chronic unless near an ulcer. The lesion offers no diagnostic challenge and is treated by surgical excision and adjustment of the denture to prevent recurrence.

Drug-Induced Gingival Hyperplasia

Early in the curriculum, students in the health sciences learn that anti-convulsants may cause gingival enlargement. Purists argue that the term gingival hyperplasia is incorrectly used because the enlargement is caused by the accumulation of extracellular matrix rather than an increase in the number of cells. Soon after the introduction of phenytoin in 1938, this adverse effect was observed. More recently, two other classes of drugs, calcium channel blockers and cyclosporine, have been implicated. The risk associated with phenytoin is in the order of 50% and for cyclosporine, approximately 25%. Among the calcium channel blockers, the risk of gingival hyperplasia varies with the class of drug, from a high of 42% with nifedipine to a low of 4% with verapamil, drug-induced gingival hyperplasia begins within weeks to months and is announced by increased bulk and granularity of the interdental gingiva. The extent of enlargement may be modest and of cosmetic concern only or it may be so florid that teeth disappear in a mass of flesh. Scrupulous dental hygiene may reduce the severity but does not completely abolish the risk. Reports suggest that discontinuation of the drug produces regression of the mass at approximately the same rate it commenced. Furthermore, these drugs exhibit synergism with respect to the hyperplasia: administration of two drugs has a more pronounced effect than administration of a single agent. The histopathology is characterized by collagen-rich, cell-poor proliferation of fibrous connective tissue covered by squamous epithelium that typically exhibits elongated, bayonet-like rete ridges. In those cases requiring treatment, surgical gingivectomy is the only option. Meticulous control of bacterial dental plaque will help blunt recurrence. Diphenylhydantoin and sodium valproate not only produce well-documented gingival effects but they also induce a state of pseudohypoparathyroidism by increasing end-organ resistance to parathyroid hormone. Children receiving these anti-convulsants during years of tooth formation are subject to dental-pitting defects, hypodontia, and delayed dental eruption.

Bone Central Giant Cell Lesion (Giant Cell Reparative Granuloma, Giant Cell Tumor)

The term "central giant cell reparative granuloma" is a controversially termed lesion, as it implies a lesion arising as a response to injury. The conspicuous fact that this lesion arises in the absence of trauma, does not histologically resemble reparative tissue, is a purposeless growth, and shows progressive growth at the expense of the host argues persuasively that this lesion is a neoplasm. The term "giant cell lesion" avoids the controversy. The giant cell lesion may not be as aggressive as its extragnathic counterpart, perhaps partially accounted for by earlier discovery and treatment. The clinical features, radiographic characteristics, and behavior of this lesion are well known. The approximate rule of two-thirds is useful: two-thirds of patients are female, two-thirds are under the age of thirty, and two-thirds of the lesions occur in the mandible. Smaller lesions do not penetrate the cortex, but as the lesion expands, the cortical plate is eroded and the expanding mass is then covered by a thin shell of reactive bone. The lesion may not cause pain until it reaches a large size. It is not possible to recognize giant cell granuloma on radiographs alone, but clues are evident: the lesions do not form a calcified product, so are always radiolucent. When small they are unilocular but as they enlarge, scalloping at the tumor–host interface may create a sense of multi-locularity but seldom to the extent seen in lesions with which it may be confused, such as ameloblastoma. Teeth may be displaced, and roots frequently are resorbed.

Histologically, this lesion consists of a proliferation of mononuclear stromal cells, putative fibroblasts, and macrophages. Varying numbers of multi-nucleated giant cells are gathered in clusters or scattered evenly throughout the stromal cells. As many as 20 nuclei may be present in one giant cell. One-third of giant cell granulomas show osteoid formation but mineralization is insufficient to appear on radiographs. It is clear the giant cells are osteoclasts. They label with monoclonal antibodies to human osteoclasts (13C2 and 23C6) and show the same immunohistochemical profile as their extragnathic counterpart. Furthermore, the giant cells excavate bone, a property that is abolished by calcitonin. The old name of osteoclastoma may be an appropriate term. There is a histologic overlap of giant cell granuloma with cherubism and brown tumor of hyperparathyroidism. The treatment for this lesion is ordinarily by vigorous curettage, a procedure complicated by the presence of teeth. The recurrence rate is approximately 20%. Resection is reserved for those too large to curette. Subcutaneous injection of calcitonin has been reported to be successful in the management of giant cell lesions of the jaws and may be an alternative to surgery, especially for large lesions.

Florid Osseous Dysplasia (FOD)

Florid osseous dysplasia is the preferred name for a condition that has many other names, each reflecting a different opinion regarding the fundamental nature of the disease and the tissue of origin, bone or cementum. It is acquired during the early adult years, is non-neoplastic and non-inflammatory, is self-limiting and generally requires no treatment. The strong propensity that FOD exhibits for middle age African American females is unexplained, and the reason it affects the jaws and is unknown in the rest of the skeleton remains a mystery. The condition may be ushered in by painless expansion of the jaws but more commonly is silent and discovered on radiographs taken for other reasons.

Both the maxilla and mandible may be involved but variants are encountered in which one jaw or one quadrant of one jaw is involved. The mandible bears the brunt of the disease. Radiographically, FOD progresses over a period of years beginning as a purely radiolucent lesion and ending as solid, dense masses in the jaws. The intermediate stage appears as a mixed radiolucent-radiodense lesion involving much of the body of the bone. Confluent sclerotic masses surrounded by radiolucent areas form an image that is virtually pathognomic. The appearance of early lesions in the vicinity of dental root tips has led to speculation that the calcified, dense material is cementum rather than bone. This accounts for other names such as cemento-osseous dysplasia and sclerotic cemental masses of the jaws. As it progresses, lesions spread far beyond the teeth and fill the surrounding bone. Teeth are not resorbed nor displaced. Florid osseous dysplasia may be the ultimate expression of a spectrum of fibro-osseous disease, the minimal form of which is the common cementoma (periapical cemental dysplasia), which also shows a propensity for African American females. Cavities resembling traumatic bone cysts are encountered in some cases of FOD. The histologic features of FOD overlap other fibro-osseous lesions so that radiographic and clinical correlation is necessary. From benign, cellular fibrous connective tissue arise trabeculae of woven bone and droplet, acellular calcifications that resemble cementum. The latter may grow to form large, globular masses that are more basophilic than bone and have prominent reversal lines. The histologic and radiographic features mimic Paget's disease of bone to some extent but in FOD, serum calcium values and alkaline phosphatase are unaltered and extragnathic lesions do not exist. When FOD is localized, it may resemble ossifying fibroma radiographically and histologically. No treatment is required for florid osseous dysplasia.

However, clinicians should be aware that sclerotic bone, regardless of the cause, is more vulnerable to infection. Invasive dental procedures such as dental extractions should take this into account. Edentulous patients pose another problem. Slow but inexorable atrophy of the alveolar bone may alter denture fit so that friction ulcers develop. This creates a portal of entry for pathogens and heightens the risk of osteomyelitis.

Cherubism

Cherubism was originally described as familial multi-locular cystic disease of the jaws in 1933. When it became apparent that the jaw lesions were not cysts, it was retermed as familial FD of the jaws, which was subsequently abandoned when it was observed that it differed histologically from FD of bone. The swollen jaws so characteristic of this disease resemble full-faced cherubs in Renaissance art, thus "cherubism." Most cases of cherubism are inherited as an autosomal dominant trait. Symptoms may appear as early as three years. Painless swelling of one or both jaws is common and failure of teeth to erupt on time or to erupt ectopically may call attention to the disorder. Expression is variable in that some children have minimal swelling, and others may experience massive enlargement. Penetrance of the gene is approximately 70% in females. Clinically normal mothers may pass cherubism to their children, and new mutations account for sporadic cases. The gene for cherubism has been mapped to chromosome 4p16.3; the candidate gene codes for a fibroblastic growth factor receptor. Mutations in this gene have been implicated in a variety of other skeletal disorders including achondroplasia, thanatophoric dysplasia type I, and Crouzon syndrome. Patients exhibiting both cherubism and the Noonan phenotype have been described. The radiographic features of cherubism are characteristic and easily recognized on panoramic films. In the early stage, bilateral multi-locular radiolucent lesions appear in the angles of the mandible and the ascending rami.

Lesions in the maxilla are more difficult to see because of the presence of the nasal cavities and the maxillary sinuses. More sophisticated imaging such as computed tomography may be required. As the condition progresses, the jaws enlarge painlessly and the radiolucent lesions advance and occupy virtually the entire volume of the jaws. Maxillary lesions impinge on the orbit and press the globe upward producing the heavenly gaze. Most patients have jaw lesions only, but occasionally a solitary extragnathic lesion may be found. The histopathologic features of cherubism resemble those of giant cell granuloma. Multi-nucleated giant cells lie in a stroma of mononuclear fibroblasts. The giant cells are osteoclasts which synthesize tartrate-resistant acid phosphatase, express the receptor for vitronectin, and are capable of resorbing bone, a property that is inhibited by calcitonin. The treatment of cherubism is determined by the severity of the disease. The established fact that this disease tends to slow with age and may completely regress in the early adult years is the rationale for treatment that does not exceed that which functional and esthetic considerations require. When treatment is required, the only option is surgical reduction by curettage and recontouring.

Fibrous Dysplasia (FD)

The hallmark of FD is the appearance of painless enlargement of bone usually before the end of the second decade of life. It may involve one bone (monostotic) or many bones (polyostotic). Polyostotic FD occurring with cutaneous cafe au lait pigmentation and endocrinopathy constitute the McCune–Albright syndrome. The cause of FD has been a mystery since its recognition more than a half century ago. The discovery of a gain-in-function mutation in the gene encoding the signal transducing G protein has provided new insight. Cells with this mutation have a proliferation advantage over those that do not. The extent of the disease is determined by the time in life when the activating mutation occurs.

Mutation early in embryogenesis accounts for the mosaic distribution of skeletal lesions resulting in polyostotic disease. If the mutation is confined to osteoprogenitor cells, the phenotype is skeletal disease only, the Jaffe phenotype. Appearance of the mutating event earlier in embryogenesis and ostensibly involving a cell ancestral to osteoprogenitor, endocrine, and pigment cell lineages results in the full McCune–Albright syndrome. Somatic mutation later in life accounts for more common monostotic presentation that accounts for approximately 70% of all cases. The fact that the lesions appear to grow without purpose and are attributed to gene mutations that have oncogene-like function suggests a neoplastic disease. However, the observation that lesions of FD eventually decrease proliferation and that growth of the lesion is arrested as the skeleton matures indicates a developmental abnormality. There is lack of agreement regarding the radiographic appearance of FD. Some authors accept a radiolucent lesion with well-defined borders as within the range of FD. The prevailing view is the FD appears as a fine-grain (ground glass), radiodense lesion with indistinct borders that blends imperceptibly with adjacent normal bone. The two views are not mutually exclusive. FD may evolve as the disease progresses, changing radiographically along the way similar to Paget's disease of bone and florid osseous dysplasia. The bone lesions of FD are characterized by the proliferation of spindle mesenchymal cells that replace and fill the normal marrow, cause resorption of native bone matrix, expand the bone and thin the cortex, and eventually replace the normal lamellated bone with new, structurally unsound woven bone. Unrestrained activity enlarges the bone and betrays the presence of the disease. Because the histopathologic features of FD are similar to other fibro-osseous lesions, microscopy alone is often insufficient for diagnosis.

It is useful to determine if there is osteoblastic rimming, a term that describes an orderly row of osteoblasts bordering newly formed bone. The absence of rimming is widely accepted as a feature of FD that helps to separate it from other lesions; however, published accounts of inherited craniofacial lesions of FD show osteoblastic rimming. The shape of the newly deposited bone trabeculae has been described as being curvilinear, an unreliable feature. The spindle cells that constitute the parenchyma are osteoprogenitor cells that resemble ordinary fibroblasts, and the nuclei are uniform in size and shape. The appearance of nuclear pleomorphism or atypical mitoses suggests the diagnosis of FD may be wrong as FD is not neoplastic. Rather, it forms a mass that may clinically and radiographically resemble a neoplasm but with time, growth ceases. A similar unexplained phenomenon occurs in other jaw disease such as cherubism. Treatment planning should take the limited growth potential into account. Surgery is the only option and should be reserved for those cases that exceed acceptable functional and cosmetic limits. The conversion of FD to osteogenic sarcoma has been reported but it is a rare event.

Langerhans Cell Granulomatosis [Langerhans Cell Histocytosis (LCH)]

Clonal expansion of Langerhans cells creates a spectrum of disease whose unknown cause and unpredictable behavior have thwarted attempts at classification. The recognition that LCH is a monoclonal proliferation and when disseminated, is aggressive and potentially fatal, suggests it is neoplastic. However, the indolent behavior of localized lesions and instances of spontaneous regression suggest otherwise. Despite monoclonality, LCH may eventually prove to be a condition whose underpinning is the loss of regulatory control of an immune response. Although generally thought of as a childhood diseases, LCH has been encountered from infancy through the ninth decade of life. Few organs are immune but bone, lung, skin, lymph nodes, and the hypothalamus/pituitary axis bear the brunt of the disease.

The clinical presentation is wide ranging. The most common is unifocal or multi-focal osseous disease, and approximately 30% have disseminated multi-system disease. In the mouth, LCH is often announced by unexplained pain in the maxilla or mandible, and the overlying mucosa may be swollen or ulcerated. The mandible is more often involved than is the maxilla. It is found chiefly in the young, and most patients are under the age of 30. The radiographic features are not diagnostic; biopsy is required for diagnosis. Lesions are invariably radiolucent, and the border may be well defined or indistinct. Lesions of LCH occur chiefly in the tooth-bearing areas of the jaws. Painful and destructive lesions around the teeth may be confused with infections of dental origin. The teeth are innocent bystanders and when incorporated in the lesions of LCH, they may be bodily displaced or roots may undergo resorption. Seldom do the microscopic features present a diagnostic problem. Sheets of mononuclear macrophages efface the normal architecture. They are often accompanied by varying numbers of eosinophils and occasional multinucleated giant cells. If the lesion is in soft tissue that is ulcerated, non-specific inflammation obscures the underlying disease. Langerhans cells are identified by a positive reaction to the anti-S100 immunoperoxidase stain. It is ordinarily not necessary to demonstrate other identifying features such as surface CD1a and Birbeck granules. Chemotherapy is the mainstay of disseminated disease, and prednisone and vinblastine are one of several regimens. For unifocal bone disease, the form most commonly encountered in the jaws, surgical curettage alone or in combination with external-beam, low-dose radiotherapy provides a cure rate of approximately 90%. The optimum dose of radiotherapy has not been established but ordinarily does not exceed 15 Gy.

Osteosclerosis

Sclerotic lesions in the maxilla and mandible are seen in a variety of well-characterized conditions including florid osseous dysplasia, Gardner's syndrome, and others. When these are eliminated, there remains localized, self-limiting sclerotic lesions of unknown origin that have been recognized by a variety of names including idiopathic osteosclerosis, dense bone islands, bone whorl, enostosis, and others. Surveys of dental radiographs reveal an incidence of about 5%. Osteosclerosis is discovered on radiographs taken for other reasons and is always asymptomatic. The most common location is the mandible and the majority is seen in the cuspid–bicuspid region. Osteosclerotic lesions may be seen in children but most are recognized in young adults. Radiographically they appear as a uniform dense lesion that sharply abuts on adjacent bone without a radiolucent halo. The size ranges from a few millimeters to several centimeters. In tooth-bearing areas, osteosclerosis may envelop a portion of the tooth root and appear to be attached. Alternately, they may partially fill the space between teeth or occupy an edentulous area. Even large lesions do not expand the jaw. The history will provide no explanation regarding cause, as there is no common denominator. Some lesions may be of developmental origin, whereas others are the result of overzealous bone repair after oral surgery or from past infections. Clinicians whose responsibilities include the jaws should be familiar with osteosclerosis, the range of its appearance, and harmless behavior.

Exostosis

Non-neoplastic bony enlargements of the jaws that have limited growth potential are collectively referred to as exostoses. Those that occur in the midline of the maxilla are known as torus palatinus, and when located on the lingual aspect of the mandible as torus mandibularis. At other sites, they have no special name. The frequency with which they occur is uncertain. An often-quoted figure for torus palatinus is 20%, for torus mandibularis approximately 10%. One survey found 29 per 1000 persons (2.9%) for all tori, a figure that seems more accurate. Palatal tori are twice as common in females as in males but there is no sex specificity for mandibular lesions. Exostoses arise early in life, as early as the first decade. The majority is present before age 40. Mandibular tori are usually bilateral and located on the lingual aspect of the mandible in the cuspid–bicuspid region. They may appear as a single nodule or as a row of confluent nodules. Their size ranges from those so small they are inconspicuous to those so large they fill the floor of the mouth. Exostoses do not present a diagnostic problem to those who are aware of their existence and are familiar with their clinical appearance. Exostoses are asymptomatic, bony hard, and covered by normal oral mucosa; thus, people are chiefly unaware of their existence. Health care workers who are unfamiliar with exostoses of the jaws are likely to overdiagnose them as tumors. Histologically they consist of medullary bone with a fatty marrow and a thin cortex. Removal is not required unless they interfere with dental prostheses.

Cysts

Periapical Cyst (Radicular Cyst, Root-End Cyst)

A periapical cyst arises at the root-end of a tooth whose pulp in inflamed or necrotic. Common causes of pulp inflammation and necrosis are dental caries, blunt trauma, and thermal injury. Regardless of cause, inflammation is originally confined to the interior of the tooth. If untreated, inflammation exits the tooth and spreads to the apical periodontal membrane and adjacent bone. With time, bone is resorbed, creating a periapical lesion consisting of inflamed granulation tissue. At this stage, the lesion is referred to as a periapical granuloma. If there is suppuration, it is a periapical abscess. If epithelial rests of Malassez lie within this smoldering lesion, they may proliferate to form a ball of epithelium that eventually becomes hollow in the center. The result is a periapical cyst. Most periapical cysts are discovered on routine dental radiographs. Radiographs reveal a round to oval, sharply circumscribed radiolucent lesion usually centered over the root tip of the offending tooth. In some cases, the cyst may lie along the side of the root. The tooth is not responsive to thermal and electrical stimulation. If the tooth responds normally to stimulation, the lesion is not a periapical cyst but another disease masquerading as one. The histologic features are rather constant. If the cyst is removed intact, the pathologist identities a central cavity, the lumen, which contains the detritus of inflammation, hemorrhage, and sloughed epithelium. The cyst wall is of fibrous connective tissue exhibiting a polymorphic inflammatory infiltrate, plasma cells, and lymphocytes. Apicular clefts identify the areas occupied by cholesterol crystals. Foreign body giant cells and hemosiderin pigment are found between these clefts. In a minority of cases, brightly eosinophilic Rushton bodies are seen in the squamous epithelium that lines the cyst lumen. The treatment of periapical cyst is tied to the treatment of the offending tooth. If the tooth is amenable to endodontic treatment, the cyst may resolve without surgical intervention. Large cysts are ordinarily removed in conjunction with the endodontic procedure. The alternative is extraction of the offending tooth accompanied by cystectomy.

Dentigerous Cyst (Follicular Cyst)

A cyst that occurs around the crown of an unerupted tooth is called a dentigerous cyst or follicular cyst. They are thought to arise as a result of the accumulation of fluid between the crown of the tooth and the dental follicular tissue that surrounds the crown. Why this happens is unknown. A cyst may develop around any impacted tooth but they are more commonly encountered around impacted third molar teeth. The risk of developing a dentigerous cyst around an unerupted tooth has been placed at approximately 1.0%. Dentigerous cysts range in size from those that are so small they may appear to be a hyperplastic follicle to those that are many centimeters, so large that they occupy large regions of the bone. Large cysts may remain asymptomatic but will cause expansion of the bone. On radiographs, they are purely radiolucent and usually are unilocular, rarely multi-locular. The associated tooth may be inverted and displaced far from its normal location. Histologically, the dentigerous cyst is lined by unremarkable stratified squamous epithelium. The cyst wall is of fibrous connective tissue and it is attached to the neck of the associated tooth. It may or may not exhibit inflammation. The treatment consists of cystectomy along with the offending tooth. Large cysts respond to marsupialization. The radiographic differential diagnosis is odontogenic keratocyst (OKC), adenomatoid odontogenic tumor, and cystic ameloblastoma.

OKC and the Nevoid Basal Cell Carcinoma Syndrome

This is the most interesting of jaw cysts. Unlike other cysts, it has a high recurrence rate estimated to be about 30%. Radiographically, OKC is a great mimic and may resemble dentigerous cyst, periapical cyst, traumatic bone cyst, and tumors such as giant cell granuloma and ameloblastoma. It is so named because of the prodigious production of keratin by the lining epithelium, so much that the cyst lumen may be virtually filled with keratin. The OKC may be discovered on routine dental radiographs or by the appearance of unexplained swelling. The radiographic characteristics are not diagnostic but the histomorphology is. The lining epithelium has a flat basement membrane, basal epithelial cells are frequently columnar or cuboidal and aligned-like dominos, a feature referred to as basal cell palisading. The surface of the epithelium is frequently undulating with a thin layer of keratin or parakeratin. Orthokeratin is sloughed into the cyst lumen where it appears as lamellated, eosinophilic strands that on gross examination may resemble toothpaste. Small daughter cysts may be found in the cyst wall. The keratocyst may be sporadic or a part of the nevoid basal cell carcinoma syndrome (Gorin's syndrome). The syndrome is transmitted as an autosomal dominant trait and is characterized by the early onset of multiple cutaneous basal cell carcinomas, multiple keratocysts, bifid ribs, calcified falx cerebri, and medulloblastoma, and a host of other lesions. The gene has been mapped to 9q22.3 and is the human equivalent of the transmembrane-patched protein involved in the determination of segment polarity in *Drosophila*. Mutations in this gene have been found in the Gorin syndrome, sporadic cutaneous basal cell carcinoma, medulloblastoma, and the epithelial cells in both sporadic and syndromic OKCs. The gene behaves as a tumor suppressor gene. OKCs are ordinarily treated by curettage but also respond to marsupialization. Peripheral osteotomy has also been advocated. In this approach, following curettage, a round bone bur is used to enlarge the bony cavity to eliminate remnants of the cyst that may be the source of a future recurrence. Chemical cautery of the cyst bed using topical application of Carnoy's solution has been recommended as an alternative to surgical osteotomy. Carnoy's solution, a mixture of absolute alcohol, chloroform, glacial acetic acid, and ferric chloride, is not readily available in the United States. A third approach using application of liquid nitrogen either by direct spray or cryoprobe followed by immediate bone grafting using cancellous bone and marrow has been used to reduce the risk of recurrence of a variety of aggressive bone lesions including OKCs.

Traumatic Bone Cyst

The traumatic bone cyst is an exception to the rule that jaw cysts have an epithelial lining. Not only does it lack an epithelial lining, but also it may be almost devoid of tissue of any type. Surgical entry into this lesion reveals an empty cavity whose only contents are a few shards of fibrous connective tissue, a small amount of fluid, or hemorrhagic debris. The absence of a history of injury in many who have a traumatic bone cyst is reason to doubt the relationship to trauma. The increased incidence in males, supposedly accounted for by their robust lifestyle, has not been supported by large series that show no sex preference. The traumatic bone cyst is a lesion of youth, fully 75% occur before the age of 30. Mandibular lesions account for more than 95% of all cases; they are rare in the maxilla. In the mandible, it is more common in the premolar–molar region. Multiple cysts in a single patient have been reported but are rare. The increased incidence of multiple cysts in black females may reflect a relationship to florid osseous dysplasia, a bone disease in which traumatic bone cyst-like cavities are known to occur. Most traumatic bone cysts are asymptomatic but occasionally there is swelling, pain, or paresthesia. Because the radiographs are not diagnostic, biopsy is required. Upon entry into the lesion, if the surgeon finds an empty cavity, then the diagnosis is established, and no further procedure is required. Even large lesions will fill with bone in 6–12 months.

Odontogenic Tumor

After tooth formation is completed at approximately the age of 18 years, remnants of odontogenic tissue remain in the jaws for a lifetime. They are called the epithelial rests of Malassez when located in the periodontal membrane and rests of Serres in the gingiva. These odontogenic epithelial rests along with the epithelial lining of cysts and basal cells of gingival epithelium are thought to be the source of many odontogenic tumors. Odontogenic tumors are diverse but generally benign, although they may be locally aggressive and grow to considerable size.

Ameloblastoma

Ameloblastoma is one of the most sinister of odontogenic tumors. It is unencapsulated, infiltrates through bone marrow, and requires excision with a wide margin of surrounding bone to prevent recurrence. This tumor is named for its resemblance to ameloblasts, the enamel-forming cells of the tooth germ. This tumor is found mainly in the middle years and occurs chiefly in the body of the mandible; only 15% occur in the maxilla. Small tumors may escape detection unless found on routine dental radiographs. Eventually they expand the jaw and may cause pain or paresthesia. Three distinct types of ameloblastoma exist. The most common type is the solid ameloblastoma, which paradoxically may develop microcystic spaces. It is this type that infiltrates bone and requires aggressive treatment. It typically appears as a multi-locular radiolucent lesion although unilocular tumors do occur. The histologic features of solid ameloblastoma are easily recognized. The tumor cells form islands (the follicular pattern) or anastomosing cords (the plexiform pattern) that are caricatures of the enamel organ. Most peripheral cells are tall, columnar cells resting on a basement membrane that abuts the surrounding fibrous connective tissue stroma. The nuclei of the tall cells migrate to the end most remote from the basement membrane, a property referred to as reverse nuclear polarity. Furthermore, the cytoplasm between the nucleus and the basal end is typically vacuolated. These two features are important identifying characteristics. In the central regions of the epithelial islands or cords, the cells are angular to fusiform to stellate in shape. The resemblance to the stellate reticulum of the epithelial portion of the tooth germ is inescapable. There are histologic variants of ameloblastoma. Acanthomatous, desmoplastic, clear cell, and granular cell variants have been described. A less common type is the unicystic ameloblastoma. It typically appears as a solitary, unilocular radiolucent lesion that may bear no relationship to teeth or alternately may be associated with an unerupted tooth, in which case it radiographically resembles a dentigerous cyst. The epithelium that lines this lesion exhibits the characteristic cytologic features of odontogenic epithelium.

This lesion has a low recurrence rate after simple curettage. In some instances, budding of the tumor cells into the wall of this cystic tumor results in a "mural" tumor. Should the infiltrating tumor cells penetrate the full thickness of the tumor wall and invade surrounding bone, it should be treated as a solid ameloblastoma.

The peripheral ameloblastoma is the third and least common type. It arises from basal cells of the gingival epithelium and clinically appears as a soft tissue mass in the gingival. The peripheral ameloblastoma is the result of neoplastic transformation of basal epithelium in the gingiva and is analogous to cutaneous basal cell carcinoma. The tumor infiltrates underlying connective tissue in a pattern that resembles basal cell carcinoma except that the tumor cells retain odontogenic characteristics. There are rare examples of ameloblastoma in which the tumor cells exhibit cytologic features ordinarily associated with malignancy. Such tumors are referred to as ameloblastic carcinoma and they are capable of metastasis. Whether the rare clear cell odontogenic carcinoma is a separate entity or a clear cell variant of ameloblastoma is unknown. There is little controversy about the treatment of large, solid ameloblastoma. Curettage is so often met with recurrence that most surgeons recommend complete excision with at least a 1.0 cm margin of bone beyond the radiographic edge of the tumor. Because mandibular tumors so often encroach on the inferior border of the mandible, it may not be possible to achieve an adequate margin in which case full-thickness resection is required. For smaller tumors in which a margin is attainable, a lesser procedure that does not interrupt the continuity of the bone may suffice. Some surgeons recommend the tumor bed be treated by peripheral osteotomy, chemical cautery, or cryotherapy as discussed under the section on OKCs.

Large tumors in the posterior maxilla present a special problem because of the presence of the maxillary sinus and proximity of other structures such as the eye. The unicystic variant is ordinarily treated by vigorous curettage unless tumor cells have penetrated the full thickness of the tumor wall, in which case it must be treated more aggressively. Peripheral ameloblastomas are ordinarily recognized when still small and have a good prognosis after simple excision with a margin free of tumor.

Adenomatoid Odontogenic Tumor

The adenomatoid odontogenic tumor accounts for approximately 5% of odontogenic tumors and is one of the most innocuous. The name derives from the histopathology, which reveals the formation of duct-like structures that impart a glandular appearance. It is a tumor of youth; most occur before age 30. Approximately 75% are found to be associated with an unerupted tooth. They occur more often in the anterior segments of the jaws and two-thirds of all cases occur in the maxilla. There is some variation in the radiographic appearance. Most are purely radiolucent but small calcifications may be seen in a minority of cases. Those that are associated with an unerupted tooth radiographically resemble a typical dentigerous cyst. The tumor is enveloped by a thick capsule of fibrous connective tissue. Within the capsule is tumor tissue that consists of oval to spindle epithelium that forms round "rosettes." In the typical case, the rosettes develop a central cavity lined by cuboidal to columnar epithelial cells that form duct-like structures. The tumor stroma is scant and acellular and may contain small areas of dystrophic calcification. Anastomosing thin strands of tumor cells often form a network at the tumor–capsule interface. The presence of a thick capsule eases curettage, and recurrences are virtually unknown.

Ameloblastic Fibroma

Ameloblastic fibroma is a tumor in which both the epithelial component and stroma are neoplastic. It is rare: only 122 cases had been reported by 1997. Clinicians and pathologists should be aware of this tumor to avoid confusing it with ameloblastoma. It is found almost exclusively in the first two decades of life; the average age is 14 years. Almost 70% are found in the posterior mandible. It is not unusual for this tumor to interfere with formation and eruption of teeth, a finding in approximately 75% of patients. Painless swelling or failure of teeth to erupt calls attention to the tumor. Small lesions less than 4.0 cm may be unilocular but larger tumors are more often multi-locular. The microscopic features are characterized by small islands and cords of epithelium growing in an ectomesenchymal stroma that resembles primitive dental pulp tissue. The peripheral epithelial cells may be columnar and exhibit reverse nuclear polarity but there is little tendency to form stellate reticulum-like tissue. Stromal hyalinization adjacent to the epithelium is presumed to be an inductive effect but hard tissue is not formed in this tumor. A granular cell variant of ameloblastic fibroma exists in which the ectomesenchymal element is converted to eosinophilic, granular cells. Additionally, there is a malignant version, the ameloblastic fibrosarcoma. In this tumor, the ectomesenchyme assumes the cytologic characteristics and behavior of a sarcoma. More than 50 cases have been reported. The ameloblastic fibroma is not encapsulated but local infiltration is minimal. Most are cured by thorough enucleation. A recurrence rate of 18% has been reported.

Myxoma

The evidence that myxoma is a tumor of odontogenic ectomesenchyme is circumstantial. The observation that most myxomas occur in tooth-bearing areas of the jaws and are so infrequently encountered in an extragnathic location has been cited as evidence of origin from odontogenic tissue. In one series of 5000 bone tumors, three examples of extragnathic myxoma were identified, all in the femur. This is not an impressive number but does cast doubt on the concept that myxoma is derived from odontogenic ectomesenchyme. Immunoperoxidase stains, usually helpful in identifying cell lineage in so many tumors, is not useful with odontogenic tumors including myxomas. Stains for vimentin and muscle-specific actin are positive but add little regarding histogenesis. Myxoma is a tumor seen principally in the second and third decades. Like many tumors of the jaws, they provoke little symptoms and may grow to a large size before discovery. Radiographically, there are no identifying characteristics, and biopsy is required for diagnosis. They are purely radiolucent and may be unilocular or multi-locular. "Wispy" trabeculae of bone may course through the tumor and are highly suggestive of myxoma but they are not pathognomonic. The microscopic features of myxoma are straightforward, and special stains are ordinarily not required. Seasoned surgeons may recognize the tumor first by the white, slippery, and gelatinous consistency. The tumor is hypocellular. Spindle, angular, or stellate myxoblasts lie randomly arranged in a pale, mucoid matrix comprised of hyaluronic acid and chondroitin sulfate. Occasional islands of odontogenic epithelium may be encountered but they are not an essential part of the tumor. Rests of Malassez may be incidentally incorporated in the tumor. Areas may be encountered in which there is transition to more cellular and collagen rich zones. The term myxofibroma has been used to describe such tumors but the behavior remains unchanged. Myxomas are unencapsulated, locally infiltrating tumors. When small, cure may be achieved by vigorous curettage. Large tumors require complete surgical excision with a margin or normal bone. In this regard, the treatment is essentially the same as for ameloblastoma.

Odontoma

Odontomas are the most common odontogenic tumors, accounting for almost 50% of all cases. Although, they are referred to as neoplasms, they behave more like odontogenic hamartomas rather than neoplasms. Odontomas are of compound and complex types. The compound type is characterized by the formation of multiple small, malformed tooth-like structures. All of the tissues that comprise a tooth, including enamel and dentin matrix and dental soft tissues, are present and are assembled in the form of imperfect caricatures of teeth. In the complex odontoma, the same tissues are present but in a tangled mass that bears no resemblance to teeth. The distinction is arbitrary since there are hybrid lesions exhibiting mixtures of the two and there is no difference in behavior. It is argued that the compound odontoma is a true hamartoma whereas the complex type is the end stage of the maturation of an ameloblastic fibroma. The issue is of academic interest only. Odontomas are found in aft regions of both jaws and most are recognized before age 20. They cause no symptoms and are discovered on radiographs taken in the course of routine dental care. Because they occur during the time of life when teeth are forming and erupting, they may impair these activities. It is common to find an impacted but otherwise normal tooth in the vicinity of an odontoma. Most odontomas are recognizable radiographically. This is especially true of compound odontomas. Multiple small dense bodies resemble a "bag of marbles." Complex odontoma does not have this identifying characteristic and removal for microscopic examination may be required to rule out other bone tumors. Odontomas may be associated with a cyst. The cyst may be mundane and lined by simple squamous epithelium, but there are a number of reports of odontoma associated with the calcifying odontogenic cyst. Approximately 15% of odontomas will be found to have ghost cells of the type encountered in the calcifying odontogenic cyst but no cyst is present. Removal is elective. These tumors seem to have a predetermined size and when this size is attained, growth ceases. Tumors that do no harm to adjacent structures or do not occupy needed space may be followed radiographically and removed it there is change, which is unlikely.

REFERENCES

1. Alani RM, Munger K. Human papillomaviruses and associated malignancies. J Clin Oncol 1998; 16(1):330–337.
2. Angelopoulos AP. Pyogenic granuloma of the oral cavity: statistical analysis of its clinical features. J Oral Surg 1971; 29(12):840–847.
3. Appleton RE, Leach H. Delayed eruption of secondary dentition associated with phenytoin therapy. Dev Med Child Neurol 1991; 33(12):1117–1118.
4. Ardekian L, et al. Clinical and radiographic features of eosinophilic granuloma in the jaws: review of 41 lesions treated by surgery and low-dose radiotherapy. Oral Surg Oral Med Oral Pathol Oral Radiol Endod 1999; 87(2):238–242.
5. Barker BF. Odontogenic myxoma. Semin Diagn Pathol 1999; 16(4):297–301.
6. Barker DS, Lucas RB. Localised fibrous overgrowths of the oral mucosa. Br J Oral Surg 1967; 5(2):86–92.
7. Barreto DC, et al. PTCH gene mutations in odontogenic keratocysts. J Dent Res 2000; 79(6):1418–1422.
8. Bouquot JE, Gundlach KK. Oral exophytic lesions in 23,616 white Americans over 35 years of age. Oral Surg Oral Med Oral Pathol 1986; 62(3):284–291.

9. Brook IM, King DJ, Miller ID. Chronic granulomatous cheilitis and its relationship to Crohn's disease. Oral Surg Oral Med Oral Pathol 1983; 56(4):405–408.
10. Carvalho YR, et al. Peripheral giant cell granuloma. An immunohistochemical and ultrastructural study. Oral Dis 1995; 1(1):20–25.
11. Corio RL, et al. Ameloblastic carcinoma: a clinicopathologic study and assessment of eight cases. Oral Surg Oral Med Oral Pathol 1987; 64(5):570–576.
12. Courtney RM, Kerr DA. The odontogenic adenomatoid tumor. A comprehensive study of twenty new cases. Oral Surg Oral Med Oral Pathol 1975; 39(3):424–435.
13. Cutright DE. The histopathologic findings in 583 cases of epulis fissuratum. Oral Surg Oral Med Oral Pathol 1974; 37(3):401–411.
14. Favara BE, et al. Contemporary classification of histiocytic disorders. The WHO Committee on histiocytic/reticulum cell proliferations. Reclassification Working Group of the Histiocyte Society. Med Pediatr Oncol 1997; 29(3):157–166.
15. Flanagan AM, et al. The multinucleate cells in giant cell granulomas of the jaw are osteoclasts. Cancer 1988; 62(6):1139–1145.
16. Gardner DG. Peripheral ameloblastoma: a study of 21 cases, including 5 reported as basal cell carcinoma of the gingiva. Cancer 1977; 39(4):1625–1633.
17. Gardner DG. Some current concepts on the pathology of ameloblastomas. Oral Surg Oral Med Oral Pathol Oral Radiol Endod 1996; 82(6):660–669.
18. Garlick JA, Taichman LB. Human papillomavirus infection of the oral mucosa. Am J Dermatopathol 1991; 13(4):386–395.
19. Geist JR, Katz JO. The frequency and distribution of idiopathic osteosclerosis. Oral Surg Oral Med Oral Pathol 1990; 69(3):388–393.
20. Greene RM, Rogers RS III. Melkersson-Rosenthal syndrome: a review of 36 patients. J Am Acad Dermatol 1989; 21(6):1263–1270.
21. Hallmon WW, Rossmann JA. The role of drugs in the pathogenesis of gingival overgrowth. A collective review of current concepts. Periodontol 2000 1999; 21:176–196.
22. Harris M. Central giant cell granulomas of the jaws regress with calcitonin therapy. Br J Oral Maxillofac Surg 1993; 31(2):89–94.
23. Harrison JD. Salivary mucoceles. Oral Surg Oral Med Oral Pathol 1975; 39(2): 268–278.
24. Howarth DM, et al. Langerhans cell histiocytosis: diagnosis, natural history, management, and outcome. Cancer 1999; 85(10):2278–2290.
25. Jones W. Familial multiocular cystic disease of the jaw. Am J Cancer 1933; 17: 946—950.
26. Kaiserling E, Ruck P, Xiao JC. Congenital epulis and granular cell tumor: a histologic and immunohistochemical study. Oral Surg Oral Med Oral Pathol Oral Radiol Endod 1995; 80(6):687–697.
27. Katsikeris N, Kakarantza-Angelopoulou E, Angelopoulos AP. Peripheral giant cell granuloma. Clinicopathologic study of 224 new cases and review of 956 reported cases. Int J Oral Maxillofac Surg 1988; 17(2):94–99.
28. Kaugars GE, Cale AE. Traumatic bone cyst. Oral Surg Oral Med Oral Pathol 1987; 63(3):318–324.
29. Kolas S, et al. The occurrance and distribution of idiopathic osteosclerosis. Oral Surg Oral Med Oral Pathol 1953; 6(9):1134–1141.
30. Leider AS, Eversole LR, Barkin ME. Cystic ameloblastoma. A clinicopathologic analysis. Oral Surg Oral Med Oral Pathol 1985; 60(6):624–630.
31. Lo Muzio L, et al. Odontogenic myxoma of the jaws: a clinical, radiologic, immunohistochemical, and ultrastructural study. Oral Surg Oral Med Oral Pathol Oral Radiol Endod 1996; 82(4):426–433.
32. Loong S, Lance J. A case of the melkersson-rosenthal syndrome apparently responsive to cyproheptadine. Med J Aust 1968; 2(16):671–672.
33. Mangion J, et al. The gene for cherubism maps to chromosome 4p16.3. Am J Hum Genet 1999; 65(1):151–157.

34. Martin RW III, et al. Multiple cutaneous granular cell tumors and neurofibromatosis in childhood. A case report and review of the literature. Arch Dermatol 1990; 126(8): 1051–1056.
35. McClure DK, Dahlin DC. Myxoma of bone. Report of three cases. Mayo Clin Proc 1977; 52(4):249–253.
36. McDonnell D. Dense bone island. A review of 107 patients. Oral Surg Oral Med Oral Pathol 1993; 76(1):124–128.
37. Melrose RJ. Benign epithelial odontogenic tumors. Semin Diagn Pathol 1999; 16(4): 271–287.
38. Mighell AJ, Robinson PA, Hume WJ. Peripheral giant cell granuloma: a clinical study of 77 cases from 62 patients, and literature review. Oral Dis 1995; 1(1):12–19.
39. Miller CS, White DK. Human papillomavirus expression in oral mucosa, premalignant conditions, and squamous cell carcinoma: a retrospective review of the literature. Oral Surg Oral Med Oral Pathol Oral Radiol Endod 1996; 82(1):57–68.
40. Neville B. Oral and Maxillofacial Pathology. Philadelphia: Saunders, 1995:362–364.
41. Nichols GE, et al. Lobular capillary hemangioma. An immunohistochemical study including steroid hormone receptor status. Am J Clin Pathol 1992; 97(6):770–775.
42. Ordonez NG. Granular cell tumor: a review and update. Adv Anat Pathol 1999; 6(4):186–203.
43. Philipsen HP, Reichart PA, Praetorius F. Mixed odontogenic tumours and odontomas. Considerations on interrelationship. Review of the literature and presentation of 134 new cases of odontomas. Oral Oncol 1997; 33(2):86–99.
44. Pierce AM, Wilson DF, Goss AN. Inherited craniofacial fibrous dysplasia. Oral Surg Oral Med Oral Pathol 1985; 60(4):403–409.
45. Podmore P, Burrows D. Clofazimine–an effective treatment for Melkersson-Rosenthal syndrome or Miescher's cheilitis. Clin Exp Dermatol 1986; 11(2):173–178.
46. Salmassy DA, Pogrel MA. Liquid nitrogen cryosurgery and immediate bone grafting in the management of aggressive primary jaw lesions. J Oral Maxillofac Surg 1995; 53(7): 784–790.
47. Schnabel P, Bohm M. Mutations of signal-transducing G proteins in human disease. J Mol Med 1995; 73(5):221–228.
48. Scully C, et al. Papillomaviruses: the current status in relation to oral disease. Oral Surg Oral Med Oral Pathol 1988; 65(5):526–532.
49. Sehdev MK, et al. Proceedings: ameloblastoma of maxilla and mandible. Cancer 1974; 33(2):324–333.
50. Shenker A, et al. An activating Gs alpha mutation is present in fibrous dysplasia of bone in the McCune-Albright syndrome. J Clin Endocrinol Metab 1994; 79(3):750–755.
51. Southgate J, et al. Study of the cell biology and biochemistry of cherubism. J Clin Pathol 1998; 51(11):831–837.
52. Stanley HR, et al. Pathological sequelae of "neglected" impacted third molars. J Oral Pathol 1988; 17(3):113–117.
53. Stewart CM, et al. Oral granular cell tumors: a clinicopathologic and immunocytochemical study. Oral Surg Oral Med Oral Pathol 1988; 65(4):427–435.
54. Syrjanen S, et al. Two different human papillomavirus (HPV) types associated with oral mucosal lesions in an HIV-seropositive man. J Oral Pathol Med 1989; 18(6):366–370.
55. Tomich CE. Benign mixed odontogenic tumors. Semin Diagn Pathol 1999; 16(4): 308–316.
56. Tyring SK. Human papillomavirus infections: epidemiology, pathogenesis, and host immune response. J Am Acad Dermatol 2000; 43(1 Pt 2):S18–S26.
57. Whitaker SB, Waldron CA. Central giant cell lesions of the jaws. A clinical, radiologic, and histopathologic study. Oral Surg Oral Med Oral Pathol 1993; 75(2):199–208.
58. Williams HK, Williams DM. Oral granular cell tumours: a histological and immunocytochemical study. J Oral Pathol Med 1997; 26(4):164–169.

59. Williams TP, Connor FA Jr. Surgical management of the odontogenic keratocyst: aggressive approach. J Oral Maxillofac Surg 1994; 52(9):964–946.
60. Willman CL, et al. Langerhans'-cell histiocytosis (histiocytosis X)–a clonal proliferative disease. N Engl J Med 1994; 331(3):154–160.
61. Zain RB, Fei YJ. Fibrous lesions of the gingiva: a histopathologic analysis of 204 cases. Oral Surg Oral Med Oral Pathol 1990; 70(4):466–470.
62. Zimmer WM, et al. Orofacial manifestations of Melkersson-Rosenthal syndrome. A study of 42 patients and review of 220 cases from the literature. Oral Surg Oral Med Oral Pathol 1992; 74(5):610–619.

6
Planning and Diagnostic Evaluation in Oral Cavity Reconstruction

Terance T. Tsue
Medical Research Service, Veterans Affairs Medical Center, Kansas City, Missouri, and Department of Otolaryngology—Head and Neck Surgery, University of Kansas School of Medicine, Kansas City, Kansas, U.S.A.

David J. Kriet, Derrick I. Wallace, and Douglas A. Girod
Department of Otolaryngology—Head and Neck Surgery, University of Kansas School of Medicine, Kansas City, Kansas, U.S.A.

INTRODUCTION

Surgical oncologic treatment of head and neck cancer has advanced considerably, but the overall cure rate has not improved proportionally (1). To increase the cure rate, new therapies and techniques have been developed and more emphasis is being placed on the improvement of the overall quality of the treatment of these oncologically challenging patients. Thus, success should be measured not only by disease control, but also by the restoration and maintenance of the patient to as normal as possible conditions. Such improvements in a patient's quality of life can temporarily offset continued frustrations with controlling head and neck cancer.

The impetus for change in head and neck cancer treatment has underscored the significance of the reconstructive portion of the surgical treatment. Enhancements in our reconstructive abilities have paralleled advances in anesthetic safety, perioperative care of medical comorbidities, and progress in adjuvant therapies. These concurrent advances have pushed the threshold of resectability higher as demands increase for larger and more complex reconstructions.

It is advantageous but not required that surgical treatment of the oral cancer patient involve a two-team approach, a direct extension of the modern multi-disciplinary approach to oncologic patient management. For high-stage lesions or those neoplasms in regions of significant functional import, this approach is not only time-efficient and minimizes caregiver fatigue, but maximizes the specific sub-specialty expertise available to the patient. In order to provide the most expeditious care, evaluation of the reconstructive aspects of the cancer patient's care must also begin at presentation. Although, the patient usually first meets the extirpative oncologic surgeon, early introduction of the reconstructive surgeon partner is paramount because the reconstructive portion of the surgery is ultimately dependent on the result of the extirpative procedure. The reconstructive surgeon's desire to preserve locoregional native tissue and organs should not compromise the extirpative surgeon's interpretation of the adequacy of oncologic resection. Maintenance of this successful, but often tenuous, balance is dependent on good communication among and interdisciplinary knowledge within the extirpative and reconstructive surgeons. In addition, given the current radiographic technology, appropriate reconstruction should not interfere with oncologic surveillance. A joint treatment plan should be discussed among the surgeons and the patient, with several layers of contingency plans, depending on both preoperative and intraoperative findings.

EVALUATION AND PLANNING

History and Physical Examination

At first referral, acute issues such as airway maintenance and hemorrhage, if compromised, need to be dealt with immediately. Any significant history or signs of immediate or impending airway compromise (i.e., stridor, cyanosis, sturgor, choking or dyspnea episodes) warrants expeditious and focused airway evaluation and possible urgent surgical airway stabilization. Similarly, sentinel or sizeable bleeding requires focused workup and treatment. A more comprehensive history and physical should wait until the patient is safe to evaluate. Malnutrition should also be recognized early and aggressively treated with proper nutritional support. Although, the age of the patient is not a contraindication, age is a factor affecting post-treatment complications (2,3). Thus, special attention should be paid to fine-tuning any medical condition, especially those that are poorly controlled (i.e., diabetes, hypertension, sepsis), preoperatively. This is also the time to recruit and inform family and friends for the necessary physical and emotional support that complements medical therapy, with the appropriate precautions in place to safeguard the patient's privacy. Understanding the patient's occupation and recreational activities are important considerations during the evaluation of extirpative and reconstructive options in the event that the patient desires to maintain a crucial skill and/or hobby.

An extensive history of symptoms and signs will not only help determine the location and T-stage of the current neoplastic problem, but will also yield information about potential synchronous primary or metastatic disease. All of these factors directly influence the types of viable reconstructive options. Complaints of unilateral conductive hearing loss, hyponasal speech, breathy voice, ptosis, trismus, chin numbness, otalgia, and contralateral symptoms are frequently indicators of deep or extensive disease that is not immediately apparent. In addition, compromised anatomy, such as after radical neck dissections, neck incisions, and previous flaps, may limit the reconstructive options (4). This information frequently requires both careful review of old operative reports and discussion with previous surgeons to supplement the patient's memory. Similarly, extensive radiotherapy can compromise the vascularity and healing, and thus the reliability of local flaps (5). Finally, previous radiotherapy can increase the risk and aggressiveness of mandibular invasion (6,7).

The history of premorbid oral cavity function, compared to oral function at presentation, is important. Not only will this suggest involved structures, but it also dictates the possible functional goal of any reconstruction. The reconstructive functional result in terms of deglutition, taste, mastication, voice, breathing, and cosmesis cannot be improved beyond the premorbid state. In patients with compromised premorbid function due to neurologic disability or prior treatments, preoperative counseling about potential reconstructive outcome is even more crucial to provide realistic expectations.

Several objective measures of oral function have been proposed (8–10). The lack of consensus, equipment, or expertise necessary for detailed measurements has made most of these assessments difficult to perform. Such measures can be useful for comparison to actual post-operative outcome. Unfortunately, such studies are frequently limited by lack of adequate numbers of patients with uniform surgical defects and premorbid conditions.

The reconstructive surgeon should also perform a complete head and neck exam. Direct visualization of the neoplasm, along with bimanual palpation, should complement the tumor mapping anticipated by the symptom history. This should also include mirror and fiberoptic evaluation of hidden structures. This initial survey allows an educated intercourse with the extirpative surgeon in terms of the anticipated surgical defect size and potential structures to be removed (mucosa, skin, and bone) and/or exposed (brain, orbit, carotid artery). A secondary survey can then focus on the anticipated fine-tuning reconstructive procedures necessary during either the primary or secondary setting to maximize functional and aesthetic outcome. This includes status of the parotid and submandibular ducts, lip vermillion, and oral commissure integrity, dental status and occlusion, exposed maxillary sinus, anticipated palatal defect, Eustachian tube dysfunction with conductive hearing loss, facial sensation, and motor nerve sacrifice. The extent of neck disease determines not only prognosis, but also the type of neck dissection. This influences changes in neck volume, contour, and potential available recipient vessels for microvascular anastomosis. A superinfected area of cutaneous involvement should be treated with antibiotics to delineate infected versus neoplastically involved tissue, promoting a more efficient resection and likely improved pain, hygiene, and healing.

A patient's past medical history directly impacts the medical fitness of a patient for the anticipated extirpative and reconstructive procedure. Adequate cardiopulmonary function and reserve must be present to tolerate the often prolonged anesthesia time and intravascular fluid shifts associated with many types of reconstructive procedures (11). Such comorbid disease can significantly lower the limits of resectability. Preoperative evaluation and clearance by a hospitalist, cardiologist and/or pulmonologist can often help to maximize cardiopulmonary preoperative function. Mental impairment can jeopardize reconstructive success and recovery, as well as limit overall rehabilitative potential. Diabetes, advanced age, vascular disease (i.e., atherosclerosis, hypertension, arteritis), poor nutritional status, hypothyroidism, previous radiation therapy, and chronic steroid usage seriously hinders healing and can guide the reconstructive surgeon to either more conservative or more aggressive reconstructive options (12). A history of cerebrovascular incidents can indicate significant carotid vascular disease. This not only increases the risk of neurologic morbidity and mandates adjustment of anesthetic management, but can also potentially compromise available arterial vessels for microvascular anastamosis. Significant sleep apnea influences perioperative airway management and can be seriously worsened post-operatively by large, bulky, and swollen reconstructions. The long-term treatment of this disorder must be re-evaluated after surgery, and often requires a prolonged tracheotomy. A history of hematologic diatheses (i.e., von Willebrand's disease, hemophilia, lupus anticoagulant abnormality, thrombocytopenia, polycythemia vera, sickle cell disease, or protein C deficiency) contraindicate extensive surgery and/or microvascular free-tissue transfer if poorly or un-treatable perioperatively (13). Paraneoplastic hypercoagulability syndromes can also cause influence anastamotic patency. In addition, the patient is advised to immediately cease activities that could cause perioperative bleeding difficulties such as smoking (vasoconstriction can compromise local skin flaps), and drinking, and taking medications (aspirin, ibuprofen, vitamin E, etc.) (14). A history of regular alcohol usage requires aggressive perioperative withdrawal prophylaxis and nutritional supplementation.

In patients requiring regional pedicled or distant free flaps for reconstruction, a donor-site specific history and exam is necessary. Detailed inquiry of a patient's handedness, footedness, occupation, and recreational activities also reveals information that can dictate the side or site of a flap harvest. The presence of a thoracotomy scar, a pacemaker, or indwelling central line may require use of the contralateral pectoralis major flap or a modified surgical approach to the ipsilateral flap harvest. Previous abdominal and pelvic surgery can obviate the use of some potential free flap vascular pedicles (i.e., rectus abdominis, iliac crest). Claudication or rest pain are indicative of significant peripheral vascular disease and warrant aggressive workup of extremity vascular pedicle adequacy. History of previous surgery or trauma to the donor-site prompts in-depth evaluation of the donor-site anatomy. This includes workup of both arterial and venous supplies as well as boney integrity.

Exam of the potential donor site for scars, asymmetries, or bony deformities can often prompt a patient's memory to an old injury or surgery. Objective evaluation of the mobility, strength, and function of the extremity should confirm the patient's history. Non-healing sores, cold fingers and toes, loss of sensation, and significant distal extremity swelling are also indicators of inadequate vascularity and frequently contraindicate the involved extremity from usage as a donor site. Unfortunately, most of these conditions are bilateral and usually require the use of a completely different, and often less ideal, donor site for reconstruction. Palpation of distal pulses (i.e., radial, ulnar, dorsalis pedis, and posterior tibial arteries), subjective Allen's tests, and ankle-arm indices can be reassuring, but adequacy determinations should be supplemented by formal vascular assessments in equivocal cases (15,16). Body habitus, especially morbid obesity, may influence perioperative recovery and healing and may require alteration in reconstructive technique or donor site (17).

Laboratory and Radiologic Studies

The reconstructive surgeon should review the laboratory and radiologic exams ordered by the extirpative surgeon during the preoperative and metastatic workup of the head and neck patient. Abnormal liver function, platelet count, blood urea nitrogen, prothrombin, and/or prothromboplastin time may lead to significant intraoperative blood loss and post-operative hematomas and possible compressive flap loss and/or infection. These abnormalities need to be investigated and corrected as much as possible preoperatively. Preoperative albumin, prealbumin, and leukocyte count can give an estimate of the level of malnourishment that can affect post-operative healing. Usually computed tomography (CT) and magnetic resonance imaging (MRI) scans of the head and neck region are the dominant radiographic studies ordered. These studies complement and confirm the history, physical exam, and endoscopic evaluation, and help to further delineate the tumor extent locally, regionally, and distantly. This is a key step for both extirpative and reconstructive reasons, as the educated estimate of the anticipated surgical defect dictates the further necessary preoperative workup for the reconstructive surgeon. CT, MRI, bone scan, and panorex findings can also to varying degrees help to indicate mandibular involvement and the need for segmental resection and subsequent bony reconstruction (18,19). MRI followed by MRA, CT angiography, Doppler, and/or angiography is used in cases of potential resection for carotid artery involvement. These data can also indicate the adequacy of the external carotid branches to support microvascular anastamosis (20). At times, the patency of the transverse cervical arterial system and viability of the dependent trapezius flap network can also be determined. The integrity of potential microvascular recipient veins in the neck can also be detected radiographically, including predicting the need for sacrifice of the internal and/or external jugular venous network. The need for venous angiography would be rare.

Radiographic evaluation of the determined potential regional and distant reconstructive flap donor sites should help supplement the physical exam in determining safe harvest. A preoperative Allen's test is crucial for maintaining adequate hand perfusion after radial or ulnar forearm free-flap harvest. In cases with an equivocal subjective Allen's test, Doppler plethysmography can objectively document adequate collateral perfusion to the donor hand (15). Since most head and neck cancer patients also are at risk for significant and progressive peripheral vascular disease due to smoking, other clinical, Doppler, MRA, and angiographic techniques have been used adjunctively to study vasculature prior to harvest of extremity free flaps (21–24). These studies can detect anatomic abnormalities, assure adequate cutaneous flap perforator supply, and document the adequacy of distal collateral arterial flow. In patients with previous trauma or surgery, plain X-ray films can document adequate boney integrity and any compromising hardware.

Treatment Planning

With the above information, the patient is presented to the multi-disciplinary Head and Neck Tumor Board to obtain a consensus opinion on treatment options. In general, the oncologic efficacy of any therapy takes preference when ranking treatment options for the individual patient. The Board's recommendations can be heavily influenced by the expected post-operative functional outcome, which is significantly dependent on the reconstructive options available. Since the best reconstructive option may not be available to every patient due to expertise, previous therapy, or anatomic abnormality, functional outcome may be compromised. Especially in cases in which oncologic efficacy has a semblance of comparability, this potential functional outcome may significantly influence a patient's decision. All treatment and reconstructive options are presented to the patient. Post-therapeutic expectations should be discussed in detail. The Tumor Board's opinion frequently obviates the need for the patient to meet the radiation and medical oncology consultants, but this is certainly an option for those who would benefit during their decision process.

Efficient post-operative recovery and early inpatient discharge also involves a multi-disciplinary approach. Therapy should begin with preoperative consultation and counseling by involved surgical colleagues (i.e., neurosurgery, ophthalmology, vascular surgery, oral surgery) and anticipated ancillary personnel (i.e., speech pathology, physical therapy, social work, prostheticist) respectively. Experienced anesthesiologists understand how judicious use of intravenous fluids, vasoconstrictors, and muscle relaxants are crucial to operative success (11). Patient positioning and padding, specific vascular access placements, body temperature, oxygenation, and ventilator parameters are also important influential factors controlled by the anesthesiologist. Well-trained teams for the operating room, intensive care, and inpatient ward with prepared OR case carts, pre-printed standard orders and clinical pathways are important for a consistent and efficient hospital recovery. The presence of both the extirpative and reconstructive surgeon guiding the preparation of the operative patient can facilitate team efforts later in the operative day. In those patients who will endure a prolonged period of enteral feedings, percutaneous or open gastrostomy tube placement is prudent for maximizing preoperative nutritional status and obviating the need for a nasogastric feeding tube. This is generally more comfortable for the patient and decreases the incidence of sinusitis, gastroesophageal reflux, and pharyngeal swelling (25). All of these factors can potentially inhibit return of post-operative deglutition. The myriad of preoperative appointments is best coordinated for the patient by a dedicated patient care coordinator.

Surgical Planning—Incisions

Reconstructive planning occurs from initial presentation and undergoes an evolving process until a final plan with possible contingencies is developed. This plan can even change intraoperatively due to unexpected oncologic findings, anatomic abnormalities, and anesthetic instability. Surgical incision planning extends beyond just the purview of the oncologic surgeon. Adequate access and visualization of the surgical field, especially for posteriorly based neoplasms, is paramount for resection. Fortunately, frequently multiple transcutaneous or transoral approaches exist that can achieve the same exposure necessary for cancer resection. The chosen surgical approach must also provide adequate access for the planned reconstruction. Visualization is necessary for safe and adequate inset suturing of the planned reconstruction flap into the surgical defect. A needle holder frequently requires more maneuverable exposure than a monopolar (Bovie) cautery, knife, scissor, or laser. In addition to recipient-site edema, initial flap bulk can be larger than the extirpated native tissue volume. Suturing gaps can lead to salivary leakage, wound infection, and potential flap or large vessel compromise. Myofascial pedicled flaps require a surgical approach that allows non-constricting passage of an often thick, muscular, vascular pedicle. These needs may require potential incision extension or new incisions.

Incision placement also depends on the quality of the native tissue. Not infrequently, surgical candidates requiring complex reconstructions have had previous cervico-facial incisions, traumatic incisions, skin-flap elevation, prolonged steroid usage, radiation therapy, and now more commonly, chemotherapy. All of these factors play a role in subsequent skin-flap viability, requiring worst-case scenario planning. Old incisions are the best initial choice, as the native vascularity is already compromised. Sub-platysmal or thicker skin-flap elevations are desirable, but are often limited by oncologic considerations. Further incisions must respect these lines of compromised vascularity, avoiding elevated areas of skin flap even partially isolated from their vascular supply. Chin incision trifurcations, and carotid endarterectomy scars are classic examples of this. Such an error, at best, will result in skin-flap loss and poor cosmesis, and it can yield large vessel, hardware, alloplast, allograft, and/or boney exposure risks. Exposure of a microvascular pedicle can result in the loss of the entire reconstruction. If detected intraoperatively, providing a well vascularized muscular or fascial bed underneath the compromised skin-flap area may result in preserving cutaneous coverage in the best case and provide a good bed for skin grafting in the worst case. Alternatively, the devascularized area should be resected and become part of the reconstructive defect. Full-thickness reconstructions from mucosa to skin add significant complexity and difficulty to the procedure. Poor incision planning and/or delayed detection usually requires a larger, secondary and/or more complicated reconstruction than anticipated. This is in addition to the morbidity of another operation with its concomitant risk to the previous reconstruction.

Further skill in incision planning involves anticipation of future potential extirpative and loco-regional flap needs, which can be quite difficult, but should be attempted in all cases. Generally, vascularity for potential local rotation and advancement flaps can be preserved, but after multiple previous surgeries and adjuvant therapy, their viability and usefulness remains in question. Preservation of potential standard regional flap pedicles is important (i.e., superior trapezius flap, deltopectoral flap, pectoralis major flap).

An improved aesthetic result can be achieved with incision placement in natural skin creases, aesthetic unit junctions, relaxed skin tension lines, old scars, or hair-bearing areas. Such considerations should be secondary to those stated above.

Primary and Neck Resection

Throughout the extirpation, there must be good communication between the extirpative and reconstructive surgeons. Frequently, both are working concurrently to minimize anesthesia time. Continuous monitoring of the patient status intraoperatively is also crucial, as any decline in the medical status of a patient, requires an immediate change in the operative plan. Unlike the aesthetic resection of a complete nasal unit, in the oral cavity, any native tissue in the oral cavity that can be spared will generally provide improved post-operative function. During the resection, unanticipated areas of resection or tissue sparing and areas of potential re-resection after frozen-section margin analysis should be accurately communicated to the reconstructive surgeon to allow for intraoperative adjustments. This information not only can affect flap cutaneous paddle size but also its shape and orientation. Having the surgeon to mark transected nerve stumps that require subsequent re-anastomosis or cable grafting can be advantageous because of the inherent difficulties in finding these areas at the end of the case. This is also pertinent when innervated free flaps are going to be inset later in the case.

In cases involving mandibulotomy, best occlusal results are obtained when the internal fixation or reconstruction plate (compressive or locking) is modeled on the buccal and labial contour spanning the anticipated mandibulotomy site. In the instance of compression- and tension-band plate placement, the two medial holes of each plate should be drilled appropriately eccentrically and neutrally positioned, respectively. Subsequent plate holes can be drilled at the time of mandibulotomy repair, because this will assure good compression across the mandibulotomy site. Similarly, in cases of segmental mandibulectomy, pre-contouring the reconstruction plate is crucial for maintaining the best occlusal relationships and temporomandibular function. Even in edentulous cases, this planning and early effort can maintain a more natural contour and good joint function. If there is involvement and/or distortion of the buccal or labial cortex of the mandible, direct plate contouring to the bone is not possible. Placement of the patient into maxillo-mandibular fixation or use of a mandibular fix bridge system (Synthes CMF, Paoli, Pennsylvania) can help maintain preoperative occlusal and joint relationships. Post-resection freehand plate contouring and fixation is difficult and often yields suboptimal symmetry and joint function. With the currently available low-profile locking reconstruction plates, the contoured plate can closely approximate the natural mandibular projection and contour without sacrificing durability and strength when used in conjunction with bone grafts (26,27). These thinner reconstruction plates are usually not visible or palpable through the external skin flap, even after some subcutaneous tissue resection. In the atrophic edentulous mandible, the older, more stout reconstruction plates (i.e., THORP; titanium hollow screw reconstruction plate) must often be set back distally one to two holes to avoid mentum over-projection and minimize tension on the overlying skin paddle. This is usually not necessary with the slimmer and lower profile reconstruction plates (2.0 mm and 2.4 mm). In addition, with the locking-plate design, less accurate contouring of the native mandible contour is necessary prior to screw fixation since it acts as an internal external-fixator device. Accurate measurement of bicortical locking screw length is paramount to minimizing readily palpable, and often bothersome, sharp lingual screw tips. This is also true for lingually placed bone grafts placed in the segmental defect. The plate should be screw-fixated at the appropriate location along the native mandibular height such that the bone graft and overlying alveolar soft tissue paddle lie even with the remaining native occlussal surface. Adequate neo-mandibular height will also facilitate maintenance of gingivo-buccal, gingivo-labial and floor of mouth sulci to preserve tongue mobility, oral competence, and adhesive surface area for dentures. Use of reconstruction plates to span segmental mandibular defects without the concomitant use of bone grafts can affect the long-term complication rate and functional effect of the reconstruction, depending upon the mandibular defect location and size and the type of plate used (28–30). Depending upon the size and location of the soft-tissue defect, removal of the reconstruction plate prior to flap inset by the surgeon may be necessary for adequate exposure to perform the inset or microvascular anastomosis.

Communication among surgeons during the neck dissection is also important. For anticipated microvascular cases, gentle dissection and sparing of arterial and venous vessels and lengthy stumps is important for maintaining anastomosis options. Although this requires extra effort and time, sparing extra vessels such as the transverse cervical pedicle and external jugular vein should usually not compromise oncologic resection. The appropriate recipient vessel size needed can be estimated from the anticipated donor site. In addition, inter-surgeon communication of anticipated defect location and microvascular pedicle length, can guide the extirpative surgeon to save potential recipient vessels in a given area of the neck, while allowing faster dissection in non-essential areas. Similarly, anticipated resection of the proximal external carotid arterial system due to neck disease should be communicated to the reconstructive surgeon so alternative recipient arterial supplies can be prepared (31). This frequently requires vein grafting and can compromise anastomotic patency (17,32). Sacrifice of the ipsilateral sternocleidomastoid muscle should also be strongly considered for cases requiring pedicled myofascial or myocutaneous flap reconstruction, as the pedicle muscle bulk is significant and can serve as carotid sheath coverage. Partial removal of the anterior sternocleidomastoid muscle can allow improved microvascular pedicle geometry and/or decrease venous pedicle compression. In cases of across-midline resections or previous ipsilateral radical neck dissections, vessels from the contralateral neck may need to be isolated and prepared. This need may prompt the extirpative surgeon to perform a full-neck dissection for oncologic reasons in a borderline indication case.

Suction drain placement at the completion of the procedure is also crucial. The best type of post-operative neck drainage remains controversial, but a balance between adequate drainage of all potential dead spaces and minimal interruption of any reconstructive flap pedicle must be maintained. A tight neck closure can apply significant pressure to a drain tube if it overlies a vascular pedicle, especially with routine post-operative swelling. Compression dressings can also compromise pedicled and free-flap pedicles. Drains should typically be placed parallel to flap pedicles and carotid sheath contents. Drain tips should be placed away from mucosal or skin suture lines to avoid salivary or air leakage. Maintenance of internal drain position with post-operative head and neck movement can be assured by loose suturing with absorbable sutures.

RECONSTRUCTIVE OPTIONS

At the very minimum, any reconstructive technique must maintain a watertight intraoral closure to prevent neck salivary contamination. The main goal of any reconstruction is to maximize both function and form. Reconstruction of function includes restoration of tongue mobility and volume, maintenance of oral competence, preservation of taste, facilitation of masticatory rehabilitation (tissue-borne or osseointegrated implants), reestablishment of intraoral sensation and an adequate respiratory conduit. These factors can help prevent or minimize aspiration. Simultaneously addressing possible trismus with coronoidectomy and/or subperiosteal masticatory muscular detachment can also help improve post-operative function. This is especially important in patients that require bulky maxillary obturators. In addition, coverage of important structures such as bone, large vessels, and brain parenchyma is vital.

Fulfillment of these goals with a minimum of incisions helps reconstruction of form. This also includes maintenance of facial soft tissue proportions, maxillary-mandibular contours, and dental occlusion. Ideally, reconstruction of form involves replacement of like with like. Unfortunately, like tissue does not necessary retain all the function of native tissue, especially in terms of sensation and motor function. The appropriate reconstruction will try to maximize both of these goals concurrently using the technically simplest method possible with the minimal amount of collateral disability at the donor site. This philosophy minimizes the procedure length, technical complexity and post-operative complication potential. This approach is especially important in the current environment of managed and limited health care resources. Fortunately, although each reconstructive challenge must be individualized to each patient, indications for specific reconstructive methods along the reconstruction

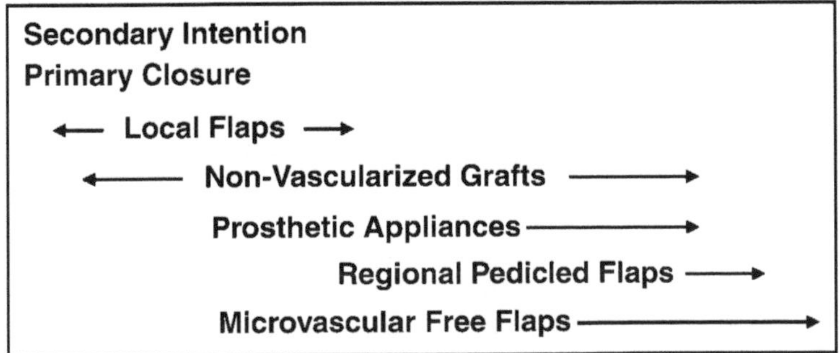

Figure 1 Oral cavity reconstruction alternatives.

spectrum are greatly overlapping (Fig. 1). Also, techniques are often used in combination to maximize the overall reconstructive outcome. Whatever reconstructive technique is implemented, it should not hinder post-operative recovery with multiple surgeries, possibly delaying or preventing necessary timely adjuvant therapy. Single-stage primary reconstructions are best for meeting this goal. Similarly, complications are always possible, and should be dealt with expeditiously.

Using primary closure or healing by secondary intention is the simplest reconstructive method requiring minimal reconstructive expertise and operative time. Often, primary closures under great tension due to size, poor native-tissue healing ability, and mobility considerations become healing by secondary intention. It is the ideal for replacing like with like, although scarred granulation tissue is not functionally equivalent to the native tissue. Also, this scar tissue generally contracts significantly, causing distortion, and has decreased pliability. In addition, aggressive granulation cannot be easily differentiated from early recurrence of carcinoma. This technique is generally limited to small to medium size defects in areas with significant mobility such as the tongue, lip and vestibule. Primary closure of larger defects is also possible, including segmental composite defects, but often with significant effects of post-operative form. Effects on function are variable (33,34).

Local tissue rearrangement techniques or direct random flaps move tissue from a site adjacent or near to the primary defect, maintaining attachment to some form of vascular supply. Generally, small to medium primary defect sites adjacent to areas of increased mobility and/or elasticity are most amenable to closure using these techniques. The uvula, palate, lateral tongue, and buccal mucosa are examples of random flap sources. These techniques also require minimal reconstructive technical expertise and operative time. Frequently this reconstructive method is used in combination with other more advanced techniques described below. Unfortunately, previous radiation therapy and/or surgical incisions can compromise the blood flow to local direct flaps, lowering their success rate and usability. This can potentially leave a larger defect to have to repair or heal. Also, the donor site may also be left with some functional impairment (i.e., tongue, palate).

Oral cavity reconstruction using non-vascularized tissue techniques can be divided into two general categories: soft-tissue coverage and skeletal jaw support. Reconstructions requiring replacement of only one tissue type have been used with success in the oral cavity (35,36). Both autograft and allograft techniques have been described for mucosal reconstruction. In complex reconstructions comprising more than one type of tissue (i.e., soft tissue and bone), these techniques require combination with vascularized techniques due to the need for recipient-bed neovascularization or protection of the graft from oral or external contamination.

For soft-tissue reconstructions, very large defects can be covered and healed with this technique, which also requires minimal technical expertise and operative time. Soft-tissue reconstructions can provide water-tight closures and are best used in concave intraoral areas that require coverage of a large surface area, but are not suitable for areas requiring replacement with bulk (i.e., floor-of-mouth, vestibule, sulci, and maxillectomy cavities). Large split-thickness skin grafts can be harvested concurrently with the extirpative procedure with minimal donor-site morbidity. Allograft usage is faster and incurs no potential donor-site morbidity. Full-thickness grafts are rarely used intraorally because of the significant mobility and contamination within the oral cavity. Graft success depends mostly on the vascular supply of the recipient bed and maintenance of low-mobility contact between the graft and recipient bed. Neovascularization of these grafts is compromised in areas with poorly vascularized tissues such as cortical bone, cartilage, tendon, fibrotic scar, irradiated or crushed tissue, or defects containing foreign bodies (i.e., reconstruction plates, alloplastic material). Large bolsters are often needed, which can temporarily compromise the airway or deglutition. Thus, this technique is not universally applicable throughout the oral cavity. In addition, there is a significant degree of contraction with split-thickness skin grafts during the healing process in mobile areas. This contraction can cause a significant amount of intraoral tethering, with concurrent loss of mobility or concavity. Allograft incorporation takes significantly longer and requires mucosalization of the surface. Collapse of two opposing raw mucosalizing surfaces of a previously bolstered concavity can cause synechia or collapse, resulting in a suboptimal result.

Non-vascularized skeletal reconstruction usually involves prosthetics or autologous bone grafts in combination with rigid fixation techniques. Both grafts and implants generally need protection from oral or external contamination for incorporation. Unfortunately, this is more troublesome in the setting of primary reconstructions and/or the poorly vascular recipient bed, although not impossible (37–40). This method is generally more successful in the setting of secondary bone reconstructions, allowing isolation of the avascular bone graft site from oral contamination via an established soft-tissue barrier. Reconstruction of composite oral defects with vascularized soft tissue and a mandibular reconstruction plate is possible, but it can have a significant complication rate on a long-term basis (28,29). Radiation dosimetry effects of reconstruction plates have not proven to be a hindrance clinically (41). Use of homograft bone is not widely practiced and use of hydroxyapatite cement or xenograft bone grafts in the jaws is currently not indicated.

The use of prosthetic maxillary obturators for reconstruction of partial maxillary alveolar and hard palate defects has a longstanding and successful history (42). Maintenance of tongue abutment against the reconstructed hard palate is important for speech and bolus preparation and transport. For limited defects, both form and function are well maintained. In addition, the recipient extirpative bed is easily evaluated for disease recurrence without being covered up by a complex reconstruction. Larger maxillary defects are less adequately reconstructed with prosthetic obturators alone due to lack of adequate skeletal support for mastication and prosthesis adherence. In these cases consideration should be given to fasciocutaneous or osteocutaneous free-tissue reconstruction (43–45). Tissue-born dentures and osseointegrated dental implants are important adjuncts to assist with post-operative mastication. The best time to place osseointegrated implants remains controversial (46). Tissue-borne dentures are best left to well after oncologic therapy is finished. Financial constraints often severely limit widespread availability of these dental restorations. Also, free cable nerve grafts are available to assist reinnervation of both facial and intraoral sensation to maximize post-operative function (37).

In general, larger and/or more complex oral cavity extirpative defects require larger and more complex reconstructions. Replacing like with like frequently requires the use of vascularized tissue reconstructions from outside the oral cavity. Regional pedicled flaps for head and neck reconstruction have been used successfully for greater than 30 years (47–49). These techniques include many different regional donor sites with capabilities to transfer skin, fascia, muscle, and bone in different combinations, although pedicled boney flaps generally have very limited usefulness and reliability in current day reconstructions. Pedicled-flap reconstructions are taught in essentially all head and neck residencies and are easy techniques to learn, but the art of successful and appropriate application requires prolonged experience (50–53). One of the advantages of the use of regional pedicled flaps is the technical ease of harvest of well-vascularized tissue that is usually outside the prior head and neck irradiation field. The reliable vascular supply can be readily identified, and the thick vascular pedicle can provide needed coverage of exposed neck structures with better healing. In contrast to simpler reconstruction techniques, large surface areas can be reconstructed, but survival difficulty can arise if too small of a skin paddle is harvested. Some flaps do require staging procedures to increase size, survivability, and overall cosmetic result. Some require other concurrent procedures at the recipient and/or donor sites such as supplemental skin grafts.

Rough handling, tension, pedicle kinking or compression, or minimization of the pedicled fasciocutaneous paddle can compromise the sometimes tenuous vascular perforators and result in partial or total flap loss. In addition, availability of donor sites is very sensitive to previous surgical incisions, trauma, and neck dissections. Concurrent harvest during the extirpative procedure is often difficult due to the closeness of the recipient and donor sites and differences in patient positioning. Pedicled flaps usually are limited in their reach, malleability, and mobility secondary to the tethering pedicle's arc of rotation. Most have a significant amount of bulk and subsequent difficulty with gravitational settling which can hinder both function and cosmesis (54). With time, this bulk tends to atrophy due to denervation. The effect on donor site cosmesis and function is also significant compared to simpler local reconstructive techniques, especially in the setting of ipsilateral compromise of trapezius function from a neck dissection.

Many challenges associated with the use of the pedicled flap in reconstruction have been minimized with the increased popularity and availability of microvascular free-tissue transfer. The numerous donor sites provide options for not only large and composite defects, but can also provide attractive reconstructions for smaller defects with complex geometry restraints (i.e., posterior-lateral oral cavity, ventral tongue-anterior floor-of-mouth). Replacement of cutaneous lining, mucosa, bone, soft tissue volume, and function (i.e., sensation, secretions, muscular movement) in various combinations are available in a single-stage reconstruction depending on the specific donor site chosen. Unfortunately, reconstructive priorities are frequent determinants of the available options. Free flaps can provide well-vascularized tissue aiding healing in the previously irradiated oral cavity. Many free flaps provide sensory reinnervation capability via transferred intrinsic nerve grafts (55–57). However, even without direct neurography, some level of intraoral flap sensation is possible (58). Frequently, flaps can be harvested concurrently with the oncologic resection to minimize total anesthetic and operative time. In most cases, adequate recipient vessels can be accessed in several places of the extirpative field. This, in combination with frequently long flap pedicles, provides relative freedom of flap placement throughout the head and neck. In addition, free-flap reliability in large centers is equivalent or better than with pedicled tissue transfer (11,59,60).

Free-tissue transfer techniques do demand sub-specialty training and involve a career-long learning process. In addition to the added expertise, microvascular reconstructions require increased health care resources, including time, equipment and personnel. The actual costs of microvascular reconstruction are comparable to other techniques (54,61,62). Free flaps are dependent on the presence of adequate recipient bed vessels for microvascular anastomosis, which may not always be readily available in the multiply operated patient. Donor-site morbidity can range from minimal to inhibiting. These issues must be weighed in balance with their success in terms of restoring oral cavity form and function. The best result often subsequently requires multiple fine-tuning operations after the initial extirpative and reconstructive procedure, taking advantage of aesthetic facial plastic techniques by a facial plastic surgeon.

CONCLUSION

Successful reconstruction in the oral cavity begins with careful planning from initial patient presentation. Close interaction and planning is necessary between the extirpative and reconstructive surgeons. No two patient situations are exactly similar and the treatment planning process must be individualized. Frequently, oral cavity reconstruction requires a combination of multiple techniques to maximize outcome. Future directions should focus on prospective evidence-based evaluation of current reconstructive techniques (32). New applications and enhancements of current techniques need to be developed, including use of bioengineered tissues, prefabricated reconstructions and minimally invasive harvest techniques (32,63–67). In parallel, further development of new reconstructive donor sites, techniques and technologies, including the use of allograft and alloplastic materials, is also important. The reconstructive surgeon must continuously strive to evaluate the outcome of each patient, and successful restoration of form and function remains a lifelong learning process.

REFERENCES

1. American Cancer Society. Cancer Facts and Figures, 2003.
2. Shaari CM, Buchbinder D, Costantino PD, et al. Complications of microvascular head and neck surgery in the elderly. Arch Otolaryngol Head Neck Surg 1998; 124:407–411.
3. Blackwell KE, Azizzadeh B, Ayala C, et al. Octogenarian free flap reconstruction: complications and cost of therapy. Otolaryngol Head Neck Surg 2002; 126:301–306.
4. Head C, Sercarz JA, Abemayor E, et al. Microvascular reconstruction after previous neck dissection. Arch Otolaryngol Head Neck Surg 2002; 128:328–331.
5. Sumi Y, Ueda M, Oka T, et al. Effects of irradiation of skin flaps. J Oral Maxillofac Surg 1984; 42:447–452.
6. McGregor AD, MacDonald DG. Routes of entry of squamous cell carcinoma to the mandible. Head Neck Surg 1988; 10:294–301.
7. McGregor AD, MacDonald DG. Patterns of spread of squamous cell carcinoma to the ramus of the mandible. Head Neck 1993; 15:440–444.
8. Matloub HS, Larson DL, Kuhn JC, et al. Lateral arm free flap in oral cavity reconstruction: a functional evaluation. Head Neck 1989; 11:205–211.
9. Marunick MT, Mathes BE, Klein BB. Masticatory function in hemimandibulectomy patients. J Oral Rehabil 1992; 19:289–295.
10. Haribhakti VV, Kavarana NM, Tibrewala AN. Oral cavity reconstruction: an objective assessment of function. Head Neck 1993; 15:119–124.
11. Haughey BH, Wilson E, Kluwe L, et al. Free flap reconstruction of the head and neck: analysis of 241 cases. Otolaryngol Head Neck Surg 2001; 125:10–17.
12. Ondrey FG, Hom DB. Effects of nutrition on wound healing. Otolaryngol Head Neck Surg 1994; 110:557–559.
13. Ayala C, Blackwell KE. Protein C deficiency in microvascular head and neck reconstruction. Laryngoscope 1999; 109:259–265.

14. Rees TD, Liverett DM, Guy CL. The effect of cigarette smoking on skin-flap survival in the face lift patient. Plast Reconstr Surg 1984; 73:911–915.
15. Nuckols DA, Tsue TT, Toby EB, et al. Preoperative evaluation of the radial forearm free flap patient with the objective Allen's test. Otolaryngol Head Neck Surg 2000; 123:553–557.
16. Manabe S, Tabuchi N, Toyama M, et al. Measurement of ulnar flow is helpful in predicting ischemia after radial artery harvest. Thorac Cardiovasc Surg 2002; 50:325–328.
17. Kroll SS, Schusterman MA, Reece GP, et al. Choice of flap and incidence of free flap success. Plast Reconstr Surg 1996; 98:459–463.
18. Ator GA, Abemayor E, Lufkin RB, et al. Evaluation of mandibular tumor invasion with magnetic resonance imaging. Arch Otolaryngol Head Neck Surg 1990; 116:454–459.
19. Tsue TT, McCulloch TM, Girod DA, et al. Predictors of carcinomatous invasion of the mandible. Head Neck 1994; 16:116–126.
20. Nagler RM, Braun J, Daitzman M, et al. Spiral CT angiography: an alternative vascular evaluation technique for head and neck microvascular reconstruction. Plast Reconstr Surg 1997; 100:1697–1702.
21. Futran ND, Stack BC Jr, Payne LP. Use of color Doppler flow imaging for preoperative assessment in fibular osteoseptocutaneous free tissue transfer. Otolaryngol Head Neck Surg 1997; 117:660–663.
22. Futran ND, Stack BC Jr, Zachariah AP. Ankle-arm index as a screening examination for fibula free tissue transfer. Ann Otol Rhinol Laryngol 1999; 108:777–780.
23. Lorenz RR, Esclamado R. Preoperative magnetic resonance angiography in fibular-free flap reconstruction of head and neck defects. Head Neck 2001; 23:844–850.
24. Blackwell KE. Donor site evaluation for fibula free flap transfer. Am J Otolaryngol 1998; 19:89–95.
25. Magne N, Marcy PY, Foa C, et al. Comparison between nasogastric tube feeding and percutaneous fluoroscopic gastrostomy in advanced head and neck cancer patients. Eur Arch Otorhinolaryngol 2001; 258:89–92.
26. Militsakh O, Wallace D, Girod D, et al. Use of 2.0 mm locking reconstruction plate system in oromandibular reconstruction [abstr]. Otlaryngol Head Neck Surg 2003.
27. Herford AS, Ellis E III. Use of a locking reconstruction bone plate/screw system for mandibular surgery. J Oral Maxillofac Surg 1998; 56:1261–1265.
28. Blackwell KE, Buchbinder D, Urken ML. Lateral mandibular reconstruction using soft-tissue free flaps and plates. Arch Otolaryngol Head Neck Surg 1996; 122:672–678.
29. Blackwell KE, Lacombe V. The bridging lateral mandibular reconstruction plate revisited. Arch Otolaryngol Head Neck Surg 1999; 125:988–993.
30. Shpitzer T, Gullane PJ, Neligan PC, et al. The free vascularized flap and the flap plate options: comparative results of reconstruction of lateral mandibular defects. Laryngoscope 2000; 110:2056–2060.
31. Harris JR, Lueg E, Genden E, et al. The thoracoacromial/cephalic vascular system for microvascular anastomoses in the vessel-depleted neck. Arch Otolaryngol Head Neck Surg 2002; 128:319–323.
32. Miller MJ. Minimally invasive techniques of tissue harvest in head and neck reconstruction. Clin Plast Surg 1994; 21:149–159.
33. McConnel FM, Pauloski BR, Logemann JA, et al. Functional results of primary closure vs flaps in oropharyngeal reconstruction: a prospective study of speech and swallowing. Arch Otolaryngol Head Neck Surg 1998; 124:625–630.
34. Chuanjun C, Zhiyuan Z, Shaopu G, et al. Speech after partial glossectomy: a comparison between reconstruction and nonreconstruction patients. J Oral Maxillofac Surg 2002; 60:404–407.
35. Schramm VL Jr, Johnson JT, Myers EN. Skin grafts and flaps in oral cavity reconstruction. Arch Otolaryngol 1983; 109:175–177.

36. O'Brien CJ, Archer DJ, Breach NM, et al. Reconstruction of the mandible with autogenous bone following treatment for squamous carcinoma. Aust N Z J Surg 1986; 56:707–715.
37. Pogrel MA. The results of microneurosurgery of the inferior alveolar and lingual nerve. J Oral Maxillofac Surg 2002; 60:485–489.
38. Greene D, Sussman S, Singer MI. Experience with segmental reconstruction of the radiated mandible with alloplastic prostheses. Laryngoscope 1997; 107:1018–1023.
39. Foster RD, Anthony JP, Sharma A, et al. Vascularized bone flaps versus nonvascularized bone grafts for mandibular reconstruction: an outcome analysis of primary bony union and endosseous implant success. Head Neck 1999; 21:66–71.
40. Kiyokawa K, Tai Y, Tanaka S, et al. A new regenerative approach to oromandibular reconstruction after the resection of head and neck malignant tumor. J Craniofac Surg 2002; 13:337–346; discussion 347–348.
41. Scher N, Poe D, Kuchnir F, et al. Radiotherapy of the resected mandible following stainless steel plate fixation. Laryngoscope 1988; 98:561–563.
42. Okay DJ, Genden E, Buchbinder D, et al. Prosthodontic guidelines for surgical reconstruction of the maxilla: a classification system of defects. J Prosthet Dent 2001; 86:352–363.
43. Futran ND, Haller JR. Considerations for free-flap reconstruction of the hard palate. Arch Otolaryngol Head Neck Surg 1999; 125:665–669.
44. Triana RJ Jr, Uglesic V, Virag M, et al. Microvascular free flap reconstructive options in patients with partial and total maxillectomy defects. Arch Facial Plast Surg 2000; 2:91–101.
45. Genden EM, Wallace D, Buchbinder D, et al. Iliac crest internal oblique osteomusculocutaneous free flap reconstruction of the postablative palatomaxillary defect. Arch Otolaryngol Head Neck Surg 2001; 127:854–861.
46. Sclaroff A, Haughey B, Gay WD, et al. Immediate mandibular reconstruction and placement of dental implants. At the time of ablative surgery. Oral Surg Oral Med Oral Pathol 1994; 78:711–717.
47. Egerton M, Zovickian A. Reconstruction of major defects of the palate. Plastic and Reconstructive Surgery 1956; 17:105–128.
48. Baek SM, Biller HF, Krespi YP, et al. The pectoralis major myocutaneous island flap for reconstruction of the head and neck. Head Neck Surg 1979; 1:293–300.
49. Bakamjian VY. Total reconstruction of pharynx with medially based deltopectoral skin flap. N Y State J Med 1968; 68:2771–2778.
50. Esclamado RM, Burkey BB, Carroll WR, et al. The platysma myocutaneous flap. Indications and caveats. Arch Otolaryngol Head Neck Surg 1994; 120:32–35.
51. Zbar RI, Funk GF, McCulloch TM, et al. Pectoralis major myofascial flap: a valuable tool in contemporary head and neck reconstruction. Head Neck 1997; 19:412–418.
52. Kierner AC, Zelenka I, Gstoettner W. The sternocleidomastoid flap–its indications and limitations. Laryngoscope 2001; 111:2201–2204.
53. Liu R, Gullane P, Brown D, et al. Pectoralis major myocutaneous pedicled flap in head and neck reconstruction: retrospective review of indications and results in 244 consecutive cases at the Toronto General Hospital. J Otolaryngol 2001; 30:34–40.
54. Tsue TT, Desyatnikova SS, Deleyiannis FW, et al. Comparison of cost and function in reconstruction of the posterior oral cavity and oropharynx. Free vs pedicled soft tissue transfer. Arch Otolaryngol Head Neck Surg 1997; 123:731–737.
55. Urken ML. The restoration or preservation of sensation in the oral cavity following ablative surgery. Arch Otolaryngol Head Neck Surg 1995; 121:607–612.
56. Urken ML, Weinberg H, Vickery C, et al. The neurofasciocutaneous radial forearm flap in head and neck reconstruction: a preliminary report. Laryngoscope 1990; 100:161–173.
57. Mah SM, Durham JS, Anderson DW, et al. Functional results in oral cavity reconstruction using reinnervated versus nonreinnervated free fasciocutaneous grafts. J Otolaryngol 1996; 25:75–81.

58. Shindo ML, Sinha UK, Rice DH. Sensory recovery in noninnervated free flaps for head and neck reconstruction. Laryngoscope 1995; 105:1290–1293.
59. Urken ML, Weinberg H, Buchbinder D, et al. Microvascular free flaps in head and neck reconstruction. Report of 200 cases and review of complications. Arch Otolaryngol Head Neck Surg 1994; 120:633–640.
60. Blackwell KE. Unsurpassed reliability of free flaps for head and neck reconstruction. Arch Otolaryngol Head Neck Surg 1999; 125:295–299.
61. Kroll SS, Evans GR, Reece GP, et al. Comparison of resource costs of free and conventional TRAM flap breast reconstruction. Plast Reconstr Surg 1996; 98:74–77.
62. Brown MR, McCulloch TM, Funk GF, et al. Resource utilization and patient morbidity in head and neck reconstruction. Laryngoscope 1997; 107:1028–1031.
63. Germann G, Pelzer M, Sauerbier M. [Prefabricated flaps, a new reconstructive concept]. Orthopade 1998; 27:451–456.
64. Kunstfeld R, Petzelbauer P, Wickenhauser G, et al. The prefabricated scapula flap consists of syngeneic bone, connective tissue, and a self-assembled epithelial coating. Plast Reconstr Surg 2001; 108:1908–1914.
65. Wadsworth JT, Futran N, Eubanks TR. Laparoscopic harvest of the jejunal free flap for reconstruction of hypopharyngeal and cervical esophageal defects. Arch Otolaryngol Head Neck Surg 2002; 128:1384–1387.
66. Chiarini L, De Santis G, Bedogni A, et al. Lining the mouth floor with prelaminated fascio-mucosal free flaps: clinical experience. Microsurgery 2002; 22:177–186.
67. Gath HJ, Hell B, Zarrinbal R, et al. Regeneration of intraoral defects after tumor resection with a bioengineered human dermal replacement (Dermagraft). Plast Reconstr Surg 2002; 109:889–893; discussion 894–895.

7
Surgical Approaches to the Oral Cavity

J. David Osguthorpe and Judith M. Skoner
Department of Otolaryngology—Head and Neck Surgery, Medical University of South Carolina, Charleston, South Carolina, U.S.A.

INTRODUCTION

The preponderance of surgery performed on the oral cavity utilizes a transoral route, such as for dental diseases, chronic tonsillitis, and sleep apnea. However, malignancy will be the primary focus of this chapter, although benign tumors such as ameloblastomas and some congenital and/or traumatic abnormalities can also require an involved surgical exposure. Approximately 70% of the neoplasms occur in dependent portions of the oral cavity, the regions most commonly bathed with food, saliva and tobacco residue. Although this chapter focuses on the surgical approaches to the oral cavity in a framework of the final reconstruction, it is necessary to appreciate the indications for certain approaches based on the primary treatment of a particular disease process.

Throughout treatment planning the extirpative and reconstructive surgeon must communicate to provide the patient with the optimal potential for cure but also the ideal reconstruction, which may provide an improved quality of life. Issues that require pre-operative planning between the extirpative team and the reconstructive team have been discussed in detail in another chapter of this text.

Therapy for benign neoplasia of the oral cavity, as elsewhere in the body, usually entails local excision with minimal, but clear, margins via a transoral approach for all but the largest or recurrent lesions. For malignant neoplasia, the issues of what is an adequate margin and how to manage the draining lymphatics add significant complexity to therapy decisions and surgical approaches. Most advocate at least a 1-cm margin of uninvolved tissue, except that which is adjacent to bone, and many favor 1.5-cm margins around poorly differentiated or less circumscribed lesions, in addition to intra-operative histologic control of such margins via frozen section studies (1–10). For tumor approaching bone, such as the mandible or the hard palate, an uninvolved and intact layer of periosteum is usually deemed adequate (1,3–5,8,10–13). If the periosteum is involved, but the outer table of the adjacent bone is grossly intact, then drilling off the outer cortex of that bone suffices. If a bony cortex is eroded, at least a 1-cm margin of grossly uninvolved bone is required although many prefer 1.5-cm, recognizing that frozen section verification of clear margins is difficult for the pathologist in this densely calcified tissue.

The marrow space can be evaluated by rolling a moistened, cotton-tipped applicator over the tissue for cytologic examination or using a curette to remove the soft marrow tissue for frozen-section analysis. The inferior alveolar neurovascular bundle can also be dissected free from the bony canal and processed for frozen-section analysis. For management of the mandible, most surgeons prefer a marginal mandibulectomy (commonly the superior half of the mandible) when the periosteum of the alveolar arch is breached by a mucosal malignancy. In cases of superficial erosion of the mandibular cortex, however, a segmental mandibulectomy is felt to be necessary (1–4,12–17).

For confirmation of adequate soft-tissue margins, the authors prefer the use of intra-operative micrographic mapping of tissue margins (as commonly practiced on cutaneous malignancy; Figs. 1–3) for all T1 or most small T2 verrucous or well-differentiated squamous cell carcinomas of the buccal, lip, or palatal mucosa. Somewhat more selective frozen section guidance of margins is required for larger lesions with deep extent.

More advanced lesions of the oral cavity require a more aggressive surgical approach with exposure beyond which can be achieved through a transoral approach. These more extensive procedures will often be combined with postoperative radiotherapy. It is in these more complex situations that careful evaluation and planning will help determine the appropriate surgical approach to accomplish all the goals of treatment and reconstruction.

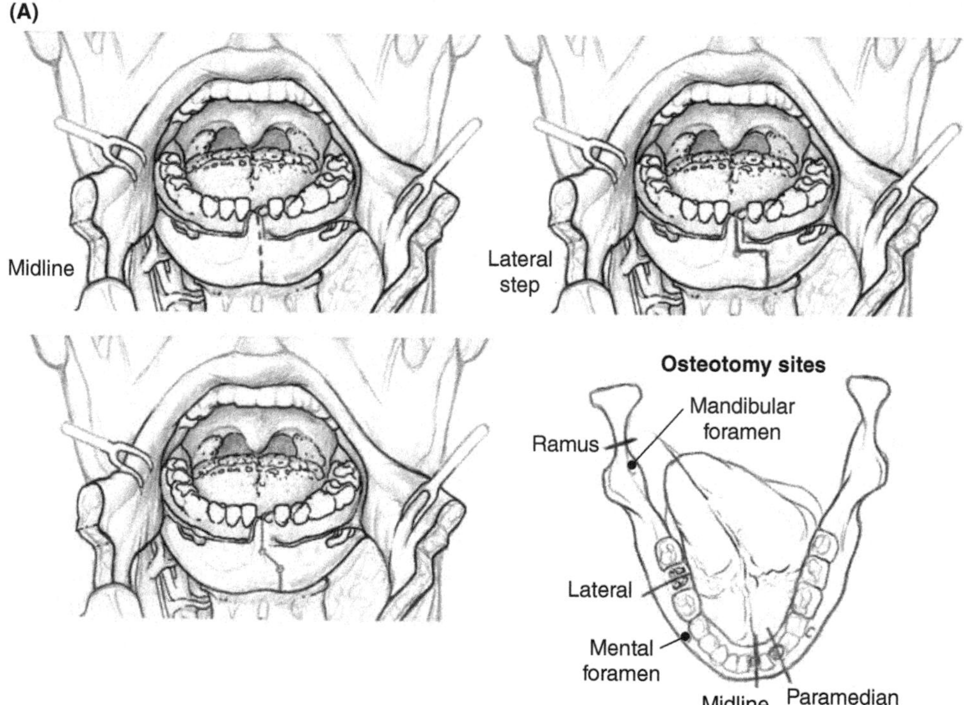

Figure 1A–B (A) Via lip split, access to the paramedian mandible is achieved. If osteotomy is desired, a stairstep cut with a side cutting burr or an oscillating saw is accomplished after preliminary placement, and then removal of a mandibular bridging plate. Placement of the osteotomy is commonly through the socket of a lateral incisor, sparing the more deeply rooted canine tooth.

(B)

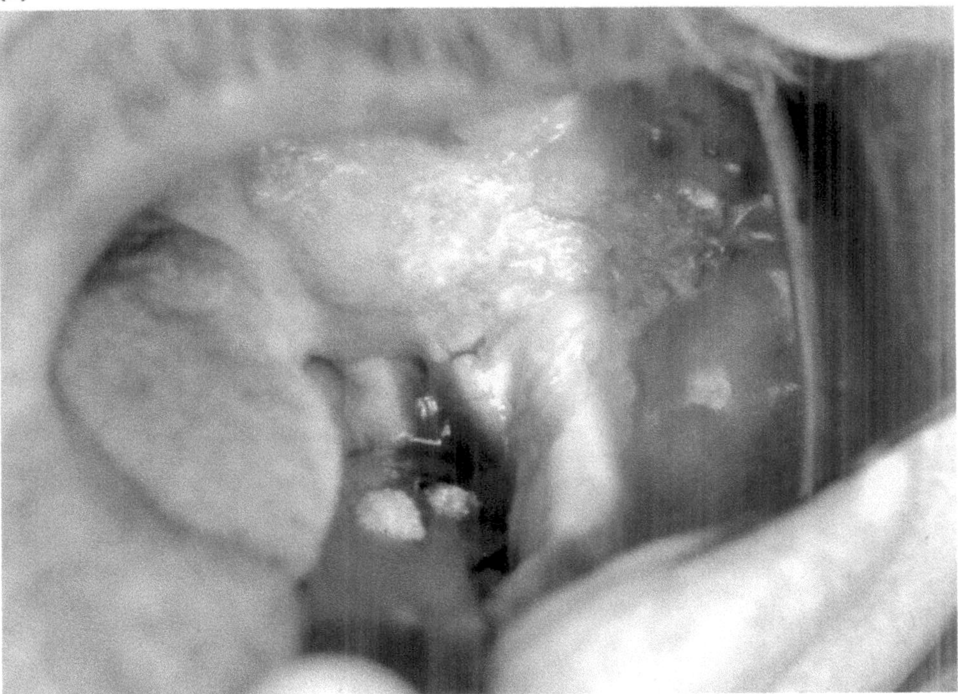

Figure 1 (**B**) Intra-operative transoral view of a 3.5 cm verrucous carcinoma of the soft palate, retromolar trigone and adjacent buccal mucosa, less than 5-mm thick.

(A)

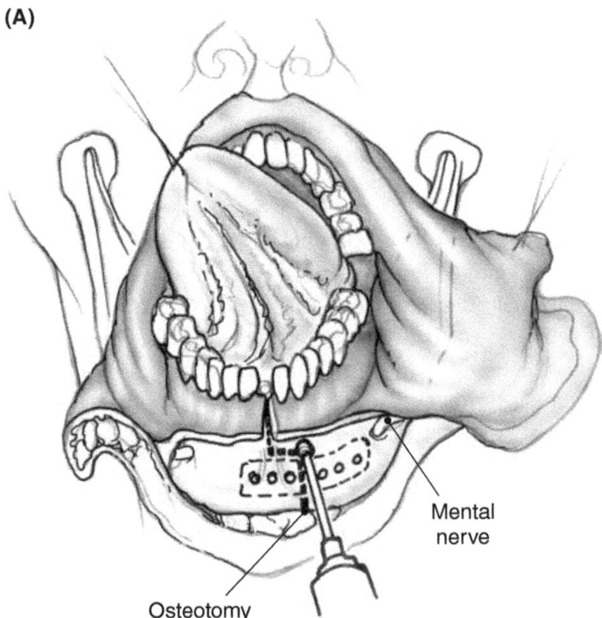

Figure 2 (**A**) Prior to mandibular osteotomy, a mandibular bridging plate is placed to assure proper alignment of dentition after the tumor resection.

(B)

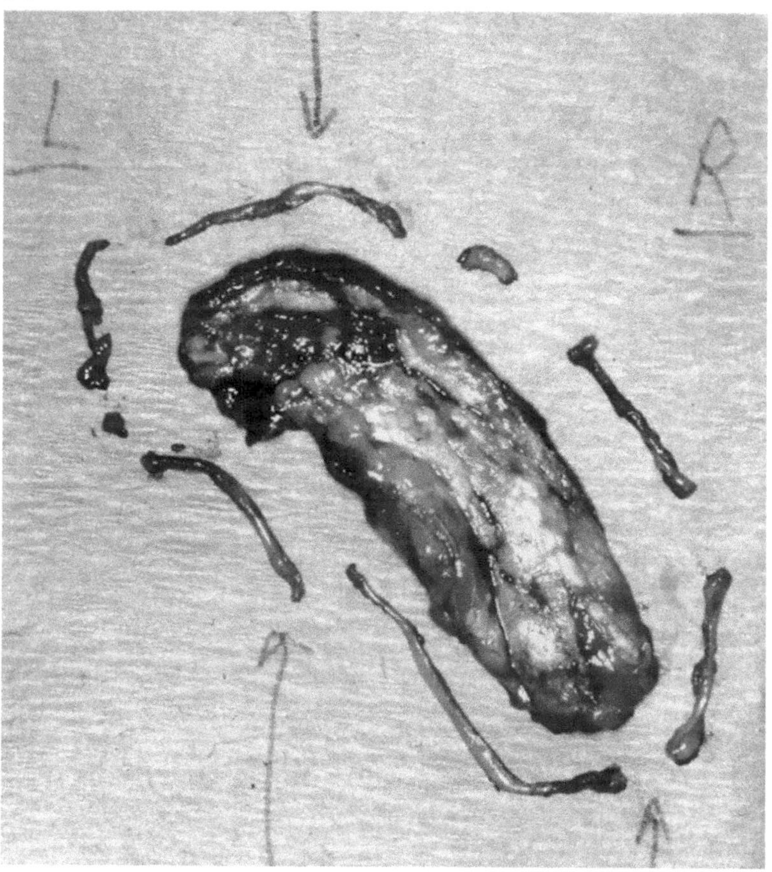

Figure 2 (**B**) En bloc specimen with margins around periphery, and entire deep margin, processed by micrographic mapping; oral defect allowed to granulate.

EVALUATION AND PLANNING

Initial approaches to oral cavity neoplasia, first described in detail in the early 1800s, involved transoral resection of relatively small lesions, limited by the patient's pain tolerance and the need to control blood and secretion aspiration while maintaining an adequate airway. With improvements in anesthesia in the early 20th century, more aggressive local interventions were tried, in combination with tracheostomy as necessary. With the advent of endotracheal intubation and an evolving understanding of the successful surgical management of metastatic adenopathy, extirpative techniques had almost reached the sophistication of current techniques by the 1950s: lip and mandibular splits to access large malignancies, combined with neck dissection(s), became commonplace (1–3,11). During the latter half of the 20th century, surgical advances have been made in the management of oral cavity neoplasia, such as the less deforming facial degloving approaches and selective neck dissections that can preserve form and function without compromising cure, and in three-dimensional planning and delivering of irradiation. That said, a preponderance of the differences in the treatment of oral malignancies between the 1950s and the

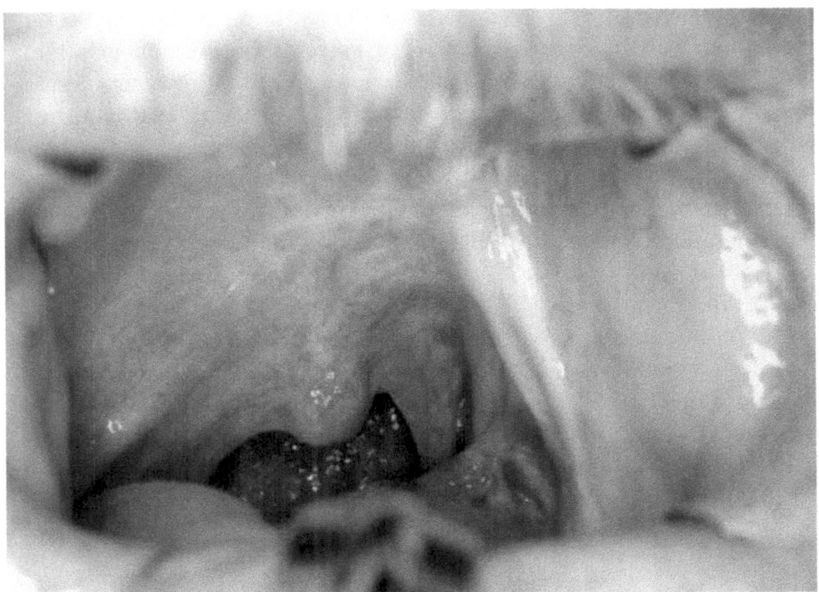

Figure 3 End result (three years postoperative) of granulation/scarring of defect from transoral resection of verrucous carcinoma (Fig. 2).

present has been the result of advances in surgical tumor-defect reconstructions, ranging from metal bridging plates and osseointegrated implants to composite free flaps.

When planning comprehensive treatment for an oral cavity neoplasm, the surgeon must consider many factors. Lesion location in the oral cavity, and its size and proximity to the mandibular or hard palatal bone are the first factors to consider (Table 1). Access is usually straightforward for anteriorly located lesions, as such are easier to inspect and palpate, and hence to excise, as the surgeon can retract adjacent normal tissues away from all but the most bulky lesions (1,2,4,7,15). Lesions abutting but not penetrating the outer cortex of bone can be excised transorally with a bony margin obtained via marginal mandibulectomy or partial hard palatectomy, or even by simply drilling off bone widely around the neoplasm. It is

Table 1 Issues Related to Head and Neck Surgical Approach

	Type of neck dissection	Location of tumor	Structures needing resection	Incisions
Type of flap reconstruction	—	X	X	—
Length of free flap vascular pedicle	X	X	X	—
Cosmesis	—	X	X	X
Functional outcome	X	X	X	—
Availability of recipient vessels for free flap	X	—	X	—
Mandibular/maxillary relationship and need for IMF, plate fixation and/or intermediate splint	—	X	X	X

Abbreviation: IMF, intermaxillary fixation.

always preferable to perform an *en bloc* resection that minimizes the chances of tumor seeding and allows histologic verification of margins on permanent section studies after specimen decalcification. Gross mandibular invasion, however, necessitates a segmental resection and some form of defect reconstruction that can range from a metal bridging plate to a vascularized osteocutaneous free-tissue transfer (13,15,16,18,19). In such cases, a transcervical (or "external") approach, in addition to the transoral exposure, is usually required. The risk of occult cervical metastases or clinical or radiographic evidence of adenopathy also mandates some form of external approach in addition to the transoral exposure of the primary tumor, with or without postoperative irradiation (10,20–23). The choice of a surgical approach and subsequent reconstruction of the oral cavity will be influenced by the plan for management of cervical nodal disease. The cervical lymphatics at greatest risk for metastatic disease are the Level I regions for primary lesions of the lips, anterior floor of mouth (FOM), anterior third of the tongue, the gingiva, and the buccal and hard palatal regions. The Level II regions are the primary at-risk site for the remainder of oral cavity locations (Fig. 4). The appropriate lymphatics should be

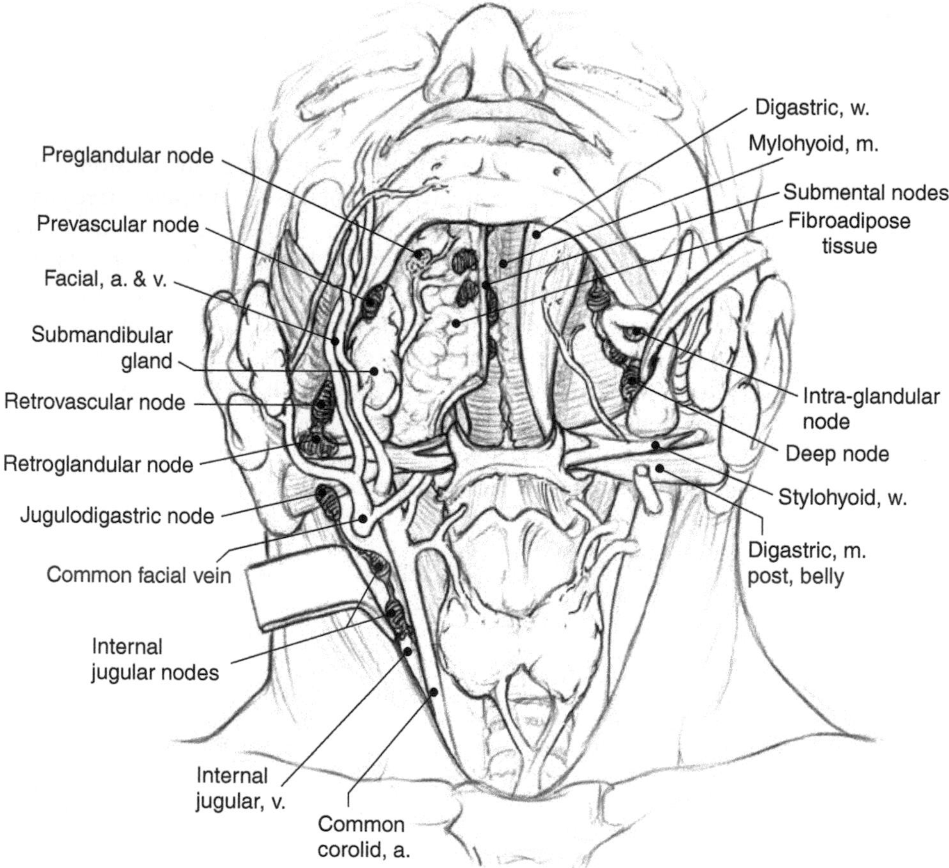

Figure 4 Lymphatics that drain the oral cavity structures (lower lip, anterior FOM and tip of tongue to submental nodes; upper lip, buccal region, lateral FOM and mobile tongue to perivascular facial or submandibular nodes; remainder of oral structures and the aforementioned nodal regions into jugulodigastric or level II nodes). *Abbreviation*: FOM, floor of mouth. *Source*: From Ref. 28.

addressed either surgically or with post-operative radiotherapy when the risk of metastasis exceeds 20% or when clinical nodal disease is evident (1,2,5,10,12,24–26). This will certainly be the case for most T2 and larger oral cavity malignancies, and for some earlier lesions. For tumors originating at or crossing the midline, both sides of the neck are at risk for metastatic disease and should be addressed (7,16,20–22,27,28). In the salvage surgery situation, the surgeon must err on the aggressive side of management as the lymphatic drainage pattern of a neoplasm is not as predictable after irradiation or surgery as before such and the patient is unlikely to have a curative option should the salvage fail (1,2,9,16). Tumor extirpation takes precedence over preservation of form and function, when the oncology surgeon manages the care of any particular patient. However, recent advances have increased the options for surgical access and reconstruction without compromising cure, with cosmetic and functional factors becoming increasingly important in the determination of the extirpative approach. Mandibular integrity is preserved when there has been no gross penetration of the mandibular cortex by tumor, and if an osteotomy is required, such as for a mandibular swing access, the osteotomy is preferentially placed anterior to the mental foramen to preserve sensation to the ipsilateral lip, and only one tooth is sacrificed at the mandibulotomy site (preferably not the functionally important canine tooth) (14,15,29).

It is critical to place the patient in proper maxillomandibular relationship by intermaxillary fixation, intermediate splint, or with pre-osteotomy plating of the mandible with rigid fixation. A helpful adjunct at the time of osteotomy is to preserve a flap of gingivae at least 1-cm proximal or distal to the osteotomy to place over the osteomy site at the conclusion of the procedure to prevent fistula formation and nonunion.

Preservation of the lingual, hypoglossal, and marginal mandibular nerves are routine unless such are directly involved with the tumor. If perineural propagation of the tumor is in question, resection of 1-cm of the nerve closest to the tumor is essential with subsequent frozen-section analysis. Then, mobilization of the proximal and distal segments of that nerve is required for a reanastomosis should there be no perineural invasion. Any of the aforementioned nerves can easily be mobilized sufficiently, without tension on the suture line, to make up for a 1-cm defect.

Preservation of the facial artery and vein becomes relevant should a platysmal myocutanous or submental island flap be part of the reconstructive option, and ample stumps of those vessels are routinely tagged by the extirpative surgeon to allow the reconstructive surgeon ready access to such vessels should a free flap be selected.

It is important to remember that any artery or vein of sufficient caliber (including external jugular vein, superior thyroid artery, facial artery and vein, and transverse cervical artery and vein) should not be ligated if possible during the neck dissection or tumor extirpation to preserve flow for possible free-tissue transfer. If ligation is mandated, an atraumatic vascular clamp may be placed at the proximal stump to avoid clotting within the vessel during the remainder of the procedure. At least 2-cm of vessel should be preserved if possible and additional length is beneficial particularly for flaps reaching superior to the hard palate.

With resection of a large tumor, reformation of the supporting elements of functionally important oral structures must be re-established, such as the tongue to the inner surface of the anterior mandibular arch or of the larynx to the inferior mandible (if the digastric and mylohyoid muscle and/or stylohyoid ligament suspensory elements have been disrupted).

Prior to beginning a resection, the extirpative surgeon needs not only to plan an oncologically sound ablation of the primary tumor, and of any draining lymphatic regions if the chance of metastasis is greater than 20%, but also should plan to minimize disruption of uninvolved structures and to minimize cosmetic deformity and functional impairment where feasible. With such considerations prior to the ablation, the reconstructive team has not only the requisite field of clear margins, but also the maximum spectrum of rehabilitative options.

RECONSTRUCTIVE OPTIONS

The surgeon's choice of approach must be communicated to anesthesia and operating room personnel prior to the patient entering the operating room. The anesthesiologist should be instructed on whether a nasotracheal or orotracheal intubation is preferred and, if the latter, on what side of the mouth should the tube be taped, or if the surgeon plans to stabilize the tube in the midline with a Crowe-Davis mouth gag or similar instrumentation. Endotracheal tube placement becomes less important if the surgeon plans to convert to a tracheostomy early in the operation for the purposes of improving access to the tumor and/or post-operative airway control during resolution of edema. Common positions around the operating table during transoral approaches for the surgeon, scrub nurse, and anesthesiologist are illustrated in Figure 5, with the surgeon positioned above the patient's head for transoral approaches, and at the patient's side for external approaches, as in Figure 6.

If the reconstructive options include the possibility of a scapular or latissimus dorsi free flap, a beanbag must be placed underneath the patient's torso and hips in

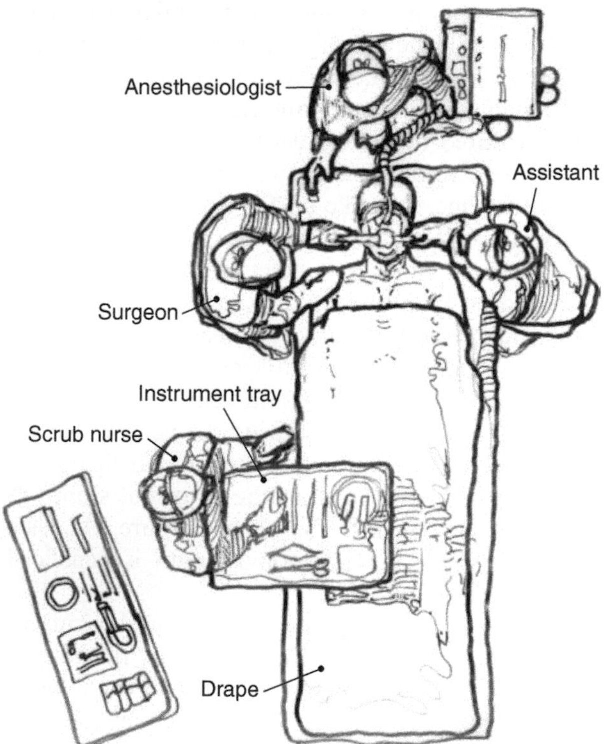

Figure 5 Positioning around operating table of nasally intubated patient, with anesthesiologist above patient's head.

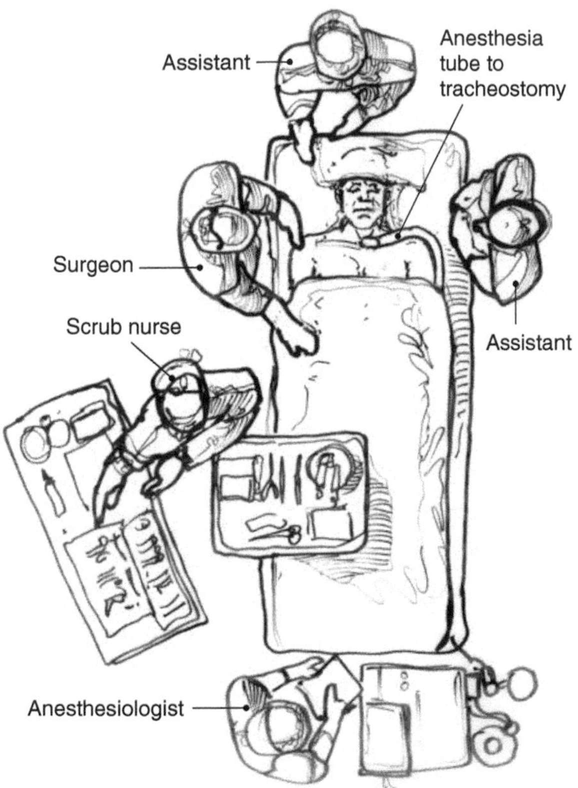

Figure 6 Optimal positioning around operating table of patient intubated via tracheostomy, with anesthesiologist at patient's feet.

order to rotate and stabilize them in a lateral decubitus position during the reconstructive phase of the procedure (Fig. 7). In addition, if the reconstructive team prefers to be seated while performing a microanastamosis, it is prudent to position the patient's head at the normal foot of the operating table which, in most operating theaters, allows sufficient room under the table near the patient's head and neck for the surgeon's legs and chair to be positioned comfortably.

For longer extirpative cases and all those in which a plastic and reconstructive team will scrub in after tumor resection, the patient should be fitted with sequential compression devices on their lower extremities, unless a fibular free flap or skin graft from a thigh donor site is needed. It is also prudent to have a urinary drainage catheter in place, and an arterial line is useful if a modest degree of patient hypotension is desired. The authors have found that such modest hypotension, plus placing the patient in a mild degree of anti-Trendelenburg to diminish the size of the neck veins, speeds the extirpation.

Surgical instrumentation for an external approach to an oral cavity lesion basically utilizes the same instruments as for a standard neck dissection, plus the addition of malleable retractors for visualization of recesses of the oral cavity and bone dividing instruments, usually an air driven drill with a side cutting burr or an oscillating saw. In cases for which an osteotomy is anticipated, the reconstructive surgeon's choice of a mandibular plating system must be available. Instrumentation for transoral access is much simpler, essentially the same as that for uvulopalatopharyngoplasty,

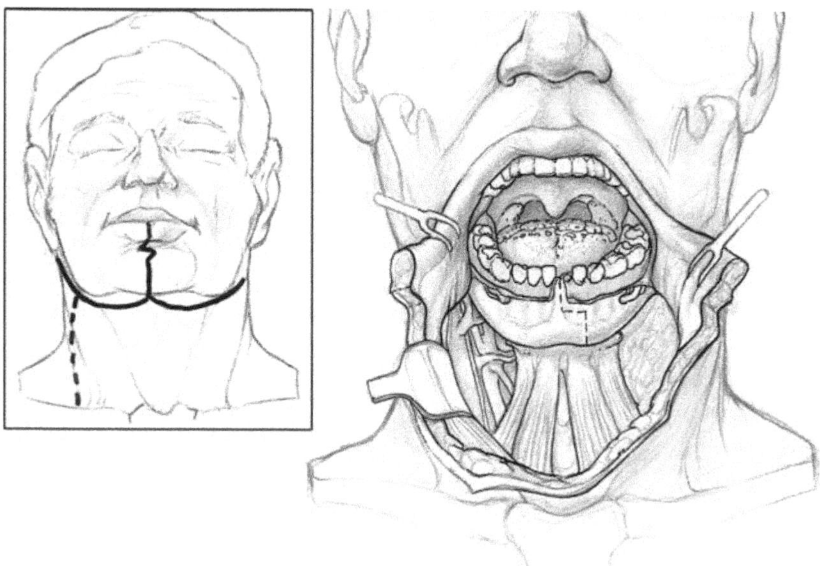

Figure 7 Defect after excision of T4N2A tumor of lip and buccal mucosa (involvement of cheek and upper neck skin) with synchronous T1 primary of FOM; note anterolateral neck dissection; repaired with latissimus dorsi free flap, providing intraoral and cheek resurfacing. *Abbreviation*: FOM, floor of mouth.

with the addition of periosteal elevators and drills when needed. The most commonly utilized instruments are illustrated in Figure 8.

Transoral Approach

A transoral excision is feasible for most T1 oral cavity or oropharyngeal malignancies, and for many T2 lesions (Table 1) (1–4,10–12). In addition, some portion of the resection of larger oral lesions is usually accomplished transorally, commonly the anterior margins of an extirpation, supplementing the lateral and posterior exposures afforded by a transcervical access. For lesions of the roof of the mouth and upper alveolar arch, the surgeon is usually positioned at the patient's head, with the patient in a Rose position as for uvulopalatopharyngoplasty; the orotracheal tube is stabilized in midline, and the tongue retracted inferiorly by a Crowe-Davis or similar mouth gag (Figs. 9 and 10).

Tumors of the buccal mucosa and lower half of the oral cavity are also accessed via a transoral route, but with the surgeon and assistant positioned at the sides of the patient's head and shoulders. In such cases, the surgeon should be on the side opposite the tumor, as visualization is progressively compromised with more posterior locations in the oral cavity and it is easier to visualize the proposed posterior margins from the contralateral side. Indeed, the surgeon must be able to visualize well around the periphery of the tumor, and be confident of access to tissue planes deep to the tumor as estimated by preoperative palpation. Computed tomography (CT) or magnetic resonance imaging (MRI) contrast enhanced studies can help delineate deep tumor extensions (13,19).

Transoral access for even small tumors is sometimes not feasible in patients with trismus, macroglossia, or similar impairments to an adequate transoral exposure. Though the standard overhead lights of surgical theaters can usually afford reasonable

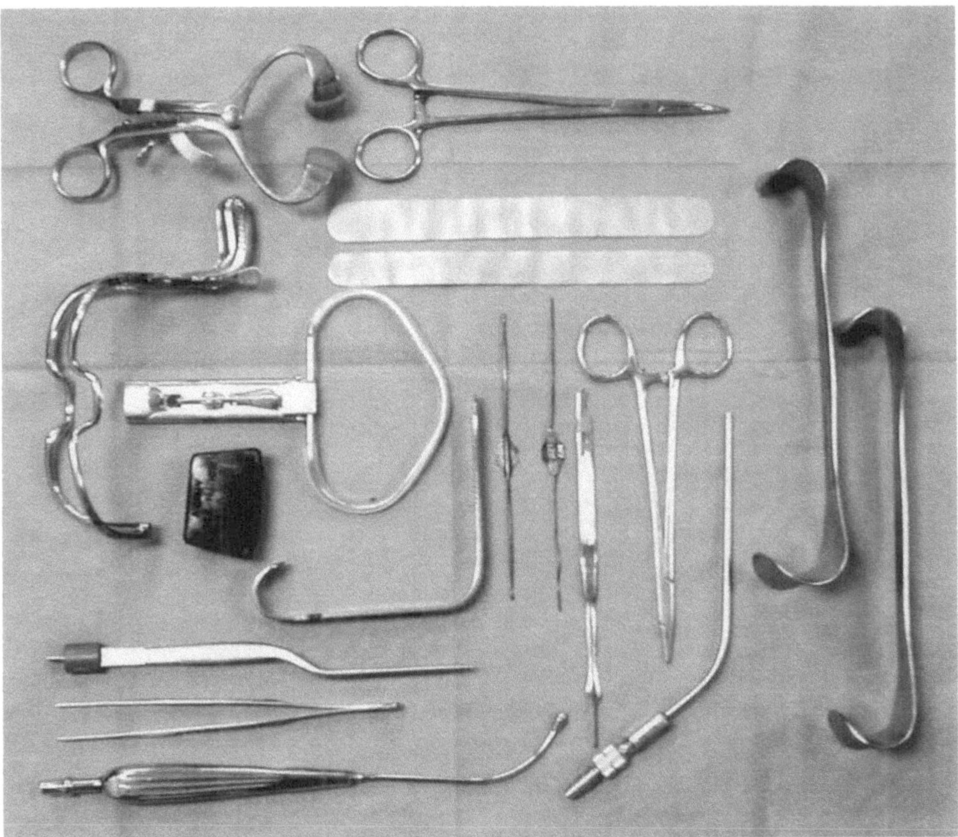

Figure 8 Instruments commonly utilized in a transoral resection of a tumor of the oral cavity.

visualization of intraoral structures, particularly anteriorly placed ones, most surgeons prefer headlights to assure adequate illumination of posterior or deep-tumor margins. Margins of at least 1-cm around all visible and palpable tumor is prudent, plus a further 3–5 mm is ideal for frozen-section analyses. The surgeon should indicate the tumor side margin with methylene blue, so the pathologist knows which is the "true" margin. A frozen-section control markedly decreases the necessity of secondary procedures for positive margins evident on a permanent section study.

Depending on size, most defects resulting from transoral tumor resections can be either closed primarily, allowed to granulate over a period of weeks, or be resurfaced with a split-thickness skin, dermal graft, or allograft such as Alloderm TM (Fig. 11) (1,3,5,12,17). Unfortunately, if 1-cm margins are obtained around a 1 cm^2 tumor, the resultant defect is 9 cm^2 which may cause significant dysfunction, particularly at the tongue-FOM junction. In cases with the potential for significant scar contracture with tethering of adjacent structures, flap reconstruction may provide improved functional outcome and prevent dysarthria.

Post-operative management of these patients depends on the size of the defect and whether a graft has been placed, and in the latter case, whether such graft has been quilted into place or secured by a bolster. For primary closures or wounds allowed to granulate, a post-tonsillectomy regimen suffices, but for larger surface areas covered with skin grafts, the patient may need to remain nasogastric-tube dependent for five

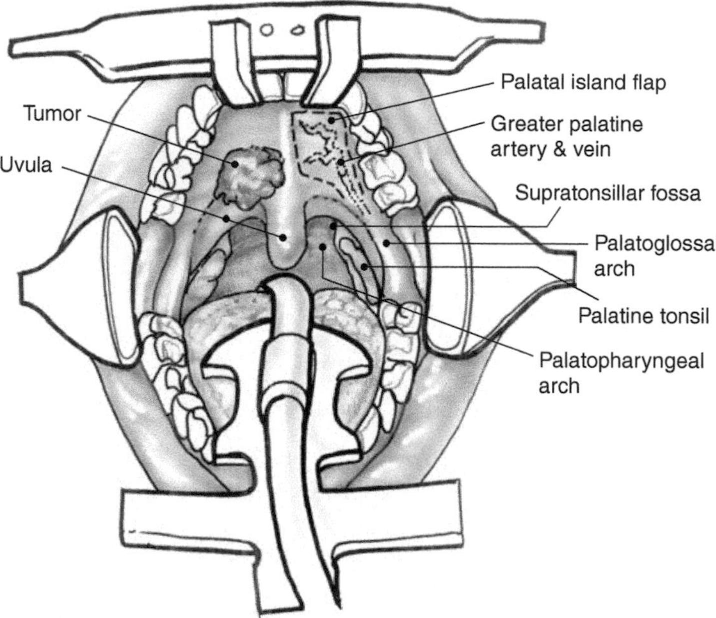

Figure 9 Illustration of transoral view of hard and partial soft palate tumor; note location of greater palatine artery and vein, on which palatal island flap is based for local reconstruction after tumor resection.

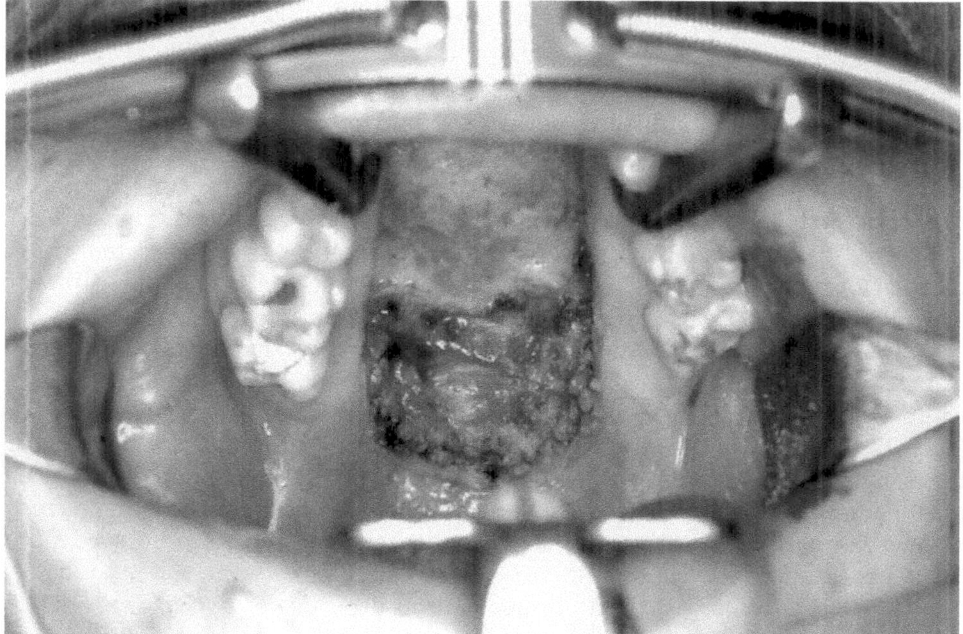

Figure 10 Transoral view of hard and partial soft palate defect after resection of a polymorphous adenocarcinoma of a minor salivary gland; note Dingman retractor stabilizes the endotracheal tube, and retracts tongue inferiorly and cheeks laterally.

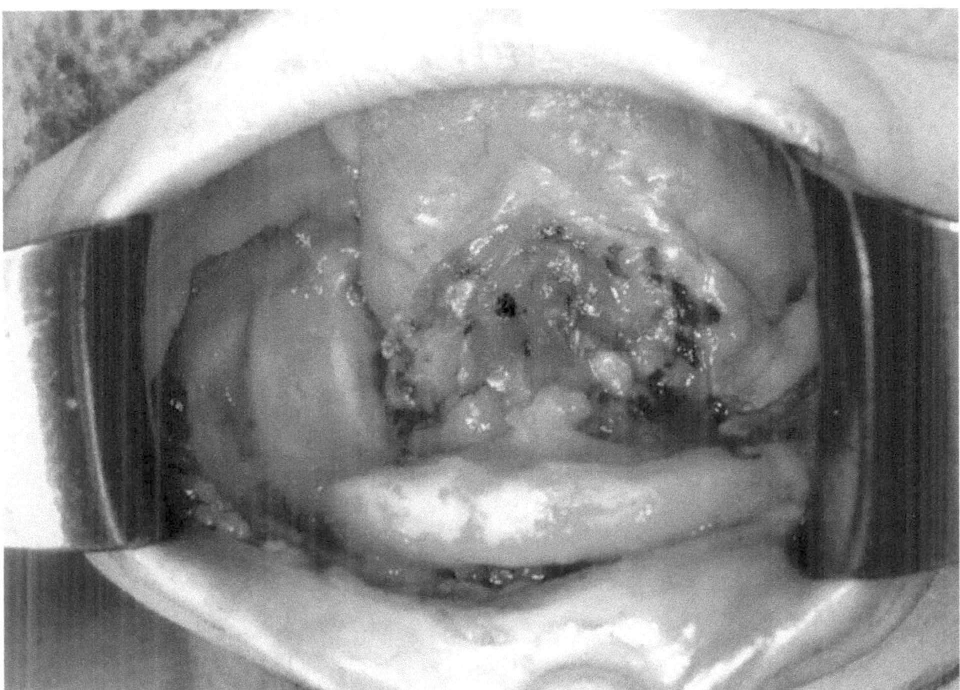

Figure 11 Intra-operative view of defect from transoral excision of superficial T2 anterior FOM and adjacent mandibular alveolar arch (periosteum not penetrated by tumor), defect closed with dermal graft stabilized by a bolster. *Abbreviation*: FOM, anterior floor of mouth.

to seven days. Most patients are prescribed post-operative intravenous antibiotics for the first 24 hours, and, thereafter, liquid oral antibiotics for one week, supplemented by saline and hydrogen peroxide combination mouthwashes.

Midline Glossotomy

The midline glossotomy is a combination of the transoral approach with a transcervical approach and can be performed either with or without a midline mandibulotomy which is usually necessary for lesions of the posterior mobile tongue or adjacent oropharynx (1,3,12,15). This procedure is accomplished with the surgeon and assistant positioned on opposite sides of the patient's neck. Although there are many options for incision placement for the "lip split" (Fig. 12), in the authors' opinion, the best cosmetic outcome is achieved via a stairstep incision through the lower lip; the stairstep begins at the vermillion border to break up any scar contraction that would later cause a notch in the lip, and then curves around the chin to make the skin incision conform with that soft tissue block of the face.

The mandible may also be divided in a stairstep fashion, halving the distance between the upper and lower borders with the horizontal portion of the osteotomy, while staying below the tooth roots in a dentulous patient (Fig. 13). Prior to mandibular division an appropriate plate should be fitted with bicortical screws at the lower border of the mandible. In the dentulous patient an additional plate with monocortical screws is place above the horizontal bone cut to function as a tension band. The plates are then removed and placed on the back table while mandibulotomy is performed. At the end of the procedure, the plates can then be rapidly

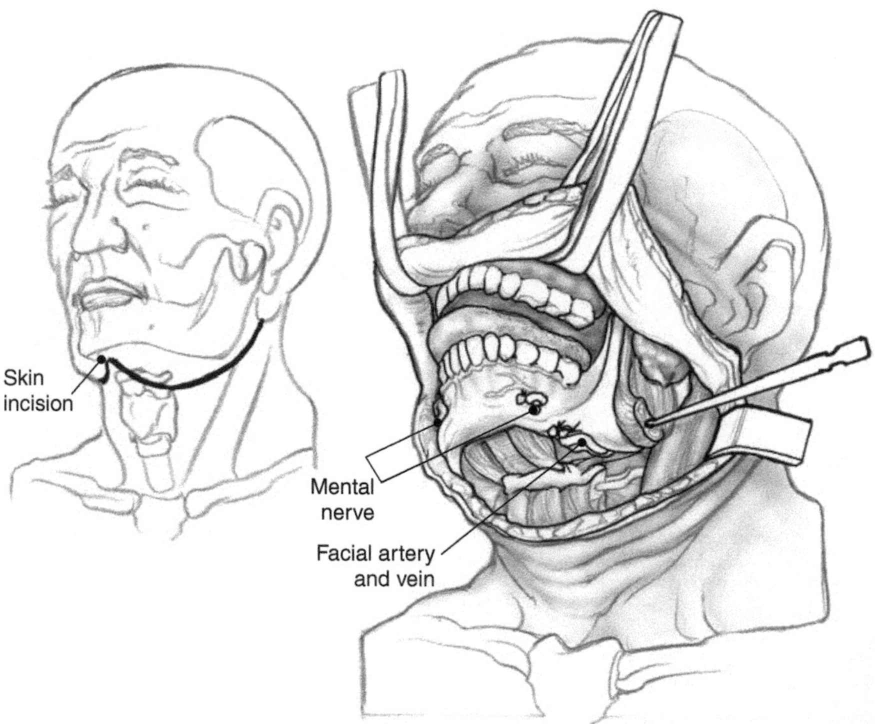

Figure 12 Neck incisions for lower facial ("cervical") degloving, placed two fingerbreadths below inferior border of mandible in its mid portion, closer to mandible near midline, avoiding damage to marginal mandibular nerve; subsequent undermining affords exposure for mandibulotomy, lymphadenectomies.

replaced, with assurance of reformation of the preoperative dental occlusion and chin contour. It is usually necessary to remove at least one of the incisor teeth to perform the osteotomy. If sharp bony edges remain after osteotomy, these edges should be rounded with a round burr to prevent trauma on the incision line post-operatively.

Dissection through the anterior FOM is kept strictly in the midline, avoiding damage to Wharton's ducts, and the possibility of submandibular obstruction and infection. The tongue is then divided along the midline raphae which is a fairly avascular plane. Keeping the incision in the midline avoids all significant nervous and vascular structures and will minimize any muscular dysfunction. This approach is carried as far posteriorly as needed to provide access to the posterior tongue, tongue base, or posterior pharynx. On closure the tongue is repaired with deep and superficial absorbable sutures.

Lip Split with Cheek Flap and Mandibulotomy

The traditional and still most commonly applied approach to advanced lesions of the oral cavity is the lip/chin split incision which is connected with the ipsilateral neck incision and combined with a either mandibulotomy or mandibulectomy (Figs. 14 and 15). This allows mobilization and retraction of the entire cheek, posterior mandibular segment and upper neck flap to expose the oral cavity. The lip split is accomplished in an identical fashion to that previously described for the

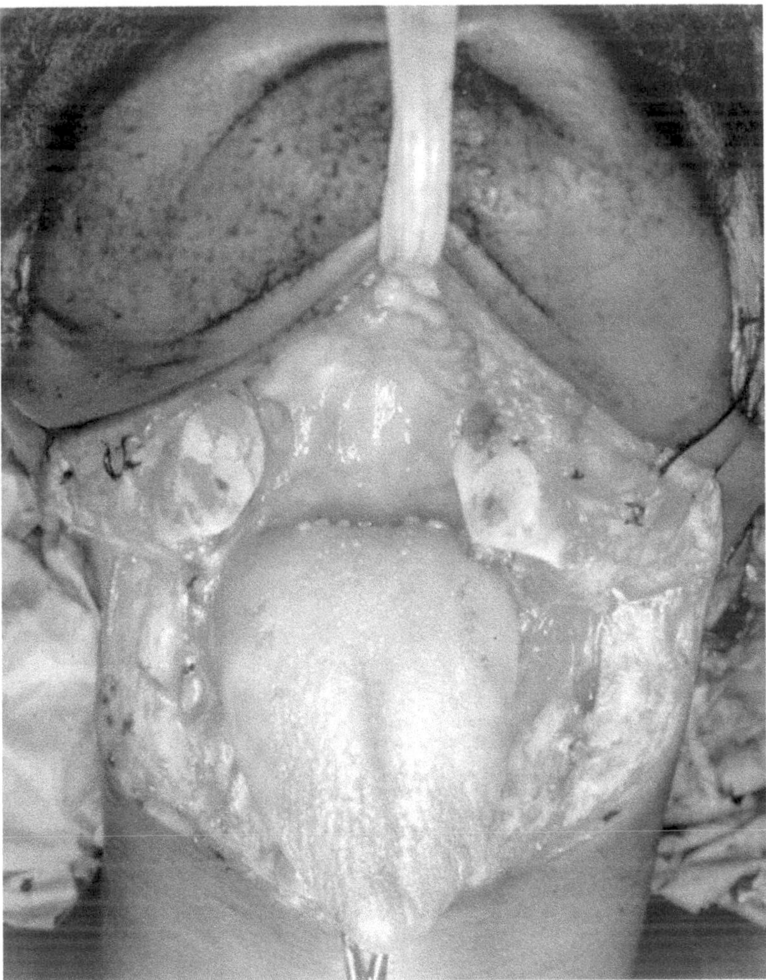

Figure 13 Lower facial degloving for T4 of anterior FOM that penetrated mandibular symphysis; note upward retraction of chin and lip, and anterior and inferior retraction of tongue, plus lymphadenectomies of levels I and II bilaterally (no positive nodes). *Abbreviation*: FOM, anterior floor of mouth.

midline glossotomy as described above. From the chin the incision curves posteriorly to connect with the upper limb of the neck incision which should be at least two fingerbreadths below the mandibular body to avoid injury to the marginal branch of the facial nerve. This incision can usually be placed in a natural skin crease and carried posteriorly and upward to the mastoid tip for maximal exposure.

Lymphadenectomy is usually accomplished first, facilitating access to the under surface of the mandible and subsequently the tumor through the submandibular and submental triangles, with preservation of the hypoglossal and/or lingual nerves when feasible. Intra-operative hemostasis is obtained in a routine fashion, but it is optimized by infiltration of a 1:100,000 or 1:200,000 epinephrine solution (the latter if greater than a 15-mL infiltration is anticipated in an average sized adult) along the anticipated resection lines, plus ligation of arteries that feed the resection area such as the ipsilateral lingual artery for a hemiglossectomy.

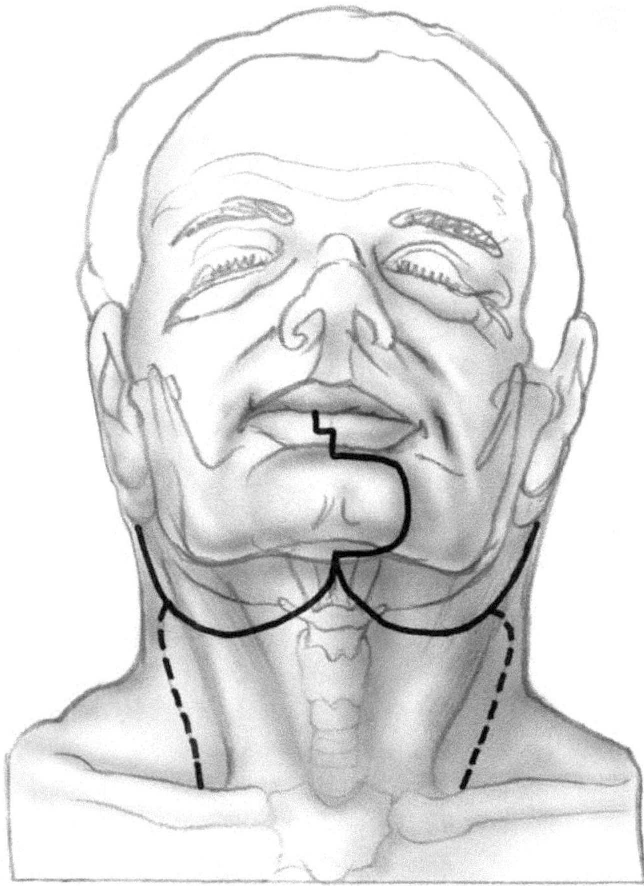

Figure 14 Lip/chin split extension of neck incision; note bridging plate and corresponding drill holes designed prior to bony resection, facilitating reconstitution of mandibular contour; stairstep osteotomy, positioned anterior to mental foramen, with preservation of the canine tooth.

To access a large FOM or mobile tongue tumor, the stairstep osteotomy is placed either near the midline after removal of one of the incisor teeth (Fig. 14). For more posterior lesions the osteotomy is placed more lateral, just anterior to the mental foramen, preserving the mental nerves to avoid post-operative lip numbness. Low profile plates should be fashioned and placed/removed prior to the osteotomy as described previously to ensure preservation of dental relationships.

Should the mandible be involved by tumor, and bone resection is anticipated, the osteotomy should be placed to allow at least a 1- to 1.5-cm tumor-free margin on the mandible. The inferior alveolar nerve almost will always be sacrificed in this situation. Application of an appropriately shaped bridging plate prior to the bony resection is mandatory (Fig. 15). If resection of the entire ramus is anticipated, drill holes are placed in the mandible distal to the resection, and a new temporomandibular joint is fashioned from a preformed metal plate with a smooth ball on one end that will fit in the glenoid fossa, a costal cartilage and rib graft, or a free flap transfer.

In closing a lip-split defect, it is crucial to approximate the oral mucosa, orbicularis muscle and skin planes in three separate layers, and to carefully align the stairstep incision at the vermillion border. Nasogastric feeding for 7–10 days

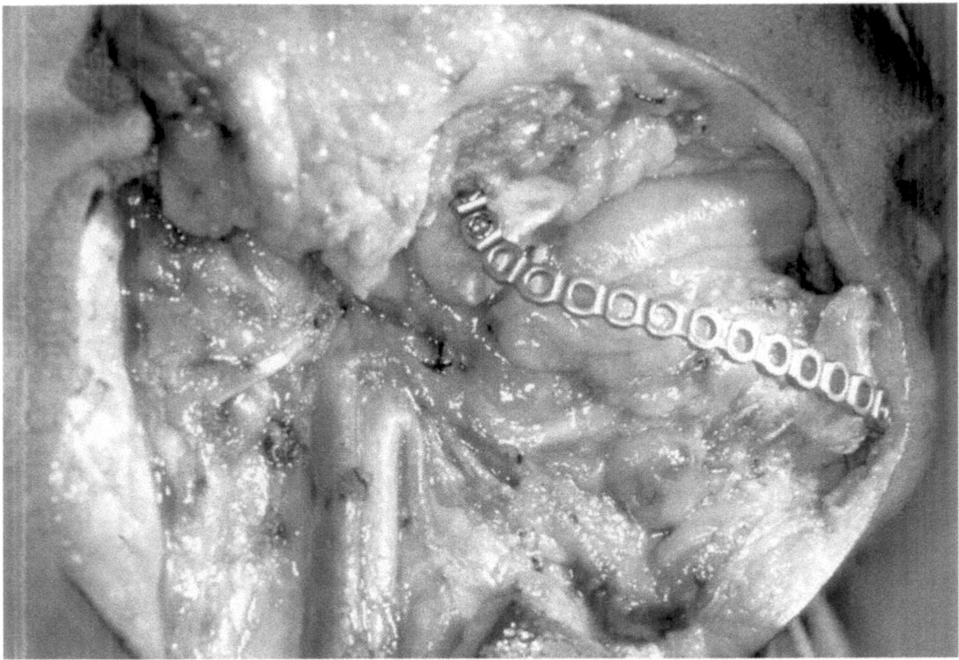

Figure 15 Lip/chin split, cheek rotation and segmental mandibulectomy for T4N2B of retromolar trigone and adjacent FOM; note metal bridging plate for attachment of fibular free flap, and radical neck dissection (spinal accessory nerve, internal jugular vein and sternocleidomastoid muscle all involved with extracapsular extension of metastases). *Abbreviation*: FOM, anterior floor of mouth.

should be anticipated, and if a longer period of time is desired, a percutaneous gastrostomy (PEG) is preferred (i.e., better tolerated) by most patients. If such is planned, the PEG should be placed prior to the sterile preparation and draping for the head and neck tumor resection, to avoid intra-operative contamination of a chest or abdominal flap donor area.

Degloving Approach to the Oral Cavity

The term "degloving" is applied to oral cavity procedures which utilize neck or mucosal incisions to access the tumor, with or without a concominant lymphadenectomy, without the necessity of a chin or lip incision. Previously, it has implied that the mandible was not divided, as in prior decades mandibulotomy was always performed after lip split and lateral cheek mobilization. However, upward retraction of the cheek and chin soft tissues after extensive undermining via a "cervical degloving," often performed bilaterally, can afford adequate room for a mandible split or resection. The lateral and inferior rotation of the proximal segment of the mandible without a lip/chin split in the authors' hands, is now the most common access for larger oral cavity tumors (Figs. 12 and 13) Table 2.

The more commonly utilized "degloving" procedure is a unilateral or bilateral transcervical approach to a mid to lower oral cavity neoplasm such as of the FOM, tongue or alveolar arch. The initial cut is basically the upper limb of a Schobinger or "apron" type of neck incision, crossing the midline below the chin in a gentle curve to

Table 2 Selection of Surgical Approach to Oral Cavity Tumor Based on Tumor Size and Location

Surgical approach	Tumor size	Location
Transoral	T1, selected T2	All Locations
Transoral, with mid facial degloving	T2–T4	Upper gingiva, hard and/or soft palate
Transoral, with limited mandibulectomy	Selected T2 or T4[a]	Lower gingiva, adjacent FOM or labial/ buccal region
Transoral with midline glossotomy	T2	Central tongue or oropharynx with/without midline mandibulotomy
Transcervical with lower facial degloving	T2–T4	Any Location with/without mandibulotomy or mandibulectomy
Transcervical with lip/chin split	T3–T4	Any location with/without mandibulotomy or mandibulectomy
Transcervical with lingual release	Any stage	Oropharynx, hypopharynx, base of tongue

[a]By virtue of limited mandibular invasion but overall tumor <4cm.
Abbreviation: FOM, floor of mouth.

the contralateral neck and, hence, onward toward the mastoid tip should a bilateral access be necessary. The neck incisions are always placed two fingerbreadths below the inferior border of the body of the mandible in its mid portion (closer to the mandible near the midline) to avoid damage to the marginal mandibular branch of the facial nerve, and can extend well below such for a substantial "apron," even to a trach site, should access to lower echelons of cervical nodes be indicated (1–4,7,30). For a standard submandibular type of unilateral apron flap, access to the Level I and Level II nodes is straightforward, although an inferiorly placed apron is often necessary to reach the Level III or IV nodes. From the neck incision, the immediate subcutaneous tissues and platysma are divided and a plane of dissection is established superiorly toward the mandible, over the lateral capsule of the submandibular gland and the adjacent anterior and posterior bellies of the digastric muscle. By staying at this depth and suture ligating the distal stumps of the facial artery and vein (only if necessary for oncologic purposes or if a free-tissue transfer and recipient vessels are unnecessary) to the overlying platysma (Hayes Martin maneuver), damage to the marginal mandibular nerve can be prevented.

Tumors of the buccal mucosa and lateral alveolar arch may commonly result in metastases along the perivascular nodes that follow the facial artery and vein (28). In such cases these nodes must be removed, and require the surgeon to visually identify, with the assistance of a nerve stimulator if desired, the marginal mandibular nerve to preserve that structure while the facial artery and vein are skeletonized of associated lymphatic structures.

Once the inferior border of the mandible is exposed, a subperiosteal plane can be established with a Freer, Lempert, or similar elevator on both the lateral and medial cortices of the mandible, recognizing that the mylohyoid muscle inserts on the medial cortex of the anterior two-thirds of the mandibular arch, and must be detached to gain access to the submucosa of the oral cavity. For oral cavity tumors near the midline, the submental triangle is stripped of its fat and nodal tissues, along with the submandibular triangle contents, accomplishing a Level I nodal dissection. Most surgeons likewise strip the adjacent Level II nodes from the jugulodigastric region even if no nodes suspicious for tumor are present which not only aids in eventual tumor staging and post-operative treatment, but allows simple circumferential exposure to branches of the external carotid artery and jugular vein for recipient vessel access. Additional nodal dissection is completed as indicated.

After removal of the relevant cervical lymphatic structures, associated fat and the submandibular gland(s), the surgeon is in close proximity underneath any oral or oropharyngeal neoplasm, and only needs to identify the hypoglossal and lingual nerves and external carotid system before proceeding to *en bloc* resection of the tumor via a combination transoral and the transcervical access.

If a bony resection is necessary, the degloving approach still frequently suffices, with exposure of the entire mandibular body and most of the ascending rami, and obviates a lip/chin split (Fig. 16). To accomplish such, the periosteum over the lateral cortex of the mandible is elevated, and, if necessary the mental nerve is divided as it exits the mental foramen on the ipsilateral side, allowing the surgeon to place one-inch Penrose drains from the neck incision through the oral cavity and out the mouth. Upward traction then can readily distract the lip and chin soft tissues superiorly, while downward traction on the mandible with a bone hook will deliver the mandible, FOM and tongue into the neck dissection field. Prior to the bony resection, the anticipated bony defect is marked, and an appropriately tailored titanium locking 2.0 or 2.4 bridging plate is bent to conform to the contours of the anticipated proximal and distal bony segments. It is most convenient to utilize a pre-

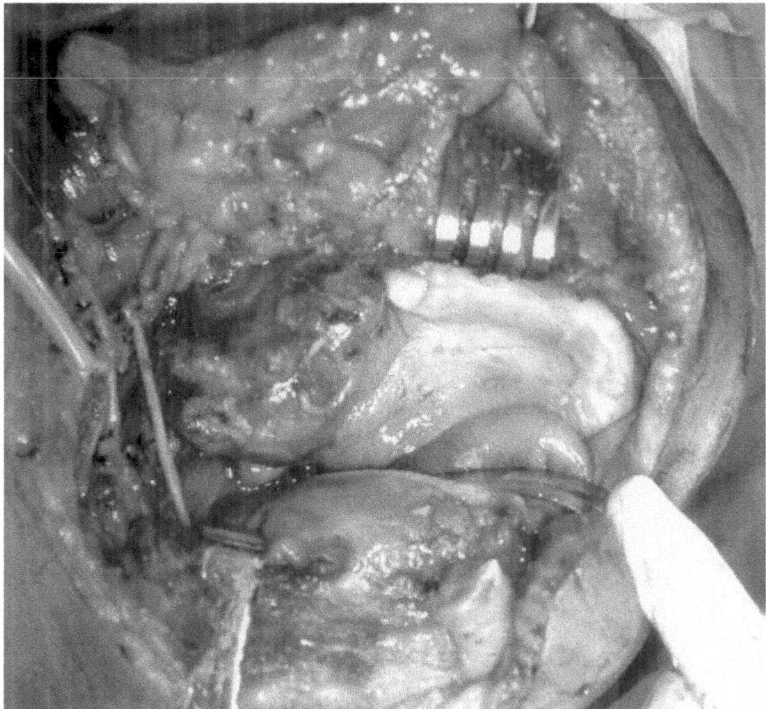

Figure 16 Lateral facial degloving for T3 of tonsil, soft palate and adjacent tongue; note intact lip and chin yet a mandibulotomy with a lateral rotation and superior retraction of the ipsilateral body and ramus; note vascular tapes around internal and external carotid arteries in the posterior field of dissection.

fabricated angulated bridging plate if the ascending ramus of the mandible is part of the proximal segment, placing four, rather than the minimum of three bi-cortical screws, in that segment as the ramus is much thinner than the body of the mandible. To maximize stability, the plate is positioned along the posterior border of the ramus, its thickest segment.

Some patients with relatively circumscribed intraoral lesions can have an extirpation without the necessity of a tracheostomy even if the mandibular contour has been disrupted (but intra-operatively reconstituted with a bridging plate). However, in most cases in which a mandibulotomy is performed or when there has been extensive mobilization of the tongue, peri-operative use of a tracheostomy is prudent, particularly when the anterior tongue attachments are separated from the mandible (base of tongue migrates posteriorly).

Midface Degloving Approach

For tumors of the hard palate mucosa that invade bone and require a wide area of bone resection, another type of "degloving," a "midfacial degloving," is an excellent way to approach the tumor, and is preferred to a lateral rhinotomy with a lip split and cheek rotation unless there is tumor spread posteriorly through the pterygoid plates and/or into the parapharyngeal space (3,12,31). Such a "degloving" involves retracting the upper lips laterally and superiorly, typically with Goulet retractors, and is performing what is essentially a bilateral Caldwell-Luc access (extended across the midline, through the pyriform apertures and the base of the septum; Fig. 17). First, the mucosa is elevated over the anterior faces of the maxillary sinuses, extending superiorly to the levels of the infraorbital nerves. The anterior face of one or both

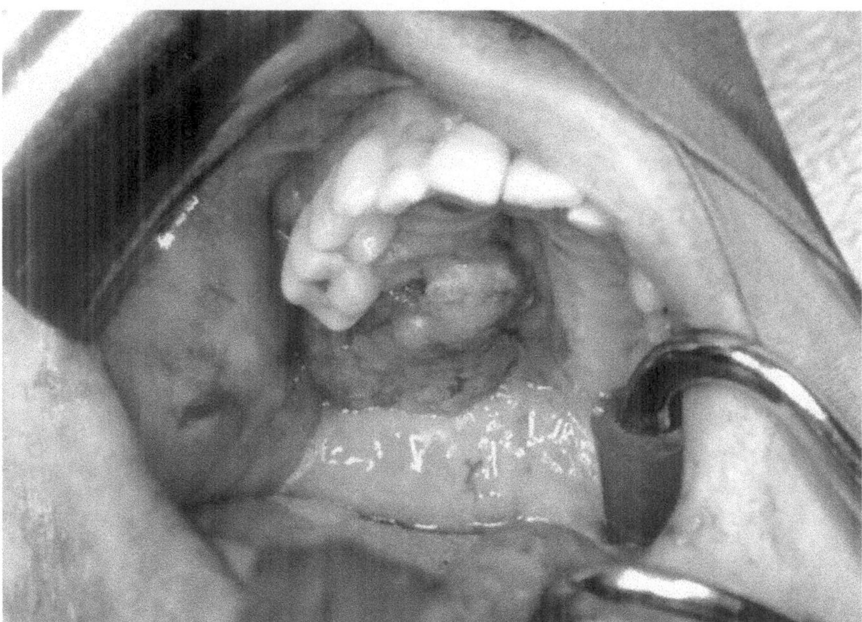

Figure 17 Well differentiated carcinoma of posterior hard palate and adjacent soft palate, eroding through hard palatal bone to floor of maxillary sinus, excised via unilateral midfacial degloving and transoral routes.

maxillary sinuses can be removed, depending on tumor location. Such allows the surgeon access to the floor(s) of the maxillary sinus(es) and adjacent nasal cavity(s), and, in most cases, a clear margin above any palatal tumor. Indeed, removal of the entire hard and soft palates can be accomplished through this straightforward midfacial degloving approach, although the reconstruction of such a defect is a significant challenge and involves placement of the initial stage of osseointegrated implants in the same surgical sitting that clear tumor margins are confirmed by frozen-section study.

If the anterior or premaxillary region does not require resection, it is helpful to leave this area intact, including the periosteum, and perform a combined transoral/transfacial (lateral rhinotomy or sublabial incision) or transoral/endoscopic approach.

Lingual Release Approach

The lingual release approach can be considered an "internal degloving" approach to the more posteriolateral aspect of the oral cavity, tonsillar fossa, and oropharynx, hypopharynx and base of tongue. Described by Bradley and Stell (32) and popularized by Stanley (33), this access is achieved via a combination of transcervical and intraoral incisions. The external cervical incision consists of a broad apron flap placed in a skin crease approximately two fingerbreadths below the mandible and extending from mastoid to mastoid. The skin flap is elevated as for a degloving approach with the elevation of the submandibular fascia to protect the marginal mandibular branch of the facial nerve (Hayes Martin maneuver). This elevation is carried across the midline to expose the inferior border of the mandible from angle to angle. The periosteum of the mandible is then encised along the lower boarder of the mandible allowing elevation on the lingual surface of the bone from angle to angle.

The intraoral incision is then made through a transoral approach. If the mandible is edentulous the incision is placed on the superior aspect of the alveolar ridge from retromolar trigone to retromolar trigone and carried into the oropharynx as needed. If the patient has dentition the mucosa of the lingual surface of the mandible can be elevated from the dental ligament at the base of the teeth or an incision can be placed 2-mm below the base of the teeth. The periosteum on the lingual surface of the mandible is then elevated to the lower border of the mandible which will include elevation of the insertion of the mylohyoid muscle from it's insertion along a ridge of bone.

At this juncture of the exposure the periosteal pocket developed intraorally is connected with the elevation started extraorally to completely free the lingual mandibular periosteum. The only remaining attachment will be that of glossal muscles to the midline genial tubercle which must be released either sharply or with electrocautery. The entire oral tongue/FOM/mandibular mucoal-periosteum complex is then passed into the neck wound by placing a suture in the tip of the tongue and pulling it medial to the mandible into the neck (pull-through technique).

The neck skin flap and mandible are then retracted superiorly while the oral cavity contents including the FOM, submandibular ducts, sublingual tissues, lingual and hypoglossal nerves and oral tongue are pulled inferiorly as a unit (Figs. 12 and 13). If the tumor to be excised involves the oropharynx, hypopharynx, or base of tongue, the mucosal incisions may be extended posteriorly to improve the exposure. Unlike the mandibular swing approach, with the lingual release method, the further posteriorly the exposure, the better the visualization in these areas. Obviously, a mandibulotomy is avoided as well. If necessary, a composite resection can be combined with this approach which is then more like the traditional degloving operations (Fig. 16).

Once the resection is performed and any needed reconstruction completed the intraoral mucosal incision must be carefully repaired via a transoral approach. This is very straight forward in the edentulous patient with simple repair of the alveolar ridge mucosa. In the dentulous patient it is useful to support the repair with mattress sutures passed around teeth rather than relying on mucosal sutures placed at the tooth root level. Resuspension of the oral cavity structures relies primarily on the mucosal repair. Reattachment of the lingual muscles to the mandible anteriorly is accomplished by placing a 2.0-suture through the muscle attachments from the genial tubercle to the intact periosteum of the mandible in the midline. This successfully resuspends the hyoid bone and supralaryngeal structures.

The lingual release approach has largely replaced the lip split/mandibulotomy approach to the posterior oral cavity and pharynx in many instances. A violation of the mandible is avoided, the lip and chin scar becomes unnecessary and posterior exposure is superior. However, performing the intraoral incisions and closure can be quite difficult in the dentulous patient with trismus and another approach should be considered.

Transhyoid Approach

Although this text is on oral cavity reconstruction more posterior and larger tumors of the oral cavity can invade the oropharynx, particularly from a mid third of tongue, retromolar trigone or tonsillar primary. Though rarely employed as a sole approach, a transhyoid exposure of the base of the tongue and inferior tonsillar region may serve as an adjunct to one of the previously mentioned accesses (1–3,34). Such is most commonly utilized in conjunction with a lower facial "degloving" and/or transoral approach. After careful identification and preservation of the hypoglossal and superior laryngeal nerves, some surgeons excise the entire hyoid bone by cutting it free of the strap and tongue base muscles, whereas others, such as the authors, merely cut along the superior surface of the hyoid, thus releasing the base of tongue, digastric and mylohyoid muscles and allowing the hyoid to drop inferiorly in the neck. The vallecula and lateral oropharyngeal mucosa are within 5 mm of the hyoid bone in most patients, so entering these regions is quickly and easily accomplished by pulling the base of tongue anteriorly into the wound and somewhat superiorly with a wide, double-pronged hook. Next, by retracting inferiorly on the hyoid, the surgeon, with the help of headlight illumination, can view the entire base of tongue, inferior tonsil, and soft palatal regions, and thereby can control the inferior aspects of an oral tumor resection. After tumor resection and reconstruction of the defect, it is prudent to resuspend the hyoid, and hence laryngotracheal complex, to the mandible, using permanent sutures around the hyoid at each lesser cornu, stabilized to small drill holes in the inferior borders of the mandible in the region of the mandibular angles, or to a similarly located bridging plate used to reconstruct a mandibular defect. If free-tissue transfer is used, confirm that there does not exist any compression by these permanent sutures on the flap or pedicle prior to closing the wound.

CONCLUSION

The extirpative surgeon has a number of options in exposing oral malignancy, and selects among these based on tumor size and location, and whether lymphadenectomy is prudent. Once an oncologically sound procedure is planned, the reconstruction should be designed to provide for optimal reconstruction based on the expected defect and functional deficits. Options include transoral exposure, midfacial or lower facial degloving, and lip splitting with mandibular rotation, the latter to which a lingual release or transhyoid adjunct can be useful in selected cases. Whatever the approach chosen, preservation of the form and function of uninvolved structures adjacent to the tumor is desirable, controlling the resection margins between such structures and the tumor with intra-operative frozen section studies. For other than small malignancies that can be encompassed by transoral excision, the head and neck reconstructive surgeon is consulted pre-operatively, meeting with the patient and then reviewing with the extirpative surgeon the alternatives in reconstruction, and later rehabilitation, of each patient based on the anticipated resection and any adjunctive therapies such as irradiation.

REFERENCES

1. Alvi A, Myers E, Johnson J. Cancer of the oral cavity. In: Myers E, Suen J, eds. Cancer of the Head and Neck. Philadelphia: Saunders, WB, 1996:321—360.
2. Civantos F, Goodwin W. Cancer of the oropharynx. In: Myers E, Suen J, eds. Cancer of the Head and Neck. Philadelphia: Saunders, WB, 1996:361—380.
3. Bailey B. Surgery of the Oral Cavity. Chicago: Year Book Medical Publishers, 1989.
4. Chhetri DK, Rawnsley JD, Calcaterra TC. Carcinoma of the buccal mucosa. Otolaryngol Head Neck Surg 2000; 123:566–571.
5. Yco MS, Cruickshank JC. Treatment of stage I carcinoma of the anterior floor of the mouth. Arch Otolaryngol Head Neck Surg 1986; 112:1085–1089.
6. Barton RT, Ucmakli A. Treatment of squamous cell carcinoma of the floor of the mouth. Surg Gynecol Obstet 1977; 145:21–27.
7. Hicks WL Jr, Loree TR, Garcia RI, Maamoun S, Marshall D, Orner JB, Bakamjian VY, Shedd DP. Squamous cell carcinoma of the floor of mouth: a 20-year review. Head Neck 1997; 19:400–405.
8. Rogers SN, Lowe D, Brown JS, Vaughan ED. The University of Washington head and neck cancer measure as a predictor of outcome following primary surgery for oral cancer. Head Neck 1999; 21:394–401.
9. Rodgers LW Jr, Stringer SP, Mendenhall WM, Parsons JT, Cassisi NJ, Million RR. Management of squamous cell carcinoma of the floor of mouth. Head Neck 1993; 15:16–19.
10. Schuller DE, Bier-Laning CM, Sharma PK, Siegle RJ, Pellegrini AE, Karanfilov B, Bellisari G, Miller R, Young DC. Tissue-conserving surgery for prognosis, treatment, and function preservation. Laryngoscope 1998; 108:1599–1604.
11. Charabi S, Balle V, Charabi B, Berthelsen A, Thomsen J. Squamous cell carcinoma of the oral cavity: the results of the surgical and non-surgical therapeutic modalities in a consecutive series of 156 patients treated in Copenhagen county. Acta Otolaryngol 1997; 529(suppl):226–228.
12. Eibling D. Transoral excision of oropharyngeal malignancy. In: Myers E, ed. Operative Otolaryngology. Philadelphia: Saunders, WB, 1997:294–303.
13. Jones AS, England J, Hamilton J, Helliwell TR, Field J, Gerlinger I, Karkanevatos T. Mandibular invasion in patients with oral and oropharyngeal squamous carcinoma. Clin Otolaryngol 1997; 22:239–245.
14. De Vicente JC, Lopez-Arranz JS. Preservation of the inferior alveolar nerve in the surgical approach to cancer of the posterior oral cavity. J Oral Maxillofac Surg 1998; 56: 1214–1216.

15. Johnson J. Mandible-splitting approaches. In: Myers E, ed. Operative Otolaryngology. Philadelphia: Saunders, WB, 1997:294—303.
16. Schwartz GJ, Mehta RH, Wenig BL, Shaligram C, Portugal LG. Salvage treatment for recurrent squamous cell carcinoma of the oral cavity. Head Neck 2000; 22:34–41.
17. Vegers JW, Snow GB, van der Waal I. Squamous cell carcinoma of the buccal mucosa. A review of 85 cases. Arch Otolaryngol 1979; 105:192–195.
18. de Graeff A, de Leeuw JR, Ros WJ, Hordijk GJ, Blijham GH, Winnubst JA. A prospective study on quality of life of patients with cancer of the oral cavity or oropharynx treated with surgery with or without radiotherapy. Oral Oncol 1999; 35:27–32.
19. Lane AP, Buckmire RA, Mukherji SK, Pillsbury HC 3rd, Meredith SD. Use of computed tomography in the assessment of mandibular invasion in carcinoma of the retromolar trigone. Otolaryngol Head Neck Surg 2000; 122:673–677.
20. Myers EN, Fagan JJ. Treatment of the N+ neck in squamous cell carcinoma of the upper aerodigestive tract. Otolaryngol Clin North Am 1998; 31:671–686.
21. Kowalski LP, Bagietto R, Lara JR, Santos RL, Tagawa EK, Santos IR. Factors influencing contralateral lymph node metastasis from oral carcinoma. Head Neck 1999; 21: 104–110.
22. Majoufre C, Faucher A, Laroche C, De Bonfils C, Siberchicot F, Renaud-Salis JL, Pinsolle J. Supraomohyoid neck dissection in cancer of the oral cavity. Am J Surg 1999; 178:73–77.
23. Tankere F, Camproux A, Barry B, Guedon C, Depondt J, Gehanno P. Prognostic value of lymph node involvement in oral cancers: a study of 137 cases. Laryngoscope 2000; 110:2061–2065.
24. Society of Surgical Oncology Practice Guidelines. Oropharyngeal and oral cavity cancer surgical practice guidelines. Oncology (Huntingt) 1997; 11:1211–1212, 1215–1216.
25. Persky MS, Lagmay VM. Treatment of the clinically negative neck in oral squamous cell carcinoma. Laryngoscope 1999; 109:1160–1164.
26. Breau RL, Suen JY. Management of the N(0) neck. Otolaryngol Clin North Am 1998; 31:657–669.
27. Hosal AS, Carrau RL, Johnson JT, Myers EN. Selective neck dissection in the management of the clinically node-negative neck. Laryngoscope 2000; 110:2037–2040.
28. DiNardo LJ. Lymphatics of the submandibular space: an anatomic, clinical, and pathologic study with applications to floor-of-mouth carcinoma. Laryngoscope 1998; 108:206—214.
29. Pinsolle J, Siberchicot F, Emparanza A, Caix P, Michelet FX. Approach to the pterygomaxillary space and posterior part of the tongue by lateral stair-step mandibulotomy. Arch Otolaryngol Head Neck Surg 1989; 115:313—315.
30. Omura S, Bukawa H, Kawabe R, Aoki S, Fujita K. Comparison between hockey stick and reversed hockey stick incision: gently curved single linear neck incisions for oral cancer. Int J Oral Maxillofac Surg 1999; 28:197–202.
31. Jones AS, Beasley NJ, Houghton DJ, Helliwell TR, Husband DJ. Tumours of the minor salivary glands. Clin Otolaryngol 1998; 23:27—33.
32. Bradley PJ, Stell PM. Surgeon's workshop: a modification of the "pull through" technique of glossectomy. Clin Otolaryngol 1982; 7:59–62.
33. Stanley RB. Mandibular lingual releasing approach to oral and oropharyngeal carcinomas. Laryngoscope 1984; 94:596–600.
34. Agrawal A, Wenig BL. Resection of cancer of the tongue base and tonsil via the transhyoid approach. Laryngoscope 2000; 110:1802–1806.

8
Lip Reconstruction

Gregory Renner
Department of Otolaryngology—Head and Neck Surgery, University of Missouri School of Medicine, Columbia, Missouri, U.S.A.

INTRODUCTION

The upper and lower lips are the principle features of the lower third of the face and also the most anterior structures of the oral cavity. Together they comprise a very distinct and important anatomic and aesthetic unit. They are very necessary for facial appearance and for control of entry, retention or exit with respect to the oral cavity. With influence from the surrounding muscles of facial expression, the lips are normally capable of many different and important motions or expressions such as smiling, frowning, blowing, kissing, and whistling. Sensory functions of the lips are also very important to help monitor contacting or transiting materials for temperature and other characteristics and to allow enjoyment in functions such as kissing. It should be the goal of any reconstructive surgery to try to respect or restore the aesthetics and functions of the lip complex in the best possible manner.

From simple to complex, there are a large variety of reconstructive options that have been devised for reconstruction of the lip (1–4). The need for lip repair goes back to the very beginnings of surgical history (Fig. 1A and B). With the exception of free flap repairs, most of the lip reconstructions favored today have their roots in surgical literature from the mid-nineteenth to the early part of the twentieth centuries (1,4). The purpose of this chapter is to describe those procedures that are currently of particular importance and try to offer guidance in choosing a method of repair.

PERTINENT ANATOMY

The lips are comprised of three principle layers (skin, muscle, and mucosa) and have no direct skeletal part. The lip complex is a very distinct anatomic and aesthetic facial unit (Fig. 2A). The inferior border of the lower lip is well marked by the gentle curving mental crease, whereas the superior border of the lip is marked even more clearly by the nasal base and bilateral melolabial (nasolabial) creases. Relaxed skin tension lines of the lips are oriented in a radiant fashion about the mouth opening, similar to the spokes of a wheel, and are reflected in older patients as labial rhytids (Fig. 2B). A principle feature of the lips is the vermilion, which is

(A)

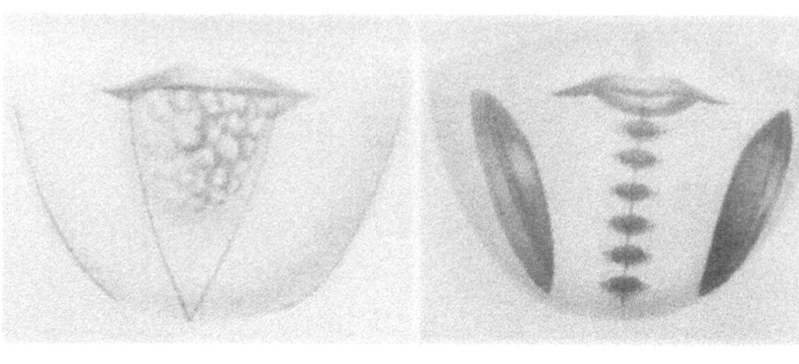

(B)

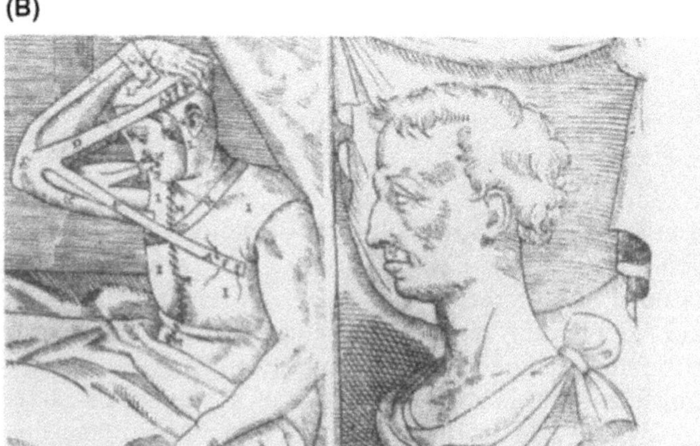

Figure 1 (**A**) Cheek relaxing incisions to allow opposing advancement flap repair of the lower lip by Celsus in the first century A.D. (**B**) Repair of upper lip with distant flap from arm by Tagliacozzi. *Source*: From Refs. 4a, 4b.

a mucosal surface specially adapted to external exposure. The mucocutaneous or anterior vermilion line is normally very well defined, though may become a little faded with solar exposure and aging. The philtrum is a structure special to the central region of the upper lip that is created by the fusion of the frontonasal and bilateral maxillary processes during embryologic development and can be difficult to duplicate in reconstruction.

The orbicularis oris is the muscle that makes up the body of both lips. It functions as a sphincter that regulates mouth opening and retention of oral materials. This muscle courses horizontally through both the upper and lower lips and connects in a crisscross or decussated fashion immediately lateral to the oral commissure on both sides. The muscles of facial expression that affect the lip lie deep in the cheeks and chin and exert their respective influence.

The upper and lower labial arteries are the principle source of blood supply to the lips. For purposes of reconstruction, it is important to understand that they derive from the facial artery on each side and course horizontally in the submucosal plane, just beyond the posterior vermilion line (the last part of the vermilion that is seen when the lips are held open). The labial arteries can actually be detected by palpation of the posterior surface of the lip in most patients. An

(A)

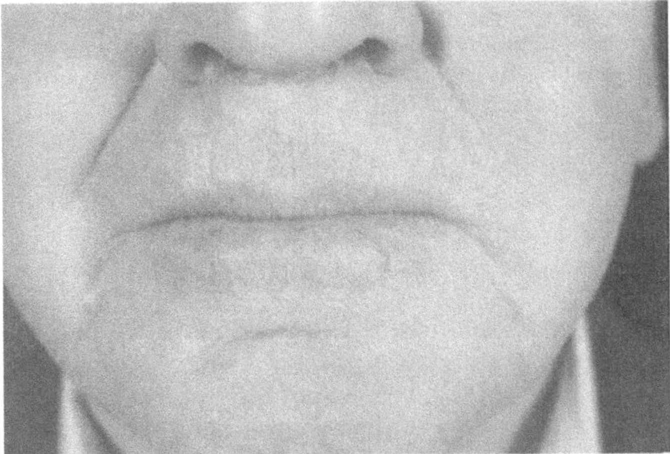

(B)

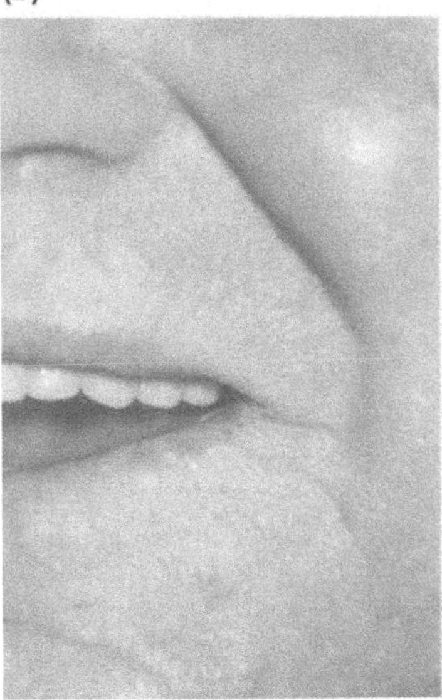

Figure 2 (**A**) Patient with normal upper and lower lips. Note strong outline for lip complex with melolabial and mental creases. Note the fine rhytids that course in a "radiant" pattern about the mouth opening. (**B**) Note progressive decrease in height of more lateral portions of upper lip. The melolabial crease passes much close to the free margin of the lip near the oral commissure.

anatomic study of the arterial structures of the lower face by Park reveals a variable pattern of anastamosing vessels across the lower lip and chin with a horizontally oriented mental branch in many as well as one or more vertically oriented labiomental branches (5).

Motor innervation to the upper lip is primarily via the buccal branch of the facial nerve and to the lower lip primarily by the marginal mandibular nerve branch. Sensory innervation of the upper lip is via the infraorbital nerve and to the lower lip via the mental nerve.

EVALUATION AND PLANNING

Aesthetics and function are both very important in lip reconstruction. The surgeon should plan to place lines of incision compatible with the creases that surround the lip, the relaxed skin tension lines respective to that part of the lip, or to the anterior vermilion line for optimal scar camouflage. Incision lines hi the central region of the upper lip may in some cases be made compatible with the vertical lines of the philtrum.

Reconstruction of smaller defects of the lip can generally be done with readjustment of tissue from within the lip complex, restoring lip with adjacent lip tissue. Restoration of an intact lip muscle sphincter is strongly preferred, unless doing so would result in an excessive microstomia. Reconstructions that produce an adynamic lip segment are generally less ideal as they are more likely to result in functional incompetence. Some patients do function reasonably well with an adynamic lip segment, particularly if the reconstructed lip is suspended or reconstructed to reduce lip laxity. The importance of maintaining muscle function is relatively greater in the lower lip. Problems with oral competence are more likely to occur in reconstructions of the lower lip and in reconstructions that involve larger portions of either lip.

In general it is best if the muscles of facial expression that surround the lip complex sustain minimal adverse change. When tissue is taken from the cheek for full-thickness lip repair, there is little appreciable gain that can be made by including facial musculature in the composite flap. In all reconstructions consideration should be given to how scar contraction will eventually affect the final result in both static and dynamic situations.

Aesthetic reconstruction of the upper lip requires some special considerations. The greatest problem in many upper lip repairs becomes how to prevent distortion of or restore the philtrum. In many cases it is not restored completely, an issue that tends to be less noted in older patients. Distortion of the nasal base can also produce a visible deformity and potentially impairment the nasal airway as well. In males, it is also important to recognize that while most of the upper lip skin is bearded, skin immediately below and lateral to the nasal ala on both sides is not. Transfer of either bearded or nonbearded skin into the wrong site can in some cases produce significant cosmetic detraction.

The bilateral melolabial (nasolabial) creases and, to a sometimes lesser extent, the mental crease are facial landmarks that tend to be very apparent. Even relatively minor distortion of their shape may be readily noted. While these are often excellent sites for camouflage of scars, they are lines that should be strongly considered and kept natural in any aesthetic lip repair. It should be recognized that the most superior part of the melolabial crease rises on both sides and does not attach to the ala until it reaches its upper margin (Fig. 2B). It is also important to recognize that as it descends, the natural melolabial crease passes relatively close to the oral commissure on both sides. Flaps designed from this region of the lip will commonly need to include some amount of cheek tissue lateral to the actual melolabial crease if they are to fit into most lip defects.

With tissue transfer, it is necessary to recognize that there is a natural disparity in thickness to lip tissue about the mouth opening. Lip tissue near the oral commissure on either side is appreciably thinner than lip tissue from the central region. Accommodation must be made for this, particularly in approximation at the free margin of the lip.

When planning for anything more than a simple lip reconstruction, it is normally helpful to consider a variety of repair methods so that the best choice can be made (Fig. 3A and B). Defects that are skin only should be addressed with repairs done similar to those in other skin areas. With full-thickness repairs first consideration is usually given to primary closure. If this is not suitable, then consideration is made for some method of flap reconstruction. A first preference is normally given to flap designs that involve movement of tissue from within the lip complex, with thoughts of confining scars to this aesthetic unit and also attempt to restore a complete, circumoral muscle sphincter. If these initial choices are likely to result in excessive microstomia, consideration should then be given to various flap designs that can provide a satisfactory restoration using tissue from the adjacent cheeks, chin or some more distant site. Reconstruction of a total lip defect presents a very serious challenge, as all available methods of repair impart some detractive consequences.

(A)

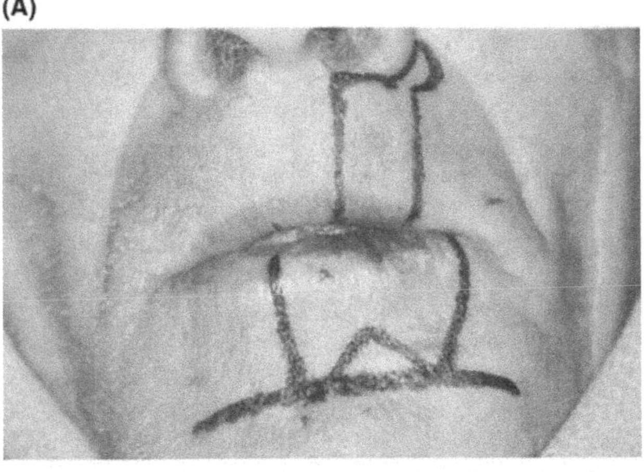

(B)

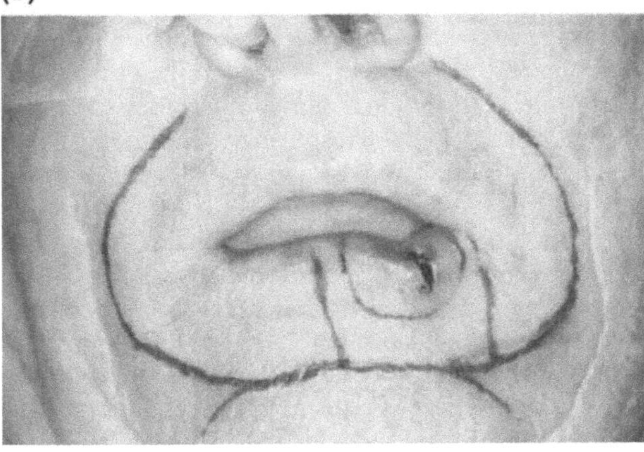

Figure 3 (**A**) Options for W-lip closure, opposing advancement flap repair, and cross-lip flap are all being considered for this patient as the lip cancer is about to be resected. (**B**) Note divergent outline planned along mental crease for possible opposing advancement flap repair versus circumoral Karapandzic flaps.

RECONSTRUCTIVE OPTIONS

Primary Cutaneous Lip Repair

Closure of a smaller cutaneous defect is best done with a basic fusiform design, with the long axis preferably placed in parallel with the relaxed skin tension line appropriate for that particular site of the lip. Orientation of the long axis in the fusiform design should be made progressively more oblique for defects that approach closer to the oral commissure on either side, similar to what is seen with the natural lip rhytids. Either end of a fusiform may be modified with an M-plasty design to limit extension of the long axis beyond a desired point, however one has to then deal with two diverging angles of closure. Defects of as much as 2 cm can generally be closed in primary fashion, though sometimes the repaired lip may appear to be somewhat tight until the wound site is fully matured. The end of a fusiform may have to be carried over the free margin of the lip in order to minimize distortion of the vermilion as the skin margins are pulled together over the lip muscle.

Skin Grafts

A skin graft may be used to restore a cutaneous defect of either lip. A full-thickness skin graft is more often preferred as they tend to offer a better match of color and thickness and undergo less eventual contraction than split-thickness skin grafts. With placement of any skin graft in the lip, this author advises that it be made large and set into the defect with a minimum of stretching, so that there will be less ultimate contraction of the grafted defect site. Any skin graft placed on the lip will require some manner of adequate immobilization until it becomes sufficiently attached to that site. A split-thickness skin graft, dermal, or allograft are the common modalities used in restoration of the buccal surface of the lip where the consequences of contraction and poorer match are not generally seen. A skin graft placed on the external surface of the lip will tend to look better if it somehow restores a full aesthetic unit rather than filling a random defect. One site in which a skin graft may offer the best means of restoration is the central portion of the philtrum (Fig. 4A and B).

Local cutaneous flap transfers may be done with a variety of designs within the confines of the lip complex. Due to the relaxed skin tension lines of the lip, vertical scar lines are better accepted than those that are more horizontal, unless they are placed along the melolabial or mental creases. Local flaps brought into the lip complex should not violate the anatomy of the outlining lip creases or distort the normal patterns of bearding.

Primary closure of a defect in the upper lip can be more difficult due to the effects of pulling on the philtrum and nasal base. Rotation/advancement of tissue from the region immediately inferolateral is an excellent option for repair of many defects, particularly if they involve the more lateral portion of the upper lip (Fig. 5A–C). Often an ideal option for local cutaneous repair within the lip complex is the use of two opposing flaps, borrowing skin of various amounts from both sides of the defect. Transfer of such flaps employs varying degrees of advancement and rotation, particularly if tissue is transferred around the oral commissure (Fig. 6A–C). It is important to consider how tissue transfer from the central region of the lip will affect the philtrum and nasal base. Continuing a release incision beneath the nasal base may actually allow a stretching out of the philtrum rather than a pulling to one side.

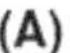

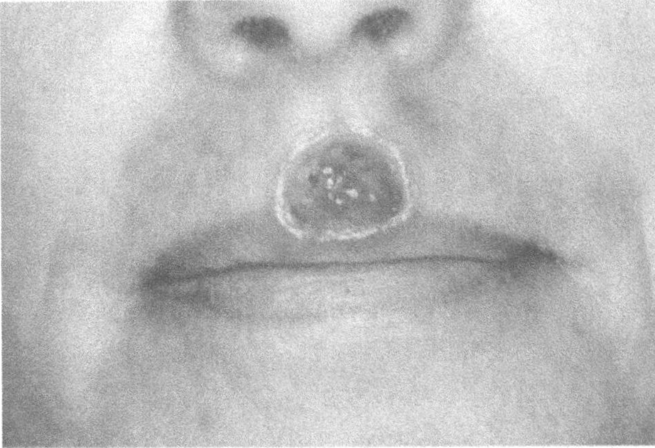

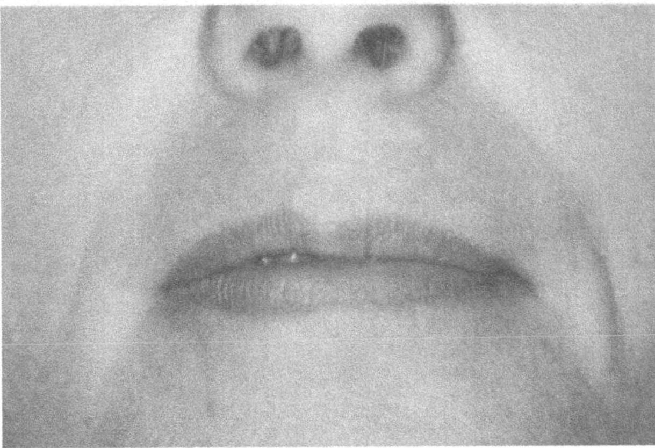

Figure 4 (**A**) Mohs defect involves lower half of philtrum with slight extension into vermilion. (**B**) Result with full-thickness skin graft at about eight months.

Transfer of cutaneous tissue in the lateral portion of the lip will occasionally result in a hooding or upturn of the oral commissure, which may resolve gradually secondary to the natural pulling of the lip musculature over time or be corrected with a later revision procedure.

Vermilion Repair

Restoration of the vermilion surface of the lip is most often accomplished with forward advancement of mucosa from the inner surface of the lip (Fig. 7A and B). The mucosal surface of the lip offers a tissue that is very similar to the vermilion, though is commonly appears to be slightly more shiny and red, particularly when compared to vermilion that has become more faded with solar exposure over time. This method of repair involves raising a composite of mucosa and submucosal tissue from the posterior or deep surface of the orbicularis oris muscle and advancing the flap forward, usually to the anterior vermilion line. While flap elevation has traditionally been done with sharp dissection, sensory function may be better preserved by raising

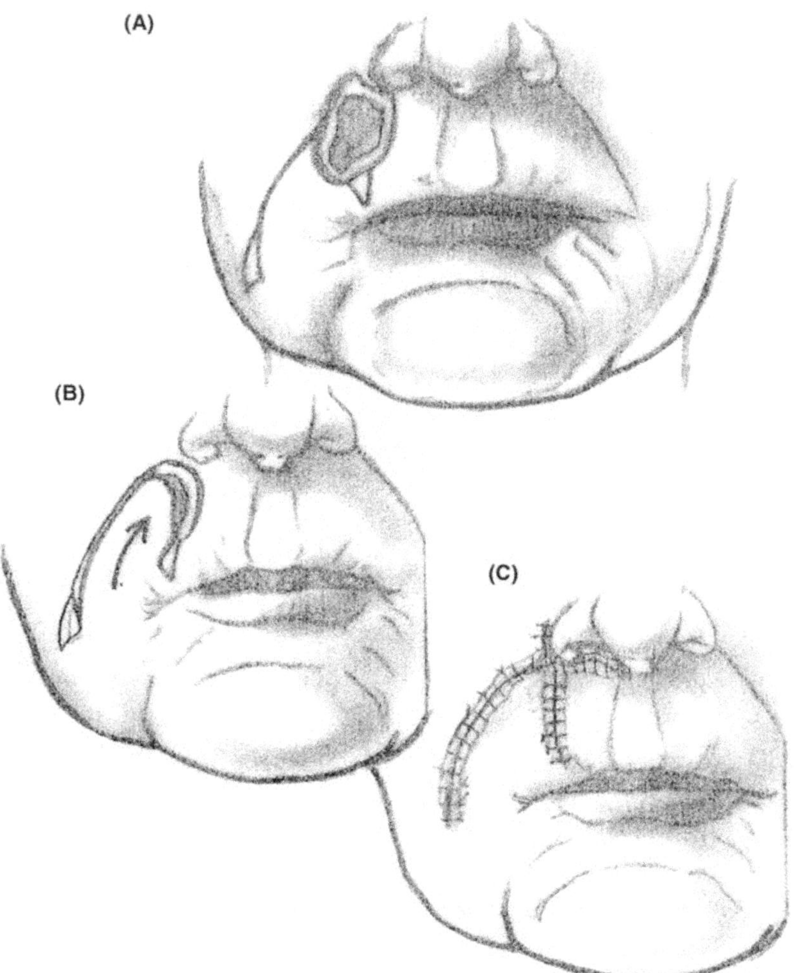

Figure 5 Illustration of labial rotation/advancement flap. (**A**) Basic outline for flap. Triangular excision may be done at distal margin, though not generally necessary. Triangle taken at base of defect to facilitate comfortable closure in the vertical plane. (**B**) Transfer of flap. Note that width of flap must be adequate to fill in more medial region of upper lip. Flap outline will normally have to extend a slight distance into the cheek to allow for this width. (**C**) Closure facilitated by smaller rotation/advancement of flap from central region of lip with care to minimize distortion of philtrum and nasal base.

the flap with a meticulous spreading technique, taking care to identify and preserve as many of the fine neural structures as possible. These structures are then freed up enough so that they can be stretched along with the flap at the time of flap transfer. This author advocates minimal flap dissection with belief that there will be less eventual flap contraction as the wound matures over time. With flap contraction the lip may become slightly thickened in appearance and whisker hairs could begin to bother the opposing lip as the anterior vermilion line gets pulled back slightly (Fig. 7C). A later, less aggressive readvancement of the mucosa could be considered, though is seldom necessary.

Restoration of the vermilion may also be done with two-staged transfer of mucosal tissue from the opposing lip. This method of transfer can be designed either as a smaller flap using a single pedicle or a much longer flap designed initially with

(A)

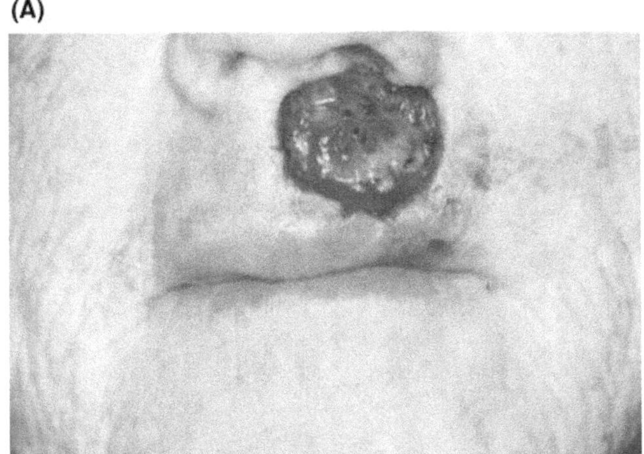

(B)

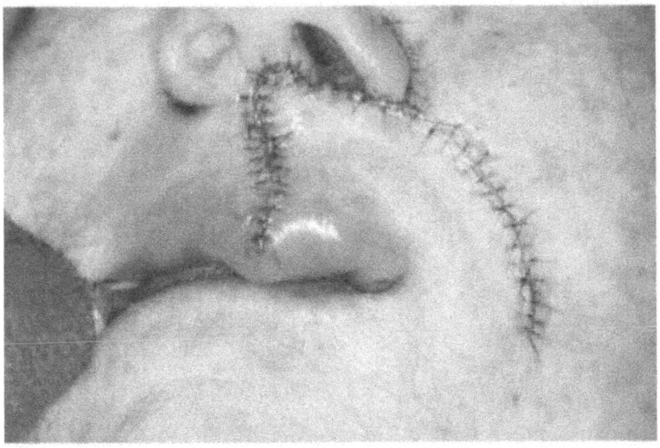

(C)

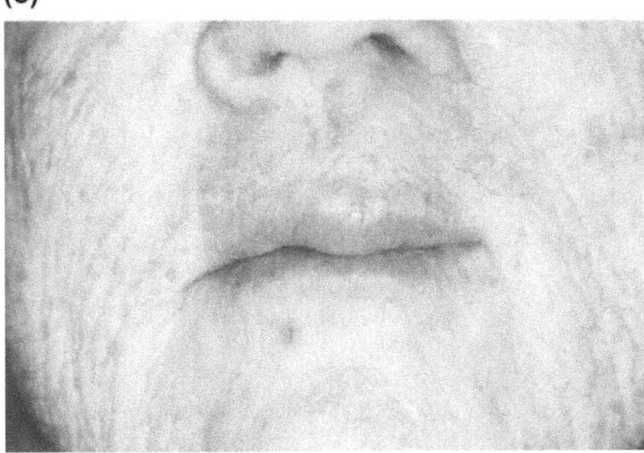

Figure 6 (**A**) Large defect of left central region of upper lip. (**B**) Typical rotation/advancement flap with some early local distortions apparent. (**C**) Result at about one year after tissues have settled. Very slight asymmetries still present, but acceptable for this case. This flap is easier to use when defect involves more lateral portion of upper lip.

(A)

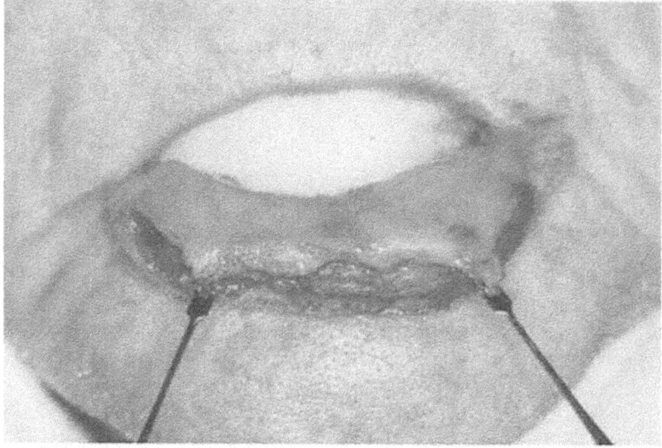

(B)

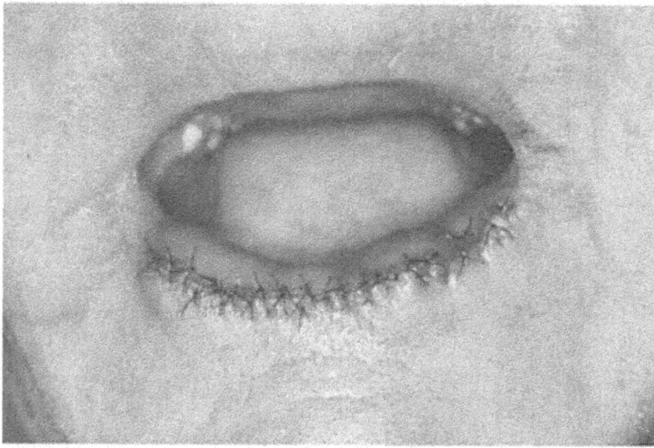

(C)

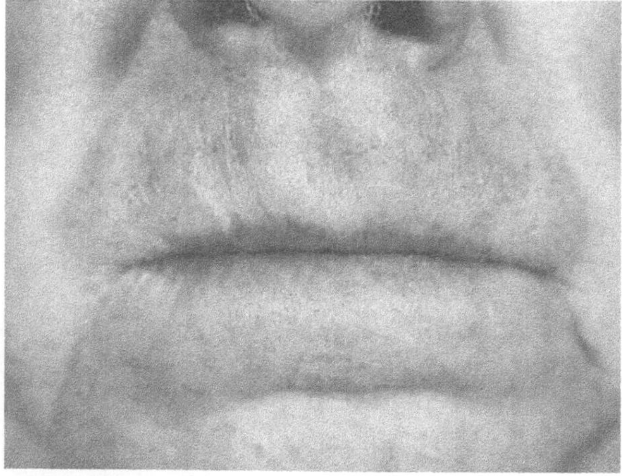

Figure 7 (**A**) Typical forward advancement of labial buccal mucosa after conservative undermining. (**B**) Immediate postoperative result. (**C**) Different patient who has had extended flap dissection and now shows later effect of contraction, causing anterior vermilion margin to be pulled back to a less favorable position.

two pedicles, one made separately at both ends, similar to the "handle" of a bucket (1,3). The anterior margin for this type of flap design is typically made immediately posterior the posterior vermilion line so that it does not produce a visible donor site scar. This type of flap can be designed relatively long and narrow because the labial artery is incorporated into the pedicle. Division of the pedicle(s) can be done safely at about three weeks. While this method of vermilion repair is more complicated than the simple mucosal advancement flap, it can include some muscle and provide a thicker unit of soft tissue when necessary. The single pedicled design can be particularly helpful when there is need to fill a more focal or "notch-like" vermilion defect (3).

Mucosal tissue can also be transferred from the tongue in a similar two-staged manner. A variety of pedicled designs are possible to accomodate to various defect situations (3,6,7). The papillated surface of glossal mucosa and the inherent awkwardness of even temporarily limiting tongue mobility make this a less desirable choice for vermilion restoration. Care must be taken to avoid impairment to speech articulation.

Buccal mucosa may be transferred as a free graft for vermilion restoration. Proper immobilization of the graft can be awkward and graft take is not always certain. When the situation is more complicated, it is acceptable to make use of a skin graft or extended portion of a cutaneous flap to provide at least initial coverage over the free margin of the lip. Replacement with some form of mucosal tissue could be then done later and with greater precision if desired.

LIP REPAIR TECHNIQUES

Technique

The V-lip procedure is designed as a triangle with two lines of incision, one on each side of a given unit of tissue that is to be excised, and the base portion being the free margin of the lip (Fig. 8A and B). The two lines of incision are angled in opposing fashion so that they meet at some distance away from the lip margin. Design for a V-lip excision and closure should be done with attempt to be as compatible as possible with the relaxed skin tension lines normal to that particular region of the lip (3). The classic V design is appropriate for excision and repair involving the central region of either lip, while a slanted V or "hound's tooth" design is more appropriate in situations involving lateral regions of the lip (Fig. 9A and B). The line of closure should be planned so that a line passing from the center of the vermilion portion of the defect to the apex of the V should match that of the relaxed skin tension line for that same location on the lip.

For cosmesis, it is ideal if the apex of a V design can be kept confined within the lip and not extend beyond either the melolabial or mental crease. With excision of bulky tumors it can sometimes be awkward to design a V comfortably around the lesion and stay confined within the lip. In these cases the V design may be modified to a W shape, in which the lateral members of the excision design do not converge so acutely (Fig. 10A). The two angles of the W should be slanted and often of varied size when excision involves more lateral regions of the lip, again with attempt to make the lines of repair as compatible as possible with the natural relaxed skin tension lines of the lip.

Closure of any full-thickness defect of the lip is best done in at least four layers: mucosa (or submucosa), muscle, subcutaneous tissue, and skin. Good approximation of all four layers will help minimize the effects of scar contracture through

(A)

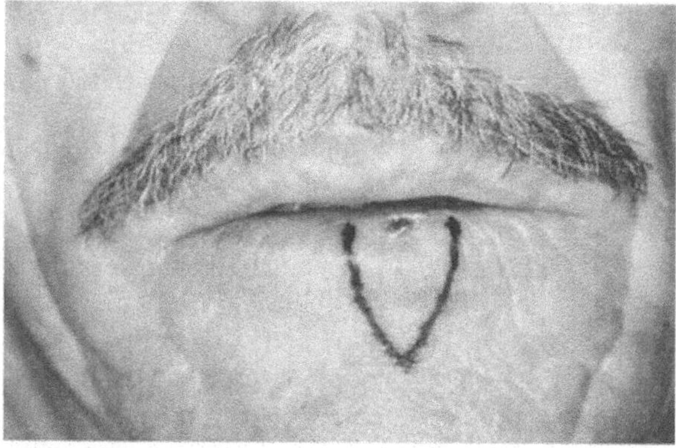

(B)

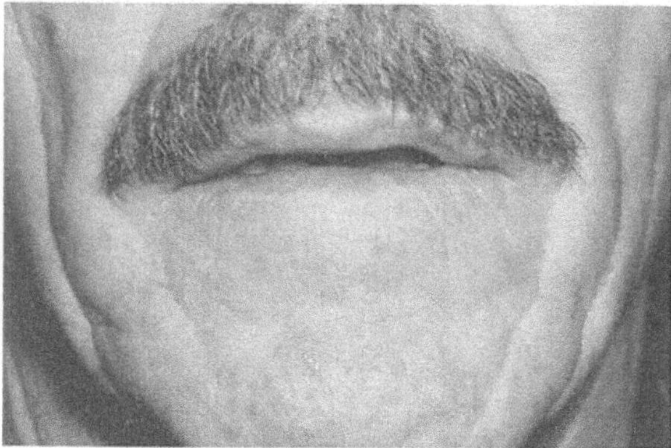

Figure 8 (**A**) Typical outline for V-lip excision. (**B**) Result at one year with good scar camouflage.

the body of the lip as the wound matures. Particular attention should be made to assuring good approximation of muscle tissue immediately beneath the vermilion, as this will minimize the chance for later development of a depressed or notched appearance along the free margin of the lip. Early identification of the anterior vermilion line on each side is very helpful as a reference point to assure proper alignment of tissues in the closure. This point does not have to be closed immediately, but clearly established as a reference point before other approximations are done (Fig. 10A). Because tissue from the lateral portion of the lip is naturally thinner, it is helpful to next identify the most appropriate site on each side that should become the posterior vermilion line, so that any disparity in width can be adjusted for early in the closure.

Advantages/Disadvantages

The V-lip procedure is the most basic technique for both lip tumor excision and good full-thickness restoration of the lip. There is no need for releasing incisions and preservation of both motor and sensory functions is expected to be near-complete. With good technique, there should be optimal matching of tissue at the free margin of the lip and the single line of scar should hide well, reflecting the natural skin tension

(A)

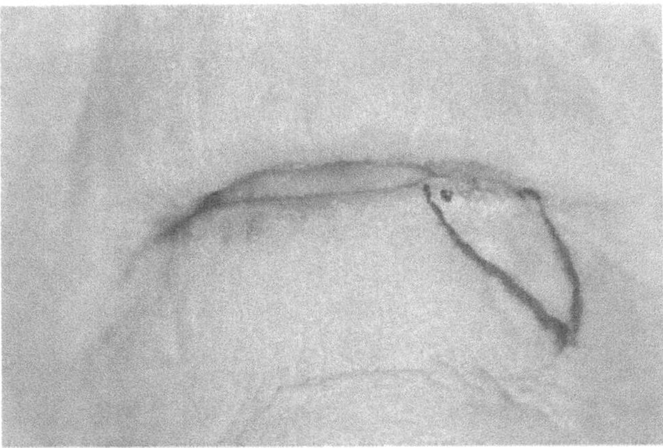

(B)

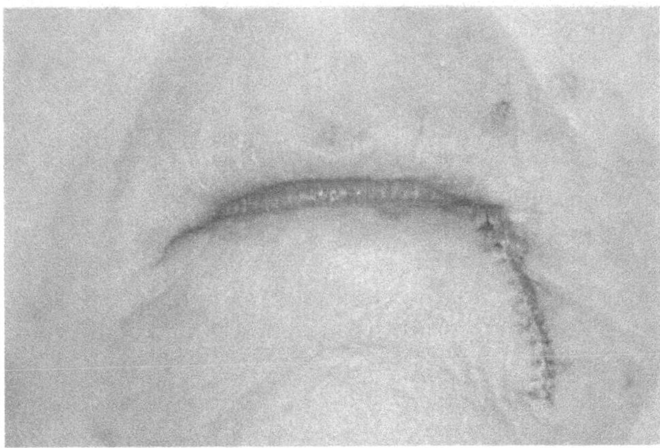

Figure 9 (A) Offset "hound's tooth" V-lip design for more lateral region of lip. (B) Result immediately after closure with orientation reasonably compatible with relaxed skin tension line for this region of lip.

line for that site on the lip. A depression is more likely to be seen in the scar line with the lip in repose if the orbicularis muscle tissue has not been fully approximated in the closure.

As with any lip tissue repair there can be issue with infection, although it is rarely a problem and patients are normally allowed to eat and drink with gentle effort immediately after the repair is done. Suture abscesses are not uncommon, particularly in those with heavy bearded or sebaceous skin. The most common faults seen with V-lip repair are contour irregularity at the free lip margin and depression of the line of scar with the lip in repose, both of which can generally be avoided with good technique. Planning the V-excision must not be done with compromise to the adequacy of proper margins for tumor resection.

Limitations

It is generally taught that V-lip excision can involve as much as one-third of the lip without producing a result that would he considered as too tight or otherwise unsightly. This tends to be truer in older patients who tend to have relatively greater

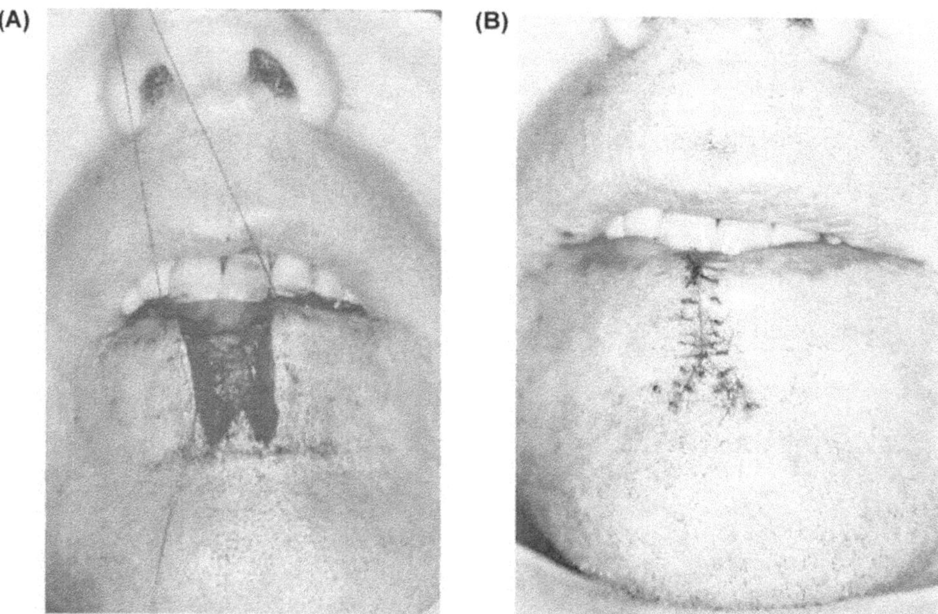

Figure 10 (**A**) Beginning of closure for defect with W design. Note suture marking the anterior vermilion line which helps to keep proper orientation as other layers are closed first. (**B**) Early closure result.

laxity and redundancy in their lip tissue. Because of the philtrum and greater variation in height across the upper lip, aesthetically there are more limits for comfortable size of V-lip excision in the upper lip.

SIMPLE LIP ADVANCEMENT FLAPS

Technique

Composite linear lip tissue transfer may be performed as a single flap or as bilateral flaps brought together in opposing fashion (1–4). The lower lip lends itself more easily to this method of repair as the anatomy is simple and the lines of flap release can usually be masked well along the mental crease. Though there is a slight curvature to the mental crease, the change is gradual and generally of little consequence as tissue is transferred to an immediately adjacent defect, particularly when it involves the central region of the lip. In some cases tissue from the central region of the lower lip may not have sufficient vertical height to restore a defect involving the more extreme lateral region of the lip without some additional tissue maneuver.

In the upper lip, it is more difficult to maintain uniform flap width if the lines of release are made within the melolabial crease, which approaches appreciably closer to the free margin of the lip as it courses laterally and downward on both sides. Because of the issue of symmetry, opposing advancement flap reconstruction is best suited to reconstruction in the central region of the upper lip. It is not necessary to extend the incisions far along the melolabial crease on either side if one makes use of a crescent-shape excision of soft tissue immediately lateral to the nasal ala on whichever side a flap will be passed from (1,3,4). This allows the cheek and lip tissue to move more in unison and an easy transfer of the lip flap beneath the base of the nose (Fig. 12A–C).

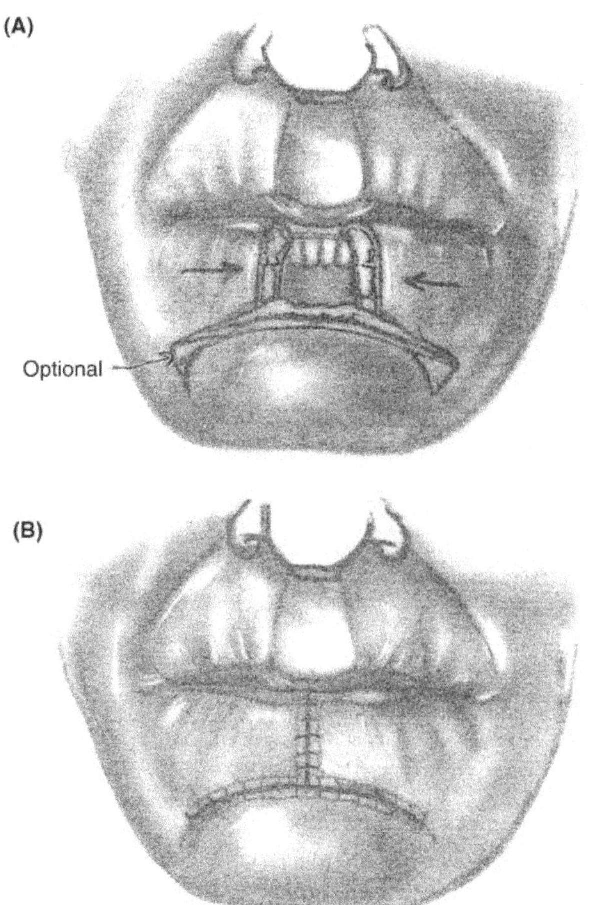

Figure 11 Illustration depicting (**A**) Plan for simple bilateral opposing advancement flap repair. Lower incision is made along course of mental crease. Burow triangular excision may be used at either end to facilitate ease of flap advancement, but is not usually necessary. (**B**) Typical closure result.

Whenever there is need for full-thickness transfer of lip tissue, consideration should be given to the method of dissection first advocated by Karpandzic, which makes a special attempt to preserve vascular and neural structures (Fig. 14) (1–3,8,9). Sharp incision is made through the skin and immediate subcutaneous tissue. As neural and vascular structures are encountered in the deeper dissection, an attempt is made to preserve as many as possible. Each is dissected in a "teasing" manner so that it can be stretched and carried along with the flap as it is transferred (Fig. 14). Sharp incision may be made separately in the labial mucosa and does not usually have to be carried out as widely as that through the skin.

Advantages/Disadvantages

The use of opposing advancement flaps is a relatively simple concept and can produce an excellent repair, particularly when used in reconstruction of the central region of either lip. A deficiency of this method in upper lip repair is that it does not truly restore the philtrum. To a limited extent, a vertical scar near the midline

(A)

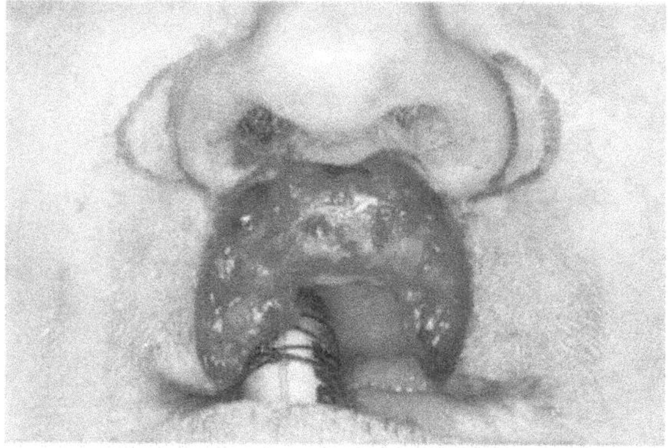

(B)

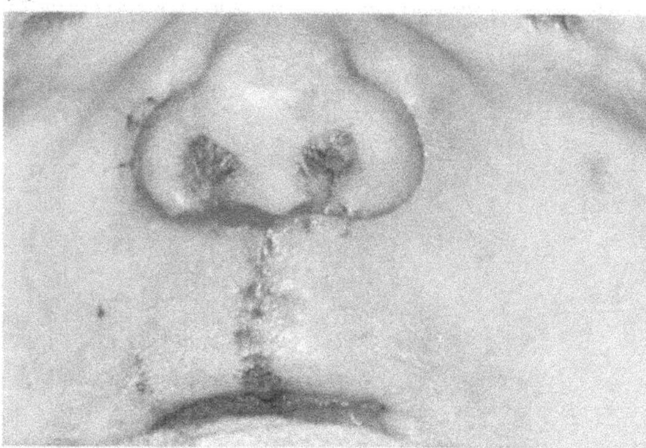

(C)

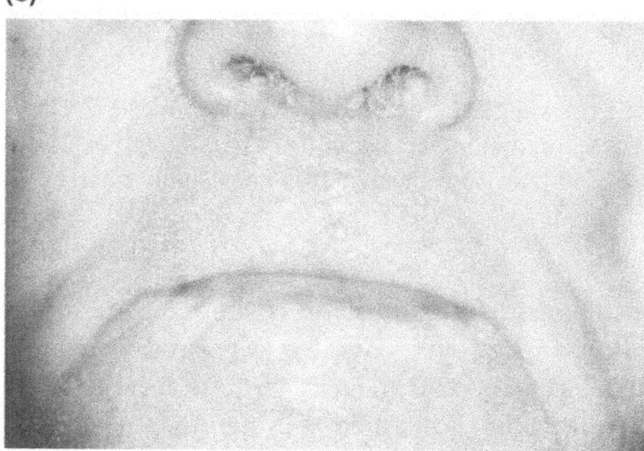

Figure 12 (**A**) Defect of central region of upper lip with plan for perialar crescent excisions that will help allow opposing advancement flap repair. (**B**) Opposing advancements completed with comfortable fit about nasal base. (**C**) Result seen at six months. While a philtrum is not really present, it does not show as a serious deformity in this patient.

can mimic as the central philtrum sulcus. In older patients lack of the philtrum seems to be less noticed.

This author strongly favors the "Karapandzic-style"neurovascular dissection technique, which allows the best possible preservation of both motor and sensory-function in the restored lip (2,3,8,9).

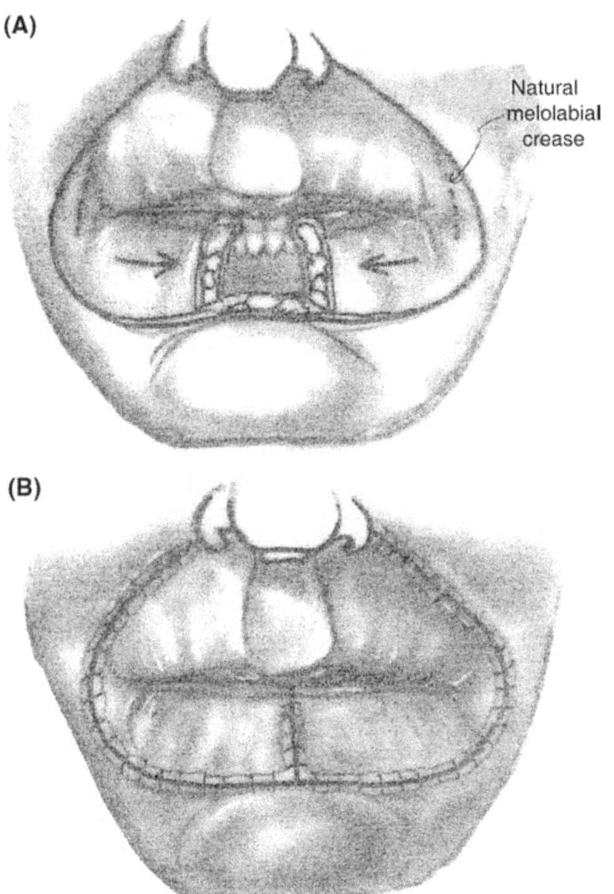

Figure 13 Illustration of bilateral Karapandzic flaps. (**A**) Typical plan for repair of lower lip defect. (**B**) Immediate closure. Note that there must be gradual change in flap width in the region of the oral commissure.

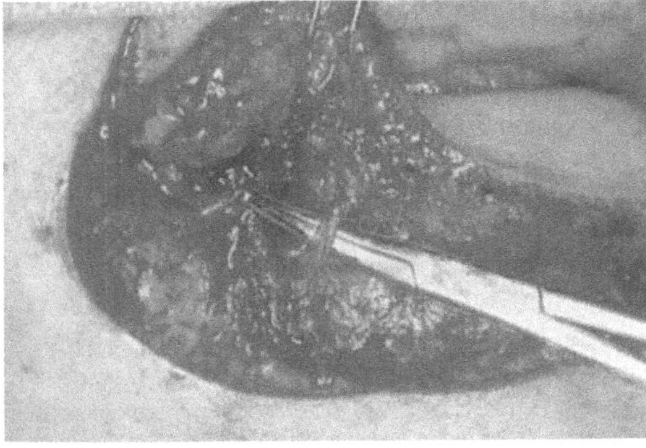

Figure 14

Limitations

This type of reconstruction is appropriate for defects of between one quarter and one half of either lip. Closure in this manner of a larger defect would likely create a lip that is too tight, especially when compared to its counterpart.

Circumoral (Karapandzic) Advancement Flaps

Technique

Expanding on the concept of opposing lip advancement flaps, von Bruns initally described the use of composite lip flaps that are passed around the oral commissure on either or both sides (1,10). It is necessary that these flaps maintain a fairly similar width throughout their length so that the all parts of the lip have adequate height after the flaps have been transferred. Because the natural melolabial crease passes close to the oral commissure on each side, outline for the flap must be extended laterally into the cheek as it passes near and around that site on each side (Fig. 15A and B). In order to accommodate for the mental and melolabial crease lines as much as possible, outline for the flap may vary slightly as it is drawn around the lip complex, as subtle and gradual differences in flap width can normally be hidden in the reconstruction.

In 1974, Karapandzic first suggested a modified method of dissection for circumoral lip advancements, with special effort to preserve neural and vascular structures (1–3,8,9). Again, sharp incisions are made through the skin and immediate subcutaneous layers and separately through the mucosa. Dissection through the deeper layers is done in a teasing fashion, with effort to preserve all neural and vascular structures. These are then dissected enough that they can be stretched along with the flap as it is transferred. The various muscles of facial expression are also carefully dissected free from the Orbicularis oris muscle and later reattached to the muscle sphincter at what would be anatomically correct sites after the flap has been transferred.

The lip flaps should be joined first and then this reconstructed lip complex can be set into the circumlabial defect in the best possible manner. Because there is now greater relative redundancy in the soft tissue surrounding the lip complex, some make use of small "pleat-like" or "Burow's triangle" excisions at various points around the reconstruction (1,5). This author finds that with use of many interrupted sutures and exacting wound margin approximation, such excisions are not usually necessary (2,3).

Advantages/Disadvantages

Karapandzic flap design can provide a satisfactory reconstruction for the lip complex. Though the flap outline necessarily extends wide from the natural lip unit border as it comes around the oral commissure on both sides, this does not tend to produce a noted deformity. As the lip flaps are brought around the corner of the mouth there is a blunting of the neocommissures. In most cases it seems that the commissure becomes more stretched out rather than an entirely new commissure being formed.

The implication from many texts is that since the orbicularis muscle sphincter is restored and muscles of facial expression become reattached at what would be now anatomically corrected sites, motor function in patients who undergo Karapandzic flaps should be fairly normal. Indeed gross motor functions such as mouth opening, closing and smiling tend to be acceptable; however, functions such as whistling or puckering may never be completely normal.

(A)

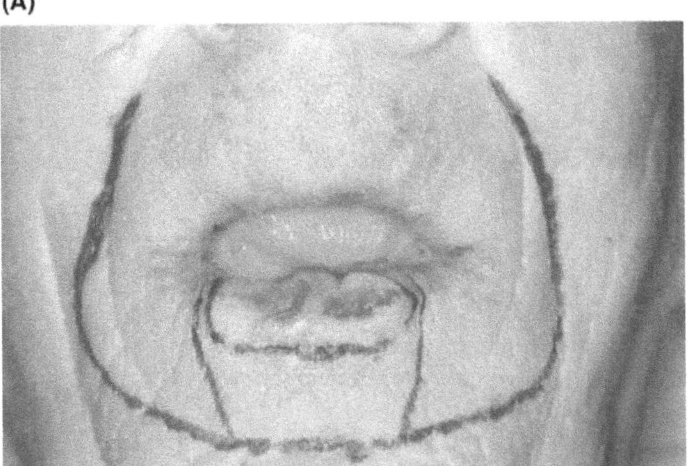

(B)

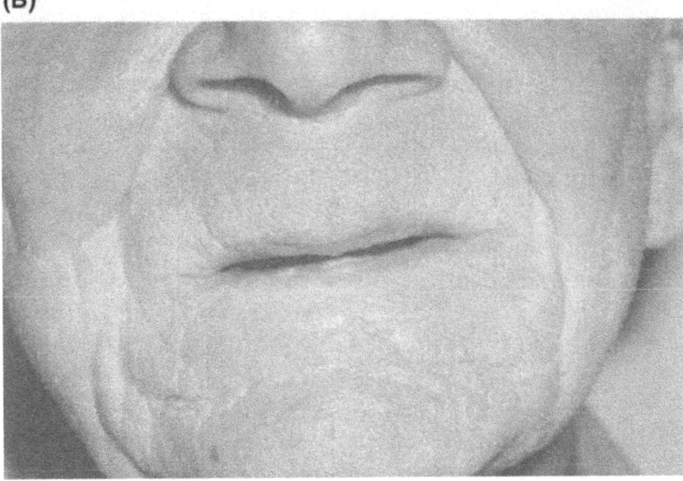

Figure 15 (**A**) Proposed plan for excision and Karapandzic flap repair. Note that outline extends wide of the lateral portion of the melolabial crease near the oral commissure to obtain adequate flap width. (**B**) Result seen at three months with smaller mouth opening, but satisfactory for this patient.

Limitations

The use of Karapandzic flaps can be an excellent way to restore the lip complex for defects of between one quarter and a little more that one half of either lip. The limit for this repair is the degree of microstomia than can be considered acceptable for any given patient. Patients who wear dentures have less tolerance for microstomia. There is some ability to enlarge the reconstructed mouth opening with either manual or prosthesis-assisted stretching over time, though accomplishing normally takes several months, considerable effort, and is uncertain. In some cases, one may attempt to increase the length of available lip tissue by recruiting some of the labial mucosa to cover over an adjacent unit of lip of cheek tissue that can be transferred into the defect along with the Orbicularis-bearing lip flaps. While this may provide additional tissue for the lip repair, it should be expected that functional results tend to be less excellent.

Cross-Lip Flaps

Technique

A composite flap may be transferred from one lip to the other in a one or two stage fashion, pedicled on the labial artery. While credit for design of cross-lip flaps has typically been given to Estlander (1874) and Abbe (1899), there are several physicians who have described cross-lip flap designs even prior to that time (1,11–13).

The classic Estlander flap is designed as a triangular flap taken from the lateral region of the upper lip and transposed around the oral commissure with a very small pedicle that is centered on the labial artery (Fig. 16) (1–3,12,14). This flap is designed for reconstruction of a defect on one side of the lower lip, which has its lateral margin involving the oral commissure, and can be used in modified form for some other situations (1,14,15). The flap is normally made half or more the size of the defect to be restored. Choice in sizing the flap can vary slightly, depending on the particular need for tissue in the repair, the feasibility of closing at least a portion of the wound primarily and the requirements for establishing optimal symmetry between the donor and recipient lips (16). After the flap is transposed around the oral commissure and into the defect of the opposing lip, closure at both sites is completed with either primary approximation or simple advancement flap type repair. The flap pedicle traverses around the oral commissure. If desired, the pedicle can be divided after three weeks or more in attempt to restore the natural angle of the oral commissure (3,17). The Estlander design may also be reversed when there is need to restore a defect of the lateral region of the upper lip that extends all the way to the oral commissure.

The classic Abbe flap is designed similarly as a triangular flap that is taken from the central region of the lower lip and transposed across the open mouth to a defect of the central region of the upper lip (Fig. 17) (1,13,14). The pedicle is also small and must include the labial artery. The pedicle in this design creates a temporary connection or bridge between the two lips that can be divided at about three weeks.

Most cross-lip flaps that are done at this time are actually a modification of both of these designs (Fig. 18). Design for cross-lip flaps that are not carried around the oral commissure can be placed at virtually any site along the donor lip and used in restoration of nearly any defect of small of intermediate size (up to, but normally less than one half of either lip) (2,3,14). Outline for a cross-lip flap can be modified

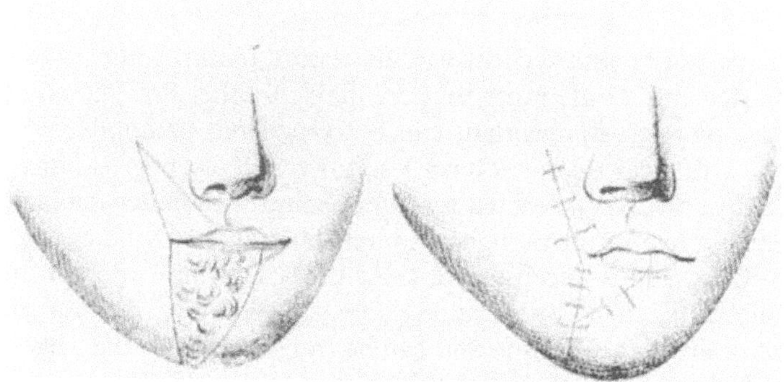

Figure 16 Original illustration of one-stage cross-lip flap by Estlander. *Source*: From Ref. 12.

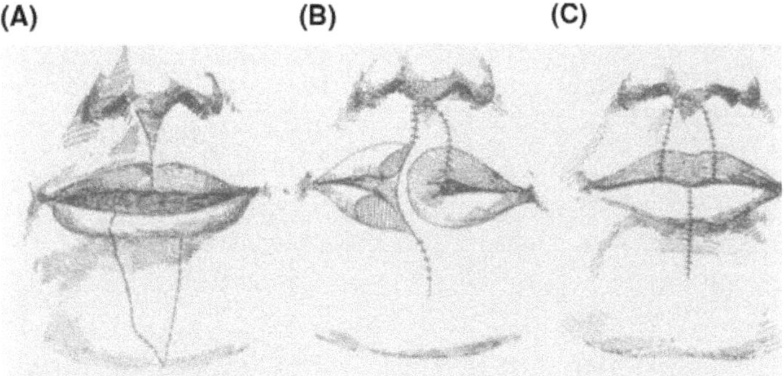

Figure 17 Original illustration of two-stage cross-lip flap reported by Abbe. *Source*: From Ref. 13.

from the classic V to a W, rectangular or other special shape, as necessary to accommodate particular needs (3,18,19). As consideration is made for shape and size of a cross lip flap, it is often helpful to consider the potential benefit of at least partial primary repair. Because it is very difficult to recreate a totally natural appearing oral commissure, this author has a strong preference for flap design that includes a temporary pedicle, even if it is placed only millimeters from the mouth corner (3).

The side of the vascular pedicle supplying the flap is not as important as the avoidance of tension, twisting, and ischemia. The principle consideration should be to how easily the flap will be able to turn into the recipient lip defect. While insetting of the flap margin that is opposite to the pedicle is relatively easy, it can be more difficult to perform properly on the pedicled side, particularly if the pedicle is of wider size. Skin incision on the pedicle side can usually be carried from the apex of the flap all the way to the anterior vermilion line in most cases. With deeper dissection care must be taken to avoid violation of the labial artery and a sufficient cuff of surrounding soft tissue so that venous drainage can be assured. Although no larger named vein passes along near either labial artery, the multiple small veins that do pass along with either artery normally prove to be sufficient for flap survival.

Advantages/Disadvantages

Cross-lip flaps can be very useful in reconstruction of many different full-thickness and even some partial-thickness lip defects (1,3,14,18,19). They make use of the relatively greater redundancy of the opposing lip to help offset the needs for a given defect closure. They also keep the reconstruction within the aesthetic lip complex and replace lip with a similar composite tissue.

A principle disadvantage is that they necessarily have to go through a phase of both motor and sensory denervation (20). Drooling or leaking from the mouth can be an issue in some, though not all patients. Electrical motor nerve potentials can be detected within several months of the flap transfer and are considered to be maximal within a year (3,20). A reasonably good amount of sensory return also normally occurs within that same time (20).

Because full-thickness scar surrounds all but the free margin of any cross-lip flap, there is a strong tendency for them to appear slightly thickened upon wound maturation. Lips are remarkably dynamic and the flap will commonly look flat while the lip is stretched in acts such as smiling, but thicker as the lip comes back to repose. Sometimes this disparity in elasticity seems to produce a slightly greater relative deformity as patient's age.

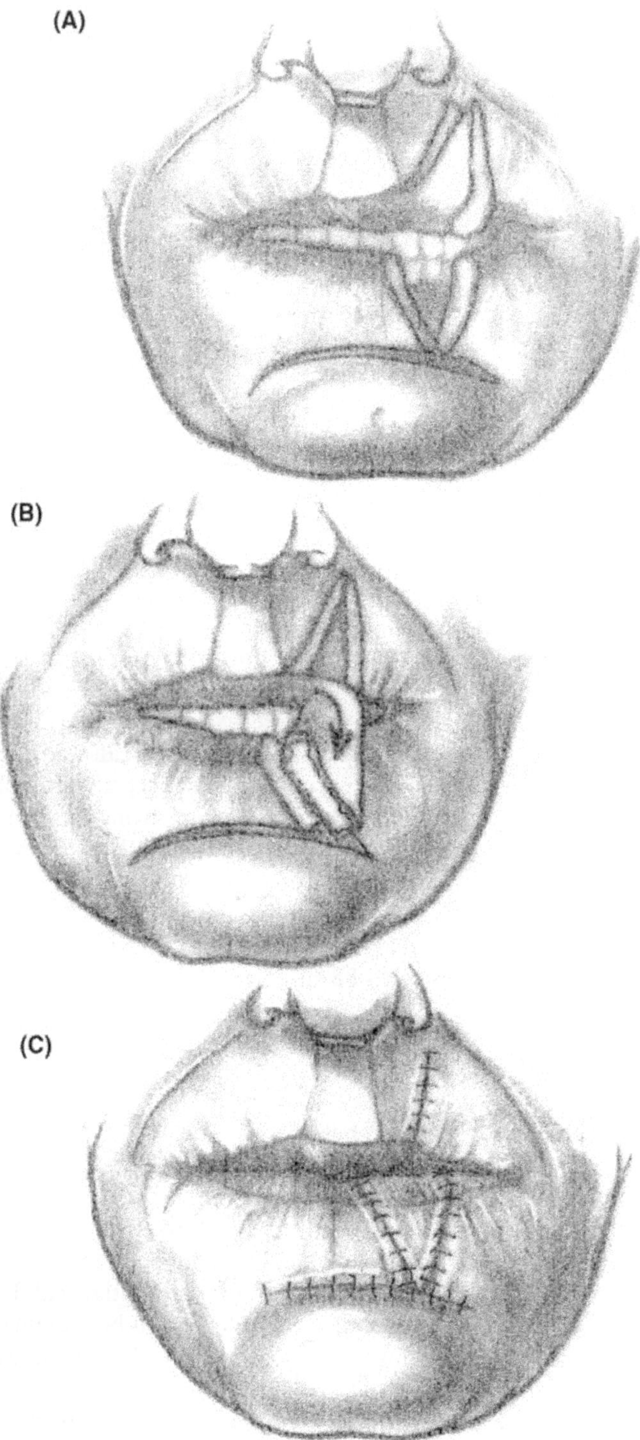

Figure 18 Illustration of two-stage cross-lip flap with no violation of ipsilateral oral commissure. (**A**) Cross-lip flap is developed. Some amount of direct closure of the recipient site may also be done either in primary fashion or with adjacent tissue advancement(s). (**B**) Flap being placed in recipient site. (**C**) Flap in place (Minimal pedicle shown in this illustration).

Limitations

Cross-lip flaps are used to reconstruct a defect of between one-fourth and one-half of either lip (16). When defects involve a wider expanse, it is normally better to find another source for lip tissue replacement to avoid undue microstomia. Kriet (21) has demonstrated that at least for the lower lip, the labial artery provides vascular supply as far inferiorly as the chin and has described the use of very large cross-lip flaps in some repairs that involve both the upper lip and low medial region of the cheek as well.

Gillies "Fan" Flap

Gillies (and Buck before him) have described a flap design that is a hybridization of the concepts of cross-lip and Karapandzic (or von Bruns) designs with a full-thickness flap taken from one lip and passed around the oral commissure to the other with a movement that can be compared to the opening of a folded hand fan (Fig. 19A–C) (1,3,4,6,22). In most cases transfer is from the upper lip to the lower lip. The unique feature of this design is that a "back-cut" type release incision is made at the proximal end of the flap to allow its release, with preservation of a vascular pedicle of larger size than that of the Estlander flap. Transfer of the flap is accomplished with a combination of circumoral advancement and rotation. While it does accomplish a reasonably good restoration of the opposite lip, there tends to be some distortion of the involved

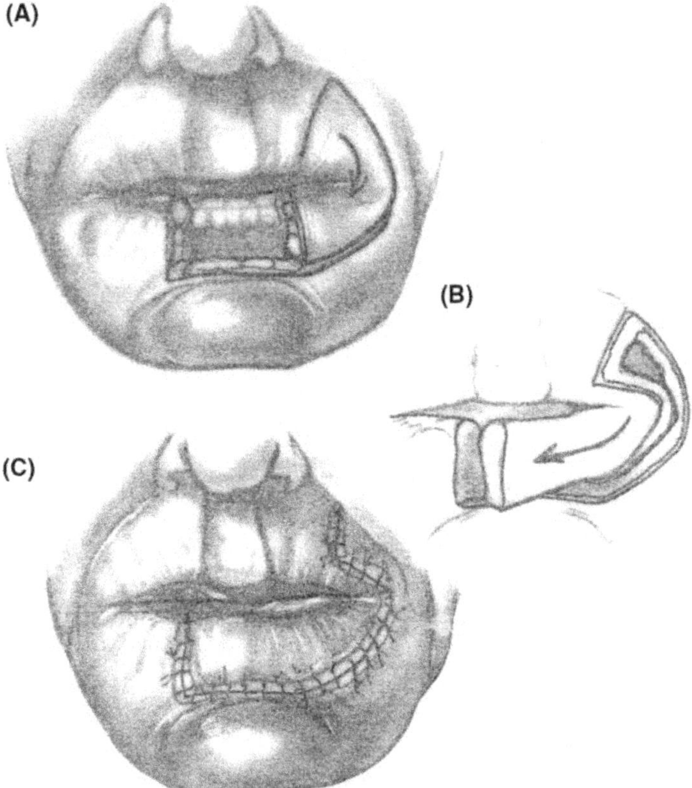

Figure 19 Illustration of Gillies fan flap. (**A**) Initial design for release of flap. (**B**) Demonstration of flap transfer. (**C**) Expected results upon transfer.

oral commissure, some distortion of the involved melolabial crease and some asymmetry along the nasal base. Variation of this design has been described (3).

Flaps from Regions Adjacent to the Lip Complex

When there is an inadequate amount of tissue remaining within the lip complex to close a given defect without creating an unacceptable microstomia, it becomes necessary to consider obtaining substitute tissue from some other site. With its relatively great tissue redundancy and immediate proximity to the lip complex, the cheek is the most common extralabial donor site for lip repair. In selected cases, flaps may also be taken from the chin region, the forehead, the scalp, the chest and other more distant sites. At the present time it is still not possible to completely restore the orbicularis oris muscle sphincter with any flap that comes from outside of the lip complex.

With extralabial flap repair, consideration must be made for the provision of both an external cutaneous surface and skin or mucosa to line the internal surface of the repair. A skin graft, whether full-thickness or split-thickness, is most often used to provide the intraoral lining for such reconstructions. It can sometimes be fairly awkward to properly secure a skin graft intraorally on the deep surface of a cutaneous flap. In some situations a skin graft can be "buried" beneath an extralabial cutaneous flap, while at the same time performing a "delay" stage, which helps to prepare the flap for later transfer of what would then become a "composite" flap.

When planning for reconstructions that employ the use of cutaneous flaps and/or skin grafts, it is advisable to consider the potential tissue and scar contractions that may later occur so that the repair does not become deficient. It is normally much easier to plan for a little extra tissue in the repair initially, even if a later reduction may be required. Attempting to add more tissue at later time may be more difficult and detract from the aesthetic result.

Melolabial (Nasolabial)

Flaps Technique

Melolabial [Melon: Greek for cheek (23)] flaps are designed to transpose tissue from that portion of the cheek that is just lateral to the lip complex. The medial border for this type of flap is planned along the melolabial crease, while the lateral border is planned further out in the cheek in a roughly parallel fashion, but tapered to connect with the medial border at the flap's distal end (Fig. 20A–C). The pedicle required for this flap may be superiorly based or inferiorly based, depending on the need.

This is basically a cutaneous flap, with a variable amount of subcutaneous tissue included to protect the subdermal vascular supply to the flap and to provide some degree of tissue thickness to the reconstruction. Blood supply within the flap is based on a random pattern only, so the length to width ratio should not exceed about 3:1 unless one or more delay stages have been included in the plan. Flap dissection should be kept superficial to the plane of the facial musculature, so that motor functions are not impaired. It is wise to design the flap with a slightly excessive width in anticipation of what later contraction will occur.

A melolabial flap may be used to restore a cutaneous defect of the lip or to help reconstruct a full-thickness deficit (1,4,24). In full-thickness reconstructions a skin graft is generally placed on the deep surface of the melolabial flap to provide an intraoral lining. The anterior edge of the graft should be carried over what is now the vermilion margin of the melolabial flap. Any graft placed should be made

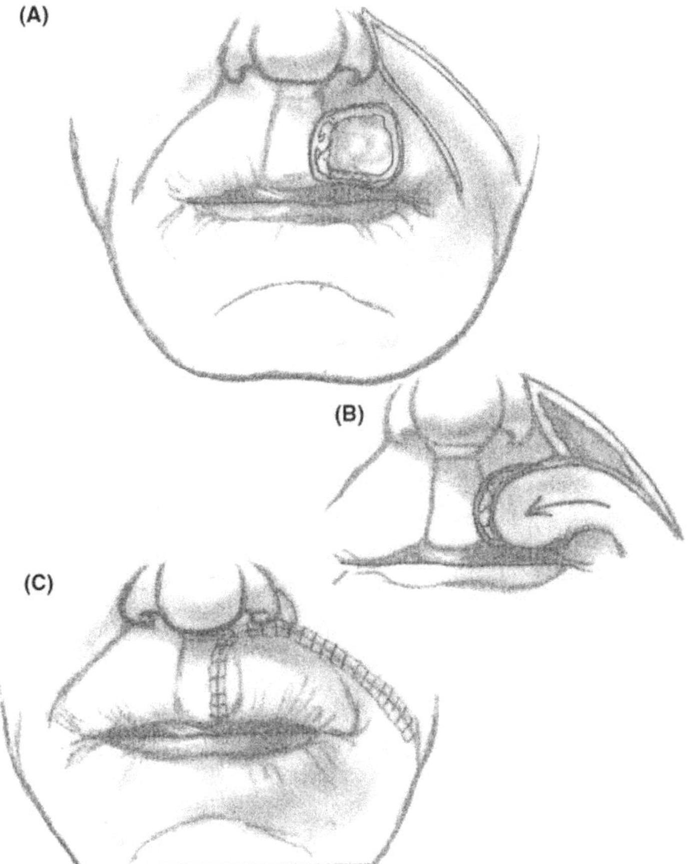

Figure 20 Illustration of an inferiorly based melolabial flap. (**A**) Initial cutaneous flap design. (**B**) Transfer of flap into defect. (**C**) Closure of lip and donor site defects with expected result.

with extra size and attached with as much redundancy as possible to minimize the affect of later contraction. If a delay stage is done prior to flap transfer, the skin graft may be attached at that time and kept "buried" until the time of "composite" flap transfer.

There are situations when bilateral melolabial flaps may be brought together in opposing, complementary fashion for reconstruction of a larger defect (1). In some selected cases it is possible, though very awkward, to make simultaneous use of bilateral melolabial flaps placed in a two-layer fashion, with one flap turned inward to provide an internal surface and the other applied over it to provide the external surface (1). Having two flaps helps to restore a more natural thickness and helps to minimize the effects of later contraction of the reconstructed lip. A number of issues, however, complicate this concept. The requirement for flap length may be a problem. One or more delay stages should be considered whenever there is concern for flap viability. Having a flap turned-in on one side interferes with the ability to attach the external-covering flap along the vertical plane at its distal margin until the pedicle of the first flap is later divided. Multiple revisions are likely to be required to deal with flap pedicles and achieve optimal cosmesis. Again it is best to plan for a fair degree of late tissue contraction with this type of reconstruction.

Advantages/Disadvantages

The relative redundancy of cheek tissue and its close proximity to the lip makes it the most readily available source of tissue for lip reconstruction. The scar line seen on closure is cosmetically well-placed along the melolabial crease. Use of this flap may produce some asymmetry of the cheeks.

The natural angle of the melolabial crease makes the inferiorly based design normally easier to set into either lip. Transposition of a melolabial flap with a superiorly based pedicle requires much more turn and consequently a greater puckering up of redundant tissue in the pedicle base. It also transgresses the upper portion of the melolabial crease. Some form of pedicle revision is almost always necessary to achieve a reasonably natural aesthetic appearance again in the upper lip.

Limitations

There can be considerable versatility in design for a transposition flap from the medial region of the cheek. Use of one or more delay stages can help allow a greater length-to-width ratio for this flap design. It is important to appreciate that there is no actual restoration of a functioning muscle sphincter in the lip reconstructed with this flap and so relative tightness can help to achieve continence with oral liquids.

Cheek Advancement (Von Burow-Bernard) Flaps

Technique

In the mid-portion of the nineteenth century doctors von Burow and Bernard separately described methods for reconstruction of a major defect of the lip with simultaneous, opposing, linear advancement of tissue flaps made from both cheeks (1–4,25,26). A number of modifications have since then been described by Webster and other physicians (1,27,28). The hallmark feature of these flaps is design for resection of triangular units of tissue from adjacent cheek sites immediately above and/or below the proximal portion of each flap (Fig. 21A and B). Resection of these triangular units facilitates a more natural advancement of each flap and minimizes the inherent distortion that such aggressive facial tissue transfer would otherwise produce (origin of term "Burow's" triangles).

In design for reconstruction of the upper lip, incisions for linear flap release are made in the horizontal plane and extended laterally from the nasal base to form the superior margin of the flap and separately from the oral commissure to form the inferior margin. A triangular (or crescent-shaped) unit of tissue is typically resected from the region immediately above the superior margin of the planned cheek flap and separately from the region immediately below the inferior flap margin (Fig. 22A and B).

In reconstruction of the lower lip there are two principle designs to choose from. In the method advocated by von Burow, a single linear flap-releasing incision is made, extending laterally from the oral commissure (1,25). A triangular unit of tissue is resected from the region immediately above this horizontal incision. A triangular unit of tissue is also resected as necessary immediately below the area of concern in the lower lip, allowing a rotation/advancement type of movement from the lower cheek region on both sides. In the modification advocated by Webster, a second and lower horizontal releasing incision is made along the course of the mental crease and carried out into the cheek on both sides, creating flaps of more rectangular design (1,27,28). A triangular resection may be done also on both sides from the

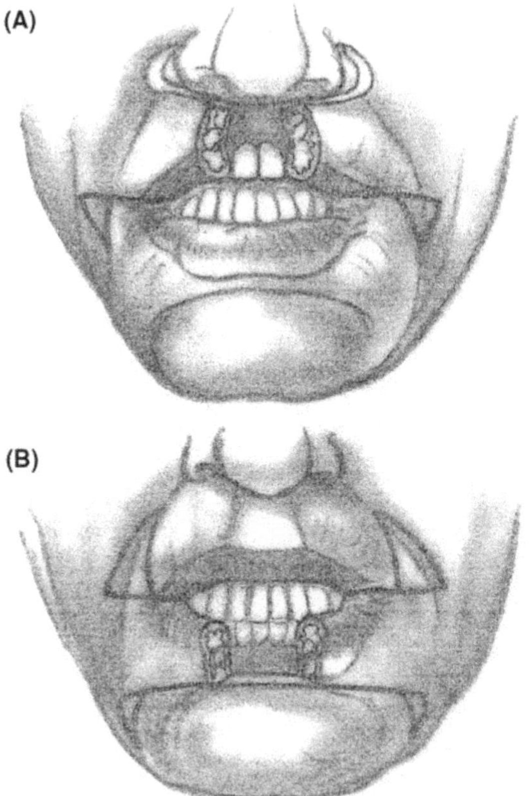

Figure 21 Illustrations of (**A**) upper lip and (**B**) lower lip reconstructions with true advancement flaps from the cheeks with triangular excisions of what will be redundant tissue.

region immediately below this second line when necessary. Flap movement with this design is a more true linear advancement, which may help minimize the tendency for later vertical insufficiency in the midline.

In all variations of this basic design incisions should be made through skin and subcutaneous tissues, but attempt to leave the facial musculature as unviolated as possible. Freeman has described a "myoplastic" modification that attempts to pull some of the adjacent Orbicularis muscle from the lateral portion of the opposite lip along with the flap as it is transferred (28).

Incisions for buccal mucosal release are made separately and should also be done with attempt to minimize violation of the facial musculature. A single linear incision extending laterally from the oral commissure may be sufficient for mucosal release. This author favors making the mucosal incision just slightly higher that the actual commissure for lower lip repair and the opposite for repair of the upper lip. This allows a small flap of mucosa to be more easily laid over the free margin of the flap, after it has been advanced, to recreate the vermilion surface.

Advantage/Disadvantages

This type of reconstruction can be used in reconstruction of as much as a complete defect of either lip. It uses tissue that is immediately adjacent to the lip complex. The general design allows for a relatively good redistribution of tissues about the mid-face. Results can be better when some meaningful remnant of lip tissue remains.

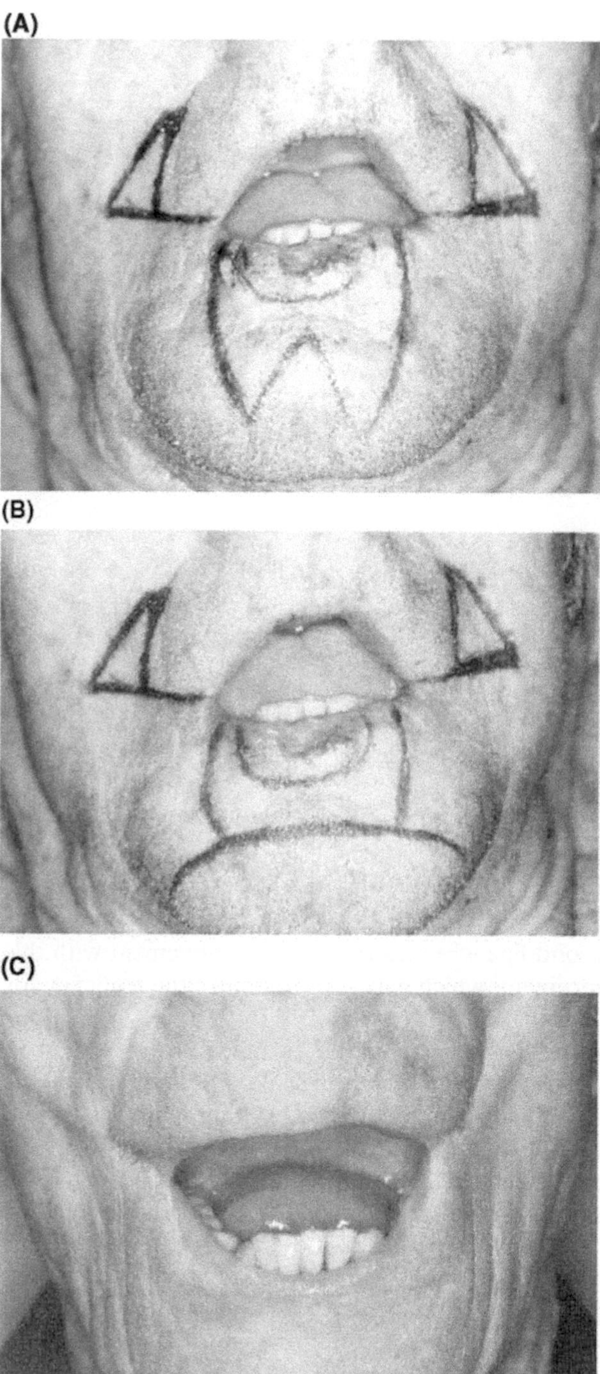

Figure 22 (**A**) Placement of incisions for planned von Burow type flap reconstruction. (**B**) Alternate plan showing Webster modification design. (**C**) Patient who had undergone von Burow type flaps to lower lip. He can wear his dentures satisfactorily, but has considerable problem with drooling and other motor problems as well. The central portion of the lower lip is found slightly deficient in the vertical plane.

The greatest drawback to this type of repair is that it fails to restore a functional muscle sphincter and that it has considerable tendency to produce impairment to many of the expressive motor functions of the lip. The simultaneous, opposing advancement of tissue from both cheeks produces considerable tightness in this type of reconstruction, which actually helps offset some of the problems with deficient motor function in the repaired lip. Without a full thickness composite of lip tissue and the tendency for contraction with wound scar maturation, there may be some gradual loss of height to the lip that is reconstructed in this manner.

Limitations

This concept of lip repair is normally used to restore a defect varying from roughly two thirds to loss of a full lip. Again, results are not as good when the repair involves a greater portion of the lip. In some cases this type of flap may be utilized on one side of the face while a simpler flap is used for the contralateral portion of the repair. Despite the use of the "Burow's" triangles the reconstructed lip commonly appears tight in contrast to the adjacent facial tissues. It must be appreciated that the flaps are not being brought together in a flat surface plane, but over a projected mid-face structure. As a general rule this concept of cheek advancement flap is not considered a first-line preference for most lip repairs.

Island Flaps

There are a variety of different flap designs that have been described that transfer flap tissue from the tissues that immediately surround the lip complex with incisions made completely around the skin paddle in "island" fashion. Use of the island design minimizes the inherent problem of bulkiness or "dog ear" deformity near the pedicle base as the flap is turned. Flaps may be designed either with a subcutaneous pedicle base that must have adequate random vascularization or axial with a more specific deep arterial tree. A number of island flap designs have been reported (1,29,30). General concerns with island flaps include issues of impairment to mid-face motor functions, orientation and appearance of donor incision lines, limitation of flap mobility and consistent flap viability.

McHugh (29) has described a method of horizontal advancement of cheek tissue as an island flap. The flap is designed in triangular fashion with an extended axis in the horizontal plane. Both the skin and mucosa are incised with upper and lower margins that meet at a distant lateral point in the cheek. This flap is based on a deep tissue pedicle and advanced into the lip complex in V–Y fashion. A blunt, teasing dissection is done to create the deep tissue pedicle, with attempt to preserve vascular and neural structures. The incision lines with this design are long and not oriented in aesthetic favor with the relaxed skin tension lines of the cheek. Change to some expressive facial motor functions would be expected.

Fugimori (30) has described a method of simultaneous opposing transposition of expanded lengths of melolabial tissue that are designed as island or what he refers to as "gate" flaps. These flaps are designed with inclusion of innervated muscle from the region immediately lateral to the melolabial crease. With no cutaneous pedicle the flaps can be transposed into the lip complex with little or no problem of "dog-ear" formation and can therefore be possibly a one-stage reconstruction. With concerns for violation to the perilabial facial musculature, extended dissection in the cheeks and consistency of skin paddle viability, this reconstruction is not done commonly.

Other Cervical-Based Flaps

Cervical-based flaps including the submental fasciocutaneous and myocutaneous flaps have been applied to many defects of the oral cavity and cutaneous perioral regions. This option may provide thicker, vascularized tissue when other flaps are not available or contraindicated. The inferior gravitational pull and potential for metastatic adenopathy remain concerns when using this flap for lip cancer defects.

The platysma myocutaneous flaps also may provide vascularized tissue when the facial artery, facial veins, and/or external jugular veins are preserved during flap elevation.

Numerous other random and pedicled cervical flaps have historically been used to reconstruct lip defects but today are well beyond the first line of reconstructive options.

Temporoparietal Scalp Flap

Technique

The scalp flap design most practical for reconstruction of the lip is taken from the temporoparietal region (4). Outline for this flap is designed as two parallel lines directed vertically on the side of the head, centered principally along the course of the posterior branch of the superficial temporal artery. The proximal end of the flap is brought down to about the level of the zygomatic arch, while the distal end is placed high in the parietal region of the scalp. The two outline incisions for the flap are brought together in a tapered fashion at the distal end. To assure an easy flap reach to the lip, it is best to plan the design with some redundant length. While flap width must be at least equal to the vertical length required for the lip repair, it is best if the flap is made a little extra wide, making accommodation for what eventual contraction will occur after the flap has been set.

Reconstruction of the intraoral lining for the lip is most often done with application of a skin graft. A split-thickness or full-thickness skin graft may be used, with results that can be fairly similar. While there should be a little less contraction when a full-thickness graft is used, the rate of graft take may be slightly less. Whichever graft is used is also brought over the free margin of the reconstructed lip to provide a modest restoration of the vermilion at the same time.

When there is question about whether the distal portion of such a flap would remain viable, the flap may be planned with an initial delay phase, in which division of the distal margin is done in one or more stages over a period of two to four weeks. Because securing a skin graft to the inner surface of the flap at the time of transfer can be technically difficult, greater consideration may be given to utilizing an initial delay stage, at which time a skin graft can be applied to the flap's deep surface in a "buried" fashion. The skin graft is then later transferred together with the scalp tissue as a composite flap. The buried graft can be brought around the edge of the flap that is to become the new free lip margin.

If greater release is found necessary as the flap is transposed, one may either extend the vertical outline at the pedicle base or create an additional releasing incision that is directed anteriorly in the horizontal plane from the pedicle base. In most cases the anterior branch of the superficial temporal artery will have to be separated, with pedicle dissection taken down to the level of the zygomatic arch. If there is concern about whether the flap would remain viable upon division of its pedicle, this could be done over a longer period in a progressive or serial fashion.

Advantages/Disadvantages

The principle advantage in using the temporoparietal scalp flap is that the anterior field of reconstruction is kept restricted to the lip unit only and minimizes scarring, deformity or impairment to the immediately surrounding mid-face region. Restoration with this flap will be adynamic, however because surrounding facial motor functions are unviolated, the overall lip function can be acceptable.

Color match of the temporoparietal scalp flap to the surrounding mid-face skin is not typically ideal. Because it is hair bearing, use of this flap is far more appropriate for males who naturally have a more bearded skin and may even choose to mask the reconstruction with a moustache or beard.

Closure of the scalp donor site can usually be done in a primary fashion. If it is done with excessive tension, there may be later loss of some hair in the closure site. Correction for this can later be done with either serial excision or much less commonly with use of a tissue expander.

Limitations

It is possible to restore an entire lip if bilateral temporoparietal flaps are connected at the top of the head and passed together in a "bucket handle" fashion (4). Functional results are much better however if the reconstruction involves a defect of only half or less of either lip. Again, the cosmesis inherent to this reconstruction is much more suited to males.

Laterally-Based Forehead Flap

The laterally-based forehead flap (referred to by some as the temporal flap) can be used to provide a large amount of soft tissue for reconstruction of larger defects of the lip region, but is seldom used in modern time (4,31). Vascular supply to the flap during its development and pedicled transfer is from the anterior branch of the superficial temporal artery.

Technique

Outline for the flap is made with two horizontally directed incisions across the forehead, one immediately above the brows and the other at some desired height across the top region of the forehead. Because vascular supply to the distal end is initially challenged with ligation across the superficial temporal artery on that side, development of the distal end is normally done with one or two delay stages. A skin graft can be placed on the underside of the flap during this time. Flap transfer is normally done in two stages with pedicle division in about three weeks or longer, with stages, if desired. The frontalis and galeal layers are normally included with the flap. Immediate cover for the forehead donor site is done with a split-thickness skin graft(s). Tissue from the flap pedicle may be returned to the forehead after pedicle division or discarded in favor of a more uniform appearance to the forehead with the grafted skin.

Advantages/Disadvantages/Limitations

This reconstruction can provide a large amount of relatively thick soft tissue for reconstruction of either lip. The principle disadvantages with this repair are that it requires multiple stages, that there is both motor and sensory loss in the forehead, and that the ultimate aesthetic result with restoration of the forehead can be considered poor. Because the skin grafts are typically more pale and draped immediately over the forehead bone, with minimal intervening soft tissue, and with loss of expression from the eyebrows, the eventual aesthetic result is commonly "mask-like" and detractive. The laterally-based forehead flap is currently considered only for major lip repair and normally after most other regional flap choices are not available.

Deltopectoral Chest Flap

Technique

The deltopectoral flap is designed to transfer cutaneous tissue from the ipsilateral shoulder to various sites of the face and can be adapted to restore a defect of either or both lips (31,32). The flap outline is made with two incisions that course transversely across the upper region of one side of the chest and connect at its distal end with a rounded outline at a desired site on the shoulder. Vascular supply to the thoracic portion of the flap is primarily from the perforating vessels that exit from the chest immediately lateral to the sternum at each intercostal space. The upper incision is placed immediately below the clavicle. The lower incision is placed inferior to the fourth intercostal space and brought across the chest in a gradually ascending fashion that passes above both the areola and axilla and onto the low, anterior portion of the shoulder. Because vascular supply to the shoulder region is more random, it is necessary to delay this flap if any appreciable amount of shoulder skin is required for extended length. The flap must be designed with sufficient laxity that it can both reach to the desired part of the face and still allow for some reasonable amount of head/neck movement while the pedicle remains intact.

Delay of the flap is typically done in two or three stages. At first the body of the flap from the sternum to the mid-anterior region of the shoulder is raised up and then reset. Dissection of the flap is done by raising of the fascia off of the superficial surface of the pectoralis major muscle. A wide initial undermining may be done in this plane beneath the proposed distal portion of the flap. Completed outline and dissection of the distal portion of the flap is later done in one or two stages, depending on how far back onto the shoulder the outline must be carried and the relative safety that is desired in assuring full viability of the flap as it is placed. Each stage is usually separated by 10–14 days. When delay is required for the distal portion of the flap, consideration may be made for initial placement of a "buried" skin graft on the flap's deep surface, with plan for later transfer of the "composite" flap.

While the skin and subcutaneous tissue of the chest generally has fair thickness, that from the shoulder is much thinner. This author has found it helpful in some cases to fold the flap over on itself to provide both an external and internal lining and a better overall thickness to the lip reconstruction. In repair of the upper lip the flap may be set into the defect with the cutaneous surface of the distal end of the flap providing the internal lining. At the time of pedicle release, the otherwise redundant portion of the flap may be saved and turned on itself to also provide the external surface, completing the lip reconstruction. When done in lower lip repair the flap would have to be folded on itself at the time of initial transfer and consideration made for what amount of contraction would occur (1,33). Folding the flap tightly could result in vascular compromise to the more distal portion. If the flap is very wide, it may be helpful to suspend some type of fascia or tendon graft from the maxilla on both sides to help provide support at the free margin of the lip, minimizing the chance for eventual contraction of the flap in the vertical plane.

Initial closure of the chest portion of the donor site can usually be done in a primary fashion, while a split-thickness skin graft is required for resurfacing of the shoulder site. What redundant portion of the pedicle is not otherwise used is commonly placed back into the chest donor site at the time of division and inset.

Advantages/Disadvantages

The deltopectoral flap can offer considerable versatility in lip repair. Since it can be made with large size, it can be adapted to many different lip defects and, in some cases, provide tissue to both lips with a single transfer. Use of this repair avoids problems of incurring additional scars, tissue loss and additional functional impairments in the region of the face associated with the lip complex.

The greatest drawback to this method of reconstruction is that it generally requires multiple stages over a period of at least several weeks. Being connected to the chest with a flap pedicle can be cumbersome and even disturbing to many patients. This flap fails to restore a functional lip muscle sphincter. Skin color with this flap tends to be lighter than that of the lower face and the flap does not usually restore a bearded skin in males.

Limitations

This flap can be used to reconstruct defects of very large size and may involve sizable areas even beyond the lip. When it is used to simultaneously reconstruct a defect involving both lips, restoration of the oral commissure is usually done at a later stage. With lack of orbicularis muscle function, any later restoration of the oral commissure should be done in a conservative manner to minimize the chance for problems with oral incontinence.

Microvascular Free Flap Lip Reconstruction

Recent advances in microvascular surgery have resulted in a variety of free flap techniques applied for restoration of more complex lip tissue defects. Free flap repair is generally considered when there is a total or near total defect of the upper, lower or both lips (Fig. 23 A–C). In patients who have been treated to the lip area with prior radiation or in patients with prior failed attempts at reconstruction, free tissue transfer should be considered. At this time the free flap most suited to restoration of a total lip defect is the radial forearm free flap, which offers a relatively thin skin paddle that can be adapted to lip repair more easily than most other free flaps. Donor site morbidity is also relatively less with this flap than other choices. Other options include the lateral arm and lateral thigh flap in thin patients.

A special problem that is encountered with reconstruction of a extensive lower lip defects is providing adequate support to maintain height and some sense of tension in this large, adynamic repair. Many surgeons have come to use the palmaris longus tendon from the forearm as a suspensory sling that is attached to the facial skeleton on both sides or to any remaining lip and the contralateral maxilla and serves to hold the flap tissue upwards across the free margin of the reconstructed lip (chap. 18, Fig. 5) (34). A much more detailed description of free flap techniques is found in other chapters of this text.

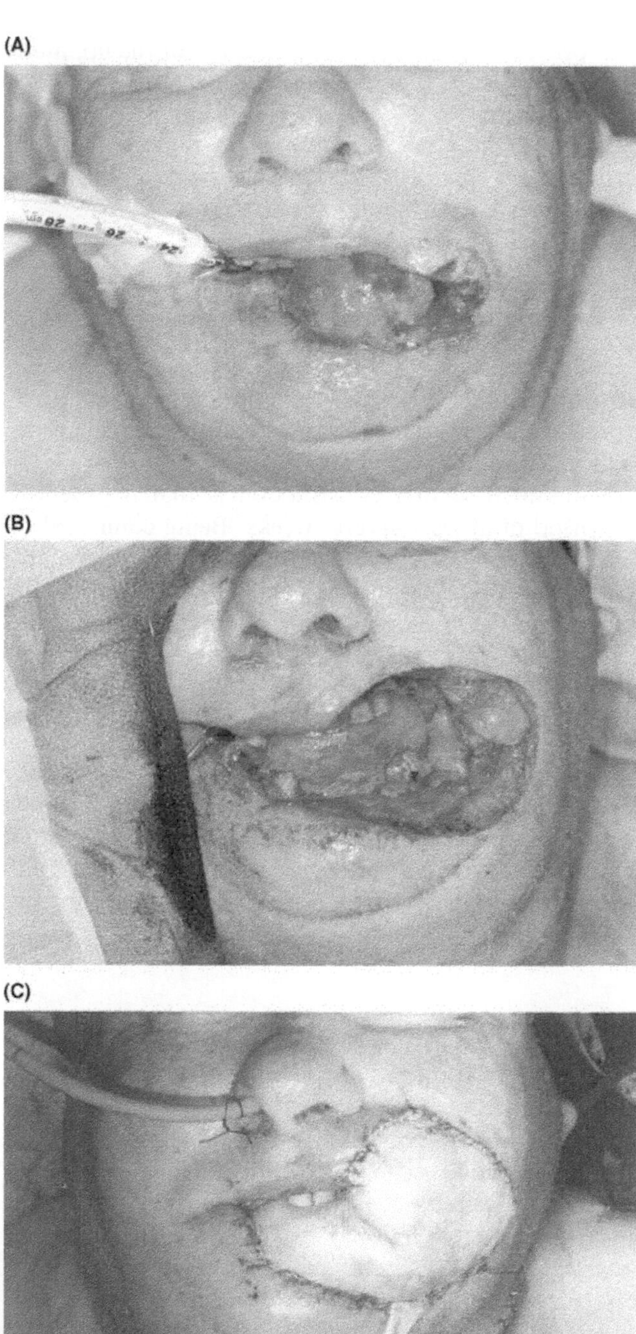

Figure 23A–C (**A**) Patient with advanced large left lower lip carcinoma extending across the oral commissure to the upper lip and deeply into the buccal mucosa. (**B**) Defect created by the resection of the carcinoma involving two thirds of the lower lip, one third of the upper lip and a large cheek/buccal defect.

Advantages/Disadvantages

A major advantage of free flap reconstruction of the lip is that it can most often be done as a one-stage procedure with both internal and external lining in one flap. Another major advantage is that very little additional scar is made in the mid-face since the tissue comes from a distant source. This also provides vascularized tissue when patients have undergone prior surgery or radiation to the area. Free flap reconstruction can be designed to provide a large volume of tissue when necessary. Addition tissue such as bone can be incorporated into the flap for combined lip and mandible reconstruction if necessary (see chap. 18 for examples). It is also possible to anastamose neural structures to the mental (less often infraorbital) nerve remnant on either side to allow for some degree of sensory restoration to the lip site.

The greatest disadvantage to free flap repair is that it requires special skills in microvascular repair and careful postoperative monitoring to assure viability. In some situations length of operating time must be considered. A multi-field operative setup is generally required and in some situations a need for patient repositioning to accommodate each part. The potential for donor site morbidities must also be considered.

The reconstruction of the lip with microvascular tissue will result in an adynamic lip which can result in oral incompetence. This can be minimized by adequately supporting and tightening the reconstructed lip. Cosmesis is clearly an issue and the color match of most microvascular donor sites is poor at best. This usually improves after radiotherapy.

Limitations

The principle limitations with free flap reconstruction of the lip are the need for special microvascular skills and the availability of suitable donor tissue. The availability and suitability of vessels in the recipient and donor sites are major considerations. The capabilities of postoperative care must be considered also.

SUMMARY

In summary, lip reconstruction presents a complex cosmetic and functional problem for both the patient and reconstructive surgeon. Multidisciplinary planning and rehabilitation is important in addressing both the oncologic and functional concerns. Postoperative rehabilitation often includes consultations with dentists, speech pathologists, maxillofacial prosthodontists, and physical therapists.

REFERENCES

1. Mazzola RF, Lupo G. Evolving concepts in lip reconstruction. Clin Plast Surg 1984; 11(4):583–617.
2. Renner GR, Zitsch RP. Cancer of the lip. In: Myers EN, Suen JY, Myers JN, Hanna EYN, eds. Cancer of the Head Neck. 4th ed. Philadelphia: Saunders, 2003.
3. Renner GR. Reconstruction of the lip. In: Baker SR, Swanson NA, eds. Local Flaps in Facial Reconstruction. St. Louis: Mosby, 1995 (2nd ed. in press 2005).
4. Webster JP. Crescentic peri-alar cheek excision for upper lip flap advancement with a short history of upper lip repair. Plast Reconstr Surg 1955; 16:434–464.

4a. Fritze HE, Reich OFG. Die Plastische, Berlin, Hirschwald, 1845.
4b. Tagliacozzi G. De Curtorum Chirgurgia per Insitionem. Libriduo. Vol. 2. Chap. 19. Venice: Bindoni, 1597.
5. Park C, Lineaweaver WC, Buncke HJ. New perioral arterial flaps: antomic study and clinical application. Plast Reconstr Surg 1994; 94(2):1268–1276.
6. Mcgregor IA. The tongue flap in lip surgery. Br J Plast Surg 1966; 19:253–263.
7. Bakamjian V. Use of tongue flaps in lower-lip reconstruction. Br J Plast Surg 1964; 17:76–87.
8. Karapandzic M. Reconstruction of lip defects by local arterial flaps. Br J Plast Surg 1974; 27:93–102.
9. Jabaley ME, Clement RL, Orcutt TW. Myocutaneous flaps in lip reconstruction: application of the Karapandzic principle. Plast Reconstr Surg 1977; 59:680–688.
10. Bruns VV. Chirurgischer atlas. Bildlische darstellung der chirurgischen krankheiten und der zu ihrer heilung erforderlichen instrumente, bandagen und operationen. II Abt: Kau- und Geschmaks-Organ.Tubingen, Laupp, 1857/1860.
11. Sabattini P. Cenno storico dell'origine e progressi della rhinoplastica e cheiloplastica. Bologna, Belle Arti, 1838.
12. Estlander JA. Eine methode aus der einen lippe substanzverluste der anderen zu ersetzen. Arch Klin Chir 14:622,1872. (Reprinted in English translation in Plast Reconstr Surg 1968; 42:361–366).
13. Abbe RA. A new plastic operation for the relief of deformity due to double harelip. Med Record 1898; 53:477–478.
14. Smith JW. Clinical experiences with the vermilion bordered lip flap. Plast Reconstr Surg 1961; 27(5):527–543.
15. Buck G. Contributions to reparative surgery: showing its application to the treatment of deformities produced by destructive disease or injury, congenital defects from arrest or excess of development, and cicatrical contractions from burns. New York: D Appleton, 1876.
16. Murray JF. Total reconstruction of a lower lip with bilateral Estlander flaps: case report. Plast Reconstr Surg 1972; 49(6):658–660.
17. Anderson R, Kurtay M. Reconstruction of the corner of the mouth. Plast Reconstr Surg 1971; 47(5):463–464.
18. Converse JM. The "over and out" flap for restoration of the corner of the mouth: case report. Plast Reconstr Surg 1975; 56(5):575–578.
19. Converse JM. The bridge flap for reconstruction of a full-thickness defect of the upper lip. Plast Reconstr Surg 1976; 57(4):442–444.
20. Smith JW. The anatomical and physiologic acclimatization of tissue transplanted by the lip switch technique. Plast Reconstr Surg 1960; 26(l):40–56.
21. Kriet JD, Cupp CL, Sherris DA, Murakami CS. The extended Abbe flap. Laryngoscope 1995; 105(9):988–992.
22. Gillies H, Millard R. The Principles and Art of Plastic Surgery. London: Butterworth, 1957.
23. Dorland's Illustrated Medical Dictionary. 26th ed. Philadelphia: WB Saunders, 1974.
24. Schewe EJ. A technique for reconstruction of the lower lip, following extensive excision for cancer. Ann Surg 1957; 146:285–290.
25. Burow CAV. Beschreibung einer neuen transplantations-methode (methode der seitlichen dreiecke) zum wiederersatz verlorengegangener teile des gesichts. Berlin, Nauck, 1855.
26. Bernard C. Cancer de la levre inferieure: restauration a l'aide de deux lambeaux lateraux quadrilatere: guerison. Bull Mem Soc Chir Paris 1853; 3:357.
27. Webster RC, Coffey RJ, Kelleher RE. Total and partial reconstruction of the lower lip with innervated muscle-bearing flaps. Plast Reconstr Surg 1960; 25:360–371.
28. Freeman BS. Myoplastic modificaiton of the Bernard cheiloplasty. Plast Reconstr Surg 1958; 21:453–460.
29. McHugh M. Reconstruction of the lower lip using a neurovascular island flap. Br J Plast Surg 1977; 30:316–318.

30. Fugimori R. "Gate flap" for the total reconstruction of the lower lip. Br J Plast Surg 1980; 33:340–345.
31. McGregor IA. Reconstruction following excision of intraoral and mandibular tumors. In: Converse JM, ed. Reconstructive Plastic Surgery. Vol. 5. Philadelphia: WB Saunders, 1977.
32. Bakamjian V, Culf NK, Bales HW. Versatility of the deltopectoral flap in reconstructions following head and neck cancer surgery. In: Sanvenero-Rosselli G, BoggioRobutti G, eds. Trans 4th Int Congr Plast Surg. Rome, Amsterdam: Excerpta Medica, 1969.
33. Delpech JM. Chirurgie Clinique de Montpelleir. Vol 2, p 587. Paris: Gabon, 1823/1828.
34. Sadove RC, Luce EA, Mcgrath PC. Reconstruction of the lower lip and chin with the composite radial forearm-palmaris longus free flap. Plast Reconstr Surg 1991; 88(2):209–214.

9
Reconstruction of the Buccal Mucosa and Salivary Ducts

Timothy M. McCulloch and D. Gregory Farwell
Otolaryngology—Head and Neck Surgery, Harborview Medical Center, University of Washington, Seattle, Washington, U.S.A.

INTRODUCTION

The oral cavity can be divided into a variety of anatomically unique sub-units. One such sub-unit is the buccal mucosal region. The buccal region has its own unique structure and design, which is necessary for normal oral function. Although a relatively passive player in speech and swallowing, it is actively involved in mastication, bolus preparation, and storage prior to swallow initiation. The major defining character of the buccal mucosa is its innate elasticity. It retains a position adjacent to the teeth during normal passive oral activity, however, it can be expanded to more than twice its size when confronted with a food bolus. This expansion may be even larger when controlling air outflow, as seen in brass and reed instrument musicians. The buccal mucosa contains approximately $40\,cm^2$ of mucosal surface on each side of the oral vestibule. The parotid gland drains through the buccal mucosa via Stenson's duct, which exits the mucosa just posterior to the maxillary molar. The buccal mucosa borders the alveolar mucosa superiorly and inferiorly, the labial mucosa anteriorly, and the anterior tonsillar pillar and retromolar trigone posteriorly. The buccal mucosa itself is littered with minor salivary glands (buccal glands) as well as connective tissue which holds it in close approximation to the buccinator muscle and posterior slips of the orbicularis oris (1). Posterior to the buccinator muscle is a relatively large fat pad, the buccal fat pad, which protects neuromuscular pathways and cushions the motion of the mandible during mastication.

In Europe and America, the buccal mucosa is a relatively rare site of primary oral cavity malignancy. However, the buccal mucosa is commonly involved secondarily from cancers arising in the structures of the jaw along the alveolar ridge, or retromolar trigone, and the tonsil through the anterior tonsillar pillar. Also labial carcinomas can extend posteriorly to involve the buccal mucosa, and on occasion skin cancers and parotid malignancies can develop direct invasion through soft tissues and secondarily involve the buccal mucosa. Chhetri et al. (2) from University of California-Los Angeles did a 20-year review of primary buccal carcinomas treated surgically at their institution and were able to identify a group of only 27 patients.

Primary buccal squamous cell carcinoma tends to occur in a somewhat older patient population. The average age of the group reviewed by Chhetri was 67-year-old with the age range extending up to 87 years of age. This may account at least in part for the common use of radiation therapy as a primary modality in buccal squamous cell carcinoma. A similar review by Strome et al. (3) evaluating the disease progression in a group of 31 patients identified very high recurrence rates in patients with stage I and II disease treated with surgery alone, even in cases where margins were deemed negative. They also support the adjunctive use of radiation therapy in buccal mucosal carcinomas. This review noted an 80% recurrence rate by five years with 72% of these recurrences found at the primary site. In a review by Nair et al. (4) 234 patients treated with primary radiation therapy were followed for a three-year period of time, with primary failure rates as high as 62% in the stage III and IV disease groups. The patients who fail radiation are a surgical challenge due to their advanced age, radiation side effects, and the necessity to resect the recurrence with wide surgical margins. This certainly limits the options of the reconstructive surgeon treating these patients.

Dysplastic hyperkeratotic lesions of the buccal mucosa are oftentimes treated surgically to alleviate symptomatology as well as to confirm a benign pathology of these potentially premalignant abnormalities. The cause of buccal mucosal leukoplakia may be traumatic, from irritation along the dental bite line, secondary to human papilloma virus, or induced by chemical irritants and carcinogens from chewing tobacco, pipe, or cigar smoking. Other non-epithelial malignant processes may also require resection of buccal mucosa, including minor salivary gland malignancies or occasionally soft tissue sarcomas such as ameloblastoma, rhabdomyosarcomas, or liposarcoma.

EVALUATION AND PLANNING

Reconstructive planning of buccal mucosal defects should be accomplished prior to tumor excision. A reconstructive plan must include multiple options depending on the final tumor resection-induced defect. It is extremely useful for the surgeon to have a variety of techniques available to deal with the potential defect, regardless of its final size. In most cases, the surgeon has to rely upon his clinical expertise to determine the extent of the mucosal defect necessary to extirpate the index tumor. The surgeon needs to consider not only the size of the mucosal defect but also what underlying structures will be included along with the excision. The resection may include important structures such as the parotid duct, the buccal fat pad, or portions of deep structures like mandible, buccinator, or masseter muscle. With deep tumors or tumors which extend into the buccal mucosa from extraoral locations, it is common that a through-and-through resection is required, including cheek skin, portions of the parotid, and facial nerve as well as the buccal mucosa. This leaves a relatively complex defect to reconstruct cosmetically and functionally.

The primary nodal drainage pattern from the buccal mucosa follows the facial vasculature and includes the perifacial nodes at the angle of the mandible, submental nodes, submandibular nodes, and some of the small nodes present in and around the tail of the parotid. Second echelon nodal involvement will include the high-level II or jugulodigastric nodal group. When tumors are extensive or lymph node dissection is required, it is reasonable for the surgeon to consider doing a parotidectomy to encompass the lymphatic drainage as well as to simplify the postoperative management of the parotid and/or the resected parotid duct. Oftentimes, as we will discuss at the end of this chapter, free tissue transfer and large cervical facial rotation flaps are required to close these complex defects.

In cases in which nodal disease is suspected or the tumor is large and infiltrative, a computer assisted tomography (CT) scan may be of assistance. Evidence of skin tethering, facial nerve deficits, or excessive pain may lead the surgeon to suspect tumor infiltration and perineural spread of disease. Such findings necessitate larger resections and secondarily larger reconstructions. With proper preoperative planning and a series of reconstructive options available most patients can be treated in a single setting with tumor extirpation and defect closure with good functional and cosmetic results.

RECONSTRUCTIVE OPTIONS (TABLE 1)

Split Thickness Skin Grafts and Acellular Human Collagen Matrix

Skin grafts are an option in many oral cavity defects, either as a temporary or permanent solution. Primary skin grafting in the oral cavity has been a longstanding method of reconstruction. Very large defects can be closed using skin grafts in either meshed or non-meshed form. Skin graft reconstructions have the advantages of simplicity and low patient donor site morbidity. Skin grafts also have the disadvantages of significant graft contracture sometimes up to 50%, as well as scar band formation along the graft mucosal margins. Schramm and Myers (5) reported in 1980, a series of moderately large oral cavity defects reconstructed with split thickness skin grafts. The authors concluded that the skin graft closures were most useful in patients who

Table 1 Reconstruction Options for Buccal Defects

Procedure	Indications
Split thickness skin grafts	Small to intermediate defects. May be successful in radiated patients
Buccal mucosal rotation flaps	Small to intermediate non-radiated defects
Buccal fat pad mobilization	Posterior defects ≤5 cm. Avoid use in radiated patients
Temporalis and temporoparietal flaps	Intermediate to large defects. Useful in radiated patients. May require additional split thickness skin graft
Cervical flaps (platysma, sternocleidomastoid)	Intermediate to large defects. Avoid in patients undergoing neck dissection or with prior radiation
Regional myocutaneous flaps	
Pectoralis major	Large and composite defects, through-and-through defects
Lower island trapezius	Large and composite defects, through-and-through defects
Upper island trapezius	Large and composite defects, through-and-through defects
Free tissue transfer	
Radial forearm free flaps	Large defects post-radiation. Repair scar contracture
Lateral arm flaps	Large defects post-radiation. Repair scar contracture. Needs reasonable neck recipient vessels
Rectus abdominus	Through-and-through defects
Trapezius flaps	Through-and-through defects
Temporizing maneuvers	
Porcine skin grafts	Temporary closure prior to final reconstruction
Avascular human collagen matrix grafts	May succeed as sole closure method in small to intermediate defects. Can skin graft or allow to epithelialized

had undergone resections which were too large to close primarily, but not large enough to require rotation of myocutaneous flaps. This article predates the wide acceptance of free tissue transfer, however, it emphasizes the utility of split thickness skin graft. They had very low morbidity from the procedure and documented successful oral cavity rehabilitation in this group of patients.

In 1987, McConnel et al. (6) evaluated three methods of oral cavity reconstruction, which included split thickness skin grafts and concluded that oral function was best retained when utilizing skin grafts compared to reconstructive flaps. Skin grafts add no bulk to the defect created and therefore oftentimes do not meet all the reconstructive goals. When placing a skin graft in the buccal mucosa, it is essential that the graft be well approximated to the underlying tissues to retain its viability (Fig. 1). Multiple sutures need to be placed throughout the graft to approximate it to buccinator, buccal fat, or associated subcutaneous tissues. Oftentimes a bolster utilizing material such as Xeroform gauze is necessary to retain approximation of the skin graft to the underlying tissues during the initial week to 10 days of healing. Large bolsters in the buccal mucosal space can be retained with stay sutures, however, they are relatively uncomfortable for the patient and can require the patient to remain in the hospital until the bolster is removed. A feeding tube may need to be placed in order for the patient to maintain nutrition and hydration. Securing a skin graft with a bolster may be simplified with the utilization of parachute or through-and-through sutures as described by Garvey et al. (2002) (Fig. 2) (7). This bolstering technique increases the skin graft contact to the underlying surface from which it obtains all its nutrient materials. In most cases, primary skin grafting is not the ideal reconstructive method. However, it can be used when faced with defects that otherwise would be impossible to close due to the unexpected size of tumor resection, or when other options are not available.

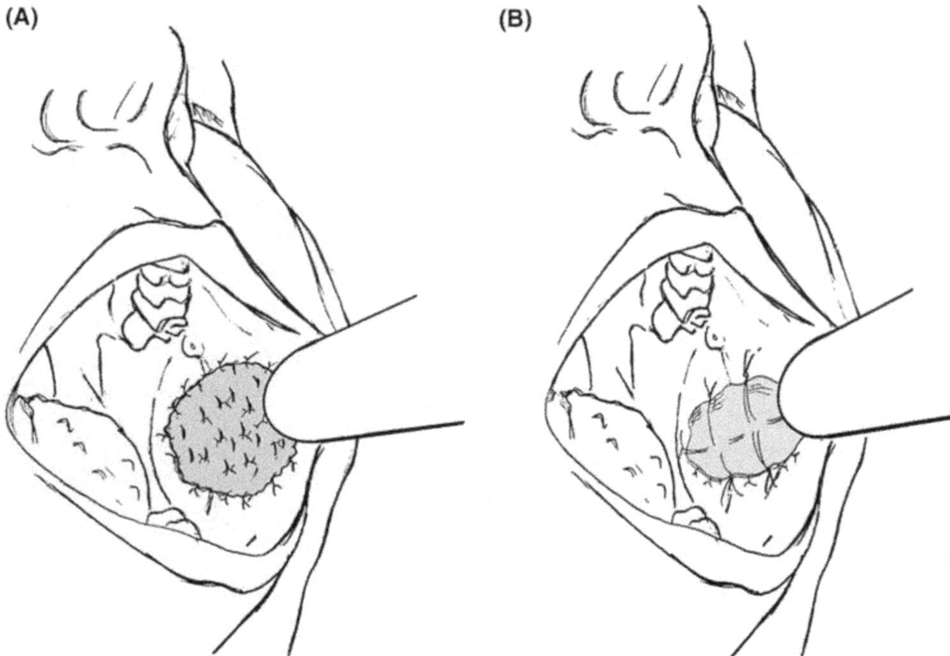

Figure 1 (**A**) Skin grafting with sutures and (**B**) bolster, held in place with stay sutures.

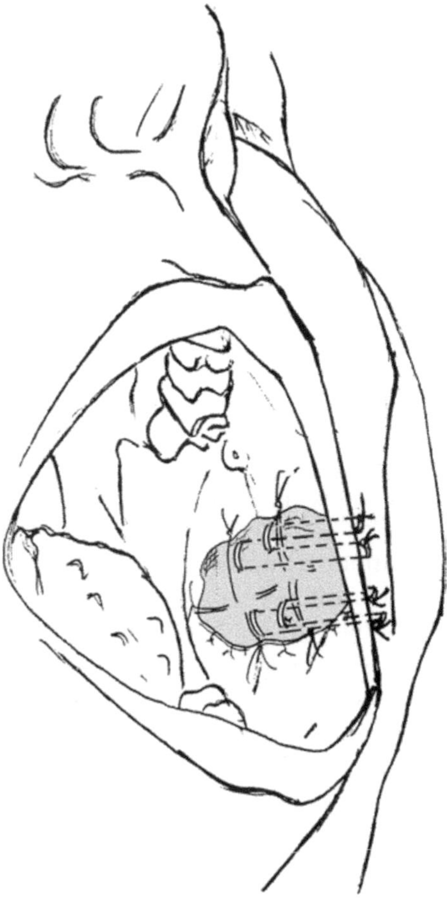

Figure 2 Skin grafting with bolster, held in place with parachute sutures *Source*: After Garvey et al., 2002 ENT Oct 80 (10) 720.

The utilization of porcine skin grafts as a temporizing maneuver in the oral cavity has also been described. A porcine skin graft can be placed temporarily over a defect to keep the underlying tissues healthy while a more extensive reconstruction is planned. These are never a permanent solution and will be sloughed by the patient spontaneously if not removed surgically (8).

The use of acellular human collagen matrix (Alloderm® Lifecell Corporation, Branchburg, New Jersey) has been described for reconstruction of mucosal defects (9,10). Large successful series with these materials as the primary and only reconstruction method are lacking. Rhee et al. (10) in a 1998 review of allograft dermal matrix reconstruction of the oral cavity evaluated 29 patients with full thickness defects reconstructed solely with allograft materials and reported a 90% success rate in wound closure and re-epithelialization. In this group of patients, the allograft is treated identical to a split thickness skin graft with re-epithelialization noted at the four week post-op time period and by eight months post-op only one of the patients had significant clinical evidence of graft contracture. Although this is a single case series, it does point out the potential utility of allograft reconstructions in the oral cavity as a sole reconstructive method or in combination with rotation flaps or skin grafting. Certainly, this case series would support the use of allograft dermal matrix materials as a short-term solution to a potential reconstructive dilemma. This product may also serve primarily as a supporting material for skin grafts, or as a temporizing maneuver until secondary reconstructions can be accomplished.

Contralateral buccal mucosal grafts may also be utilized to repair defects within the buccal mucosa. The disadvantage of a contralateral mucosal graft is the bilateral mucosal injury, limiting the patient's ability to function during the week to 10 days of rehabilitation. Primary free buccal mucosal grafts have been utilized in reconstruction of other regions throughout the body, primarily the urethra, with very high success rates. The harvesting techniques are simple and straightforward, and relatively large grafts can be obtained (11). In some cases a buccal mucosal graft may be a better alternative to a skin graft or a local buccal flap and certainly should be considered when facing these intermediate sized defects.

Local Tissue Flaps

There are many reconstructive options when dealing with small mucosal defects of the buccal mucosa. The surgeon needs to consider not only a successful closure of the defect created but also long-term preservation of function. Although, the primary function of the buccal mucosa, as outlined previously, is somewhat limited, patients will notice scar bands within the buccal mucosa. Large scar bands may significantly limit the patient's ability to open the jaw, masticate, and mobilize food across the masticatory surfaces of the teeth. Preserving the elasticity of the buccal mucosa is certainly advantageous to the patient's long-term quality of life. As in all cases, the ideal reconstruction material is that which mimics the resected material to the greatest degree.

When dealing with small buccal mucosal defects even as large as 3 cm in diameter, the ideal material for reconstruction is adjacent buccal mucosa utilizing flap rotation and local tissue transfers identical to those used in facial skin reconstruction (Fig. 3). Rhomboid flaps, rotation flaps, advancement flaps, and z-plasties can easily be utilized taking advantage of the elasticity of the native buccal mucosa to close a variety of small mucosal defects. After healing has completed, the most common finding is a relatively normal appearing buccal mucosa, and in most cases there is little or no scar formation or motion restrictions.

When designing a small rotation flap to close a buccal mucosal defect, the flap itself need not be as large as the defect it is closing. As is the case with rotation flaps covering the facial skin, the flap itself can be 2/3 to 1/2 the size of the defect. This occurs by taking advantage of surrounding tissue mobility to close a portion of the defect primarily. Therefore a 3 cm circular defect could be closed easily with a 1.5–2 cm rotation flap. Also, small areas of the buccal mucosa can be left open to heal by secondary intention with the expected result of mucosalization and normalization of function over a period of two to four weeks, not unlike the tonsillar fossa heals after tonsillectomy. The blood supply to the buccal mucosa is relatively random, and therefore the flaps can be based inferiorly, superiorly, posteriorly, or anteriorly without the likelihood of vascular compromise. Ideally flaps should be based inferiorly to take advantage of some improved arterial inflow, but more so to take advantage of venous outflow and decreased flap congestion (12). Unfortunately, patients who have undergone previous radiation therapy are not good candidates for local flaps for a variety of reasons. Perhaps first and foremost is a lack of elasticity of the tissues within the buccal mucosa after radiation therapy, and secondarily the need to take wide margins oftentimes leaves little or no mucosa for reconstructive purposes.

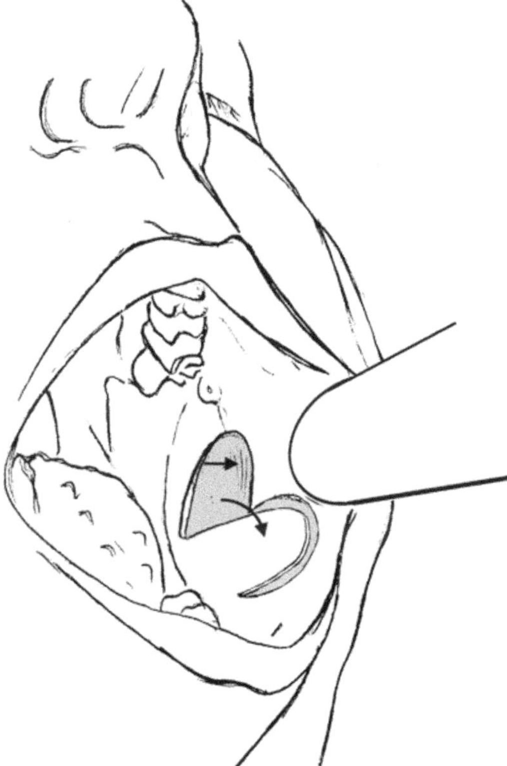

Figure 3 Transposition flap based posterior-inferior, used to close anterior mucosal defect.

Flap design is important as a poor design may induce tension lines with flap rotation, leading to displacement of the oral commissure posteriorly, or may pull the buccal mucosa into the bite line, causing the patient to chew the buccal mucosa during any masticatory effort. Even with these limitations, local tissue rearrangement is by far and away the ideal method of closing small buccal defects when the patient is in a non-radiated state and the margins are known to be adequately free of disease. Additional intraoral flaps have been described, including lateral tongue flaps and palate rotation flaps, which can reach the buccal mucosa and adequately close small buccal mucosal defects. However, the small amounts of tissue transferable by these techniques and the relative morbidity induced at the donor site markedly diminish the utility of these particular flaps in the current era of reconstructive surgery (13).

Buccal Fat Pad Grafts

The utilization of the buccal fat pad to reconstruct the buccal mucosa and areas around the retromolar trigone and anterior tonsillar pillar has been discussed in the literature for decades (14). The ability of the buccal fat pad to cover posterior mucosal defects can be extremely useful to the reconstructive surgeon. The buccal fat pad can be mobilized with gentle dissection and then rotated into the oral cavity to reach the central buccal region (Fig. 4). The buccal fat pad can cover a defect as large as 3 cm

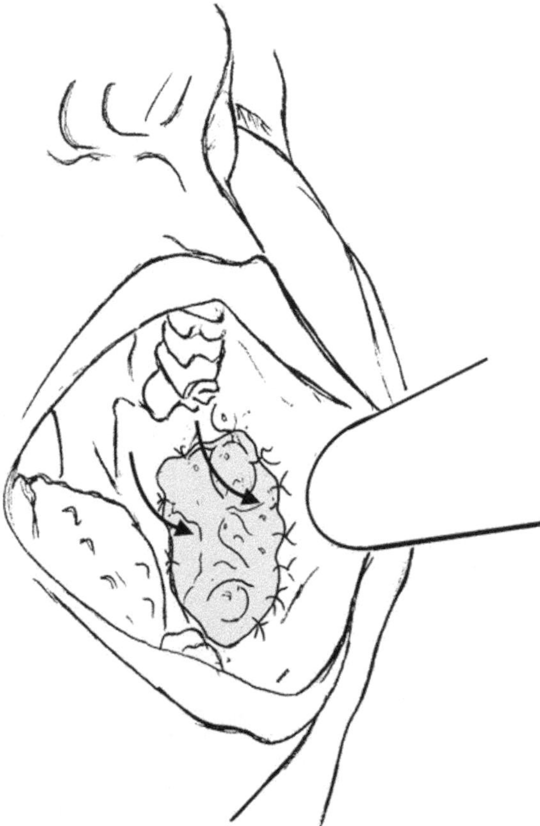

Figure 4 Buccal fat rotation of closure of a large posterior mucosal defect.

and will adequately cover small areas of exposed bone along the mandible or maxillary alveolar mucosa. In most cases, the fat does not require secondary grafting, although it will support a graft such as contralateral buccal mucosa or skin grafting if felt necessary. In most cases the exposed buccal fat will mucosalize over in a three to four week time period producing an intraoral closure without functional deficits. The primary limitation of the buccal fat graft is its immobility beyond approximately the central buccal mucosa region and the fact that mobilization of the buccal fat pad into the oral cavity in very thin individuals can leave evidence of hollowing in the central midface. However, most patients are unlikely to notice this small cosmetic deficit. In a review article by Rapidis et al. (14) published in 2000, buccal fat pad grafts were described as capable of covering defects in the retromolar trigone and buccal mucosal area measuring up to $7 \times 5 \times 2$ cm. The technique of harvesting the buccal fat pad is recommended to consist of essentially blunt and gentle scissor dissection in the region of the buccal fat. If the buccal fat is not exposed during the surgical resection of the primary tumor, an incision can be made above and posterior to the mandibular second molar, providing access to the buccal fat. Gentle traction allows luxation of the fat pad anteriorly to the site requiring repair. It is recommended that attempts be made to maintain thecapsule of the buccal fat as the blood supply of the fat resides within its capsule. The blood supply of the fat pad comes from the transverse facial artery as well as random blood supply through the surrounding soft tissues. In attempt to maintain as much blood supply as possible, it is recommended that a wide base be preserved (15). Over time, the buccal fat pad graft will heal by epithelialization and scar formation, usually leaving little functional or cosmetic deficit. Rapidis et al. (14) recommend avoiding the use of the buccal fat pad in the previously irradiated patient due to secondary fibrosis of the fat pad and decreased mobility.

Temporalis and Temporoparietal Fascia Flaps

A variety of flaps have been described from the temporalis, temporoparietal, or even forehead region in order to reconstruct buccal mucosa defects. These flaps are based on the vascularity obtained through the superficial and deep temporal arteries, which allow mobilization of superiorly positioned flaps to an intraoral location as they are rotated on their inferiorly based arterial pedicles. Laterally based forehead flaps were described in the mid-1960s and utilize large sections of skin along the forehead based superficially on the branches of the superficial temporal artery and then rotated through a precoronoid infrazygomatic tunnel into the oral cavity to be sewn in the buccal mucosal region (16). The forehead defect is then closed utilizing a split thickness skin graft. Certainly this technique, although of historic interest, is rarely utilized in the current era (8,17). The temporoparietal fascia flap, however, does have utility even today. The temporoparietal fascia flap is based on the superficial temporal artery, which carries a blood supply to both the superficial and deep temporal fascia. The superficial temporal fascia can be harvested off the temporalis muscle in a subcutaneous plane nearly to the vertex of the head (temparoparietal-galeal flap). This large flap can be relatively robust if carefully dissected (Fig. 5). The temporoparietal fascia flap elevation and mobilization techniques are well described in previous publications (18–20). Again, having an inferiorly based pedicle allows it to be rotated through an infrazygomatic tunnel into the oral cavity to reline buccal, palatal, or retromolar trigone defects. It is a relatively well vascularized flap, however, it does not contain mucosal or skin lining. Therefore, the options are either secondary intentioned healing or skin grafting over this vascularized flap. Perhaps its primary utility comes in previously irradiated patients in which the radiation field does not extend up into the temporoparietal region. This does provide a new blood supply to support healing.

The temporalis muscle can be rotated independently or in combination with temporoparietal fascia. The temporalis muscle is a muscle with a dual blood supply. However, its primary blood supply, the deep temporal artery, comes from below. The muscle originates on the coronoid process and extends up into the temporal fossa. Dissecting it out of the temporal fossa provides a large bulk of muscle which is relatively well vascularized as long as the deep temporal artery remains intact. Transferring the muscle into the oral cavity requires the creation of a subzygomatic tunnel and is limited by the muscular connections to the coronoid process of the mandible (21,22). A good description of the surgical technique and the potential utility of the temporalis muscle flap was provided by Hanasono et al. (23) in 2001. This article emphasizes the necessity for deep dissection in the infratemporal fossa region to mobilize the flap, including sectioning of the coronoid process to allow adequate rotation into the oral cavity without potential restrictions or impingements. The utility of this flap is limited due to the defect it creates in the temporal fossa, as well as its limited rotation and the availability of better reconstructive options in most cases.

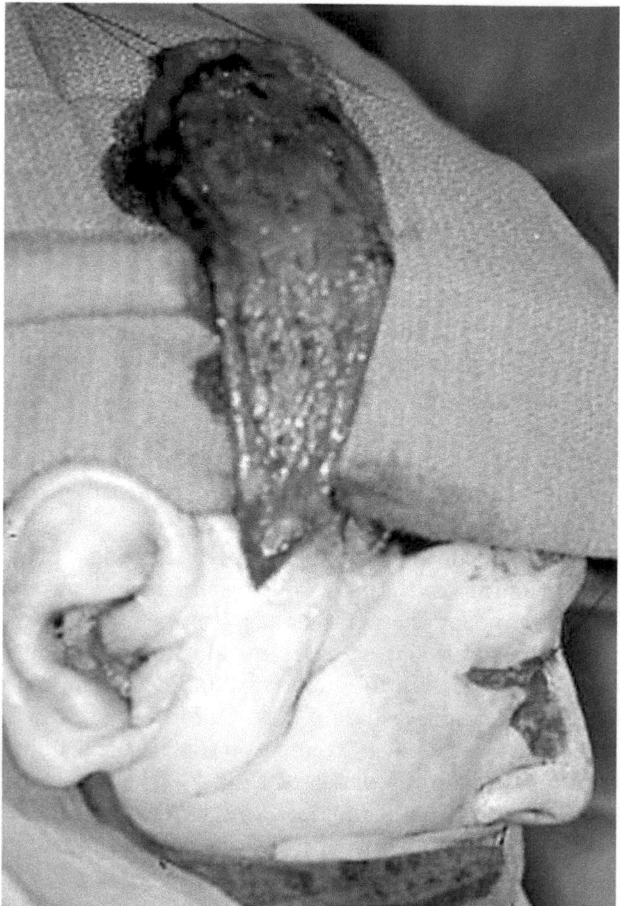

Figure 5 Temporoparietal flap after dissection prior to rotation into the oral cavity.

Cervical Pedicled Flaps (Sternocleidomastoid, Platysma, and Infrahyoid Myocutaneous Flaps)

Techniques have been described to utilize cutaneous tissues from the neck region to reconstruct oral cavity defects including the buccal mucosal region. The primary flaps described consist of a sternocleidomastoid flap, a platysma myocutaneous flap, and a submental myocutaneous rotation flap (Fig. 6). The sternocleidomastoid muscle has three primary blood supplies, one at its origin, one at its insertion, and a blood supply off the external carotid artery, which comes primarily from branches off the superior thyroid artery. This complex blood supply allows rotation of the sternocleidomastoid muscle. An inferiorly based skin paddle designed over the top of the sternocleidomastoid muscle can be harvested to incorporate the subcutaneous tissues directly over the muscle and then the muscle and skin paddle can be elevated from the surrounding tissues of the neck retaining the superior blood supply intact. This inferiorly based myocutaneous skin paddle can then be rotated up under the mandible through the floor of the mouth and then onto the buccal mucosal surfaces. This sternocleidomastoid flap is rotated primarily on a superior vascular pedicle, which consists of a blood supply from the occipital and posterior auricular arteries (24).

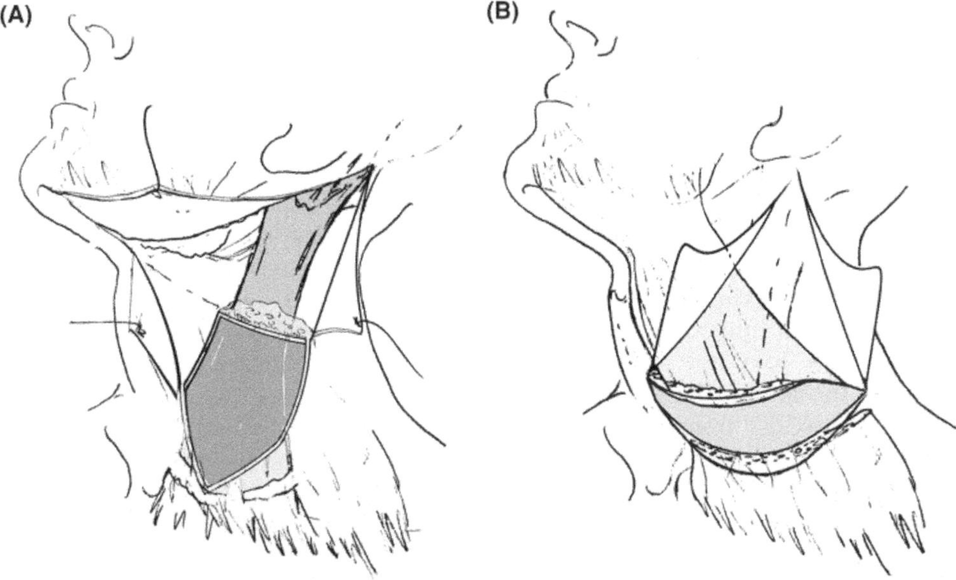

Figure 6 (**A**) Sternocleidomastoid muscle flap and (**B**) Platysma flap elevated prior to rotation into oral cavity.

When utilizing the sternocleidomastoid muscle flap in reconstructing the buccal mucosa, it is essential that the patient be either edentulous or have no posterior molars intact. Rotating this flap into the buccal region requires it to extend over the top of the masticatory regions of the mandible and may limit its utility in buccal mucosal reconstructions. Certainly in patients who have undergone composite resection along with buccal mucosal excision this flap may be useful to reconstruct a posterior composite defect.

The platysma myocutaneous flap, which is a thinner, more pliable flap based on the platysma muscle and overlying skin, can be rotated into the oral cavity through the floor of mouth similar to the sternocleidomastoid muscle. The platysma flap is based on a random blood supply derived from a variety of neck terminal arteries. When using this flap to reconstruct the buccal mucosa, the primary contributing arterial blood supply comes from a submental branch of the facial artery and the superior thyroid artery. The flap includes a skin paddle overlying the platysma muscle itself, as well as the fascia veins and arterial blood supply from the fascia, which overlies the sternocleidomastoid muscle. Attempts should be made to leave the superior thyroid artery contributions intact as the fascia over the sternocleidomastoid muscle is elevated in a lateral to medial direction. When mobilization does require sacrifice of the superior thyroid arterial blood supply, attempts should be made to maintain a wide superior flap base (25–28). This may be ideal in the edentulous patient in which the mandible needs to be wrapped with muscle for intraoral coverage. In a patient in which the mandible remains intact, a supramandibular plane may be appropriate; however, this can put the marginal mandibular branch at risk. Additionally, increasing the torsion of the pedicle may decrease the viability of the cutaneous paddle once it is sutured into the buccal space. Like the sternocleidomastoid flap, this platysma flap would be suitable in patients who have undergone composite resection where the mandible has been resected.

Small submental or submandibular flaps can also be designed to take advantage of the redundant tissues in the submental region. These flaps are laterally based primarily off the superior thyroid artery and adjacent strap muscles (29,30). As with the two previously described flaps these flaps are rotated through the floor of the mouth to gain access to the buccal mucosal space. The cosmetic defect left from these submental flaps is very minimal due to the ability to close this area primarily. The major concern with any of the cervical rotation flaps is the skin coverage loss in the neck region. In patients who have undergone neck dissections as part of the oncologic procedure the removal of skin or skin supported structures such as the platysma can lead to complications in the neck during the time of healing. These flaps are perhaps best utilized in patients who are not to undergo a neck dissection, and who certainly have not had previous radiation therapy to the neck. Metastatic disease to the neck will limit the utility of these flaps as the neck dissection will render the flaps avascular from either an arterial or venous standpoint. However, when these flaps are created in non-radiated non-dissected neck the success rates are reported close to 90% (29,26).

Regional Myocutaneous Flaps

Regional myocutaneous flaps can be utilized in buccal reconstruction in a limited number of cases. The primary utilization of such flaps would be after composite resection in which the flap can be elevated off the chest or back, rotated through the neck into the buccal mucosa without crossing the mandible. The retention of the mandible significantly limits the ability to retain vasculature to the skin paddle of large flaps rotated from the chest. In the absence of an intact mandible, the vascular pedicle is not bridged across a bony surface and will thus most likely survive its transposition into the oral cavity (31). The pectoralis major flap has been a workhorse flap for the reconstruction of all head and neck tumors since the late 1970s early 1980s when it was first co-described by Baek et al. (32,33) and Arian et al. for its uses in head and neck. The limitations of this flap include its bulk as well as its potential limited reach in patients with anatomically long necks and short chest wall. Other limitations include the female patient due to breast tissue, and patients with large amounts of adipose tissue, which significantly affects the blood supply to the skin paddle. The pectoralis myofascial flap, which does not contain a skin paddle, can oftentimes be utilized in place of a myocutaneous flap. The myofascial flap has increased limitations with regard to length, however, in most patients will reach above the mandible into the lower portions of the buccal mucosal region. Some limitations with regard to covering mucosa along an intact mandible or rotating the flap around an intact mandible have been outlined recently in article by Dr. Zbar et al. (34). In early publications, the pectoralis major flap was commonly used to reconstruct buccal mucosal defects after composite resection. Additional regional flaps have been described which can reach the buccal mucosal region including the upper trapezius flap and the lower island trapezius flap (35). Modifications of lower island trapezius flap as discussed by Netterville et al. (36) has increased the survival rate of these flaps allowing elevations to more superior locations on the head and neck. These flaps will reach the buccal mucosal region and, like the pectoralis major flap, are best utilized in a patient after composite mandibular resection has been completed. In most cases a better reconstructive option will exist, including free tissue transfer. The surgical techniques for elevating regional myocutaneous flaps have been well described in a variety of texts and articles over the last two decades. Reiterating the techniques of flaps in this chapter is redundant. However, it should be noted that attempts to utilize myocutaneous flaps in head and neck reconstruction can have a relatively high complication rate. The complication rate is certainly increased when attempts are made to reach superior locations in the oral cavity. In almost all cases in this modern era the buccal mucosal reconstructions are likely to be better accomplished with other options. However, it is useful for the reconstructive surgeon to realize that regional myocutaneous flaps are occasionally a vital option when faced with either failed free tissue transfer or the need to reconstruct defects after recurrent cancer in which the reconstructive options become limited.

Free Tissue Transfer and Buccal Mucosal Reconstruction

As in all areas of the head and neck reconstruction surgery, free tissue transfer has become one of the primary methods of reconstruction. The free tissue transfer options are multiple and allow for larger and more complex defects to be successfully closed. The most common reconstructive method for the buccal mucosa would be the radial forearm free flap (Fig. 7). The radial forearm allows the harvesting of a large vascularized skin paddle, which easily can replace the entire buccal mucosal

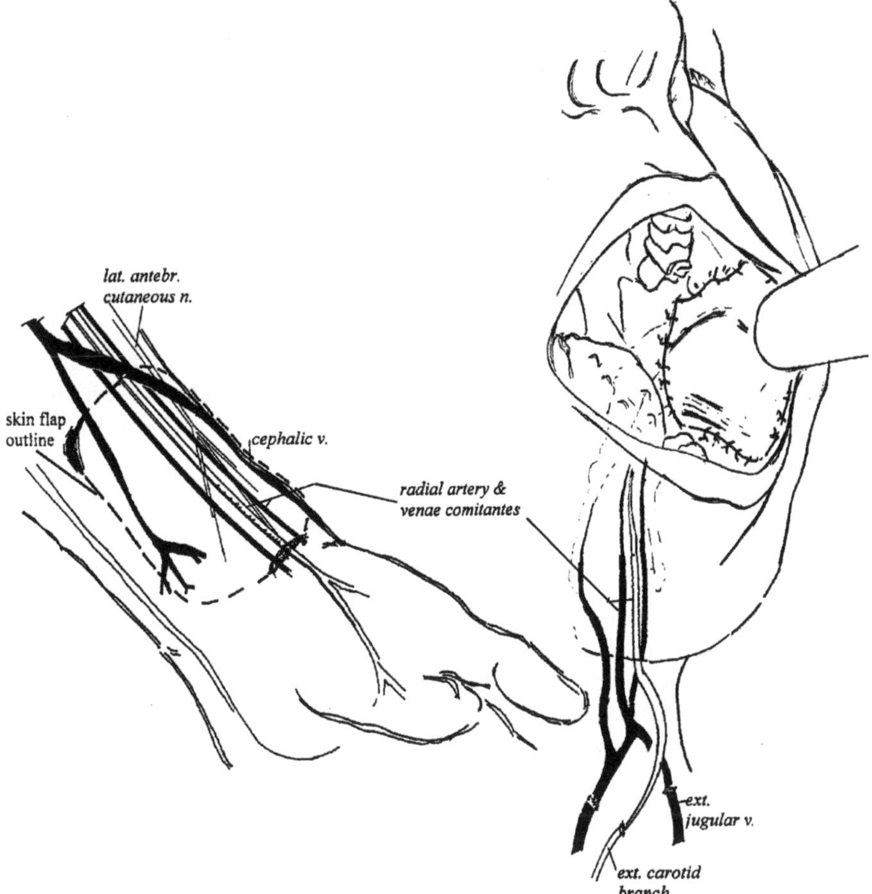

Figure 7 Radial forearm free flap repairing large buccal mucosal defect.

region (37). It is an extremely reliable flap with both a large artery and dual venous outflow. Success rates with radial forearm free flaps in this current era are close to 95% (38). The major disadvantages of this type of technique are the length of time required in surgery, the necessary rehabilitation of the forearm after surgery, and the requirement of microvascular expertise to accomplish this reconstruction. An additional functional limitation is the absence of a normal mucosal lining in the area where the reconstruction was utilized. Any large defect reconstructed with non-mucosal tissues can lead to an absence of elasticity, increased oral dryness in the reconstructed area, and decreased mobility with secondary retention of food products, saliva, or mucous buildup along the reconstructed material. Additional problems occur with scar contracture along the junctions of normal and reconstruction tissue. If a patient is not undergoing post-operative radiation therapy, hair growth on the flap may present a cosmetic nuisance.

The limitations of the reconstruction need to be weighed against the extraordinary advantages of free tissue transfers. It is useful in patients who have undergone previous radiation therapy in that it brings in non-radiated tissue to the region. It also allows for larger resections of radiated tissue to ensure completely adequate margins in tumors with margins that are oftentimes difficult to clear. It does not compromise local tissues that are absolutely necessary for cosmetic and functional reasons within the head and neck. Free tissue transfer techniques can be expanded to close very complex defects including through-and-through defects in which buccal mucosa as well as skin are resected as part of a larger composite resection.

Lateral Arm, Latissimus Dorsi, Rectus Abdominus, and Lateral Thigh Flaps

In addition to the radial forearm free flap other free tissue transfers can be utilized to reconstruct the buccal mucosa. The lateral arm flap may be a reasonable option in that its slightly increased bulk can also fill in a buccal defect that may arise from resection of buccinator muscle and/or buccal fat which if left unreconstructed leads to hollowing of the midface. The lateral arm flap is a well-described flap based on the lateral aspect of the upper forearm which after harvesting leaves little or no cosmetic deficit (39). The microvascular techniques required to elevate and inset this flap are somewhat more complicated than the standard radial forearm free flap due to the fact that the arterial and venous vessels are somewhat small. The pedicle is also slightly shorter and therefore vasculature within the mid to upper neck must be in place in order to utilize this free tissue transfer flap. The anterolateral thigh flap will function in a similar capacity (40). Other larger free tissue transfer flaps such as the latissimus dorsi or the rectus abdominus flap can be utilized to reconstruct very large defects, which include the buccal mucosa but may also include mandibular and floor of mouth resections. These flaps can be folded upon themselves, especially the latissimus dorsi flap, to allow cutaneous closure of both buccal as well as cutaneous defects (41) (Fig. 8). The bulk of this flap is sometimes useful in order to hide the hollowing effects of mandibular or posterior mandibular resection and aggressive composite resections up into the infratemporal fossa region. Even after significant resections and reconstructions, patients who have intact tongue mobility and sensation are frequently able to swallow soft foods and liquids and maintain an oral diet. However, even with these advanced reconstructive techniques, the ability to masticate after such large reconstructions is oftentimes lost.

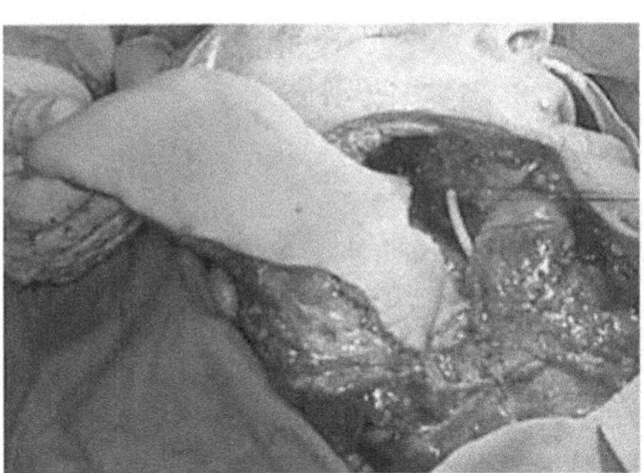

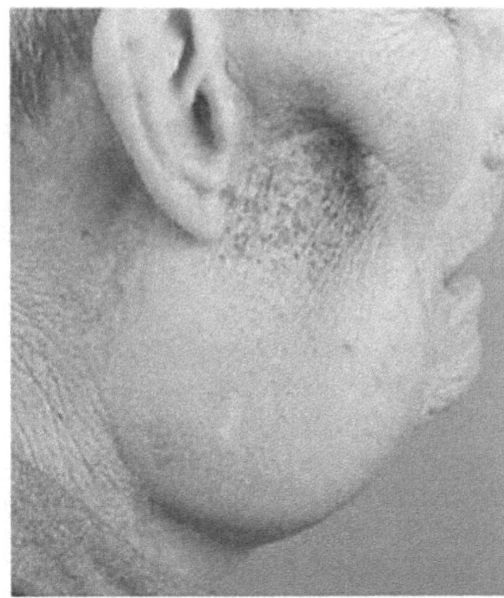

Figure 8 Latissimus free flap used to close through and through defect after resection of buccal mucosa, deep tissue, mandible and skin.

A variety of other free tissues have been described for reconstruction of buccal and oral defects. These include jejunum, colon, and mesentery. The goals of these mucosally lined flaps are to replace tissue with like tissue. Although they may produce less drying in the oral cavity, they certainly lack the mobility characteristic of the normal buccal mucosa, and require harvesting through an intra-abdominal incision. This increase in morbidity in the operative and post-operative periods is typically not worth the limited advantages (42). The techniques of free tissue transfer are well described in a variety of texts and articles and will not be discussed in detail in this particular chapter.

Combined Flaps

In an attempt to prevent cosmetic as well as functional deficits, it is not uncommon to combine flaps when complex defects are created after surgical extirpation of tumor. Cervical facial skin defects can be closed utilizing such techniques as cervical facial rotation flaps with the intraoral defect being closed utilizing free tissue transfer from radial forearm, lateral arm, or rectus muscle. Combining local mucosal flaps, buccal fat rotation and or free grafts may cover many if not all superficial defects.

Reconstruction of the Parotid (Stensen's) Duct

Dealing with the parotid and buccal mucosal reconstruction is essential, especially in cases in which the parotid duct is actually excised. The parotid duct is approximately 4 cm in length extending from its arborization within the parotid to a common duct overlying the masseter muscle and then penetrating the buccal mucosa via Stenson's duct just posterior to the second maxillary molar. The resection of this duct in a non-irradiated patient requires the remaining ductules within the gland to find a different route of egress. If no reconstruction is completed the most common event is the formation of sialoceles, or salivary collections in the subcutaneous periparotid tissues. Additionally, symptoms of duct obstruction will occur, which include salivary swelling, perisalivary soft tissue edema, possible infection, pain, and trismus.

The simplest reconstruction technique involves cannulating the duct, identifying its course toward the parotid gland, and then reanastomosing the duct remnant to the reconstructed oral mucosa in any appropriate location (Fig. 9). The duct should be slightly marsupialized and held open with suture to decrease the risk of stenosis and secondary duct obstruction symptomatology. If larger amounts of the duct require resection such that primary anastomosis is impossible, there are techniques described utilizing vein grafts to reconstitute the duct prior to positioning it within the reconstructed buccal mucosa (43). Mainly these reports are experimental only and large series in humans are not available for review. Certainly parotidectomy is an option that needs to be considered in patients in which large amounts of the duct require resection. This eliminates the need to reconstruct the duct and also increases the margin of resection, including the periparotid lymph nodes as part of the dissection. This may be useful in eliminating the metastatic disease from the buccal mucosa. Access to the parotid gland is oftentimes necessary as part of a planned neck dissection or as part of the resection of the buccal mucosa, especially when larger lesions are identified. Removing the parotid gland and safely identifying the branches of the facial nerve can also eliminate the potential inadvertent risk of cutting the essential branches of the nerve during the tumor resection. After parotidectomy, there is a lower risk of secondary infection from parotid drainage, less risk of sialocele formation, and more available space for reconstructive tissues. In many patients

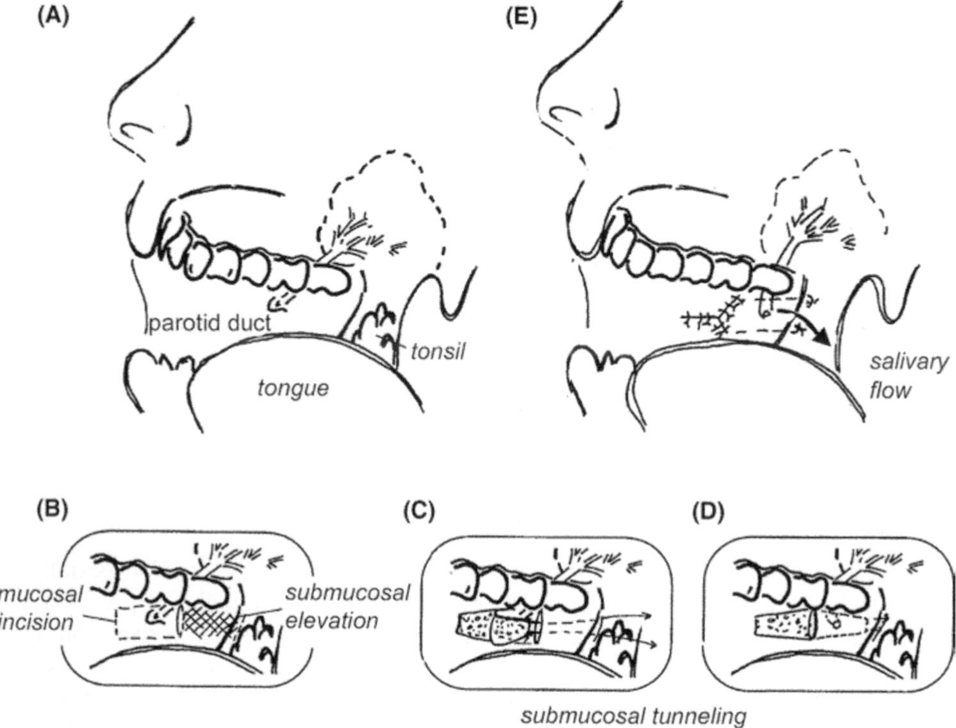

Figure 9A,E Parotid duct posterior reattachment and marsupialization. (*B–D*) Mucosal incisions and rerouting steps (b,c,d)

in which post-operative radiation therapy is planned, the function of the parotid gland itself will be limited and therefore preservation of its function is not essential.

SUMMARY

The most important part of buccal mucosal reconstruction is the ability of the surgeon to have multiple options available at the time the reconstruction is envisioned. As alluded to at the beginning of this chapter, resection of buccal lesions can be more complex than initially anticipated viewing the index lesion in a standard clinic exam. The surgeon should have in place a plan for either a small, medium, or large defect dependent on what the final tumor resection creates (44). The various reconstruction options, advantages, and limitations are outlined in Table 1. In a non-radiated patient, for small defects think first about primary closure or local flaps. For intermediate size and posterior defects think about buccal fat rotation. For large defects and in all radiated patients consider free tissue transfer. The poor local control sited in the review articles may in part be due to a failure of the oncologic surgeon to obtain wide clear margins, lacking a good technique to close the resultant defect. Free tissue transfer should eliminate this fear and hopefully increase cures rates while improving functional outcomes.

REFERENCES

1. DiFiore MSH. Atlas of Human Histology. 4th ed. Philadelphia: Lea & Febiger, 1979: 106–107.
2. Chhetri DK, Rawnsley JD, Calcaterra TC. Carcinoma of the buccal mucosa. Otolaryngol Head Neck Surg 2000; 123(5):566–571.
3. Strome SE, To W, Strawderman M, Gersten K, Devaney KO, Bradford CR, Esclamado RM. Squamous cell carcinoma of the buccal mucosa. Otolaryngol Head Neck Surg 1999; 120(3):375–379.
4. Nair MK, Sankaranarayanan R, Padmanabhan TK. Evaluation of the role of radiotherapy in the management of carcinoma of the buccal mucosa. Cancer 1988; 61:1326–1321.
5. Schramm VL Jr, Myers EN. Skin grafts in oral cavity reconstruction. Arch Otolaryngol 1980; 106(9):528–532.
6. McConnel FM, Teichgraeber JF, Adler RK. A comparison of three methods of oral reconstruction. Arch Otolaryngol Head Neck Surg 1987; 113(5):496–500.
7. Garvey CM, Panje WR, Hoffman HT. The 'parachute' bolster technique for securing intraoral skin grafts. Ear Nose Throat J 2001; 80(10):720–723.
8. Kudo K, Yokota M, Fujioka Y. Immediate reconstruction using a scalp-forehead flap for the entire upper lip defect with the application of lyophilized porcine skin to surgical wounds. A case report of a malignant melanoma in the upper lip and oral mucosa. J Maxillofac Surg 1983; 11(6):275–278.
9. Sinha UK, Chang KE, Shih CW. Reconstruction of pharyngeal defects using AlloDerm and sternocleidomastoid muscle flap. Laryngoscope 2001; 111(11 Pt 1):1910–1916.
10. Rhee PH, Friedman CD, Ridge JA, Kusiak J. The use of processed allograft dermal matrix for intraoral resurfacing: and alternative to split-thickness skin grafts. Arch Otolaryngol Head Neck Surg 1998; 124(11):1201–1204.
11. Eppley BL, Keating M, Rink R. A buccal mucosal harvesting technique for urethral reconstruction. J Urol 1997; 157(4):1268–1270.
12. Whetzel TP, Saunders CJ. Arterial anatomy of the oral cavity: an analysis of vascular territories. Plast Reconst Surg 1997; 100(3):582–587; discussion 588–590.

13. Komisar A, Lawson W. A compendium of intraoral flaps. Head Neck Surg 1985; 8(2): 91–99.
14. Rapidis AD, Alexandridis CA, Eleftheriadis E. Angelopoulos Associate Professor. The use of the buccal fat pad for reconstruction of oral defects: review of the literature and report of 15 cases. J Oral Maxillofac Surg 2000; 58(2):158–163.
15. Marx RE. Discussion. J Oral Maxillofac Surg 1988; 46(10):105.
16. Millard DR. Forehead flap in immediate repair of head, face, and jaw. Am J Surg 1964; 108:508.
17. McGregor IA. The temporal flap in intraoral cancer; its use in repairing the post-excisional defect. Br J Plast Surg 1963; 16:318–335.
18. Temporoparietal fascia flap. In: Hoffman HT, Funk G, McCulloch TM, Graham SM, Dawson C, Fitzpatrick K, Karnell MP, eds. Iowa Head and Neck Protocols: Surgery, Nursing, and Speech Pathology. San Diego: Singular Publishing Group, 2000:393–403.
19. Abul-Hassan HS, Ascher GVD, Acland RD. Surgical anatomy and blood supply of the fascial layers of the temporal region. Plast Reconst Surg 1986; 77:17–24.
20. Cheney ML, Varvares MA, Nadol JB. The temporoparietal fascial flap in head and neck reconstruction. Arch Otolaryngol Head Neck Surg 1993; 119(6):618–623.
21. Antonyshyn O, Gruss JS, Birt BD. Versatility of temporal muscle and fascial flaps. Br J Plast Surg 1988; 41(2):118–131.
22. Koranda FC, McMahon MF. The temporalis muscle flap for intraoral reconstruction: technical modifications. Otolaryngol Head Neck Surg 1988; 98(4):315–318.
23. Hanasono MM, Utley DS, Goode RL. The temporalis muscle flap for reconstruction after head and neck oncologic surgery. Laryngoscope 2001; 111(10):1719–1725.
24. Yugueros P, Woods JE. The sternocleidomastoid myocutaneous flap: a reappraisal. Br J Plast Surg 1996; 49(2):93–96.
25. Coleman JJ III, Jurkiewicz MJ, Nahai F, Mathes SJ. The platysma musculocutaneous flap: experience with 24 cases. Plast Reconst Surg 1983; 72(3):315–323.
26. Esclamado RM, Burkey BB, Carroll WR, Bradford CR. The platysma myocutaneous flap indications and caveats. Arch Otolaryngol Head Neck Surg 1994; 120(1): 32–35.
27. Hurwitz DJ, Rabson JA, Futrell JW. The anatomic basis for the platysma skin flap. Plast Reconst Surg 1983; 72(3):302–314.
28. Platysma flap. In: Hoffman HT, Funk G, McCulloch TM, Graham SM, Dawson C, Fitzpatrick K, Karnell MP, eds. Iowa Head and Neck Protocols: Surgery, Nursing, and Speech Pathology. San Diego: Singular Publishing Group, 2000:388–392.
29. Zhao YF, Zhang WF, Zhao JH. Reconstruction of intraoral defects after cancer surgery using cervical pedicle flaps. J Oral Maxillofac Surg 2001; 59(10):1142–1146.
30. Wang HS, Shen JW, Ma DB, Wang JD, Tian AL. The infrahyoid myocutaneous flap for reconstruction after resection of head and neck cancer. Cancer 1986; 57(3): 663–668.
31. Bhathena HM, Kavarana NM. The folded, bipaddled pectoralis major composite flap in oral cancer reconstruction. Br J Plast Surg 1989; 42(4):441–446.
32. Baek S, Biller HF, Krespi YP, Lawson W. The pectoralis major myocutaneous island flap for reconstruction of the head and neck. Head Neck Surg 1979; 1(4):293–300.
33. Ariyan S. The pectoralis major myocutaneous flap. A versatile flap for reconstruction in the head and neck. Plast Reconstr Surg 1979; 63(1):73–81.
34. Zbar RI, Funk GF, McCulloch TM, Graham SM, Hoffman HT. Pectoralis major myofascial flap: a valuable tool in contemporary head and neck reconstruction. Head Neck 1997; 19(5):412–418.
35. Cummings CW, Eisele DW, Coltrera MD. Lower trapezius myocutaneous island flap. Arch Otolaryngol Head Neck Surg 1989; 115(10):1181–1185.
36. Netterville JL, Wood DE. The lower trapezius flap. Vascular anatomy and surgical technique. Arch Otolaryngol Head Neck Surg 1991; 117(1):73–76.

37. Savant DN, Patel SG, Deshmukh SP, Gujarati R, Bhathena HM, Kavarana NM. Folded free radial forearm flap for reconstruction of full-thickness defects of the cheek. Head Neck 1995; 17(4):293–296.
38. Haughey BH, Wilson E, Kluwe L, Piccirillo J, Fredrickson J, Sessions D, Spector G. Free flap reconstruction of the head and neck: analysis of 241 cases. Otolaryngol Head Neck Surg 2001; 125(1):10–17.
39. Gellrich NC, Schramm A, Hara I, Gutwald R, Duker J, Schmelzeisen R. Versatility and donor site morbidity of the lateral upper arm flap in intraoral reconstruction. Otolaryngol Head Neck Surg 2001; 124(5):549–555.
40. Cipriani R, Contedini F, Caliceti U, Cavina C. Three-dimensional reconstruction of the oral cavity using the free anterolateral thigh flap. Plast Reconstr Surg 2002; 109(1):53–57.
41. Clovutivat V. Reconstruction of cheek and buccal mucosa with latissimus dorsi musculocutaneous flap. Ann Acad Med Singapore 1980; 9(3):342–346.
42. Smith G, Brennan P, Scott P, Ilankovan V. Outcome after radial forearm, gastroomental, and jejunal free flaps in oral and oropharyngeal reconstruction. Br J Oral Maxillofac Surg 2002; 40(4):330.
43. Heymans O, Nelissen X, Medot M, Fissette J. Microsurgical repair of Stensen's duct using an interposition vein graft. J Reconstr Microsurg 1999; 15(2):105–107; discussion 107–108.
44. Lutz BS, Wei FC. Microsurgical reconstruction of the buccal mucosa. Clin Plast Surg 2001; 28(2):339–347, ix.

10
Ventral Tongue and Floor of Mouth

Brian B. Burkey
Department of Otolaryngology—Head and Neck Surgery, Vanderbilt University, Nashville, Tennessee, U.S.A.

C. W. David Chang
Department of Otolaryngology, University of Missouri, Columbia, Missouri, U.S.A.

INTRODUCTION

The floor of mouth (FOM) is a common site requiring reconstruction following tumor extirpation. Regarding frequency of lesions occurring in the oral cavity, the FOM is second only to the oral tongue. Squamous cell carcinomas comprise the majority (90–95%) of these lesions (1). Other neoplasms include minor salivary gland tumors, sarcomas, and lymphoid tumors. For further details on pathologies of the oral cavity, see chapters 4 and 5: Pathology and Pathophysiology of the Oral Cavity–Neoplastic Diseases and Benign Lesions and Tumors of the Oral Cavity, respectively.

The FOM encompasses an area between the tongue and the lingual surface of the mandible. The bulk of the FOM bed is composed of the genioglossus and the mylohyoid muscles. Both the lingual and the hypoglossal nerves cross through this region. The submandibular (Wharton's) duct courses between these nerves. Anteriorly, the distal extent of the submandibular ducts is marked by two papillae, which lie on either side of the lingual frenulum. The mucosa overlying the FOM is redundant and quite extensible, permitting maximal tongue mobility. The mucosa drapes laterally to create a gingivolingual sulcus that lies in a more dependant position compared to the anterior FOM. For more information on the anatomy of the oral cavity, review chapter 2: Applied Anatomy of the Oral Cavity and Related Structures.

EVALUATION AND PLANNING

Evaluation of a FOM lesion demands a thorough head and neck exam. Classically a bimanual examination is used to palpate the size and extent of FOM lesions. Lymphatic drainage of anterior FOM is primarily in the submandibular and submental regions, whereas the lateral FOM may drain to the jugular nodal chain. Degree of tongue mobility and lesion mobility will provide clues as to the extent of tongue and FOM musculature involvement. A CT-scan may be helpful to assess mandible invasion, although this is better determined intraoperatively. Because greater than

20% of patients with FOM lesions may have synchronous tumors elsewhere in the aerodigestive tract, it is imperative to fully evaluate each patient with triple endoscopy. Chapter 6: Planning and Diagnostic Evaluation in Oral Cavity Reconstruction provides more instruction on examination and evaluation of the oral cavity.

RECONSTRUCTIVE OPTIONS

This chapter will discuss various reconstructive modalities involving the FOM and ventral tongue without the need for osseus replacement (Table 1). Historically, a multiplicity of techniques have been utilized. The options presented here form a collection of the most commonly performed methods.

Tumor size and characteristics will determine the extent of resection and influence the type of reconstruction modality used. Tumors lying adjacent to the mandible but not breaching the bony cortex can be safely removed via a marginal mandibulectomy. More osteo-invasive masses may require a segmental mandibulectomy for adequate oncologic margins. Care must be taken during resection to spare the lingual and hypoglossal nerves, if possible. Wharton's duct may need to be rerouted and reimplanted to prevent obstructive sialadenitis, inflammation or infection of the salivary gland or duct, if the papilla is excised during the course of tumor extirpation. Chapter 7: Surgical Approaches to the Oral Cavity provides background for these techniques.

The primary goals of FOM reconstruction include the need to preserve or restore normal speech, mastication and swallowing function and provide a barrier between the oral cavity and neck. The occasional, small defect resulting from benign disease may be a candidate for primary closure. However, the majority of FOM defects will require the interposition of soft tissue to recreate the native anatomic configuration of structures and to maintain near-normal tongue mobility. Other reconstructive possibilities such as the dorsalis pedis free flap, pectoralis major pedicled flap, and the buccal myomucosal flap be rarely employed for FOM defects and will not be discussed.

Split-Thickness Skin Graft

Oncologically sound resection of cancerous lesions along the FOM frequently involves the removal of a considerable amount of tissue. The resulting defect, if closed primarily, would result in functional disability due to restriction of mobile tissue, specifically the lingual tongue. If left to close by secondary intent, the unpredictable formation of subsequent scarring and granulation tissue would likewise

Table 1 Common Reconstructive Techniques for the Floor of the Mouth and Ventral Tongue Defects

Split-thickness skin graft
Allograft
Platysma flap
Submental flap
Nasolabial flap
Radial forearm free flap
Lateral arm flap

cause oral impairment. Placement of a split-thickness skin graft (STSG) provides a fast and simple means of reconstruction while preserving residual function.

Anatomy and Surgical Technique

Generally, free-skin grafts exist as full-thickness grafts and split-thickness grafts. Full thickness grafts consist of dermis, epidermis, and other appendages from the donor site including hair follicles, the latter being undesirable in oral reconstruction. STSGs are composed of the epidermis and only part of the dermal layer, leaving adnexal remnants, pilosebaceous follicles, and glands at the donor site. Epithelial cells left within these units multiply and emerge to resurface the donor site. However, donor sites of full-thickness grafts cannot re-epithelialize and must be closed primarily, covered with a STSG, or left to granulate. Full-thickness grafts can be harvested from natural creases, such as the axilla or groin, or areas of skin redundancy such as the post-auricular area, the supraclavicular region, and the upper eyelid, leaving minimal cosmetic deformity.

The STSG can be harvested from various areas but most commonly has been taken from the lateral thigh, which provides a large and relatively inconspicuous surface area. A power-driven dermatome (Brown dermatome) is used to cut the graft, and STSGs can be harvested in various thicknesses, typically 0.016–0.018 in. At this depth, the cleavage plane is below the papillary dermis but is superficial to the reticular dermis. In theory, a thinner graft has a greater chance of survival but exhibits a greater degree of contraction due to its paucity of underlying dermal scaffolding (3). The graft is best designed slightly (~25%) larger than the defect to compensate for subsequent post-operative contracture. A template of foil or paper can be used to shape the graft.

Survival of the graft requires rapid neovascularization from the recipient bed. During the initial 48–72 hours after grafting, the STSG survives by plasmatic imbibition, whereby vital nutrients from the bed diffuse into the overlying skin graft (4). During this time, capillaries bud to vascularize the graft. For this process to occur successfully, three principles must be observed. First, the recipient bed itself must be well vascularized. Second, the donor skin must well approximate the recipient bed. Finally, the graft must be rendered immobile to prevent shearing of newly formed capillaries. Poor recipient sites, such as bare cortical bone, lack good vascularity. Preservation of the periosteum is ideal for skin graft survival over bone. Alternatively, the bone may be prepared by superficial cortical removal with a fine diamond or cutting burr to improve vascularity. Histologically, the grafted skin maintains its characteristic keratinizing epithelium, and does not transform into mucosa (5). Radiated tissue represents a poor recipient bed and split-thickness skin grafts, in these circumstances, is not optimal and in many cases, is contraindicated or likely to fail.

Prior to graft placement, the recipient bed must exhibit adequate hemostasis. If an underlying hematoma develops, it becomes a barrier to capillary in growth. The skin graft must be large enough to completely line the defect without tension, which can result in "tenting" and inadequate contact between the bed and the graft. Likewise, redundancy of the graft may result in the graft folding upon itself with poor tissue approximation and graft failure. Quilting stitches may be used to insure coaptation (6). The graft is inset into the cavity and sutured in place along the cut mucosal edges of the defect. Multiple silk sutures are sewn adjacent to the graft to fasten a bolster over the STSG. The bolster, commonly made of cotton balls soaked in mineral oil and wrapped with antibiotic impregnated gauze (Xeroform), is fashioned to conform to the contours of the defect and is placed over the graft as a pressure dressing. This serves to prevent blood and serum accumulation beneath the graft and to provide graft immobilization. Small through-and-through slits may be cut sparingly throughout the graft to allow the escape of underlying fluid. The bolster is removed after 5–7 days, and during this time, the patient may be fed via nasogastric tube, if necessary. Aggressive oral hygiene should be maintained with appropriate oral rinses and wound care until healing is complete. Antibiotics should be considered due to the potential for surrounding salivary contamination.

Indications (Table 2)

Indications for the use of a STSG vary widely among surgeons. Regarding the minimum size of defect, agreement is fairly universal that a skin graft should be used for FOM lesions that just exceed resection dimensions that could be closed primarily without impeding function. In contrast, some proponents of skin grafting suggest that the defect size is not a restriction provided that the resection does not involve extreme loss of bulk, as in cases of segmental mandibulectomy or total or near-total glossectomy (7–9). For example, Schramm et al. (9) describes using STSGs, even when the defect is in continuity with a neck dissection. In his work with these high-risk patients, only two (7%) patients developed fistulae in their series, one of whom was a debilitated, chronic alcoholic who had previously undergone radiation therapy. Teichgraeber et al. (10) also described no ill effects in patients with in-continuity defects. Typically, in our experience through-and-through defects are more reliably reconstructed with vascularized flaps.

STSG survival has been described to be greater than 90% overall. In a later paper by Schramm and colleagues (8), 48 patients with superficial squamous cell carcinoma of the anterior FOM (including 19 with marginal mandibulectomy) had reconstruction with a STSG. Only two patients had partial loss of the graft and no complete losses were encountered. Alvi et al. (7) reported only one graft loss in their series of 18 patients who had marginal mandibulectomy. None of the patients in this study had prior radiation therapy. Pre-operative radiation therapy is a relative contraindication to STSG reconstruction when used to resurface irradiated bone (8). Prior radiation may impede survival of the skin graft, risking the mandible to osteomyelitis, sequestration, and pathologic fracture (11). We and other surgeons avoid use of STSG in any previously irradiated area such as the mandible (10,12).

Functional results of STSGs are controversial. Replacement of tissue volume lost from tumor extirpation with adynamic bulk provided by a flap is not necessarily desirable. Being quite thin and low profile, a skin graft does not interfere with tongue movement, as would functionless, bulky tissue. Proponents argue that with anterior FOM lesions, speech and swallowing are virtually left unimpaired unless resection involves the anterior portion of the tongue (8). In patients who underwent oral resection with

Table 2 Split-Thickness Skin Graft

Advantages	Disadvantages
Unlimited source	Postoperative graft contracture
Fast, easy to perform	Avascular, less predictable "take"
	Not well suited for coverage over irradiated mandible

marginal mandibulectomy and STSG reconstruction, Alvi et al. (7) found 94% could tolerate a soft or regular diet and 94% had intelligible speech at last follow up. McConnel et al. (13) found that STSG reconstruction provided the best oral function in patients with T2 or T3 tongue and/or FOM lesions when compared to tongue flap and pectoralis major flap reconstruction. In addition, a STSG will not blunt the alveolar-lingual sulcus, as would bulky tissue, allowing room for the use of dentures.

However, it is generally agreed that STSGs undergo a considerable amount of contracture, as much as 30–50%. Because of this shrinkage, late post-operative tethering of the tongue and resultant impaired mobility is likely. To compensate, the surgeon must use a generous amount of graft material that will easily resurface the defect. However, care must be taken not to use such an overly redundant piece that cannot be in complete contact with the surgical bed.

Acellular Allograft Dermal Matrix (Table 3)

Contracture and donor site morbidity, two disadvantages of STSG technique, can potentially be avoided through the use of an acellular allograft dermal matrix, which also results in a mucosally covered graft (Alloderm, Lifecell Corporation, Branchburg, New Jersey). This material is derived from human allograft skin, processed to reduce the immunogenicity of its biomaterial components. Rhee et al. (14) found that the use of Alloderm instead of STSG in primary oral reconstructions of 29 patients (four of whom had FOM defects) resulted in only one case of contracture, which was observed in the area of tumor recurrence. In this study, the rate-of-take was 90% despite the authors' strict definition of failure as any evidence of incomplete graft re-epithelialization. The allograft dermis serves as scaffolding that permits the migration of peripheral cells to resurface the defect while preventing contracture.

The surgical technique for the application of Alloderm in the oral cavity is identical to that of skin grafting for recipient bed preparation, securing the graft and post operative care. The material is available in various thicknesses for a number of applications, however, in the oral cavity it is important to utilize the thinnest material available (0.007–0.03 in). Many surgeons now consider Alloderm as first-line grafting material for oral cavity applications that require skin grafting.

Platysma Myocutaneous Flap

Introduced in 1978 by Futrell et al. (15) the platysma myocutaneous flap provides thin, pliable, and relatively hairless tissue which may be optimal for reconstructing FOM defects. It is particularly useful for defects that are continuous with the neck

Table 3 Acellular Alloplastic Dermal Graft

Advantages	Disadvantages
Unlimited source	Limited postoperative graft contracture
No donor site morbidity	Avascular, less predictable "take"
Results in non-keratinized mucosal covering	Not well suited for coverage over irradiated mandible

dissection. Because of its somewhat tenuous survival in some series, this flap has enjoyed only limited popularity. Because of its relative ease of elevation and low donor-site morbidity, the platysma flap should not be overlooked as a reconstructive option for both functional and cosmetic reasons.

Anatomy and Surgical Technique

The platysma is a thin muscle that lies in continuity with the superficial muscular aponeurotic system superiorly and extends inferiorly to below the clavicle. Development of this muscle varies in each individual, but rarely is this muscle absent (16). The long, broad shape of this muscle permits the harvesting of a myocutaneous flap with a fairly long pedicle.

The blood supply to the platysma flap is essentially random, although the submental artery is the major nutrient source (17). This artery branches from the facial artery, usually anterior to the submandibular gland, and courses beneath the inferior border of the mandible. In cadaveric studies, anastomoses of the distal submental artery with the lingual, inferior labial, and contralateral facial arteries were observed. This network in turn is connected by a rich anastomotic arterial web over the nasolabial and cheek region (18,19). Therefore, retrograde filling of the submental artery may be possible even if the ipsilateral facial artery is sacrificed during the neck dissection. However, for optimal survival of this flap, these vessels should be preserved. The transverse cervical, thyroid, occipital, and post auricular vessels also supply the platysma, although their connections are usually severed during flap elevation. The major venous drainage for the platysma is the external jugular vein followed by the submental vein (19).

Neck incisions must be carefully planned to preserve the vasculature of the platysma flap (Fig. 1). A low apron neck incision should be used, and upper neck incisions should be avoided, as they would divide the muscular pedicle. A horizontal supraclavicular skin ellipse large enough to accommodate the FOM defect is outlined here. Typical dimensions of the skin paddle are not much larger than $7 \times 10\,\mathrm{cm}$ or approximately $70\,\mathrm{cm}^2$. An incision through both the skin and platysma is made along the inferior margin of the skin paddle. The incision along the superior border of the paddle is made through the skin only. Dissection superior to the paddle is elevated along a subcutaneous plane. Some surgeons advocate leaving as much subcutaneous fat as possible adjacent to the platysma to reduce risk of injuring the muscle and its vasculature during dissection (16). Inferior to the paddle, the myocutaneous flap is dissected along a subplatysmal plane and raised superiorly to the inferior mandibular margin, taking care not to injure the submental artery or the marginal mandibular branch of the facial nerve. The submental artery is usually not visualized during the procedure. Preservation of the external jugular vein along the deep surface of the flap has been advocated to facilitate proper venous drainage (17,20–24).

The myocutaneous flap can be inset through the defect or in a tunnel created beneath the mandible. The muscular pedicle should not be twisted but rather folded back upon itself as the skin paddle is delivered to the oral defect. The flap is sewn into place using absorbable sutures. The donor defect is closed primarily.

Indications (Table 4)

The reliability of the platysma flap has always been in question. The reported flap survival rates range from 80% to 95%; although, flap morbidity—which includes

(A)

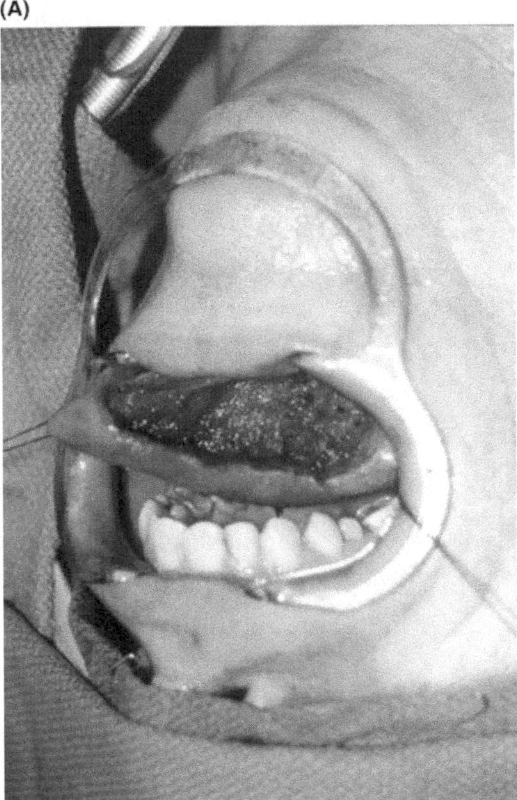

Figure 1A–E Platysma flap repair. (**A**) After tumor resection, a ventro-lateral tongue defect remains.

partial skin necrosis, epidermolysis, and fistula formation—varies widely from 10% to 50% (16,18,20–28). Some authors have reported that prior radiation therapy, radical neck dissection, and ligation of the facial artery are contraindications to the use of the platysma flap; however, these issues remain controversial. Historically the platysma flap is less robust than other reconstructive options and surgeons have sought various exclusionary criteria to improve success rates and reduce complications.

Preservation of the facial artery as a requirement for adequate flap perfusion has both proponents and detractors. Conley et al. (27) reported that ligation of the facial artery resulted in flap loss in 40% of their patients. Others have avoided use of this flap in patients requiring a radical neck dissection, as it would involve the sacrifice of the facial artery (16,20). However, McGuirt et al. (18) refuted this contraindication: in a series of 20 patients, of which 19 had sacrifice of the facial artery, no flap loss occurred. A 50–60% skin paddle necrosis with no underlying platysma muscle loss was noted in one patient. Also observed were two cases of fistulae and two cases of intraoral wound separation, both of which did not require surgical intervention. Ruark et al. (24) reported no flap loss and a complication rate of only 19% in their series of 41 patients, all of whom had facial artery ligation. Also included in their study population were patients who required a lip-splitting approach for tumor extirpation, which theoretically would partially disrupt

(B)

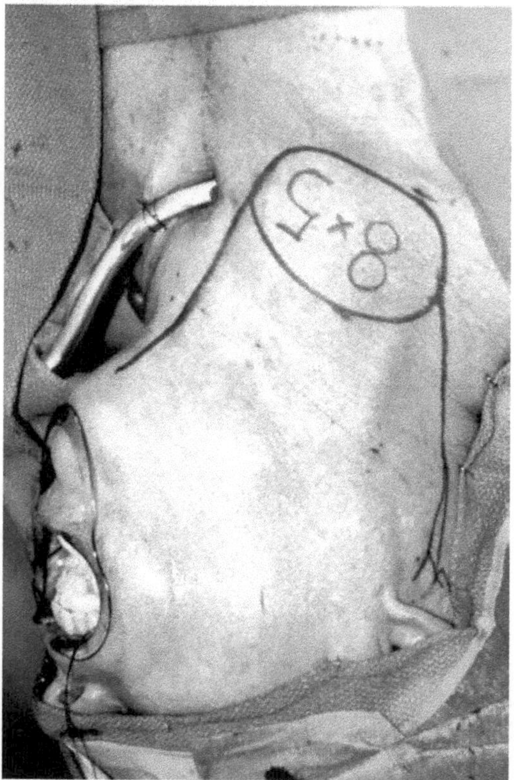

Figure 1 (**B**) An apron neck incision incorporating the platysma flap is planned.

collateral blood supply. Other authors have reported similar findings of flap survival despite radical neck dissection and/or facial artery sacrifice (26,28).

Previous radiotherapy has been examined as a possible contraindication for use of this flap. As the platysma flap is located within the radiation field of head and neck cancer patients, radiotherapy may result in post-radiation arteritis and atrophy of underlying muscle, jeopardizing its function as a vascular pedicle; however, evidence for this assertion is inconclusive. Verschuur et al. (20) reported partial necrosis of the flap in two of their patients early in their study and subsequently excluded irradiated patients as candidates for platysma flap reconstruction. Other studies have likewise excluded previously irradiated patients (28). In contrast, numerous other reports conclude that radiation has no effect upon complication rate or flap viability (16,25,26).

Similarly, previous neck dissection has been looked upon as a contraindication for flap reconstruction. Scarring and fibrosis from previous surgery has been cited as reasons that may compromise platysma vascularity. However, again McGuirt et al. (18) argues that as long as previous incisional lines do not violate the muscular pedicle, use of the platysma flap was acceptable. In their study, two patients who previously received radical neck dissections had no post-operative complications.

Venous drainage appears to be a problem widely noted after transfer of this flap. Some authors have noted discoloration of the flap with temporary venous congestion early in the post-operative period that spontaneously resolves (12,22,25). As

(C)

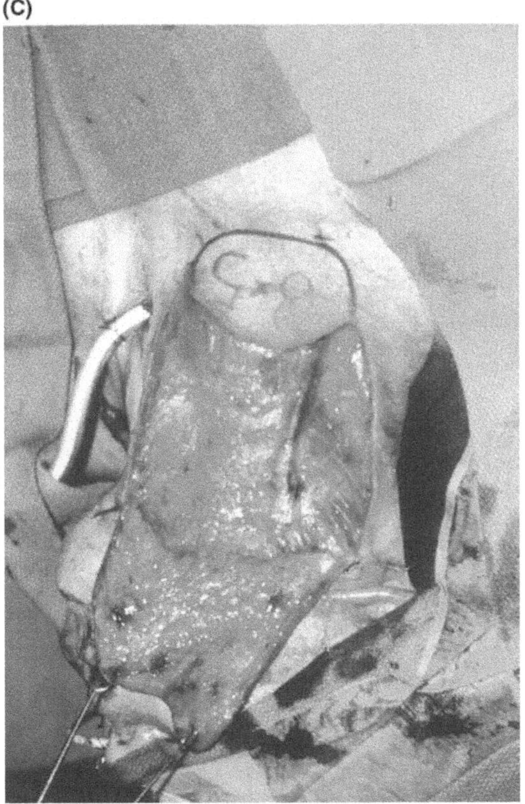

Figure 1 (C) Superior to the flap, the skin is raised along a subcutaneous plane.

the external jugular vein is the primary venous return for the flap, its preservation may alleviate this problem. Venous valves do not appear to impede flow, because the vessels do not usually distend during flap elevation, suggesting adequate outflow (17,24). Presently, conclusive evidence does not exists to show increased flap survival with the retention of the external jugular vein.

One of the greatest advantages of the platysma flap lies in its convenience. The donor site is in close proximity to the oral cavity and is indeed often already draped into the surgical field. The donor site is usually easily closed, especially in elderly patients who have a significant amount of skin laxity. Post radiation skin changes in the neck however may hinder proper mobilization of the surrounding skin (24). Cosmetic deformity is minimal because the donor site can be hidden within a relaxed skin tension line of the neck. The flap itself provides thin pliable tissue with minimal bulk. This facilitates recreation of the lingual-alveolar sulcus, preventing ankyloglossia and restriction of tongue mobility.

As the above discussion suggests, it is difficult to establish a consensus regarding contraindications for use of the platysma flap. Many literature attests to the robustness of the flap under varying circumstances. However, we look upon previous radiation therapy, previous neck surgery, and ligation of the facial artery as potential insulting factors that decrease the chances of flap survival. Thus, avoidance of these factors is optimal. In our experience, the platysma flap is finicky and is best used in ideal situations. Otherwise, an alternative method of reconstruction should be sought.

(D)

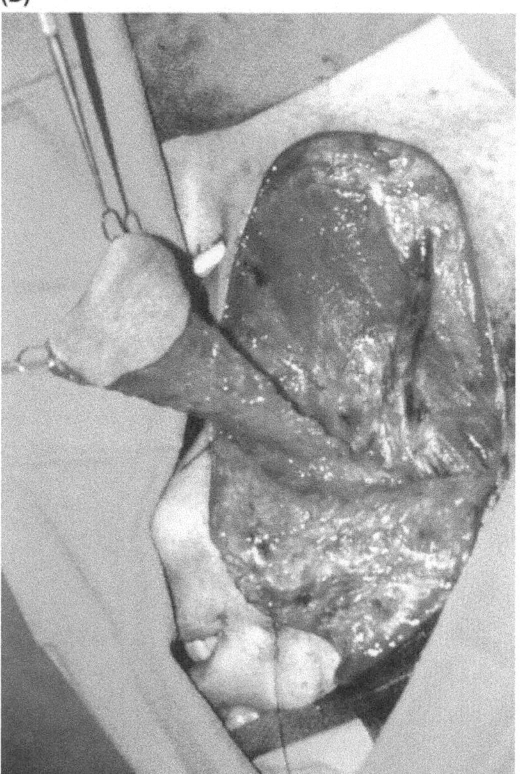

Figure 1 (**D**) The underlying platysma is then freed and the flap is mobilized into position.

Submental Island Flap

The submental flap attempts to capitalize on the advantages of the platysma flap, notably its accessibility and the minimal functional and cosmetic morbidity of the donor site, while seeking to improve flap reliability. As introduced by Martin et al. (29) in 1993, the flap may be used as a pedicled island flap or as a free flap. For reconstructing FOM defects, its proximity is sufficient for use as a pedicled flap.

Anatomy and Surgical Technique

The arterial blood supply to the submental flap is axial and provided directly by the submental branch of the facial artery. From cadaveric studies, we know that the submental artery typically arises 5.0–6.5 cm from the origin of the facial artery and has a diameter of 3–5 mm (29). The artery runs deep to the anterior belly of the digastric muscle in 70% of patients (30). Perforating branches then pierce the muscle to feed the overlying musculocutaneous region, which has been measured from injection studies to supply a skin flap ranging from 4×5 to 10×16 cm (29,30).

Typically the flap is raised as an elliptical-shaped musculocutaneous flap (Fig. 2). Superiorly, the border lies at least 1 cm behind the mandible to keep the scar hidden. The lateral extent lies just beneath the angles of the mandible. The inferior limit is assessed by the "pinch" test, which determines by the amount of skin that can be taken in the flap and still allow primary closure. A larger skin paddle can be harvested from elderly patients due to greater skin laxity.

(E)

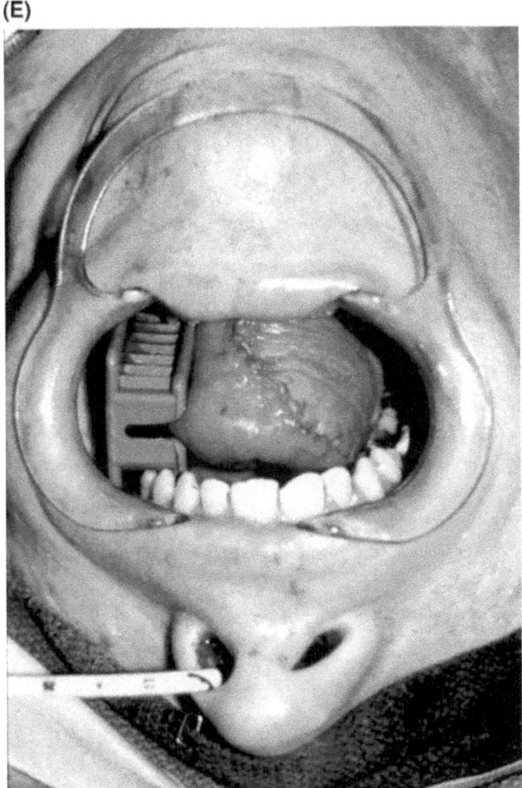

Figure 1 (E) The inset platysma flap provides adequate resurfacing of the ventral tongue.

During dissection of the flap, the ipsilateral anterior belly of the digastric muscle is taken with the flap because it is closely associated with the submental artery as previously mentioned. Although in their original paper, Martin et al. (29,31) did not perform this technique, in a subsequent review, Martin and colleagues advocated inclusion of the digastric muscle in the flap. In addition to the ipsilateral digastric muscle, skin, subcutaneous tissue, and platysma are included in the flap. Ideally, it is raised as thick as possible to insure maximal vascular preservation. Care must be taken to identify and preserve the marginal mandibular nerve when dissecting along the superior flap border.

The pedicle consists of the submental artery and vein. Mobilization of the flap is achieved by dissecting its arterial supply to the origin of the facial artery. The length of the submental vein is the limiting factor in pedicle length, although an

Table 4 Platysma Flap

Advantages	Disadvantages
Very thin, pliable; approximates thickness of mucosa	Flap survival possibly compromised by previous XRT, surgery, facial artery sacrifice
Simple elevation	Tenuous survival
Little cosmetic/functional donor-site morbidity	Random blood supply
	May be hair-bearing in men
Located in the surgical field	

(A)

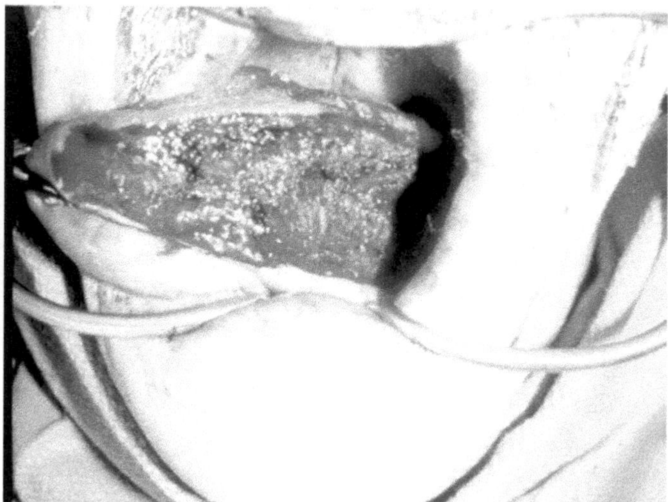

(B)

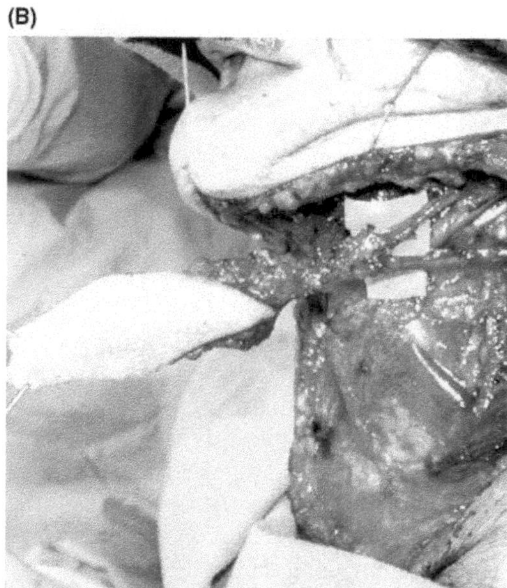

Figure 2A–D Submental flap repair. (**A**) The floor of mouth and lateral tongue defect involves a moderate amount of tissue loss. (**B**) After flap elevation, the pedicle, which is composed of the submental artery and submental vein, can be visualized against the blue background.

8-cm pedicle is possible with venous modification (29). With such close proximity to the donor site, pedicle length is usually not a concern in FOM reconstruction.

The facial artery will require proximal dissection through the submandibular gland to provide adequate pedicle length and mobilization. Removal of the submandibular gland also facilitates passage of the widely based flap into the oral cavity even if not removed for oncologic purposes. The donor site is closed primarily. A minor degree of undermining may be necessary to facilitate closure. The overlying skin can be sutured to the hyoid to recreate the cervicomental angle.

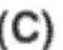

(C)

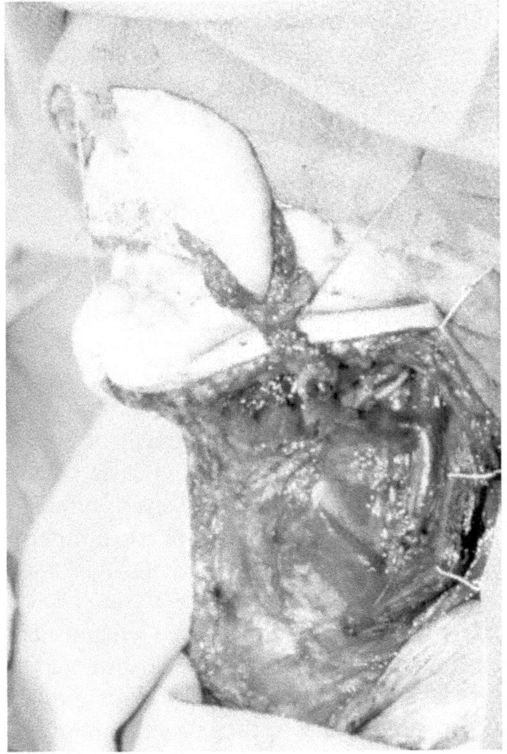

Figure 2 (C) The large arc of rotation and pedicle length demonstrate the ease with which the flap can reach virtually all areas of the oral cavity.

(D)

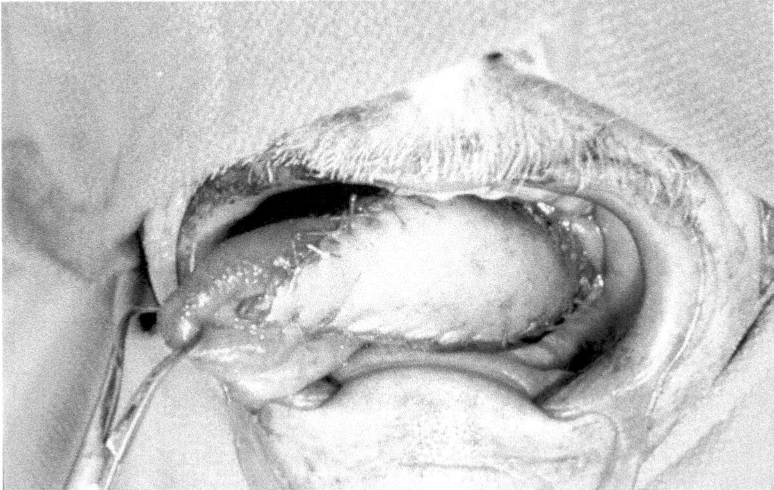

Figure 2 (D) The flap provides a mild amount of bulk.

Indications (Table 5)

Because the submental island flap receives direct vascularization by a named artery, it tends to be more robust than the platysma flap. Martin et al. (29) presented eight cases in which this flap was used and reported only one post-operative hematoma. The digastric muscle was not taken with the flap in this population. Yilmaz et al. (32) used the flap for reconstruction in 14 cases (none for FOM defects). In only three cases in which the digastric muscle taken, all flaps survived. Vural et al. (33) described its use in nine patients (two with FOM defects) and reported one partial loss. In their series of 12 patients, Sterne et al. (34) reported one hematoma, one partial loss (<5%), and one case of complete flap loss, which occurred in a flap that was raised in a reverse flow manner. These articles attest to the reliability of the flap and its constant vascular pedicle, which has been borne out in the current authors' experience.

The harvesting of the submental flap leaves little cosmetic concern. The donor site incision is relatively inconspicuous on the undersurface of the submental triangle. Furthermore the excision of excess skin may also have the added benefit of eliminating submental rhytids and excess adipose tissue. Unfortunately the close proximity of the submental flap to the lymphatic outflow of the oral cavity is a detriment. The submental (Ia) and submandibular (Ib) regions comprise the lymphatic drainage basin for anterior FOM and tongue malignancies. Use of the submental flap may compromise a thorough neck dissection, as nodal remnants may be elevated with the flap or left adjacent to the arterial pedicle. The flap should be used when nodal disease is of low concern; otherwise other reconstruction options should be sought. This caveat severely limits its use in many head and neck oncology cases. Other disadvantages to the submental flap include possible injury to the marginal mandibular nerve and its hair-bearing quality in males, which is undesirable in FOM reconstruction.

Nasolabial Flap

The nasolabial flap provides soft tissue bulk to fill small to moderate-sized FOM defects, especially those involving loss of underlying muscle. Use of a nasolabial flap has been historically described in the Hindu works of Sushrata in 600 BC, and Esser introduced an inferiorly based cutaneous nasolabial flap transferred in two stages in 1918 (35). Multiple variations of this flap have since been developed, three of which will be discussed here.

Random Cutaneous Nasolabial Flap, Staged Repair

Classically, the nasolabial flap is a random flap of cutaneous and subcutaneous tissue harvested from a site incorporating the nasofacial and melolabial folds and trans-

Table 5 Submental Island Flap

Advantages	Disadvantages
Constant vascular pedicle	Risk of marginal mandibular nerve palsy
Reliable	Hair-bearing in males
Inconspicuous donor site	Compromises Ia and Ib neck dissection
Correction of submental rhytids and excess adipose tissue	

ferred in one or two stages (Fig. 3). For use in reconstructing the FOM, an inferiorly based pedicle is chosen. The medial aspect of the flap follows the nasofacial fold and 3–4 mm medial to the melolabial fold in its inferior third (36). Superiorly, the flap extends to no closer than 5–7 mm inferior to the medial canthus to avoid ectropion of the lower lid. The lateral limb of the incision is placed to provide a 2–3 cm base and a length-to-width ratio between 2:1 and 3:1. The inferior aspect of the flap extends to a level parallel to the inferior alveolus, but can be lower if more length

(A)

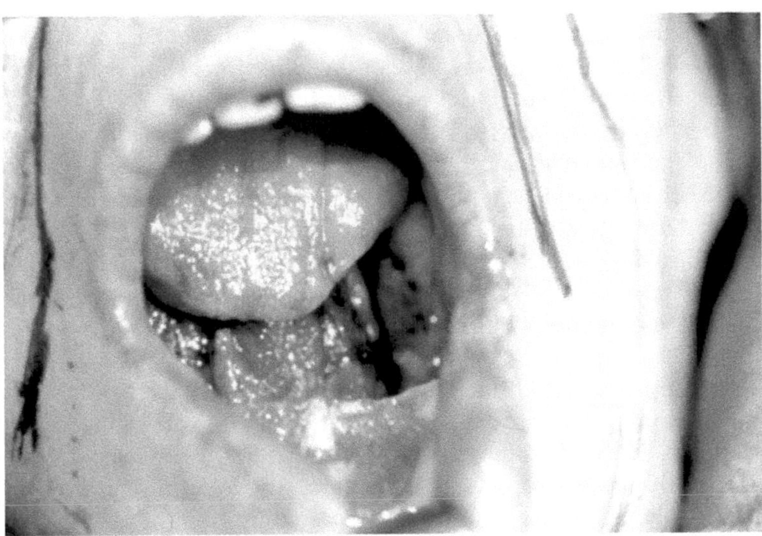

(B)

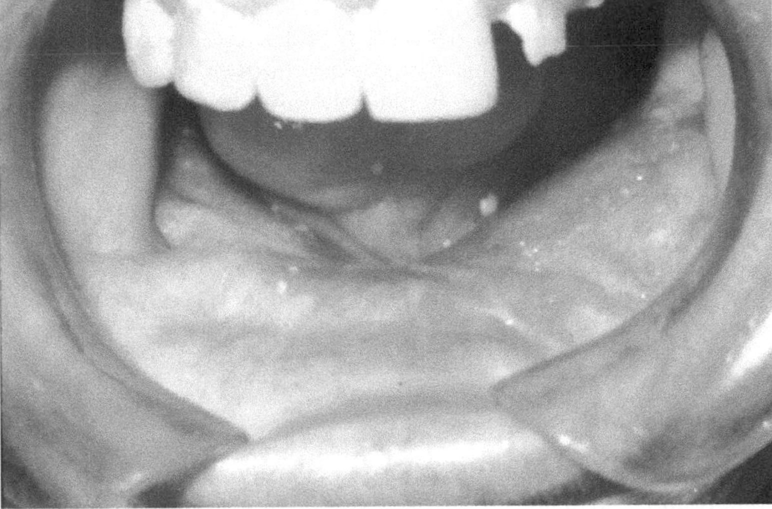

Figure 3 Nasolabial flap repair. (**A**) A large anterior floor of mouth defect with marginal mandibulectomy is to be reconstructed with bilateral nasolabial flaps as outlined. (**B**) Six months postoperatively, the nasolabial flap repair provides excellent contour and preserves tongue mobility.

is required. The flap is raised in a plane between the subcutaneous fat and the superficial fascia enveloping the underlying mimetic facial musculature. Flaps as large as 3.5×9 cm can be created, provided that enough skin laxity is present at the donor site for acceptable closure. Central FOM defects will require more flap length than lateral defects. Bilateral flaps can be raised if the defect is too large to be adequately managed with a unilateral flap.

Created in this manner, the flap exhibits random vasculature and is not a true axial flap, having no underlying artery that nourishes the flap along its entire length. Interestingly, cadaver studies of the flap do show small vessels of the subdermal plexus to be generally oriented along the long axis of the flap (37). This organization ensures good perfusion of the flap even to its most distal apex and may promote its reliability. Contributing vessels to the subdermal plexus include the facial, transverse facial, and labial arteries. When dissecting the base of the flap, effort should be made to preserve perforating vasculature entering the base.

To transfer the flap into the oral cavity, a transbuccal tunnel is created posterior to the orbicularis oris. The tunnel should be constructed wide enough to prevent strangulation of the pedicle. The pedicle is then draped over the mandible and inset into the FOM defect. Alternatively, to circumvent pedicle compression between the maxilla and mandible, the pedicle can be passed through a notch cut into the mandible. This maneuver may be impossible to safely execute in the elderly, atrophic edentulous jaw. In dentulous patients, a bite block may be necessary to prevent injury to the pedicle.

The donor site is reapproximated primarily, recreating the nasofacial and melolabial fold. Further undermining will ease closure and decrease asymmetry when using a unilateral nasolabial flap. The flap is allowed to heal for two to three weeks, during which neovascularization of the flap from the FOM occurs. After waiting this period, the pedicle is severed and the orocutaneous fistula is repaired.

One-Stage Cutaneous Nasolabial "Island" Flap

The classical nasolabial flap can also be performed as a single-stage procedure, avoiding the creation of an orocutaneous fistula, and the donor site is closed completely at the end of the case. The flap is similarly raised as described above, however, the inferior 2 cm at the base of the pedicle is de-epithelialized at a depth sufficient to remove all hair follicles. The flap is then inset and the donor site closed. The de-epithelialized portion of the flap traverses through the transbuccal tunnel. An alternative technique involves dissecting a tunnel under the mandible via another external incision at the lower border of the mandible. This allows the pedicle to pass under rather than superficial to the mandible, but this technique is rarely required in the authors' experience (38).

Myocutaneous Nasolabial Flap

Because of the random blood supply of the cutaneous flap, viability of the distal aspect may be compromised in a long thin flap. Alternatively, the flap may be harvested as a myocutaneous flap to preserve the underlying angular artery and its muscle perforators which travels along its length (39). As the facial artery lies deep to the facial muscles, dissection of this flap necessitates severing the zygomaticus major, zygomaticus minor, and levator labii superioris muscles. As well, the venous anatomy of this region is not constant. Thus, flap congestion and facial weakness make this option less favorable than the above two variants.

Indications (Table 6)

As a random cutaneous flap, the nasolabial flap is quite reliable, likely owing to its unique vasculature. Reliability of the flap ranges from 90% to 100%, and previous radiation therapy, neck dissection, or ligation of facial artery does not appear to adversely effect survival (36,40–47). However, a review of 224 cases by Varghese et al. (47) did correlate greater flap morbidity with facial artery ligation and previous radiation therapy. They also confirmed that postoperative radiotherapy did not affect long-term flap survival. Although the myocutaneous nasolabial flap is less commonly used, the few published articles report 100% success (39,48).

For FOM defects of moderate size, especially those involving partial resection of the mylohyoid, the nasolabial flap provides adequate bulk while remaining thin and pliable enough to permit tongue mobility. The harvest and inset of the flap is relatively easy to perform and provides an excellent reconstructive option, particularly in situations where more lengthy procedures with higher donor-site morbidity are not possible or contraindicated. In addition, as the donor site of the skin paddle is usually out of the radiation field, its survival is not as jeopardized as is platysma flap in previously irradiated patients. Perhaps the major threat to myocutaneous nasolabial flap survival arises from biting the pedicle. Various authors report partial flap necrosis attributed to inadvertent ligation by mastication (44,47).

Size is a limitation of the myocutaneous nasolabial flap. However, for the purposes of this chapter, most defects resulting from resection limited to the FOM can be adequately covered with bilateral nasolabial flaps if necessary. Generally a unilateral flap can cover an approximately 15 cm^2 area (46). Anteriorly FOM lesions are more likely to require two flaps, because considerable distance must be traversed for the flap to reach the defect. In men, the hair-bearing portion of the face limits the inferior border of the flap.

Although the nasolabial flap is located in a natural facial crease, closure of a large donor site can create minor complications. In addition to facial asymmetry caused by unilateral flaps, excessive tension can result in nasal flaring and upper lip distortion (41). In the myocutaneous flap, the underlying facial musculature is cut, resulting in potential impairment of mimetic function of the face. Hagan and Walker (39), who initially described the myocutaneous flap, claim minimal disruption of facial dynamics in 20 flaps procedures, although no formal functional evaluation was presented. However, because the myocutaneous flap is based on an arterial pedicle, the excised donor tissue is made elliptical in shape; as it does not need to rely on nutrient support from a wide base, and the donor defect therefore can be closed

Table 6 Nasolabial Flap

Advantages	Disadvantages
Relatively easy to perform	Potential cosmetic deformity
Donor site away from normal radiation fields	Facial weakness (esp. myocutaneous flap)
High success rate	Limited size
Can be used to cover exposed bone	Vulnerable pedicle
	Hair-bearing tissue in men

with less deformity. Other noted disadvantages include intraoral hair growth and obstructive sialadenopathy (41).

Although the nasal labial flap is an asensate flap, postoperative nerve growth can provide for acquired sensation. Civantos et al. examined sensory recovery in nasolabial flaps used for oral reconstruction in seven patients (49). After 12–18 months, the nasolabial flap in all four patients with FOM defects regained sufficient tactile sensitivity to discriminate between dull and sharp touch. Two of the four patients could discriminate between points 15 mm apart.

Radial Forearm Free Flap

For extensive soft-tissue reconstruction in the oral cavity, the radial forearm free flap (RFFF) is immensely popular. Originally designed by Yang et al. (50) in 1978 and first utilized for oral reconstruction by Soutar et al. (51) the RFFF provides thin, pliable, and predominantly hairless tissue with reliable vascularity.

Anatomy and Surgical Technique

More anatomic details and specifics of surgical methods are covered in subsequent chapters in this text. Briefly, the vascular supply of the RFFF is provided by the radial artery, which sends septocutaneous perforators to the volar skin via the lateral intermuscular septum, between the flexor carpi radialis and the brachioradialis. The radial artery is large, typically with a diameter of 2–4 mm near the antecubital fossa (52). Pedicle lengths of more than 12 cm can be easily achieved. Venous outflow is provided by a deep system through paired venae comitantes and a superficial system. These two networks both drain into the median cubital vein.

The skin paddle can be situated virtually anywhere along the volar surface of the arm (Fig. 4). A thinner flap with a longer pedicle can be obtained with a distally planned flap. The fasciocutaneous paddle can be quite large and encompass the entire forearm if necessary. Closure of the donor site is accomplished using a split thickness skin graft.

The RFFF is potentially sensate. Sensory reinnervation can be achieved by nerve anastomosis with the median and/or lateral antebrachial cutaneous nerves.

Indications (Table 7)

Numerous articles in the medical literature describes the reconstruction of various defects with the versatile RFFF. With particular regard to FOM defects, Evans et al. (53) reviewed 155 RFFF patients, of whom 95 required FOM coverage. An overall success rate of 97% was achieved, including cases of salvage with a second RFFF. A fistula rate of less than 8% was observed. These rates are similar to those found by Moscoso et al. (54) in their literature review.

The skin paddle provided by the RFFF is ideal for intraoral reconstruction. The tissue is thin and pliable; well suited to be shaped to fit most defects. Because it lacks significant bulk, the flap can fold upon itself, allowing continuous resurfacing of the ventral tongue and the FOM with a single bilobed flap. The low profile flap also enables near-normal speech and swallowing performance in patients with FOM–ventral tongue defects after reconstruction (55). The volar surface of the arm provides a good donor site as it presents abundant and relatively hairless skin.

Donor site complications are uncommon but potentially serious if adequate precautions are not taken. Delayed healing or partial loss of split-thickness skin graft

(A)

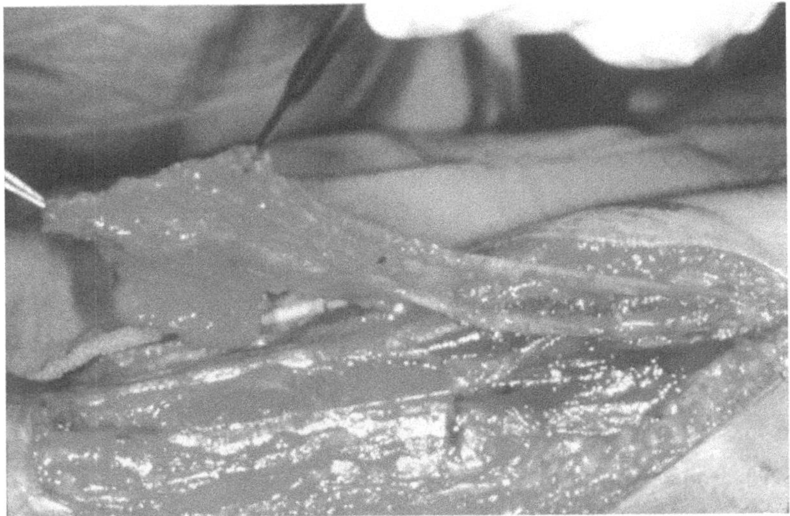

(B)

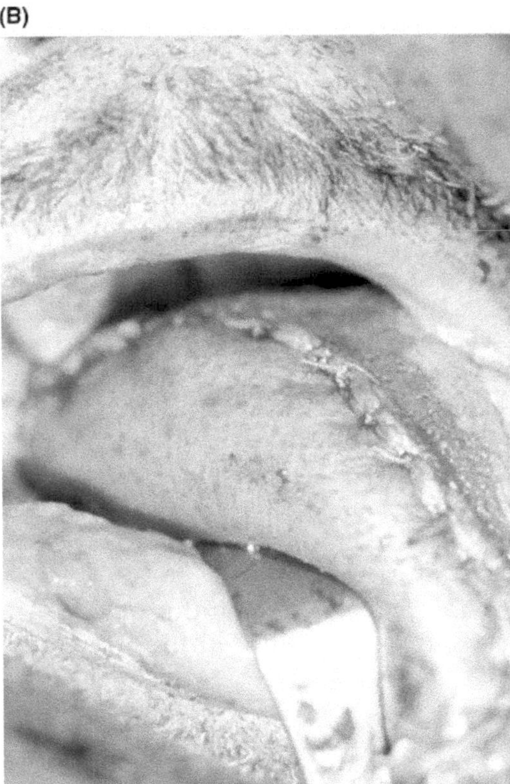

Figure 4 Radial forearm free flap repair. (**A**) The flap is raised from the volar surface of the arm. The radial artery is clearly shown. (**B**) and (**C**) The flap is supple enough to easily span the junction between the floor of mouth and the lateral tongue without impeding tongue mobility.

(C)

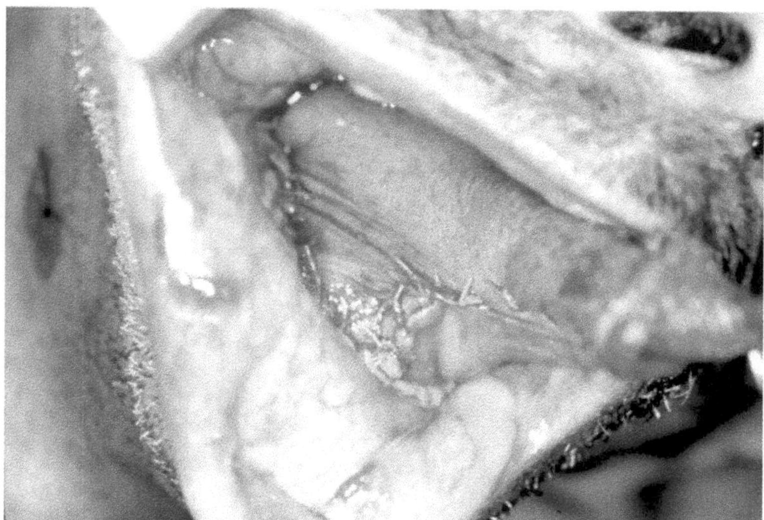

Figure 4 (*Continued*)

can occur. During flap elevation, care must be taken to preserve the paratenon over the tendons to facilitate skin graft take. Vascular compromise to the distal extremity is a dreaded complication. As the radial and ulnar arteries are the main conduits to the hand, the ulnar artery must have the ability to perfuse the hand before the radial artery is ligated. This can be pre-operatively evaluated with the Allen's test either subjectively or, preferably, objectively with Doppler imaging and/or photoplethysmography (56,57). Lack of evidence of flow from the ulnar artery to the palmar arches mandates that another flap source be considered.

Overall, the RFFF presents the most versatile option in oral cavity reconstruction, with the highest flap survival and functional success. However, this should be weighed against the potential morbidity of donor site complications, extra operative time, and technical expertise required in free tissue reconstruction. The reconstructive surgeon must weight these factors with respect to each patient.

Lateral Arm Free Flap

Although the RFFF has widespread use in head and neck reconstruction, the lateral arm free flap (LAFF) remains a suitable but less-frequently used alternative. Use of this

Table 7 Radial Forearm Free Flap

Advantages	Disadvantages
Thin, almost hairless tissue	Requires microvascular expertise
Large flap available	Time consuming
Reliable arterial supply	Potential donor site morbidity
Large vessel caliber	
Long vascular pedicle	
Sensate capability	

flap potentially provides abundant vascularized tissue without the risk of vascular compromise to the donor arm. The LAFF has been used successfully in applications for extremity and phalanx reconstruction. The limitations in head and neck reconstruction are often secondary to short pedicle length, excess soft tissue bulk, and small vessel size.

Anatomy and Surgical Technique

The LAFF, initially described by Song et al. (58) in 1982, is a septocutaneous flap based on the lateral intermuscular septum of the arm and the posterior radial collateral artery (PRCA) which courses through it. The arterial source originates from the profunda brachii artery, which runs in the humeral spiral groove along side the radial nerve. This vessel then bifurcates into the anterior radial collateral artery and the PRCA. The latter runs in along the septum between the brachialis and the brachioradialis anteriorly and the triceps posteriorly, ending in an arborization of fasciocutaneous branches near the epicondyle and the olecranon.

The skin paddle supported by this network of vessels is classically described as located on the upper arm as far distally as the epicondyle. The cutaneous area supplied in the upper arm varies from 8 × 10 cm to 14 × 15 cm (59,60). Extension of the LAFF beyond the epicondyle into the forearm has been used successfully. Dye studies and cadaveric dissections have shown that a vascular plexus from the PRCA extends well below the epicondyle, providing another 6–10 cm of additional length (61–64). Whether vascularization of the forearm skin extension is through random subcutaneous vessels or through a constant arterial branch of the PRCA is presently unclear.

Venous return occurs via paired venae comitantes accompanying the PRCA. These vessels combine to form a single venous conduit at the spiral groove of the humerus. Venous diameter averages 2 mm (59). A subcutaneous plexus system also supplies the flap, draining into the cephalic vein. The LAFF is also a potentially sensate flap. Neural supply is via the posterior cutaneous nerve of the arm.

Indications (Table 8)

The LAFF complements the RFFF in the reconstructive armamentarium of the head and neck surgeon. The vascular supply is anatomically reliable, although paired, parallel PRCAs have been described (65). In addition, harvesting the flap does not compromise vascular supply to the remainder of the arm. This feature is particularly poignant in situations which the negative results of an Allen's test, preclude the use of the RFFF for reconstruction.

At the same time, the vascular supply poses limitations to the use of the LAFF. The arterial vessels are smaller than those encountered in the RFFF, therefore increasing the difficulty of the anastomosis. However, with meticulous microvascular work, excellent results can be obtained. Civantos et al. (66) reported 100% survival even with extension of the flap beyond the epicondyle.

Table 8 Lateral Arm Flap

Advantages	Disadvantages
No risk of extremity ischemia	Short pedicle length
Large skin paddle	Small vessel diameter
Low donor site morbidity	Thicker flap
Sensate capability	More difficult dissection

The short vascular pedicle length of the LAFF is considered to be a limitation for use in reconstruction. Pedicle length can be increased by dividing the medial attachment of the triceps muscle from the humerus and dissecting the profunda brachii artery to its origin at the brachial artery. Combined with more distal placement of the skin paddle, pedicle length can be increased from 2–6 cm to 9–14 cm (67).

Elbow mobility is generally unaffected by flap harvest (66,68). Because the antebrachial cutaneous nerve is often sacrificed during flap harvest, patients have an area of anesthesia over the lower arm, but this is generally well tolerated.

Overall, the LAFF presents a reliable alternative to the RFFF where RFFF use is contraindicated. The thicker skin paddle may be cumbersome in the anterior oral cavity, but it is perfectly tailored for tongue base defects. It is technically more difficult to raise than the RFFF and so should be assigned to a secondary role in which large defects mandate free tissue transfer.

CONCLUSION

The head and neck surgeon has a wide armamentarium from which to choose the most suitable reconstructive method for the patient (Table 9). Although, small sized defects can potentially be closed primarily, resection of virtually any symptomatic tumor with oncologically safe margins will result in significant mucosal loss. Given the already narrow dimensions of the FOM and ventral tongue region, coapting the incisional margins primarily will likely lead to ankyloglossia and obliteration of the natural gingivolingual sulci.

In reconstructing the FOM and ventral tongue, three goals should be kept in mind. First, replacement of resected tissue with tissue of similar properties would be ideal. By matching tissue size, shape, thickness, and pliability, maximal oral function can be preserved. Second, recreation of native contours should be attempted. Salibian et al. (69) recommend that the anterior FOM under the tongue be made shallower than the lateral sulci to enhance salivary drainage and to prevent pooling. Adherence to the first two principles, will hopefully lead to an excellent functional result as demonstrated by tongue mobility, proper swallowing, and articulate speech. Third, the donor site should leave the patient with minimal morbidity.

Fortunately, when dealing with lesions restricted to the FOM and minor extension to the ventral tongue, the body of the tongue has not been severely affected. Therefore the emphasis of reconstruction is not so much on replacement of bulk, rather the focus is on providing thin pliable tissue that will neither obstruct nor tether the tongue. Each technique described in this chapter provides relatively thin

Table 9 Comparison of Flap Characteristics

	Size of graft	Bulk	Difficulty
Skin graft	+++	+	+
Allograft	+++	+	+
Nasolabial	+	++	++
Platysma	++	++	++
Submental	++	+++	++
Radial forearm	+++	++	+++
Lateral arm	+++	+++	+++

tissue with the possible exception of the lateral arm flap. However, comparative studies are difficult to interpret as few show direct comparison of these techniques.

The choice of the reconstructive procedure also depends upon the medical condition of the patient and the health care resources available. Free-flap reconstructions are considerably more time consuming to perform, requiring not only microvascular expertise and intensive care facilities but also a patient that has the stamina to undergo an extended procedure. In areas of limited resources, reconstruction with a local or regional pedicled flap may be the best solution.

A flap can also be combined with a STSG to provide closure of the defect. Spanning the junction between the FOM and the ventral tongue with a single flap may present excessive bulk. Instead the FOM can be repaired with the flap while the ventral tongue is resurfaced with a STSG, providing the reconstructive surgeon multiple options for optimal repairs (70).

PROBLEM-BASED DISCUSSION

The following are cases in which the reconstructive techniques presented in this chapter are described.

CASE 1. A 71-year-old male with a history of T2N0M0 squamous cell carcinoma of the larynx treated eight years ago with radiation therapy presents with an erythematous and tender oral lesion. The patient reports the sore has been growing over the past several months but has recently rapidly enlarged. Examination reveals a 2.0×1.3 cm lesion located in the right anterior-lateral aspect of the FOM near Wharton's duct. The mass does not appear to encroach upon the mandible. It abuts against but does not involve the undersurface of the tongue. Biopsy is positive for a second primary squamous cell carcinoma

After definitive resection, multiple options are available for reconstruction. The defect will be larger than the lesion itself after adequate margins are taken. Primary closure is a possibility but would likely result in significant ankyloglossia as it would draw the root of the anterior tongue forward to the gingiva. A STSG would provide sufficient coverage and could be quickly performed. However, post-operative contracture of the graft may again result in tethering. The platysma flap and submental flap are good modalities but they may introduce hair-bearing tissue in a male. In addition, post radiation changes in the neck may compromise the viability of a platysma flap. The nasolabial flap would be perfect in this case, especially since it would provide tissue not previously irradiated. With the slightly lateral location of the lesion, a single nasolabial flap may provide sufficient coverage.

CASE 2. A 67-year-old female is referred after her primary care physician discovered that she no longer wears her lower dentures because of discomfort and improper fit. An ulceration measuring 2.7×3.2 cm is evident on the lateral FOM adjacent to the mandible. Biopsy reveals squamous cell carcinoma. Clinically, no nodes are palpable in the neck. A preoperative CT scan does not reveal obvious mandibular invasion, which is confirmed intraoperatively. However, as the lesion involves the periosteum, a marginal mandibulectomy is required for an oncologically sound extirpation.

The defect remaining after such a composite resection may be sizable, even though only a margin of the mandible is removed. A STSG cannot resurface bare cortical bone absent periosteum. Although graft survival is possible over marginal mandibulectomy defects, we prefer to reconstruct with vascularized tissue to avoid issues of osteomyelitis or, in cases of a previously irradiated mandible, osteoradionecrosis. As this patient has an edentulous mandible, maximal vascularization needs to be preserved to prevent fracture development in the area of the marginal mandibulectomy. Either the platysma or the submental flap would perform well in this case, as they provide generous amounts of tissue. However if palpable submental nodes are detected and a neck dissection is indicated, harvesting a submental flap may compromise thorough removal of the level I nodal packet. In cases of prior radiation, use of the platysma flap is not ideal. The nasolabial flap can still be considered, although a bilateral flap harvest may be required for defect coverage. A RFFF would only be necessary in an irradiated patient with nodal disease.

CASE 3. A thin 64-year-old man presents with a 5-month history of progressive soreness of his mouth. Because the gentleman does not seek medical assistance regularly, he has not brought this to the attention of a specialist until recently, when the pain prevents adequate oral food intake. He reports a significant history of alcohol and tobacco use. Clinical examination reveals a large area of indurated, friable mucosa stretching from the left lateral FOM, across the midline to the right anterior floor. The tumor encroaches on the junction between the mouth floor and the ventral surface of the tongue. Leukoplakia is evident throughout the entire FOM and along the undersurface of the tongue. Intraoperatively, a large region encompassing the entire FOM was removed to achieve adequate margins. Regions of carcinoma in situ dictated mucosal resection along the ventral tongue, fortunately sparing the musculature of the lingual tongue. Bilateral selective neck dissections were performed.

In this case, a sizable surgical defect remains for reconstruction. Again no single reconstructive option is indicated, although some modalities are better than others. Because of large area involved, use of a STSG or a platysma flap is not recommended. Skin grafting a large area will result in significant functional compromise secondary to contraction. A platysma flap generally cannot adequately resurface defects that span from one mandibular angle to the other due to geometry of pedicle location, although a bilateral flap could be entertained given enough skin laxity. Nasolabial flaps likewise would have difficulty in providing enough coverage, especially since the ventral tongue is involved. If the patient is able to tolerate a long operation, a bilobed RFFF could be used. As it provides thin, pliable tissue, the flap could span the junction between the FOM and ventral tongue and minimally interfere with lingual function. If a negative Allen's test precludes the use of the RFFF, a LAF or a submental flap could be entertained although their increased bulk is suboptimal. Again a submental flap may compromise a thorough lymph node dissection. Another possible option is to reconstruct the FOM with one modality and resurface the tongue with a STSG. This reduces the complexity of the flap and enables the use of smaller flaps (eg. nasolabial flap).

REFERENCES

1. Peters G, Johns M. Management of carcinoma of the anterior floor of mouth without mandibular invasion. In: Stiernberg C, ed. Surgery of the Oral Cavity. Chicago: Year Book Medical Publishers, 1989:91–96.
2. Kolson H, Spiro RH, Rosewit B, Lawson W. Epidermoid carcinoma of the floor of the mouth. Analysis of 108 cases. Arch Otolaryngol 1971; 93:280–283.
3. McGregor I, McGregor A. Fundamental Techniques of Plastic Surgery and Their Surgical Applications. New York: Churchill Livingston, 1995.
4. Converse JM, Uhlschmid GK, Ballantyne DL Jr. "Plasmatic circulation" in skin grafts. The phase of serum imbibition. Plast Reconstr Surg 1969; 43:495–499.

5. Petruzzelli GJ, Johnson JT, Myers EN, Kline JM. Histomorphometric analysis of intraoral split-thickness skin grafts. Head Neck 1992; 14:119–124.
6. McGregor IA. "Quilted" Skin Grafting in the Mouth. Br J Plast Surg 1975; 28:100–102.
7. Alvi A, Myers EN. Skin graft reconstruction of the composite resection defect. Head Neck 1996; 18:583–543; discussion 543–544.
8. Schramm VL Jr, Johnson JT, Myers EN. Skin grafts and flaps in oral cavity reconstruction. Arch Otolaryngol 1983; 109:175–177.
9. Schramm VL Jr, Myers EN. Skin grafts in oral cavity reconstruction. Arch Otolaryngol 1980; 106:528–532.
10. Teichgraeber J, Larson DL, Castaneda O, Martin JW. Skin grafts in intraoral reconstruction. A new stenting method. Arch Otolaryngol 1984; 110:463–467.
11. Johnson J. Reconstruction of floor-of-mouth defects: split-thickness skin grafts. In: Stiernberg C, ed. Surgery of the Oral Cavity. Chicago: Year Book Medical Publishers, 1989:128–133.
12. Burkey BB, Coleman JR Jr. Current concepts in oromandibular reconstruction. Otolaryngol Clin N Am 1997; 30:607–630.
13. McConnel FM, Teichgraeber JF, Adler RK. A comparison of three methods of oral reconstruction. Arch Otolaryngol Head Neck Surg 1987; 113:496–500.
14. Rhee PH, Friedman CD, Ridge JA, Kusiak J. The use of processed allograft dermal matrix for intraoral resurfacing: an alternative to split-thickness skin grafts. Arch Otolaryngol Head Neck Surg 1998; 124:1201–1204.
15. Futrell JW, Johns ME, Edgerton MT, Cantrell RW, Fitz-Hugh GS. Platysma myocutaneous flap for intraoral reconstruction. Am J Surg 1978; 136:504–507.
16. Cannon CR, Johns ME, Atkins JP Jr, Keane WM, Cantrell RW. Reconstruction of the oral cavity using the platysma myocutaneous flap. Arch Otolarygol 1982; 108: 491–494.
17. Hurwitz DJ, Rabson JA, Futrell JW. The anatomic basis for the platysma skin flap. Plast Reconstr Surg 1983; 72:302–314.
18. McGuirt WF, Matthews BL, Brody JA, May JS. Platysma myocutaneous flap: caveats reexamined. Laryngoscope 1991; 101:1238–1244.
19. Uehara M, Helman JI, Lillie JH, Brooks SL. Blood supply to the platysma muscle flap: an anatomic study with clinical correlation. J Oral Maxillofac Surg 2001; 59:642–646.
20. Verschuur HP, Dassonville O, Santini J, Vallicioni J, Poissonnet G, Laudoyer Y, Demard F. Complications of the myocutaneous platysma flap in intraoral reconstruction. Head Neck 1998; 20:623–629.
21. Papadopoulos ON, Gamatsi IE. Platysma myocutaneous flap for intraoral and surface reconstruction. Ann Plast Surg 1993; 31:15–18.
22. Mazzola RF, Benazzo M. Platysma flap for oral reconstruction. Clin Plast Surg 2001; 28:411–419.
23. Saito H, Tsuda G, Ohtsubo T, Noda I, Fujieda S, Saito T. Platysma myocutaneous flap including the external jugular vein with special reference to neck dissection. ORL J Otorhinolaryngol Relat Spec 1998; 60:218–223.
24. Ruark DS, McClairen WC Jr, Schlehaider UK, Abdel-Misih RZ. Head and neck reconstruction using the platysma myocutaneous flap. Am J Surg 1993; 165:713–718; discussion 718–719.
25. Manni JJ, Bruaset I. Reconstruction of the anterior oral cavity using the platysma myocutaneous island flap. Laryngoscope 1986; 96:564–567.
26. Esclamado RM, Burkey BB, Carroll WR, Bradford CR. The platysma myocutaneous flap. Indications and caveats. Arch Otolaryngol Head Neck Surg 1994; 120:32–35.
27. Conley JJ, Lanier DM, Tinsley P Jr. Platysma myocutaneous flap revisited. Arch Otolaryngol Head Neck Surg 1986; 112:711–713.
28. Persky MS, Kaufman D, Cohen NL. Platysma myocutaneous flap for intraoral defects. Arch Otolaryngol 1983; 109:463–464.

29. Martin D, Pascal JF, Baudet J, Mondie JM, Farhat JB, Athoum A, Le Gaillard P, Peri G. The submental island flap: a new donor site. Anatomy and clinical applications as a free or pedicled flap. Plast Reconstr Surg 1993; 92:867–873.
30. Faltaous AA, Yetman RJ. The submental artery flap: an anatomic study. Plast Reconstr Surg 1996; 97:56–60; discussion 61–62.
31. Pistre V, Pelissier P, Martin D, Baudet J. The submental flap: its uses as a pedicled or free flap for facial reconstruction. Clin Plast Surg 2001; 28:303–309.
32. Yilmaz M, Menderes A, Barutcu A. Submental artery island flap for reconstruction of the lower and mid face. Ann Plast Surg 1997; 39:30–35.
33. Vural E, Suen JY. The submental island flap in head and neck reconstruction. Head Neck 2000; 22:572–578.
34. Sterne GD, Januszkiewicz JS, Hall PN, Bardsley AF. The submental island flap. Br J Plast Surg 1996; 49:85–89.
35. Esser J. Deckung von gaumendefekten mittels gestielter naso-labial-haultlappen. Deutsch Zeitschrift fur Chirurgie 1918; 147:128.
36. Ducic Y, Burye M. Nasolabial flap reconstruction of oral cavity defects: a report of 18 cases. J Oral Maxillofac Surg 2000; 58:1104–1108; discussion 1108–1109.
37. Hynes B, Boyd JB. The nasolabial flap: Axial or Random? Arch Otolaryngol Head Neck Surg 1988; 114:1389–1391
38. Piggot TA, Logan AM, Knight SL, Milner RH. The facial artery island flap. Ann Plast Surg 1987; 19:260–265.
39. Hagan WE, Walker LB. The Nasolabial musculocutaneous flap: clinical and anatomical correlations. Laryngoscope 1988; 98:341–346.
40. Ioannides C, Fossion E. Nasolabial flap for the reconstruction of defects of the floor of the mouth. Int J Oral Maxillofac Surg 1991; 20:40–43.
41. Mutimer KL, Poole MD. A review of nasolabial flaps for intra-oral defects. Br J Plast Surg 1987; 40:472–477.
42. Morgan RF, Chambers RG, Jaques DA, Hoopes JE. Nasolabial flap in intraoral reconstruction. Review of 55 cases. Am J Surg 1981; 142:448–450.
43. Gerwitz HS, Eilber FR, Zarem HA. Use of the nasolabial flap for reconstruction of the floor of the mouth. Am J Surg 1978; 136:508–511.
44. Rokenes HK, Bretteville G, Lovdal O, Boysen M. The nasolabial skinflap in intraoral reconstruction. ORL J Otorhinolaryngol Relat Spec 1991; 53:346–348.
45. Napolitano M, Mast BA. The nasolabial flap revisited as an adjunct to floor of mouth reconstruction. Ann Plast Surg 2001; 46:265–268.
46. Roth J, Patete M, Goodwin WJ. Use of the melolabial flap in intraoral reconstruction. Otolaryngol Head Neck Surg 1996; 114:12–17.
47. Varghese BT, Sebastian P, Cherian T, Mohan PM, Ahmed I, Koshy CM, Thomas S. Nasolabial flaps in oral reconstruction: an analysis of 224 cases. Br J Plast Surg 2001; 54:499–503.
48. Cao C, Kuang M, Yang M. One stage repair of intraoral defects after radical operation of oral carcinoma by facial vessels pedicled naso-labial myocutaneous flap. Zhongguo Xiu Fu Chong Jian Wai Ke Za Zhi 1998; 12:159–161.
49. Civantos FJ, Roth J, Goodwin WJ, Weed DT. Sensory recovery in melolabial flaps used for oral cavity reconstruction. Otolaryngol Head Neck Surg 2000; 122:509–513.
50. Yang GF, Chen PJ, Gao YZ, Liu XY, Li J, Jiang SX, He SP. Forearm free skin flap transplantation: a report of 56 cases. Br J Plast Surg 1997; 50:162–165.
51. Soutar DS, Scheker LR, Tanner NS, McGregor IA. The radial forearm flap: a versatile method for intra-oral reconstruction. Br J Plast Surg 1983; 36:1–8.
52. Soucacos PN, Beris AE, Xenakis TA, Malizos KN, Touliatos AS. Forearm flap in orthopaedic and hand surgery. Microsurgery 1992; 13:170–174.
53. Evans GR, Schusterman MA, Kroll SS, Miller MJ, Reece GP, Robb GL, Ainslie N. The radial forearm free flap for head and neck reconstruction: a review. Am J Surg 1994; 168:446–450.

54. Moscoso JF, Urken ML. Radial forearm flaps. Otolaryngol Clin N Am 1994; 27: 1119–1140.
55. Jacobson MC, Franssen E, Fliss DM, Birt BD, Gilbert RW. Free forearm flap in oral reconstruction: functional outcome. Arch Otolaryngol Head Neck Surg 1995; 121: 959–964.
56. Song R, Gao Y, Song Y, Yu Y. The forearm flap. Clin Plast Surg 1982; 9:21–26.
57. Nuckols DA, Tsue TT, Toby EB, Girod DA. Preoperative evaluation of the radial forearm free flap patient with the objective Allen's test. Otolaryngol Head Neck Surg 2000; 123:553–557.
58. Song R, Song Y, Yu Y. The upper arm free flap. Clin Plast Surg 1982; 9:27–35.
59. Katsaros J, Schusterman M, Beppu M, Banis JC Jr, Acland RD. The lateral upper arm flap: anatomy and clinical applications. Ann Plast Surg 1984; 12:489–500.
60. Rivet D, Buffet M, Martin D, Waterhouse N, Kleiman L, Delonca D, Baudet J. The lateral arm flap: an anatomic study. J Reconstr Microsurg 1987; 3:121–132.
61. Kuek LB, Chuan TL. The extended lateral arm flap: a new modification. J Reconstr Microsurg 1991; 7:167–173.
62. Brandt KE, Khouri RK. The lateral arm/proximal forearm flap. Plast Reconstr Surg 1993; 92:1137–1143.
63. Lanzetta M, Bernier M, Chollet A, St-Laurent JY. The lateral forearm flap: an anatomic study. Plast Reconstr Surg 1997; 99:460–464.
64. Tan BK, Lim BH. The lateral forearm flap as a modification of the lateral arm flap: vascular anatomy and clinical implications. Plast Reconstr Surg 2000; 105:2400–2404.
65. Sullivan MJ, Carroll WR, Kuriloff DB. Lateral arm free flap in head and neck reconstruction. Arch Otolaryngol Head Neck Surg 1992; 118:1095–1101.
66. Civantos FJ Jr, Burkey BB, Lu FL, Armstrong W. Lateral arm microvascular flap in head and neck reconstruction. Arch Otolaryngol Head Neck Surg 1997; 123:830–836.
67. Hamdi M, Coessens BC. Distally planned lateral arm flap. Microsurgery 1996; 17: 375–379.
68. Vico PG, Coessens BC. The distally based lateral arm flap for intraoral soft tissue reconstruction. Head Neck 1997; 19:33–36.
69. Salibian AH, Allison GR, Rappaport I, Krugman ME, McMicken BL, Etchepare TL. Total and subtotal glossectomy: function after microvascular reconstruction. Plast Reconstr Surg 1990; 85:513–524; discussion 525–526.
70. Butler CE. Skin grafts used in combination with free flaps for intraoral oncological reconstruction. Ann Plast Surg 2001; 47:293–298.

11
Reconstruction of Partial Glossectomy Defects

Judith M. Skoner, Joshua Hornig, and Terry A. Day
Department of Otolaryngology—Head and Neck Surgery, Medical University of South Carolina, Charleston, South Carolina, U.S.A.

INTRODUCTION

The tongue plays a vital role in daily life including speech, swallowing, breathing, and mastication. Most tongue defects are a result of surgical resected carcinomas, specifically squamous cell carcinoma; although, traumatic defects are not uncommonly seen following gunshot wounds. The tongue is intimately related to the mandible, dentition, neck, and larynx making it difficult to assess one area without consideration of the effect on the other. Not only does the tongue function in speech and swallowing, but protection of the airway, taste, and breathing can be affected by the loss of tongue function. As swallowing begins in the oral cavity, sensation provides important cues to coordinate respiration with speech and swallowing, maintain oral competence, sweep the bolus to the oropharynx, and trigger protective laryngeal reflexes. The ideal tongue reconstruction would provide identical size, shape, sensation, taste, mobility, and coordinated articulation and swallowing function in a single procedure. Unfortunately, this option does not yet exist although animal models of tongue transplantation (1), free tissue transfer advances (2), and historic efforts at creating a "new tongue" (3) provide a framework upon which the reconstructive surgeon can enhance future research and surgical techniques.

The reconstruction of the tongue and partial glossectomy defects requires an in-depth knowledge of the anatomy, physiology, and quality of life issues surrounding problems related to tongue dysfunction. This single organ is not amenable to the previous concept of "fill the hole" and requires customized reconstructive and rehabilitative efforts to provide the best functional and cosmetic outcome. Inherent in achieving the ideal outcome is cooperation among surgeons, dentists, prosthodontists, speech pathologists, radiation oncologists, nurses and the many other specialists involved in the care of patients with tongue dysfunction. Although, the following text provides a generalized approach to defects of the tongue, it is worth mentioning at the outset that each patient and defect requires an individualized approach to result in the best tongue function.

RECONSTRUCTIVE OPTIONS

On occasion, despite thorough preoperative evaluation and planning, an oncologic resection yields a defect different from that anticipated preoperatively. In oral and oropharyngeal cancers, stage does seem to have a predictive value when considering post-operative speech and swallowing function (4). This situation merely emphasizes the importance of flexibility and customization in head and neck reconstruction. It is the responsibility of the reconstructive surgeon to consider the various methods available at each level along the "reconstructive ladder," and to accordingly tailor the reconstruction to each unique defect and overall set of patient circumstances. A variety of approaches, procedures, and tissues are available for reconstruction of the oral tongue (Table 1).

In order to determine the most suitable method of reconstruction following tongue resections, the defect itself must be clearly defined. Functional deficits corresponding to the anatomic resection may then be identified and appropriately addressed. Urken and colleagues describe a classification scheme for glossectomy defects, based on size and location, to provide a framework by which to approach functional reconstruction (5). The mobile tongue, critical in oral competence, speech and articulation, is considered separately from the base of tongue, critical in airway protection and the pharyngeal phase of deglutition. Respectively, each of these two regions is then addressed within the context of the following defects: one-quarter glossectomy, hemiglossectomy, three-quarters glossectomy, total mobile tongue resection, total tongue base resection, and total glossectomy. By defining a tongue defect, the goals of reconstruction are more clearly delineated. This information then allows the surgeon to consider all potential means by which to achieve those goals, and ultimately, to choose the optimal reconstruction for a particular defect.

Although, each patient and situation is unique, and it is crucial to identify the individual subtleties, there are some general concepts by which to approach tongue reconstruction. The mobile portion of the tongue, anterior to the circumvallate papillae, is primarily responsible for speech articulation, mastication, and the oral

Table 1 Common Procedures and Flaps for Oral Tongue Reconstruction

Primary closure
Secondary intention healing
Allograft or autograft
Cervical based flaps
Submental flap
Platysma flap
Regional pedicled flaps
Pectoralis myocutaneous flap
Deltopectoral fasciocutaneous flap
Other
Free tissue transfer
Radial forearm fasciocutaneous free flap
Lateral arm fasciocutaneous free flap
Ulnar fasciocutaneous free flap
Anterolateral thigh fasciocutaneous free flap
Scapula fasciocutaneous free flap
Abdominal muscle sparing perforator free flaps
Other

phase of deglutition. Despite this area representing a small percentage of the oral cavity, surgical resection may result in significant speech and swallowing impairment (6). The tip of the tongue provides approximation to the palate, enhancing articulation, and oral phase of swallowing. Thus, anterior tongue resections result in decreased tongue motion with varying degrees of compromised speech and swallowing, especially if the resection crosses the midline. The functional goals in this area of reconstruction, therefore, are to preserve and maximize mobility of the residual tongue, and to minimize post-operative scarring, contracture and tethering of the neotongue. The base of tongue, posterior to the circumvallate papillae, assists in airway protection and is responsible for the piston-like action of propelling a food bolus through the pharynx. Volume, shape and motion are critical features of the tongue base that facilitate function. Accordingly, reconstruction of this area should provide adequate volume, or bulk, without compromising residual tongue mobility.

This chapter will discuss reconstructive options for partial glossectomy defects primarily involving the anterior or mobile tongue. Management of more extensive tongue base defects, subtotal/total glossectomy, and composite defects will be addressed in subsequent chapters. Various approaches to tongue reconstruction are presented based on defect size and location, from the very basic to the most comprehensive. Although, numerous techniques beyond those described here may be used to reconstruct the oral cavity, discussion will be limited to those methods the authors consider to offer the best overall reconstruction of partial glossectomy defects at this time.

Partial Glossectomy Defects (Less Than 25% of the Anterior Mobile Tongue)

Following reconstruction of defects involving 25% or less of the anterior mobile tongue, functional disturbances tend to be minimal. There are four common options for reconstruction after resection of one-fourth or less of the mobile tongue, including: healing by secondary intention; primary closure; auto and allografting, and; local tissue rearrangement. These are highlighted in Table 2, which provides insight into the better options for a particular size of the defect.

Allowing a wound to granulate and *reepithelialize secondarily* offers advantages of ease and decreased operative time, while yielding an excellent eventual result in the aftermath of a small defect. However, exposed resection surfaces are easily irritated in the rarely static oral cavity, especially with speech, mastication, swallowing, and intact dentition. The healing time course, therefore, may be protracted, with bleeding and/or pain until reepithelialization is complete. Consideration of secondary intention healing is not the same as secondary reconstruction and delay in definitive reconstruction is often not appropriate following oral cancer resection (7). Studies have revealed some insight into the process of secondary intention healing following surgical wounds (8,9). Also, regardless of size, an anterior tip or ventral defect left to heal by secondary intention may result in functionally unacceptable scarring to the floor of mouth mucosa, with subsequent tethering of the tongue, and thus, is best managed by other means. Conversely, laterally located defects are very amenable to secondary reepithelialization after a limited resection. Thus, secondary intention healing is best suited for the appropriately tolerant patient, with a small lateral mobile tongue defect, in whom minimizing operative time is a priority (10).

Primary closure is another reasonable option for management of a lateral defect limited to no more than 25% of the mobile tongue alone (Fig. 1). This technique is easily and expeditiously accomplished, and may be performed with minimal disturbance in

Table 2 Reconstructive Options for the Oral (Anterior) Tongue

	<10% of anterior mobile tongue	10–25% of anterior mobile tongue	25–50% of anterior mobile tongue	>50% of anterior mobile tongue	100% of anterior mobile tongue
Primary closure	+++	++	+	0	0
Secondary intention healing	++	++	+	0	0
Skin/allografting	++	+++	+++	0	0
Local flap	++	++	++	+	0
Regional flap-SM, plat	0	+++	+++	++	+
Regional flap-PMC	0	0	+	+	++
Free tissue transfer	0	++	+++	+++	+++

0, poor option; +, fair option; ++, good option; +++, best option.
Abbreviations: SM, submental flap; Plat, platysma flap; PMC, pectoralis myocutaneous flap.

post-operative oral function due to preservation of tongue protrusion and mobility. The incised surfaces are sutured together using a two layer closure of resorbable suture material, the ventral approximating the dorsal, thereby decreasing discomfort associated with an open granulating wound. Theoretically, the immediate sensate recovery, mucosal lubrication, and natural swallowing opportunity may afford the patient an improved result based on its utility in other sites (11). A potential disadvantage of this technique is cosmesis, as primary closure of a lateral defect can create a narrow neotongue that becomes more 'serpent-like' in appearance with increasing defect size. Nevertheless, in most circumstances, primary closure is still a preferred method of

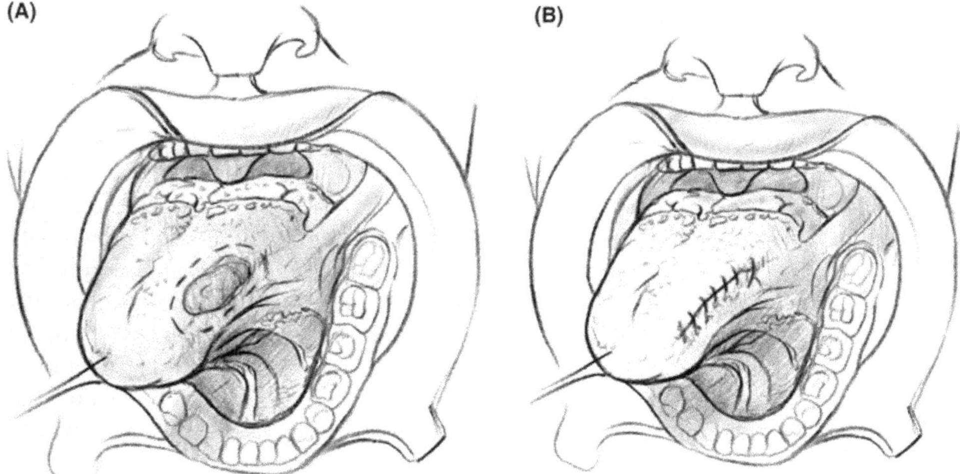

Figure 1 Primary closure. (**A**) Example of a left tongue cancer with dashed line representing planned resection margins. (**B**) Graphic depicting primary closure of the defect after resection.

reconstruction for the small lateral mobile tongue defect. Primary closure of anterior tip or ventral tongue defects of any size, however, results in a broadened tongue that may be significantly shortened with limited protrusion. Additionally, such defects often approach or involve floor of mouth mucosa, and primary closure at this location may lead to tethering of the reconstructed tongue and further motion impairment.

Several tips can be applied to primary closure including the intraoperative decision of a "vertical" or "horizontal" closure of the tongue resulting in a scar that either parallels (vertical) the midline of the tongue or is perpendicular to the midline (horizontal) resulting in significantly different shape and function. The preservation of mobility is preferred over cosmesis thus making the resultant mobility the primary consideration in deciding which direction to close the defect based on the location. Studies have suggested the importance of tongue motility in eventual articulation and speech intelligibility (12). When primary closure negatively affects the mobility and requires sutures that may compromise the lingual vessels or lingual and hypoglossal nerves, slight undermining of the mucosa, and submucosa of the tongue while leaving the muscle layer intact will provide adequate closure without compromising the native muscle or nerves. Primary closure is the preferred method used by the authors for less than 25% glossectomy defects when it does not result in limitation of tongue mobility.

Skin and allo-grafting is a more suitable reconstruction for limited anterior tip or ventral tongue defects, to maintain the mobility so critical to optimum oral functioning (Fig. 2). The most commonly used skin graft in oral cavity reconstruction is split-thickness, typically 0.015–0.018 inch, consisting of the stratified keratinized epidermis and a variable amount of dermis. Preferentially harvested from the lateral thigh, these thin grafts display excellent "take," or survival, but can contract over time. The utility of these skin grafts with limited donor site morbidity and adequate healing in the non-irradiated patient has withstood the test of time (13–15). Dermal grafts, usually 0.010–0.014 inch thick, tend to take as well as split-thickness grafts and, yet, display less contraction. These autografts are harvested from the donor bed deep to an elevated split-thickness graft, the latter of which is left attached at one end to be later redraped and sutured over the donor site. Although thicker grafts contract very little, "take" tends to decrease with increasing graft thickness, and therefore, for limited mobile tongue defects, full-thickness grafts offer no substantial gain over dermal or split-thickness. The skin graft depends on a clean healthy recipient bed and immobilization in order to allow proper exchange of nutrients and transport of metabolic waste. Meshing or pie-crusting may be performed to increase graft size and may prevent hematoma formation or separation of the graft if not secured to the underlying tissue with bolster. Once the graft is secured to the defect using absorbable suture, proper graft to recipient bed approximation and immobilization are best achieved with a bolster dressing over the graft for five to seven days.

Skin graft reconstruction of small defects involving the anterior tip or ventral tongue, facilitates mobility, while preserving cosmesis as well as the integrity of adjacent subsites such as the floor of mouth, anterior lingual sulcus and lateral sulcus. Skin grafting offers these advantages as well as versatility, ease of harvest with a short operative time requirement, low complication rate and minimal donor site morbidity. There are potential disadvantages to skin grafting, including the necessary bolster and its associated awkwardness, donor site discomfort and scar, lack of bulk desirable in larger defect reconstruction, and delayed contracture which can lead to decreased tongue mobility over time (19). Some patients may require

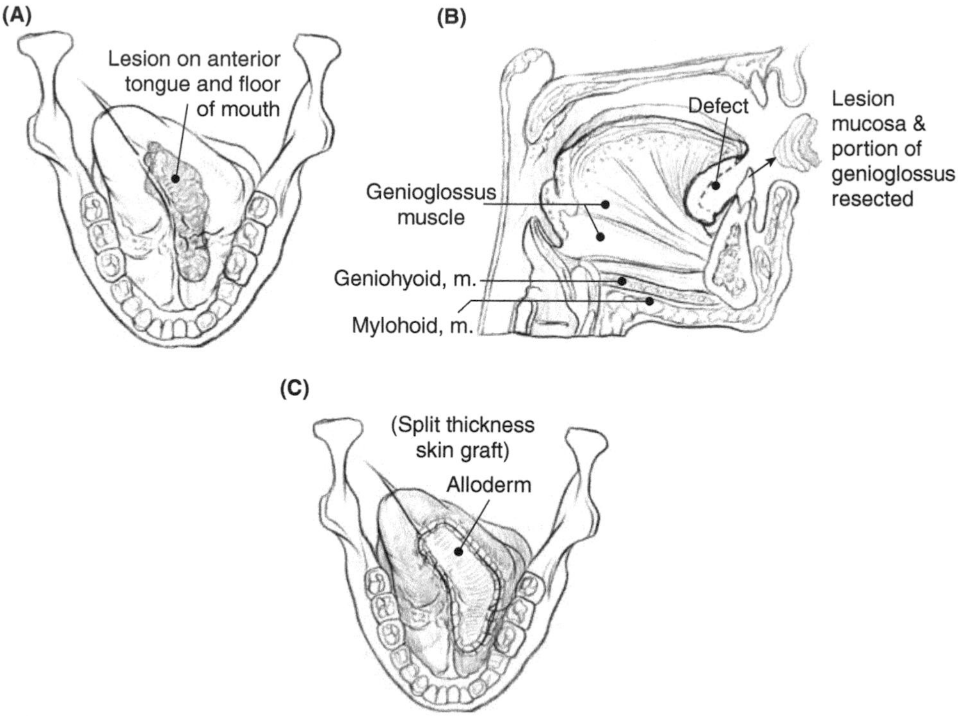

Figure 2 Skin Graft Closure. (**A**) Superior view of tongue and oral cavity revealing cancer on the ventral surface of the tongue into the floor of mouth. (**B**) Sagittal section view following removal of the tumor and deeper tissues resulting in a defect of the tongue and floor of mouth. (**C**) Superior view of skin or allograft in place following suturing to reconstruct the defect following cancer resection.

temporary tube feedings to prevent tongue mobility during this healing phase. The authors recommend this technique for anterior defects when primary closure would result in tethering of the tongue.

An additional option which is gaining acceptance is the use of *allograft* materials to cover tongue defects (16). Particularly, in circumstances when there is limited or poor quality skin available for harvest, when any donor site morbidity is unacceptable, or when operative time is to be even further minimized, an acellular dermal matrix (Alloderm^{TM}, LifeCell Corporation, Branchburg, New Jersey, U.S.A.) obtained from cadaveric harvest is now commercially available to be used as a substitute for autograft skin. This homograft material has the same indications, applications and advantages as standard skin grafts, but with no donor site morbidity. The primary disadvantage of homografts is cost, in addition to those drawbacks previously mentioned for skin grafting, with the exception of donor site issues. However, some argue that the cost of the operative time saved and decreased donor site morbidity offset the added expense of the graft material. When utilized under the appropriate circumstances, autogenous or homologous skin grafting remains a valuable technique in the reconstructive surgeon's armametarium. There does remain some concern over the use of allograft material in patients previously treated with radiation therapy although no large studies have compared this technique to other methods.

Moving up the reconstructive ladder, tongue flaps are *local tissue rearrangements* widely utilized in the past for a variety of oral cavity and oropharyngeal reconstructions. Posterior hemitongue advancement, described for anterior/lateral mobile tongue defects, is possible because of the lateral orientation of the lingual neurovascular supply. A relatively avascular median fibrous septum facilitates rapid, safe division of the tongue into two separate halves; the intact posterior tongue ipsilateral to the defect is then advanced forward and secured to the contralateral anterior tongue. Any advancement or rotational flap created from normal remnant tongue, however, introduces the potential for oral disability by recruiting otherwise intact tissue for reconstruction. Some authors, therefore, advocate abandoning the use of tongue flaps altogether, citing counterproductivity in sacrificing a structure we strive so diligently to reconstruct (19). The use of such flaps and reconstructive modalities in defects of this size is usually unnecessary except in cases where vascularized tissue is needed or in secondary reconstructions.

There will be certain situations when primary closure or grafting is not sufficient or in recurrent cancers previously operated and radiated that may require regional or distant flap reconstruction. The *regional flaps* for tongue reconstruction differ greatly from the majority of head and neck reconstructive options due to the immense need for mobility of thin, pliable tissue making the pectoralis major myocutaneous flap and deltopectoral flaps a last resort. When available, the platysma flap or submental flap are ideal for size, shape and thickness for tongue reconstruction. The problem with sound oncologic technique and prior radiation or neck dissection, however, frequently limits their use and availability. When the anterior mobile tongue is involved alone, it is not ideal to repair this with a bulky regional flap unless all other options have been exhausted.

Platysma Flap

The platysma flap has enjoyed a renewed popularity in recent years despite being used successfully decades ago in head and neck reconstruction (17). A myocutaneous flap based on branches of the facial, submental, occipital, posterior auricular, and transverse cervical arteries and with venous drainage from branches of the facial vein, internal and external jugular vein (18–20). The flap can be based superiorly, anteriorly or posteriorly for use in the oral cavity although venous drainage has been shown to be most reliable when the external jugular vein is preserved (19). The flap should be considered only on an undissected or non-irradiated neck when the vasculature remains intact although prior chemotherapy, large defects, and nodal disease may complicate outcomes (21). Complications frequently include venous congestion, epidermolysis, and wound separation although minor complications may occur in over one-third of patients (18,21,22). The flap planning, marking and incisions must be performed before any approach through the neck is begun. This is not a flap available for consideration after the neck dissection unless preoperative planning included this flap at the time of surgery. The major advantage of the flap is that it can be harvested near the field of a cancer resection and provides thin, mobile myocutaneous coverage for oral and pharyngeal defects. Unfortunately, this may also be a disadvantage since the blood supply and drainage are within areas of potential radiation and regional metastatic disease. Although, the flap is primarily supplied by the submental branch of the facial artery, it has been harvested successfully following ligation of this artery during radical neck dissection. The flap is ideally suited for oral cavity and tongue defects although a number of variations and numerous other defects may be reconstructed with this flap (23–25). The primary disadvantage is that there is a high rate of partial flap necrosis with venous congestion and epidermolysis. Although, the skin paddle often has partial necrosis, there is a low fistula rate when used for mucosal coverage (21). The flap technique requires that the distal flap incision be performed initially with a subplatysmal flap elevation taking care not to injure the arterial and venous branches from the facial vessels. The proximal incision around the elliptical cutaneous paddle in the lower neck is elevated in a supraplatysmal plane.

The flap is then tunneled into the oral cavity, floor of mouth, or cheek either deep or superficial to the mandible depending upon the defect location and pedicle orientation.

Submental Flap

The submental flap has re-emerged as a useful flap in oral and tongue reconstruction particular for reconstruction after trauma or tumors without regional metastatic disease and is an axial flap based upon the submental artery and vein.

Although described for use in burn reconstruction, the flap has been reported to have a wide variety of uses in the head and neck region including use in the oral cavity for tongue defects (26–28).

The flap has pedicle length up to 8 cm and can be harvested as a myocutaneous flap using the digastric muscle or as a fascial, fasciocutaneous, or even osteocutaneous flap (29). It has the obvious advantage of being convenient to the head and neck region with excellent color match. The scar is usually hidden inferior to the mandible and provides an improved cervicomental angle in most cases. The major disadvantage is that inadvertent harvesting of lymphatics of level IA during the flap harvest may compromise lymphadenectomy and allow for locoregional recurrence in squamous cell carcinoma. In these cases, a thinned flap is practical to prevent the inclusion of lymphatics in the flap. The technique includes an elliptical incision in the submental region that can extend laterally with a length up to 18 cm and width up to 7 cm (29). The incision is carried through the subcutaneous tissue to the contralateral anterior belly of the digastric muscle. Deep dissection to the mylohyoid is necessary and the ipsilateral (to the pedicle) anterior digastric may be included in order to incorporate additional blood supply if the flap is particularly large. The distal branch from the facial artery can be identified on the exterior surface of the submandibular gland and can be followed along its course or maintained in a bed of surrounding adipose and connective tissue. The flap is then mobilized and rotated into position as necessary.

When primary closure, grafting and the submental or platysma flap are not available, it is best to move up the ladder directly to the radial forearm, lateral arm or lateral thigh flap to allow for remaining movement to the tongue providing articulation and swallowing function to remain. The *regional pedicled flaps* including pectoralis major, trapezius, latissimus and deltopectoral flaps should be used only as a last resort in these cases but may be more appropriate when the defect involves adjacent or surrounding structures in addition to the mobile tongue. In these cases, it may be beneficial to close the tongue defect with a separate technique than the adjacent site.

Secondary intention, primary closure and/or skin grafting are thus preferred reconstructive options for glossectomy defects involving 25% or less of the anterior/mobile tongue. Subsequent chapters will address tongue reconstruction when performed for composite defects.

Hemiglossectomy Defects (Less Than 50% of the Anterior Mobile Tongue)

Following hemiglossectomy, functional disturbances tend to be more significant than with smaller defects despite reconstruction of the tongue. Studies have shown adequate swallowing rehabilitation following free tissue transfer but persistent articulatory deficits (30). There are fewer options for reconstruction after hemiglossectomy although the same techniques used for partial glossectomy or 25% defects have been described, including: healing by secondary intention; primary closure; auto and allografting, and; local tissue rearrangement. The variety of options are listed in Table 2 providing several options for each sized defect. Unfortunately, the size of the defect, the loss of the bulk of the remaining tongue leaving significant "dead space" and tethering of the remaining tongue have led most reconstructive surgeons to apply free tissue transfer to most of these defects although the thin, regional flaps including platysma and submental flaps may afford similar functional outcomes.

Allowing a wound to granulate and *reepithelialize secondarily* is a reasonable approach for smaller defects but when hemiglossectomy is performed, the large defect and potential large area of tethering place this as a secondary option.

Primary closure remains an option for management of the hemiglossectomy but results in an unusual shape to the neotongue which does not have normal function. This narrow neotongue is unable to facilitate the movement of food beyond the oral cavity in many situations and often deviates into the occlusal line resulting in repeated trauma to the tongue. Additionally, such defects often approach or involve floor of mouth mucosa, and primary closure of a full hemiglossectomy wound will result in severe tethering of the reconstructed tongue and further motion impairment. The loss of bulk on the side of the defect will allow food to collect and result in problematic swallowing function.

Skin and allo-grafting would be considered a more suitable reconstruction for hemiglossectomy defects but still does not provide the fullness in the oral cavity that is helpful in swallowing. This technique remains popular and successful results can be obtained in addition to the longstanding discussion about the ability to "monitor" the site for potential recurrent disease. The bolster placement may provide temporary swallowing and breathing difficulty due to mass effect and edema making tracheotomy placement and feeding tube placement a consideration. See the partial glossectomy section for technical issues on grafting. Allograft coverage of these defects is similar to split thickness skin grafts and recent reports suggest similar success rates.

The use of *tongue flaps* is not appropriate in hemiglossectomy defects. Local flaps and mucosal flaps also are not helpful in reconstructing the defect or in functional outcomes.

Regional flap reconstruction of hemiglossectomy is an option that should be given consideration although the bulk of the pedicled pectoralis, trapezius, latissimus and deltopectoral is often excessive. The trapezius, latissimus and non-delayed deltopectoral flap are tenuous due to the distance and potential for distal ischemia in an area at great length from the donor site. Additionally, when the mandible remains intact and/or is exposed, the decision to rotate these flaps into position either

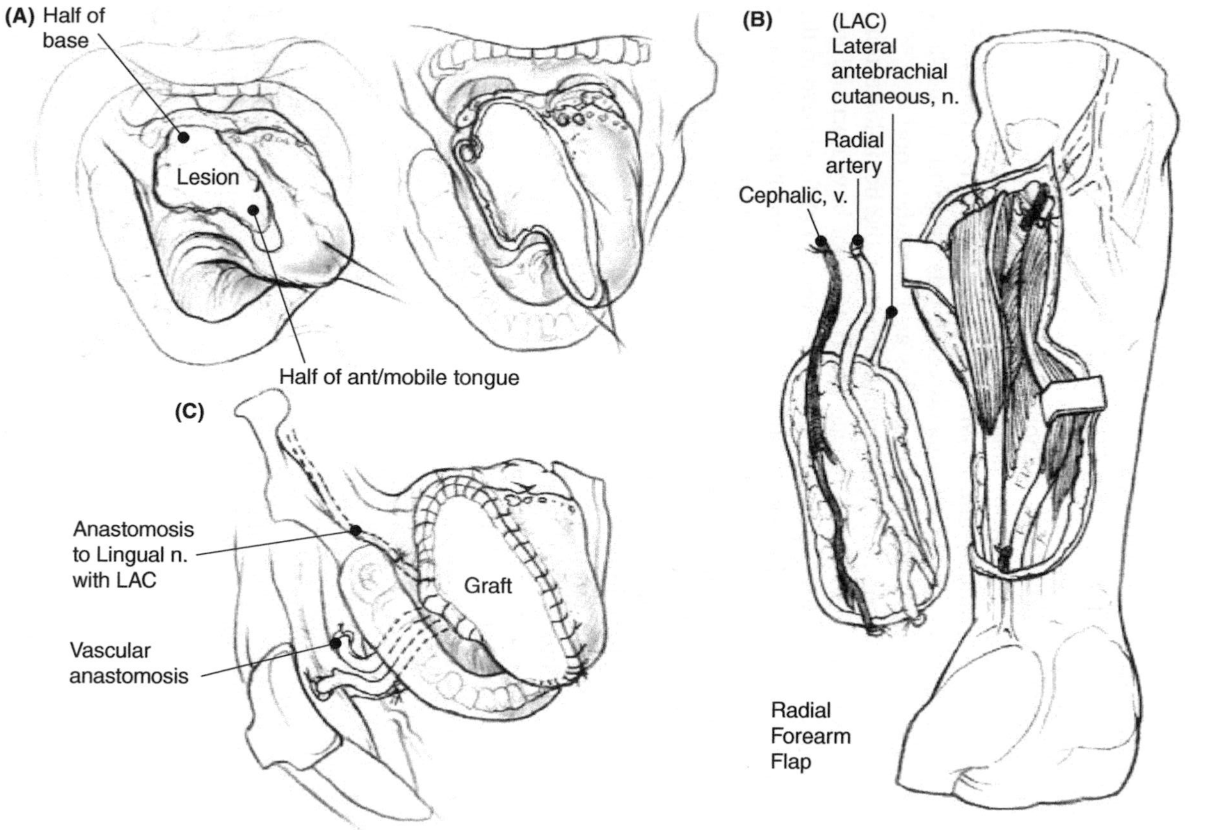

Figure 3 Radial forearm free flap reconstruction. (**A**) Large cancer of the right lateral border of tongue before and after resection. (**B**) Volar aspect of the right arm depicting the harvest of the radial forearm fasciocutaneous free flap. (**C**) View of the reconstructed tongue with the radial forearm free flap showing microvascular anastamosis in the neck and lingual nerve graft.

through a tunnel over or under the mandible may result in pedicle ischemia due to the tension at the level of the mandible. The pectoralis flap has adequate reach to this area but remains bulky for months after surgery at which time debulking can be performed. Studies have confirmed successful tongue reconstruction with the pectoralis myocutaneous flap although large prospective, controlled studies will likely not be possible and thinner free tissue transfers have the opportunity to improve function (30–32). When available, the platysma flap or submental flap are more appropriate for size, shape and thickness in tongue reconstruction. The problem with prior radiation or neck dissection, however, frequently limits their use and availability.

Free tissue transfer often is necessary for the hemiglossectomy defect affording the patient a functional, aesthetic and comprehensive reconstruction of the defect. The gold standard for hemiglossectomy defects remains the thin, pliable flaps that may include the radial forearm fasciocutaneous flap, lateral arm flap, anterolateral thigh flap, and abdominal perforator flaps (2,33,34). When primary closure, grafting and the submental or platysma flap are not indicated or available, it is often necessary to consider free tissue transfer to improve tongue mobility thus preserving articulation and swallowing function (5,35,36). The radial forearm free flap (Fig. 3) will be described in detail here as it has performed well in this area and has historically been the most commonly used free flap for larger defects of the mobile tongue although the aforementioned options may provide similar functional outcomes and can result in less donor site morbidity (35,37,38). The forearm flap also has been shown to provide sensation similar to the native tongue resulting in improved sensory input in the reconstructed tongue (39).

Soft tissue free flap reconstruction often using the radial forearm flap is thus the authors' preferred reconstructive choice for hemiglossectomy defects.

Radial Forearm Fasciocutaneous Flap (Fig. 3)

General

The radial forearm fasciocutanous free flap has achieved great success in oral tongue reconstruction since its introduction in the late 1970s (38,40). In all head and neck reconstructive sites, it appears to be the most commonly used flap (37,41). The ulnar artery based forearm flap may also be applied to oral tongue defects and has similar features to the radial based flap (42,43).

Indications

The radial forearm flap is ideally suited for the majority of anterior tongue defects following partial glossectomy. The potential addition of bone provides anatomic reconstruction of areas requiring thin bone but allows the use of the thin, pliable soft tissue for the mobile tongue aspect of the defect. The most common use of the radial forearm flap is in the oral cavity and pharynx although a multitude of indications in the head and neck are reported. The radial forearm fasciocutaneous flap is ideally suited for partial to near total glossectomy defects due to the thin, pliable, sensate skin covering. The flap usually mucosalizes over a period of 3–12 months making it difficult to differentiate from surrounding tongue surface and also may regenerate sensate potential with or sometimes without nerve grafting (39,44–47).

Anatomical Considerations

Surgeons performing harvest of the radial forearm flap should have extensive knowledge and experience with the volar aspect of the forearm to the antecubital fossa including the muscular, vascular and neurologic structures of this area. The vascular structures proximal and distal to this area should be assessed prior to harvest. The brachial artery divides into the radial and ulnar arteries near the antecubital fossa with the important radial recurrent artery the initial branch of the radial artery. The ulnar artery runs deep to the flexor carpi ulnaris but may be identified superficial in the distal forearm. The palmar arch is the critical component of flow to the hand through these vessels which usually communicate via the palmar arches in the hand. If there is not a patent arch, the flap is usually contraindicated without a vascular graft. The skin, bone and fascia of the flap are supplied via small perforators easily identified during the dissection. During dissection, the deep periosteal perforators are seen to extend through the flexor pollicis longus muscle to the radius. The anatomic location of the radial and ulnar arteries, superficial veins and vena comitantes, flexor carpi radialis, brachioradialis and palmaris longus tendons and muscles, and the radial and median nerves can be assessed during the procedure. During the harvest of bone, the insertion of the brachioradialis tendon is often the distal extent of bone harvest.

Advantages/Disadvantages

Although the radial forearm has many advantages, occasionally, the few disadvantages outweigh the advantages. The flap is reliable with a pedicle that has good caliber and length (38). The soft tissue component is thin and pliable with sensate potential adding to the benefit in individuals with expected return of swallowing function. The two team approach is straightforward and the flap is easily contoured and shaped to a particular defect. The entire skin flap is well vascularized throughout its length allowing for the use of split paddle or even three paddle skin coverage. In tongue reconstruction, the skin color match is not relevant and the majority remucosalize over time to provide nice cosmesis. The major disadvantage of the use of this flap remains the donor site although specialized techniques may improve on the unsightly scar and potential morbidity of this site (48–56). It is important that aggressive physical therapy be instituted, otherwise, limitation in range of motion of the wrist can occur due to scarring and fibrosis.

Pre-operative Evaluation

The major focus of this evaluation is the flow to the hand and palmar arch in addition to the skin overlying the forearm. Any compromise of vascular flow, including prior arterial lines, blood draws and needle sticks can interfere with the viability of flaps of this region. The standard test prior to harvest includes the Allen's Test which is performed to assess the patency of connection of the superficial and deep palmar arches in the hand. The use of both a subjective and objective Allen's Test is reported although indeterminate flow patterns can be further evaluated with Doppler examination when necessary (57). The test is performed by asking the patient to firmly make a fist repeatedly for several times while the examiner is simultaneously compressing the radial and ulnar arteries. Following complete blanching of the hand despite the patient's cessation of making a fist, the ulnar artery compression is released while firm pressure remains on the radial artery (thus duplicating the effect following ligation of the vessel). The return of blood flow to the digits, particularly the index finger and thumb, is assessed to confirm that rapid (less than five seconds) return of flow occurs. If repeated tests indicate a problem with the patency, the other arm should be examined and consideration of Doppler studies arranged to fully evaluate the system prior to harvest. The authors routinely use Doppler examinations to fully evaluate the patency of the arch in addition to the quality of flow in each vessel. The brachioradialis, flexor carpi radialis, palmaris longus, radial nerve, radial artery pulse, capillary refill, antecubital fossa, cephalic, and basilic veins should all be examined and identified prior to the planned donor site harvest (period). Ideally, the patient's non-dominant extremity is that designated for the harvest site.

Techniques

Harvest:

The patient, nursing staff and anesthesiologists should understand that the arm should not incur intravenous or arterial lines or needle sticks. A second nursing and surgical team is ideal for the two team approach. Prior to incisions, the arm is marked to identify landmarks including the radial artery, superficial veins and radial nerves. A tourniquet can be applied to the upper arm prior to sterile prep or applied sterilly after the prep but is not inflated until the arm is exsanguinated and the procedure is ready to begin. The arm is extended on the armboard which is at 90° to the table allowing surgeons to sit opposite each other during the dissection. The thigh should be prepared for skin graft harvest or appropriate allograft material available for coverage of the donor site. The skin coverage necessary is marked overlying the volar aspect of the forearm centered on the donor artery. A curvilinear incision extends to the antecubital fossa for extended length pedicle if necessary. The skin and underlying fascia is then elevated identifying the distal radial nerve branches which may divide into two to five small branches at the wrist. Care is taken to divide the fascia at the brachioradialis and dissect deep to the vascular pedicle or the pedicle can be separated from the cutaneous paddle if dissection does not proceed deep at this point. The dissection is then started from the ulnar aspect and elevated toward the pedicle taking care to remain superficial to the ulnar artery and median nerve. Preservation of the paratenon fascia overlying the tendons of the flexor carpi radialis, palmaris longus and brachioradialis muscles is crucial to prevent tendon exposure. Some authors advocate performing a suprafascial dissection allowing improved healing of the graft over the tendon. The deep osseous branches are ligated when bone is not harvested, and carefully preserved when an osteocutaneous flap is harvested. The distal and proximal incisions are connected around the periphery of the flap leaving the flap connected only proximally by the venous, neural and arterial systems and by only the radial artery distally. The cutaneous nerves are immediately deep to the subcutaneous tissue proximally and usually run alongside the distal branches of the cephalic and basilic venous system. At this point, separation of the brachioradialis and flexor carpi radialis (FCR) allows visualization of the proximal radial artery and paired venae comitantes to the antecubital fossa. The deep and superficial systems will merge into a plexus of veins in the antecubital fossa and beyond, often allowing the surgeon to perform fewer venous anastamoses but allowing flow through both systems. When all of the proximal vessels are skeletonized and ready for ligation, the distal radial artery is then clamped with a temporary clamp while the tourniquet is released confirming flow to the digits through the palmar arches. It is then safe to ligate the distal radial artery and transfer the flap when the recipient site is prepared. The forearm should be closed with a split thickness skin graft although allograft material is gaining popularity (58). A prefabricated forearm splint is placed to secure the graft material for five to seven days and monitoring of the vascular supply to the hand continues throughout the post-operative period.

Complications following radial forearm flap harvest may include skin graft loss, sensory deficits, hand cold intolerance and motor strength deficits (51,52,56), although there have been rare cases of anomalous forearm vascular supply which must be considered prior to the radial forearm harvest to prevent ischemia to the hand (59–61). Preservation of the paratenon cannot be overemphasized as this is the enveloping fascia that allows vascular ingrowth from adjacent tissues and grafts (48,51,54,62,63). When this is removed, it is helpful to advance adjacent muscle or adipose to cover any exposed tendon prior to grafting.

Physical and occupational therapy with wrist and hand range of motion exercises should commence within weeks following the procedure to ensure adequate motor function.

The branches of the radial nerve should be identified early in the dissection to prevent accidental transaction or trauma and permanent numbness although some patients do have resultant sensory loss when these branches are preserved (51).

The contraindications to the radial forearm flap include generalized coagulopathic states and other medical conditions which prevent all free tissue transfers, while contraindications unique to this flap include anomalous palmar arch anatomy, radial or ulnar agenesis or thrombosis and prior surgery or trauma to the forearm area. Patient function, occupation and avocation may also preclude the use of this donor site.

Post-harvest grafting techniques have included split thickness skin graft, dermal graft, purse-string with grafting, wound-vac assisted closure and allograft materials, although controversy remains as to the best type of material and technique (55,58,63–65).

Subtotal Glossectomy Defects (50–100% of the Anterior Mobile Tongue)

When the entire anterior tongue requires resection, the primary problems incurred are articulation difficulties and oral bolus manipulation of foods. The pharyngeal swallow and prevention of aspiration are not nearly as problematic in these anterior defects as occurs in base of tongue resections. The key to functional and aesthetic anterior total tongue reconstruction includes the use of a flap that can be "hinged" on the base of tongue providing some movement to this "static" anterior neotongue. It is also crucial to provide enough bulk to allow for the anterior neotongue to approach the palate to assist in both speech and swallowing. In fact, the shape of the reconstructed tongue and flap may play a role in swallowing outcomes (66). Unfortunately, it is not as easy to generalize to a particular flap that is ideal for all of these defects; rather it often depends upon the individual patient and, their respective body habitus and associated surgical defects.

In relatively healthy or obese individuals, the radial forearm flap provides excellent filling of complete anterior glossectomy defects and is "light" enough to allow for the posterior tongue to "carry" the neotongue in various directions. The flap is often folded upon itself anteriorly to provide a tongue tip and is more flattened posteriorly at the insertion into the base of tongue. Anti-gravity sutures to the palate or mandible in some cases provide upward pull and prevents the traditional falling of the flap tissue inferior and posteriorly. In very thin individuals or when there is associated loss of floor of mouth support, a thicker flap may be necessary including the lateral arm, lateral thigh or anterolateral thigh flaps. These are preferred over regional flaps and allow exact positioning of the flaps, a feature that regional flaps are limited by their pedicle location. In all free tissue transfers for these defects, the pedicle should emerge from the posterior insetting of the flap directly into the recipient vessels.

Other Defects

When there is a ventral anterior tongue defect possibly involving the floor of mouth resulting in loss of the anterior tip or ventral tongue, other techniques may provide the best functional outcome. Please see chapter 10 for details on this area but when the anterior tongue is absent, it is often best to perform a posterior based release and advancement to allow the tongue to protrude and reach the upper incisors and palate. This can be performed with a 2–3 cm midline split of the tongue with lateral releasing incisions and primary closure or even skin or allografting of the ventral surface. Another successful technique includes the use of primary closure for the dorsum and tip with lateral releasing incisions in the ventral tongue, which often results in a diamond shaped defect which can then be grafted. The importance of this separate cannot be overemphasized as this is the most common site of tethering and preventing articulation of certain sounds as well as oral manipulation of certain foods.

In those defects involving the base of the tongue in addition to the oral tongue, consideration has been historically given to total glossectomy and total laryngectomy. More conservative options seem to be available with the use of free tissue transfer to provide a defect-based placement of similar tissue in combination with partial anterior glossectomy and/or supraglottic laryngectomy. It is not necessary for each patient with a partial or total base of tongue resection to undergo laryngectomy to prevent aspiration. The majority of patients requiring partial base of tongue resection can be functionally rehabilitated if there remains a single hypoglossal nerve, lingual artery and lingual vein. Thicker flaps such as a lateral arm, scapula fasciocutaneous, lateral thigh, rectus or latissimus may provide the bulk necessary in these situations. It is important that laryngeal suspension and placing the flap to overhang the glottis be performed to prevent aspiration and facilitate for adequate laryngeal elevation for swallowing.

In summary, anterior mobile tongue reconstruction should focus primarily on tongue mobility related to articulation and swallowing. The reconstructive modality that optimizes these important functional abilities should be considered before all other options.

REFERENCES

1. Day TA, Tarr C, Zealear D, Burkey BB, Sullivan CA. Tongue replantation in an animal model. Microsurgery 2000; 20(3):105–108.

2. Haughey BH, Taylor SM, Fuller D. Fasciocutaneous flap reconstruction of the tongue and floor of mouth: outcomes and techniques. Arch Otolaryngol Head Neck Surg 2002; 128(12):1388–1395.
3. Conley J, Sachs ME, Parke RB. The new tongue. Otolaryngol Head Neck Surg 1982; 90(1):58–68.
4. Colangelo LA, Logemann JA, Pauloski BR, Pelzer JR, Rademaker AW. T stage and functional outcome in oral and oropharyngeal cancer patients. Head Neck 1996; 18(3):259–268.
5. Urken ML, Moscoso JF, Lawson W, Biller HF. A systematic approach to functional reconstruction of the oral cavity following partial and total glossectomy. Arch Otolaryngol Head Neck Surg 1994; 120(6):589–601.
6. Pauloski BR, Logemann JA, Rademaker AW, McConnel FM, Heiser MA, Cardinale S, Shedd D, Lewin J, Baker SR, Graner D, et al. Speech and swallowing function after anterior tongue and floor of mouth resection with distal flap reconstruction. J Speech Hear Res 1993; 36(2):267–276.
7. Salibian AH, Allison GR, Strelzow VV, Krugman ME, Rappaport I, McMicken BL, Etchepare TL. Secondary microvascular tongue reconstruction: functional results. Head Neck 1993; 15(5):389–397.
8. Greene CH, Debias DA, Henderson MJ, Fair-Covely R, Dorf B, Radin AL, Young-Seidman WL. Healing of incisions in the tongue: a comparison of results with milliwatt carbon dioxide laser tissue welding versus suture repair. Ann Otol Rhinol Laryngol 1994; 103(12):964–974.
9. Elshal EE, Inokuchi T, Yoshida S, Sekine J, Sano K, Ninomiya H, Ikeda H. A comparative study of epithelialization of subcutaneous fascial flaps and muscle-only flaps in the oral cavity. A rabbit model. Int J Oral Maxillofac Surg 1998; 27(2):141–148.
10. Sabri A. Oropharyngeal reconstruction: current state of the art. Curr Opin Otolaryngol Head Neck Surg 2003; 11(4):251–254.
11. Logemann JA, Pauloski BR, Rademaker AW, McConnel FM, Heiser MA, Cardinale S, Shedd D, Stein D, Beery Q, Johnson J, et al. Speech and swallow function after tonsil/base of tongue resection with primary closure. J Speech Hear Res 1993; 36(5):918–926.
12. Bressmann T, Sader R, Whitehill TL, Samman N. Consonant intelligibility and tongue motility in patients with partial glossectomy. J Oral Maxillofac Surg 2004; 62(3):298–303.
13. Rhee PH, Friedman CD, Ridge JA, Kusiak J. The use of processed allograft dermal matrix for intraoral resurfacing: an alternative to split-thickness skin grafts. Arch Otolaryngol Head Neck Surg 1998; 124(11):1201–1204.
14. Butler CE. "Tongue sandwich" bolster for skin graft immobilization. Head Neck 2002; 24(7):705–709.
15. Fister HW, Sharp GS. The intra-oral use of the free split-thickness skin graft in commando-type procedures. Am J Surg 1963; 106:709–711.
16. McGregor IA, McGrouther DA. Skin-graft reconstruction in carcinoma of the tongue. Head Neck Surg 1978; 1(1):47–51.
17. Futrell JW, Johns ME, Edgerton MT, Cantrell RW, Fitz-Hugh GS. Platysma myocutaneous flap for intraoral reconstruction. Am J Surg 1978; 136(4):504–507.
18. Coleman JJ III, Jurkiewioz MJ, Nahai F, Mathes SJ. The platysma musculocutaneous flap: experience with 24 cases. Plast Reconstr Surg 1983; 72(3):315–323.
19. Uehara M, Helman JL, Lillie JH, Brooks SL. Blood supply to the platysma muscle flap: an anatomic study with clinical correlation. J Oral Maxillofac Surg 2001; 59(6):642–646.
20. Agarwal A, Schneck CD, Kelley DJ. Venous drainage of the platysma myocutaneous flap. Otolaryngol Head Neck Surg 2004; 130(3):357–359.
21. Verschuur HP, Dassonville O, Santini J, Vallicioni J, Poissonnet G, Laudoyer Y, Dernard F. Complications of the myocutaneous platysma flap in intraoral reconstruction. Head Neck 1998; 20(7):623–629.
22. Mazzola RF, Benazzo M. Platysma flap for oral reconstruction. Clin Plast Surg 2001; 28(2):411–419.

23. Ariyan S. The transverse platysma myocutaneous flap for head and neck reconstruction: an update. Plast Reconstr Surg 2003; 111(1):378–380.
24. Bauer T, Schoeller T, Rhomberg M, Piza-Katzer H, Wechselberger G. Myocutaneous platysma flap for full-thickness reconstruction of the upper and lower lip and commissura. Plast Reconstr Surg 2001; 108(6):1700–1703.
25. Ozcelik T, Aksoy S, Gokler A. Platysma myocutaneous flap: use for intraoral reconstruction. Otolaryngol Head Neck Surg 1997; 116(4):493–496.
26. Horster W, Schmid E. Contour improvement in burns using submental bipedicled-flap plasty. Fortschr Kiefer Gesichtschir 1979; 24:35–38.
27. Wu Y, et al. Submental island flap for head and neck reconstruction: a review of 20 cases. Asian J Surg 1981; 21:247–252.
28. Pistre V, Pelissier P, Martin D, Lim A, Baudet J. Ten years of experience with the submental flap. Plast Reconstr Surg 2001; 108(6):1576–1581.
29. Martin D, Pascal JF, Baudet J, Mondie JM, Farhat JB, Athourn A, Le Gaillard P, Peri G. The submental island flap: a new donor site. Anatomy and clinical applications as a free or pedicled flap. Plast Reconstr Surg 1993; 92(5):867–873.
30. Hsiao HT, Leu YS, Lin CC. Tongue reconstruction with free radial forearm flap after hemiglossectomy: a functional assessment. J Reconstr Microsurg 2003; 19(3):137–142.
31. Knuuttila H, Pukander J, Maatta T, Pakarinen L, Vilkman E. Speech articulation after subtotal glossectomy and reconstruction with a myocutaneous flap. Acta Otolaryngol 1999; 119(5):621–626.
32. Su WF, Hsia YJ, Chang YC, Chen SG, Sheng H. Functional comparison after reconstruction with a radial forearm free flap or a pectoralis major flap for cancer of the tongue. Otolaryngol Head Neck Surg 2003; 128(3):412–418.
33. Agostini V, Dini M, Mori A, Franchi A, Agostini T. Adipofascial anterolateral thigh free flap for tongue repair. Br J Plast Surg 2003; 56(6):614–618.
34. Yamamoto Y, Minakawa H, Yoshida T, Igawa H. Tongue reconstruction after hemiglossectomy with the lateral arm free flap. J Reconstr Microsurg 1994; 10(2):91–94.
35. Huang CH, Chen HC, Huang YL, Mardini S, Feng GM. Comparison of the radial forearm flap and the thinned anterolateral thigh cutaneous flap for reconstruction of tongue defects: an evaluation of donor-site morbidity. Plast Reconstr Surg 2004; 114(7):1704–1710.
36. Shpitzer T, Guttman D, Gur E, Feinmesser R, Ad-El D. Transoral reconstruction of the mobile tongue, using radial forearm free flap. Microsurgery 2003; 23(1):18–20.
37. O'Brien CJ, Lee KK, Stern HS, Traynor SJ, Bron L, Tew PJ, Haghighi KS. Evaluation of 250 free-flap reconstructions after resection of tumours of the head and neck. Aust N Z J Surg 1998; 68(10):698–701.
38. Evans GR, Schusterman MA, Kroll SS, Miller MJ, Reece GP, Robb GL, Ainslie N. The radial forearm free flap for head and neck reconstruction: a review. Am J Surg 1994; 168(5):446–450.
39. Kuriakose MA, Loree TR, Spies A, Meyers S, Hicks WL Jr. Sensate radial forearm free flaps in tongue reconstruction. Arch Otolaryngol Head Neck Surg 2001; 127(12):1463–1466.
40. Yang G, Chen B, Gao Y. Forearm free skin flap transplantation. National Med J China 1981; 61:139.
41. Haughey BH, Wilson E, Kluwe L, Piccirillo J, Fredrickson J, Sessions D, Spector G. Free flap reconstruction of the head and neck: analysis of 241 cases. Otolaryngol–Head Neck Surg 2001; 125(1):10–17.
42. Christie DR, Duncan GM, Glasson DW. The ulnar artery free flap: the first 7 years. Plastic Reconstruct Surg 1994; 93(3):547–551.
43. Sieg P, Bierwolf S. Ulnar versus radial forearm flap in head and neck reconstruction: an experimental and clinical study. Head Neck 2001; 23(11):967–971.
44. Dubner S, Heller KS. Reinnervated radial forearm free flaps in head and neck reconstruction. J Reconstructive Microsurg 1992; 8(6):467–468; discussion 469–470.
45. Shindo ML, Sinha UK, Rice DH. Sensory recovery in noninnervated free flaps for head and neck reconstruction. Laryngoscope 1995; 105(12 Pt 1):1290–1293.

46. Urken ML, Weinberg H, Vickery C, Biller HF. The neurofasciocutaneous radial forearm flap in head and neck reconstruction: a preliminary report. Laryngoscope 1990; 100(2 Pt 1):161–173.
47. Badran D, Soutar DS, Robertson AG, Reid O, Milne EW, McDonald SW, Scothorne RJ. Behavior of radial forearm skin flaps transplanted into the oral cavity. Clin Anatomy 1998; 11(6):379–389.
48. Bardsley AF, Soutar DS, Elliot D, Batchelor AG. Reducing morbidity in the radial forearm flap donor site. Plastic Reconstructive Surg 1990; 86(2):287–292; discussion 293–294.
49. Bootz F, Biesinger E. Reduction of complication rate at radial forearm flap donor sites. Orl; J Oto-Rhino-Laryngology & its Related Specialties 1991; 53(3):160–164.
50. Kolker AR, Coombs CJ, Meara JG. A method for minimizing donor site complications of the radial forearm flap. Ann Plastic Surg 2000; 45(3):329–331.
51. Richardson D, Fischer SE, Vaughan ED, Brown JS. Radial forearm flap donor-site complications and morbidity: a prospective study. Plastic Reconstructive Surg 1997; 99(1):109–115.
52. Schoeller T, Otto A, Wechselberger G, Lille S. Radial forearm flap donor-site complications and morbidity. Plastic Reconstructive Surg 1998; 101(3):874–875.
53. Smith AA, Bowen CV, Rabczak R, Boyd JB. Donor site deficit of the osteocutaneous radial forearm flap. Ann Plastic Surg 1994; 32(4):372–376.
54. Swanson E, Boyd JB, Manktelow RT. The radial forearm flap: reconstructive applications and donor-site defects in 35 consecutive patients. Plastic Reconstructive Surg 1990; 85(2):258–266.
55. Wolff KD, Ervens J, Hoffmeister B. Improvement of the radial forearm donor site by prefabrication of fascial-split-thickness skin grafts. Plastic Reconstructive Surg 1996; 98(2):358–362.
56. Skoner JM, Bascom DA, Cohen JI, Andersen PE, Wax MK. Short-term functional donor site morbidity after radial forearm fasciocutaneous free flap harvest. Laryngoscope 2003; 113(12):2091–2094.
57. Nuckols DA, Tsue TT, Toby EB, Girod DA. Preoperative evaluation of the radial forearm free flap patient with the objective Allen's test. Otolaryngology-Head Neck Surg 2000; 123(5):553–557.
58. Sinha UK, Shih C, Chang K, Rice DH. Use of AlloDerm for coverage of radial forearm free flap donor site. Laryngoscope 2002; 112(2):230–234.
59. Jones BM, O'Brien CJ. Acute ischaemia of the hand resulting from elevation of a radial forearm flap. Br J Plastic Surg 1985; 38(3):396–397.
60. Funk GF, Valentino J, McCulloch TM, Graham SM, Hoffman HT. Anomalies of forearm vascular anatomy encountered during elevation of the radial forearm flap. Head Neck 1995; 17(4):284–292.
61. Heden P, Gylbert L. Anomaly of the radial artery encountered during elevation of the radial forearm flap. J Reconstructive Microsurg 1990; 6(2):139–141.
62. Turk AE, Chang J, Soroudi AE, Hui K, Lineaweaver WC. Free flap closure in complex congenital and acquired defects of the palate. Ann Plastic Surg 2000; 45(3):274–279.
63. Swift RW, Wheatley MJ, Meltzer TR. A safe, reliable method for skin-graft coverage of the radial forearm donor site. J Reconstructive Microsurg 1997; 13(7):471–473.
64. Lauer G, Schimming R, Gellrich NC, Schmelzeisen R. Prelaminating the fascial radial forearm flap by using tissue-engineered mucosa: improvement of donor and recipient sites. Plastic Reconstructive Surg 2001; 108(6):1564–1572; discussion 1573–1575.
65. Winslow CP, Hansen J, Mackenzie D, Cohen JI, Wax MK. Pursestring closure of radial forearm fasciocutaneous donor sites. Laryngoscope 2001; 110(11):1815–1818.
66. Kimata Y, Sakuraba M, Hishinuma S, Ebihara S, Hayashi R, Asakage T, Nakatsuka T, Harii K. Analysis of the relations between the shape of the reconstructed tongue and postoperative functions after subtotal or total glossectomy. Laryngoscope 2003; 113(5):905–909.

12

Reconstruction of the Base of Tongue and Total Glossectomy Defects

Mark K. Wax and Dana S. Smith
Department of Otolaryngology—Head and Neck Surgery, Oregon Health and Science University, Portland, Oregon, U.S.A.

INTRODUCTION

Reconstruction of the tongue base may be required for a variety of lingual defects. Occasionally, it is needed following traumatic injury or surgical excision of benign neoplasms. However, malignant tumors comprise the vast majority of those defects that require tongue reconstruction. Malignancies of the tongue base make up approximately 30% of oropharyngeal cancer (1). The other major subsite in the oropharynx is the tonsil. When the tonsil is the primary site, the tongue base may be secondarily involved in over 50% of cases. Thus, in almost 70% of cases of cancer of the oropharynx, there will be involvement of the tongue base.

Today early stage tumors are treated by either surgery or radiation, depending on the preference of the attending physician. Other methods, such as photodynamic therapy or cryotherapy, have also been reported but are not used by many. While there have been many advances in our understanding of tumor biology and treatment, the morbidity and mortality from tongue cancer remain significant. Five-year survival rates for stage 1 and 2 disease remain at 80% (2). With adequate surgical or radiation therapy, local control can be obtained in 90–95% of these patients. Advanced stage disease (stage 3 or 4) significantly lowers the five-year survival rate to between 30% and 50%. Local control with combined modality treatment is higher at 60%. Unfortunately, the vast majority of tongue base tumors present at an advanced stage (3).

Treatment of oropharyngeal carcinoma has undergone a paradigm shift over the last decade. In the past, oropharyngeal cancer was primarily a surgical disease. In the last decade, more and more centers have come to utilize organ preservation protocols with radiation and chemotherapy in attempts to avoid surgical excision. Unfortunately, significant numbers of patients with advanced stage disease will continue to require surgical salvage. Treatment requires resection of significant portions of the tongue base, or even total glossectomy. Reconstruction in these patients is complicated by the surrounding tissue exposure to radiation and/or chemotherapy. The advent of free tissue transfer has not only cut down on the morbidity of the surgical ablation but also has improved the rehabilitative potential of these patients.

Unfortunately, improvements in diagnosis and the ability to find and identify these tumors at an earlier stage have not shown any promise. Thus, improvements in reconstruction have led to the greatest advance in decreasing morbidity and improving rehabilitation.

Anatomy and Physiology of the Tongue

The tongue is primarily composed of striated muscle covered by stratified squamous epithelium (4). The tongue has intrinsic musculature and is comprised of complex interlacing fibers in longitudinal, transverse, and vertical orientation. In addition it possesses four paired extrinsic muscles: the genioglossus, the hyoglossus, the styloglossus, and the palatoglossus (5). All intrinsic and extrinsic muscles except the palatoglossus are innervated by paired hypoglossal nerves. The palatoglossus is innervated by the vagus nerve. These muscles act in a concerted fashion, giving the tongue the capacity for a myriad of movements that allow alterations of position and shape (4). The multitude of fibers that comprise the tongue rests on the mylohyoid muscular sling. This sling serves as a dynamic platform upon which the muscle acts. When the mylohyoid is tense, the tongue can act as a solid force that moves food around the mouth. When the mylohyoid is relaxed, the tongue can "sink" into the submental area to increase its mobility.

The tongue is divided into the oral tongue and the tongue base by the circumvalate papillae. This division is important from an oncologic point of view. Anteriorly, the oral tongue drains to ipsilateral lymph nodes, whereas, posteriorly, the tongue base drains bilaterally to the lymphatic system of the neck. The circumvalate papillae also demarcate the boundary between the oral cavity and the oropharynx. Posteriorly and inferiorly, the tongue base extends to the base of the epiglottis, and includes the pharyngoepiglottic and glossoepiglottic folds (6). The palatine tonsils and tonsillar pillars bound the lateral borders of the tongue base. Paired lingual tonsils are located on the dorsum of the tongue base. The tongue has the regular sensory function (such as fine touch, two-point discrimination, vibration, and temperature), as well as the specialized sensory functions of taste. The lingual nerve provides sensory innervation to the oral tongue. Taste is provided by the chorda tympani. The glossopharyngeal nerve provides regular sensation to the majority of the tongue base. The superior laryngeal nerve, a branch of the vagus nerve, innervates the epiglottis and a small area of the posterior tongue base (5). Paired lingual arteries supply the arterial vasculature to the tongue.

Any discussion of tongue reconstruction must take into account the specialized features that it serves. These include deglutition, airway protection, and articulation. Deglutition can be divided into preparatory, oral, pharyngeal, and esophageal phases (7). The oral tongue assists in mastication during the preparatory phase as food is manipulated into a semisolid or liquid bolus. In the oral phase, the food bolus is pushed posteriorly by the mobile tongue. The tongue is then pulled posteriorly by the styloglossus and the palatoglossus. This closes the nasopharynx and upper oropharynx and forces the bolus posteriorly. The pharyngeal phase begins as the bolus passes the anterior palatine arch (8), followed by laryngeal closure and elevation. The intrinsic laryngeal muscles close the endolarynx in a purse-string fashion and the epiglottis prolapses over the endolarynx. The palatopharyngeus, stylopharyngeus, and suprahyoid muscles (mylohyoid, digastric, geniohyoid, and genioglossus) pull the larynx anterosuperior under the tongue base, generating negative pressure in the hypopharynx (4). The esophageal phase then begins with cricopharyngeal relaxation, followed by a peristaltic wave that propels the bolus from the pharynx into the esophagus.

The oral tongue is necessary for the preparatory and oral phases of deglutition. The base of tongue is critical to the creation of a driving force that propels the food bolus through the pharynx in the pharyngeal phase of deglutition (9). Resection of any part of the tongue has the potential to seriously disrupt deglutition. Therefore, it is common for patients to experience significant dysphagia after tongue resection. This is especially so when the tongue base is resected (10). It is not clear what critical volume of tongue base remnant is required to maintain normal swallowing function. The pharyngeal constrictors are able to partially compensate for loss of tongue-base bulk, but some bulk at the tongue base is necessary to allow deglutition (4).

Resection of any part of the tongue may cause aspiration, especially during the early postoperative period (4). Patients who have tongue-base resections are at high risk for aspiration whereas those who have total glossectomy almost always have some degree of aspiration. Tongue-base resection puts the patient at a particular risk for aspiration during the pharyngeal phase of deglutition. The bulk of the base of tongue protects the laryngeal inlet. The loss of bulk combined with the loss of laryngeal elevation due to resection of the suprahyoid musculature results in aspiration (11). In addition, ptosis of the floor of mouth after total glossectomy may lead to funneling of oral secretions directly into the hypopharynx, increasing aspiration risk (1). The risk may be further increased if loss of laryngeal innervation via the superior laryngeal nerve occurs.

Articulation is a function in which normal tongue bulk and movement are essential. Any resection of normal tongue has the potential to interfere with articulation. Total glossectomy can be devastating, because speech intelligibility may be severely affected. A decrease in the ability of the patient to articulate often results in social isolation and decreases quality of life tremendously.

Resection of the tongue base often necessitates severing the motor or sensory supply to the distal oral tongue. This results in loss of bulk and decreased motion of the oral tongue. Loss of motor function to the residual tongue may be more critical in leading to functional tongue impairment than the actual volume of tongue resected (4).

After adequate resection of the tumor, healing of the wound is the next consideration. Complicating healing in this patient population is the prevalence of pretreatment with radiation to local tissues and/or chemotherapy. The goal of the reconstruction is to allow for quick healing that minimizes morbidity at the ablative site, as well as at the donor site. Once healing has occurred, the long-term goal of tongue reconstruction is restoration of lost function and preservation of remaining tongue function. It is important to consider these goals in any reconstructive planning. The effects of any method on airway protection, deglutition, and speech must be carefully considered. The ideal reconstruction would replace coordinated motor function, sensation, and bulk of the defect while resulting in no mobility impairment to the residual tongue; however, achievement of all of these aims simultaneously is rarely possible, so selection of the best reconstruction modality often involves a compromise between competing aspects which optimizes overall tongue function.

EVALUATION AND PLANNING

Evaluation should include a thorough history and physical examination focusing on the head and neck as well as pertinent laboratory and radiological tests as needed. Pertinent medical history includes systemic diseases, general health, neurological, and functional status, and substance abuse habits. Pulmonary status is critical; deficits such as chronic obstructive pulmonary disease may mandate laryngectomy with a different reconstruction due to a low tolerance of aspiration in the postoperative period. Poor pulmonary status and/or cardiac status may preclude the extended operative time necessary for free-tissue transfer. Compromised neurological status in the form of altered mentation, local sensory deficit, or motor deficit is also important. For instance, a previous stroke affecting swallowing function may result in unacceptably high postoperative aspiration risk if laryngectomy is not performed with the reconstruction. Systemic diseases such as diabetes, obesity, hypercholesterolemia, and collagen vascular diseases may be relative contraindications to free-tissue transfer due to the likelihood of microvascular disease, whereas hypercoagulable states are absolute contraindications to free tissue transfer (12). Surgical history should be obtained, with careful attention to previous oncologic resections, failed reconstructions, and operations that may have affected possible free-tissue transfer donor sites or vascular anastamotic sites in the neck. If a forearm flap is being considered for reconstruction, handedness should be established. A history of radiation therapy or steroid dependence should be elicited, as these will affect postoperative healing.

On physical examination, the oral tongue may be directly visualized and palpated. The base of tongue should also be palpated and visualized with flexible fiberoptic nasopharyngoscopy. A full cranial nerve examination should be performed with special attention to deficits in lingual sensation or motor function. The neck should be palpated to evaluate lymphadenopathy. Potential free-tissue transfer donor sites should be inspected. If a radial or ulnar forearm free flap is considered, an Allen's test should be performed; Doppler ultrasonography or angiography is generally unnecessary if this is normal. General body habitus should be inspected for signs of malnutrition, such as temporal wasting.

Laboratory studies include complete blood count, coagulation panel, and basic metabolic panel. Hepatic function studies are also obtained to screen for liver metastasis, to assess nutritional status, and to detect hepatic insufficiency secondary to alcoholic cirrhosis or chronic hepatitis, all of which may cause coagulopathy.

Classification of Tongue Resection Defects

Tongue base	**Small (less than 25% of the base of tongue)**
	Partial (25% to 75% of the base of tongue)
	Subtotal/Total (greater than 75% of the base of tongue)
Mobile tongue	Quarter glossectomy
	Hemiglossectomy
	Total anterior tongue resection
Subtotal/total	**Without laryngectomy or mandibular resection**
Glossectomy	With laryngectomy
	With mandibular resection

Figure 1 Tongue defects classified for reconstruction purposes. Items in bold text are discussed in this chapter.

<u>Classification of Reconstructive Techniques</u>

Healing by secondary intention

Primary closure

Skin graft/acellular allograft dermal matrix

Local flap reconstruction

Regional flap transfer

Distant tissue transfer

Figure 2 Reconstructive techniques classified by ascending complexity. Items in bold are employed in base-of-tongue and total glossectomy reconstruction.

Radiological studies include a neck computed tomography scan with contrast to evaluate the extent of the primary mass, bony invasion and neck lymphadenopathy. A Panorex is obtained if mandibular resection and bony reconstruction is expected with the glossectomy. A plain chest radiograph is obtained to screen for pulmonary metastasis. Positron emission tomography scanning and/or computerized tomography of the chest may be obtained depending on the status of the neck and the expectation of metastatic disease.

Preoperative speech pathology evaluation is always undertaken. A clinical swallowing evaluation is performed and, if necessary, a modified barium swallow is obtained to further evaluate swallowing function and aspiration risk. Preoperative articulation deficits are also assessed.

Prior to surgical resection, direct laryngoscopy and esophagoscopy are performed to rule out synchronous aerodigestive tract malignancy. Gastrostomy tube placement is also performed if it is likely the patient will have a long period of inadequate oral intake postoperatively. Ideally this is performed at least one week prior to tongue resection to optimize nutritional status; if this is not possible, a nasogastric feeding tube may be placed instead during the interim.

RECONSTRUCTIVE OPTIONS

Historically, tongue resection caused profound morbidity due to its marked effects on functional abilities and quality of life. This led to significant reluctance to pursue major surgery for tongue cancer. Many potentially resectable tumors were treated by radiotherapy with surgery reserved for salvage treatment (13). Advances in reconstruction techniques have steadily improved functional outcome after tongue resection. In the past, a great variety of local tongue flaps were used for reconstruction of defects. However, the use of these flaps caused significant restriction of the residual tongue's mobility, and are now of historical interest only (4). In the 1960s, the deltopectoral, forehead, and temporalis flaps were popularized for head and neck reconstruction. Their use in tongue reconstruction was an improvement but was still accompanied by much morbidity (13). Tongue prostheses have also been used after total glossectomy (14). However, results were poor. The later use of the sternocleidomastoid (15,16), trapezius, pectoralis major (3), and latissimus dorsi (17) pedicled flaps represented a significant advance by allowing one-step reconstruction of glossectomy defects (13). Finally, free-tissue transfer techniques from a plethora of

Base-of-Tongue and Total Glossectomy Reconstructive Techniques

Small Base-of-Tongue Defects

1. Primary closure
2. Radial forearm fasciocutaneous free flap
3. Ulnar forearm fasciocutaneous free flap

Partial Base-of-Tongue Defects

1. Radial forearm fasciocutaneous free flap
2. Ulnar forearm fasciocutaneous free flap
3. Lateral arm fasciocutaneous free flap
4. Pectoralis major myocutaneous pedicled flap

Subtotal / Total Base-of-Tongue Defects

1. Radial forearm fasciocutaneous free flap
2. Ulnar forearm fasciocutaneous free flap
3. Lateral arm fasciocutaneous free flap
4. Rectus abdominis myocutaneous free flap
5. Latissimus dorsi myocutaneous free flap
6. Latissimus dorsi myocutaneous pedicled flap
7. Pectoralis major myocutaneous pedicled flap

Subtotal / Total Glossectomy Defects

1. Rectus abdominis myocutaneous free flap
2. Latissimus dorsi myocutaneous free flap
3. Latissimus dorsi myocutaneous pedicled flap
4. Anterolateral thigh fasciocutaneous free flap
5. Scapular / parascapular myocutaneous free flap
6. Lateral thigh fasciocutaneous free flap
7. Lateral arm fasciocutaneous free flap
8. Pectoralis major myocutaneous pedicled flap

Figure 3 Reconstructive techniques for base-of-tongue and total glossectomy defects listed in order of the authors' general preference.

donor sites have greatly increased the reconstructive options for tongue defects. Although the cost of free flaps is slightly higher than pedicled flaps, this is more than offset by intangible costs and improved function (18).

Current reconstructive options after base-of-tongue resection and total glossectomy will be discussed according to the extent of the tongue defect (Fig. 1). Tongue-base defects are divided into small resection (involving less than 25% of the base of tongue), partial resection (involving 25–75% of the base of tongue), and subtotal/total resection (involving greater than 75% of the base of tongue). Total glossectomy is divided into glossectomy with and without laryngectomy. Glossectomy with laryngectomy is beyond the scope of this chapter and text.

In general, all tongue defect reconstructive options should be considered sequentially (Fig. 2). Healing by secondary intention causes significant scarring with a resultant distortion of the residual tongue, thus should be avoided. Primary closure can be used for small base-of-tongue lesions. Local tongue flaps, as previously mentioned, as well as skin grafting and acellular allograft dermal matrix, lead to functionally poor results with dead space, pooling of secretions, and mobility restriction and should be avoided. Pedicled muscular or myocutaneous flaps can

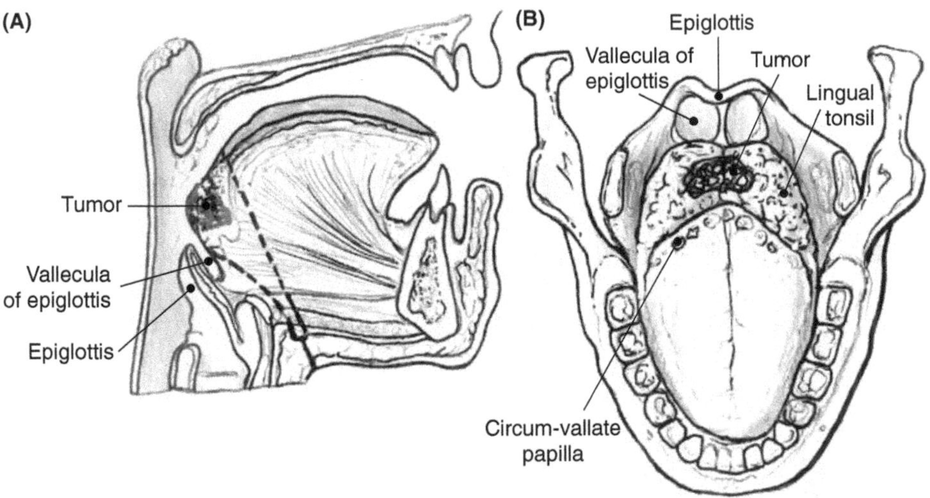

Figure 4A–D (**A**) This sagittal view of the tongue demonstrates a small <25% tumor of the tongue base. (**B**) This view demonstrates the same tongue base tumor as seen in **A**. Note that <25% of the tongue base is involved. The tumor is well circumscribed by normal appearing tongue tissue. (*Continued next page.*)

be used for larger base-of-tongue and total glossectomy defects, although free fasciocutaneous or myocutaneous flaps are generally preferable due to the number of available donor sites with diverse tissue characteristics, offering a better match for a given defect requirement.

The authors' preferred methods for base-of-tongue and total tongue reconstruction are explained for each defect type (Fig. 3). Further aspects of pedicled myocutaneous, free fasciocutaneous, and free myocutaneous flaps are then discussed individually by reconstructive technique.

Small Tongue Base Defects

For small base-of-tongue defects (a less than 25% defect), the preferred method of reconstruction is primary closure (Fig. 4). In these defects, there is minimal loss of base-of-tongue bulk. Additional bulk is not necessary for good apposition of the remaining tongue base to the soft palate and pharyngeal walls during the pharyngeal phase of deglutition. The defect is also small enough that primary closure can be accomplished with minimal tension. Primary closure is preferable to healing by secondary intention, skin grafting, or acellular allograft dermal matrix, as all of these tend to cause scarring and contraction, which limits function of the residual tongue. Another complication of these methods of reconstruction is that significant pooling of secretions and an increase of aspiration risk may occur. Although primary closure for small tongue-base defects usually allows good mobility of the residual tongue, it occasionally causes some degree of tethering of the residual tongue. If this is likely with primary closure, then a radial forearm or ulnar forearm fasciocutaneous free flap is the preferred reconstructive technique. Both of these have thin, pliable tissue, which will minimize restriction of mobility of the residual tongue. Superior functional results in speech and swallowing have been demonstrated for primary closure of small tongue-base defects compared to distal and free-flap reconstruction (19).

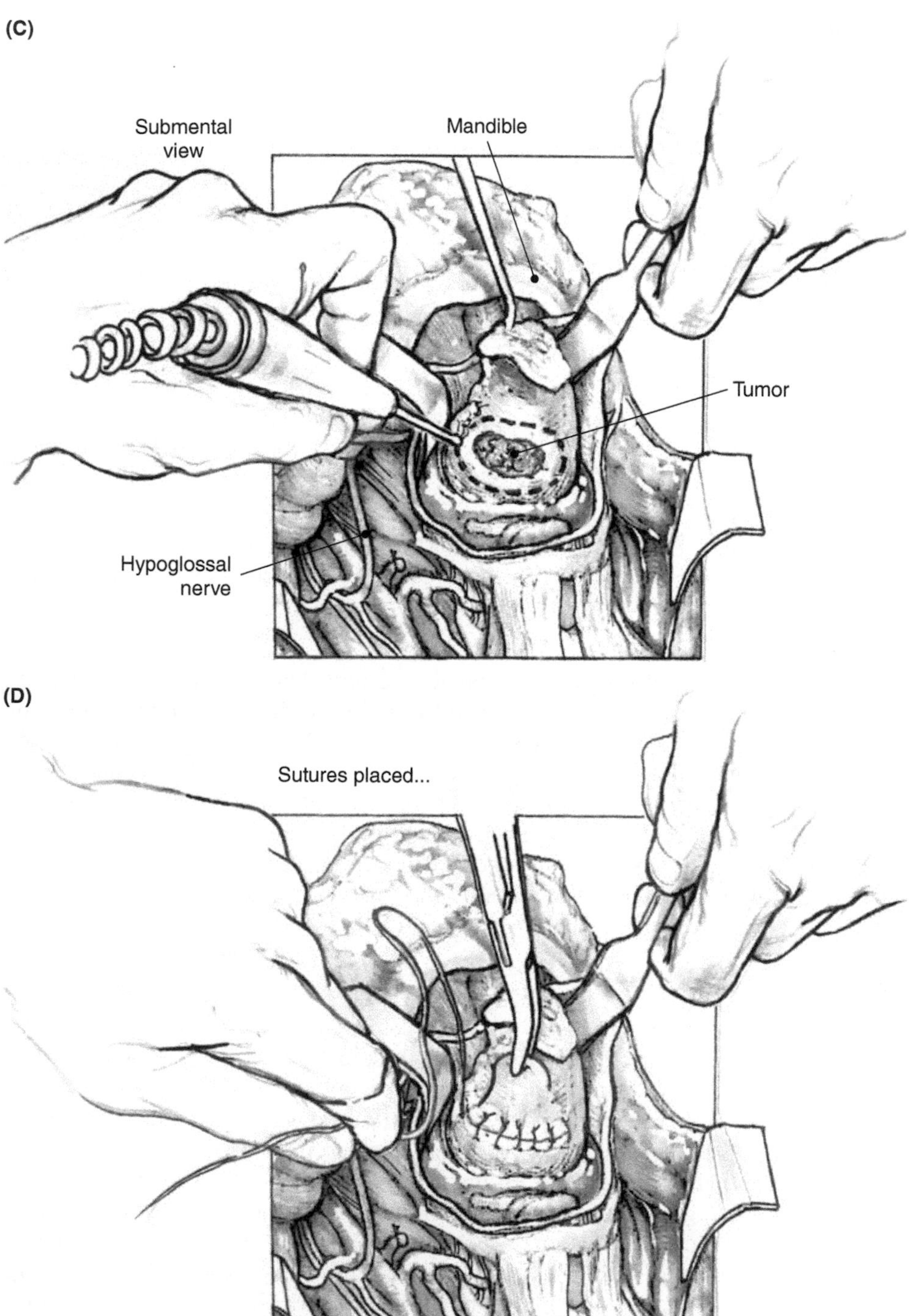

Figure 4 (C) Exposure has been obtained through a suprahyoid pharyngotomy, and the tumor is being excised with an adequate cuff of normal tissue. (D) Tumor has been resected with negative margins. Since it is relatively small, a single-layer closure using 3.0 synthetic braided suture in a vertical mattress fashion has allowed for primary closure.

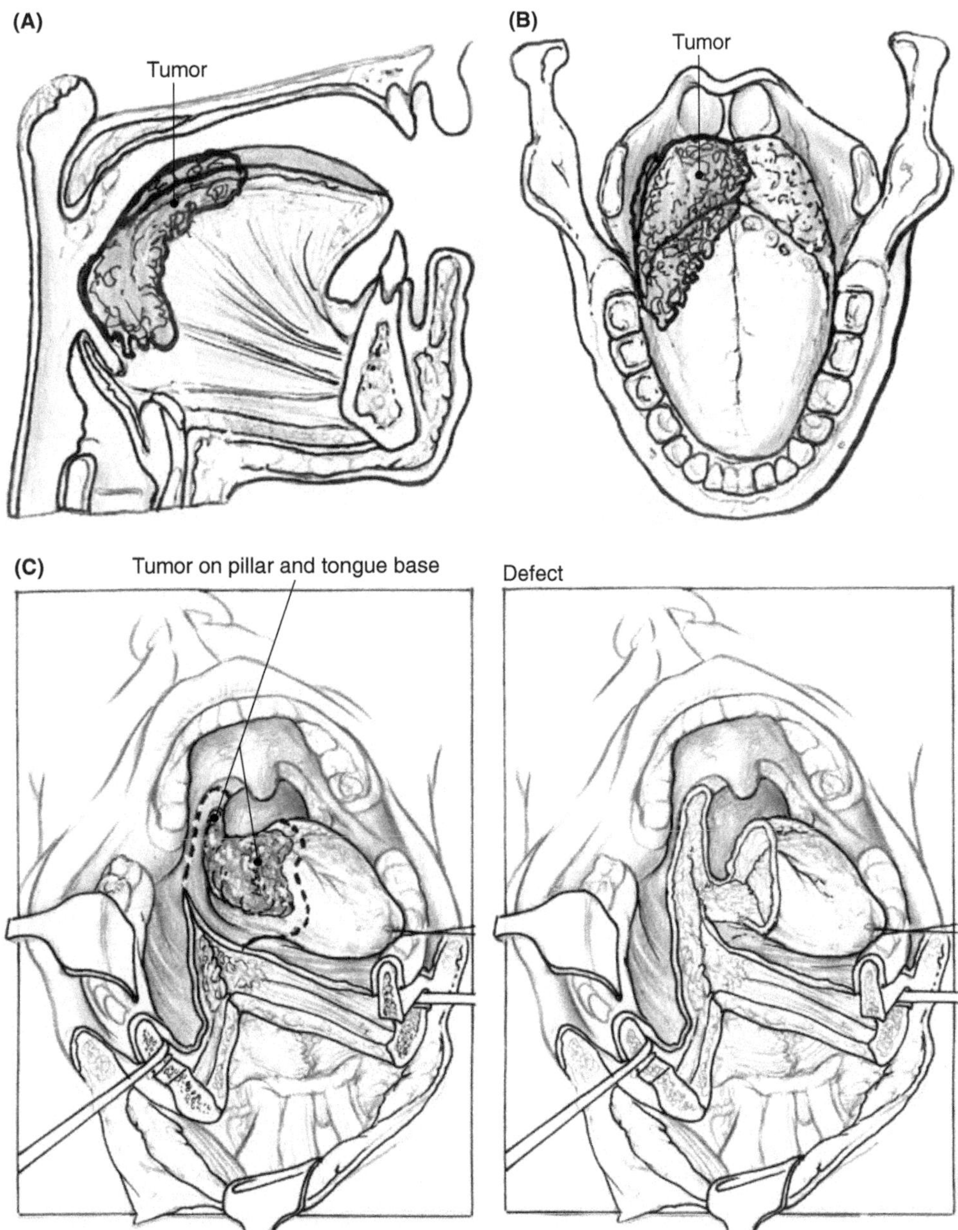

Figure 5A–G (**A**) In this rendering, the tumor occupies approximately 50% of the base of tongue with extension into the oral tongue. This lateral view demonstrates how a clear margin can be obtained in the vallecula. Removal of the tumor will require resection of some of the oral tongue. The resection will also involve some of the deep musculature of the tongue base. (**B**) This view demonstrates the same tumor as in **A** with slight extension across the midline anteriorly into the oral tongue. (**C**) After surgical removal of the tumor, a defect has been created that involves approximately 65% of the base of tongue, part of the epiglossal fold, tonsillar fossa, and mobile tongue. (*Continued next page.*)

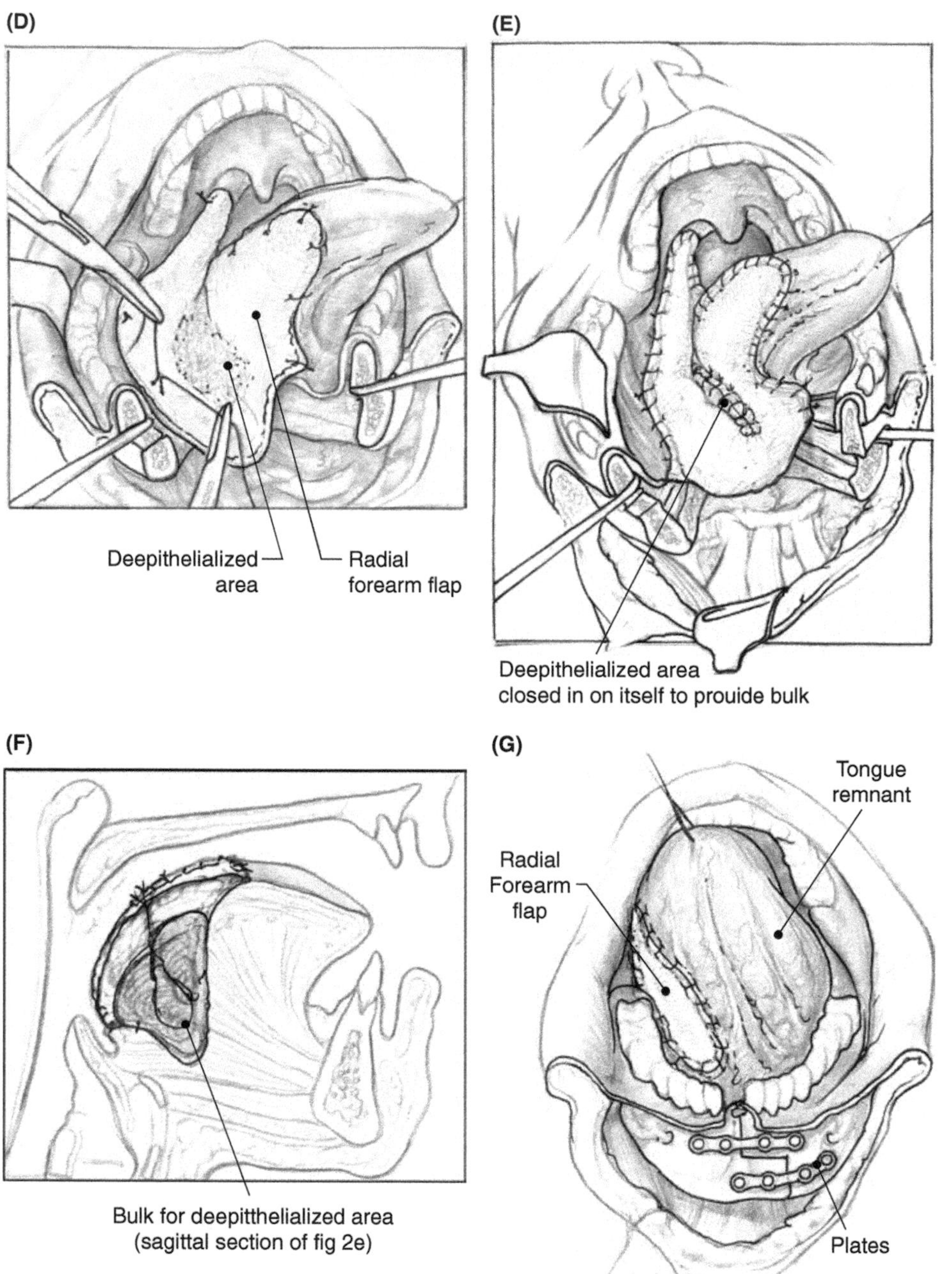

Figure 5 (**D**) A radial forearm fasciocutaneous free flap has been laid into the defect. It will be used to obtain a watertight closure. A central portion of the flap is going to be deepithelialized, then primarily closed. This will allow for increase in bulk to reconstruct the base of tongue defect. (**E**) The center part of the radial forearm flap has been deepithelialized and folded inferiorly to reconstruct the depths of the base of tongue. This will provide bulk to the flap. (**F**) Lateral view of the reconstructed tongue demonstrates how the deepithelialized portion of the radial forearm flap adds bulk to the reconstruction. (**G**) The radial forearm flap has been sewn in. Vessels have been anastomosed. Mobility of the tongue has been maintained. The mandible has been reconstructed with 2.0-mm plates.

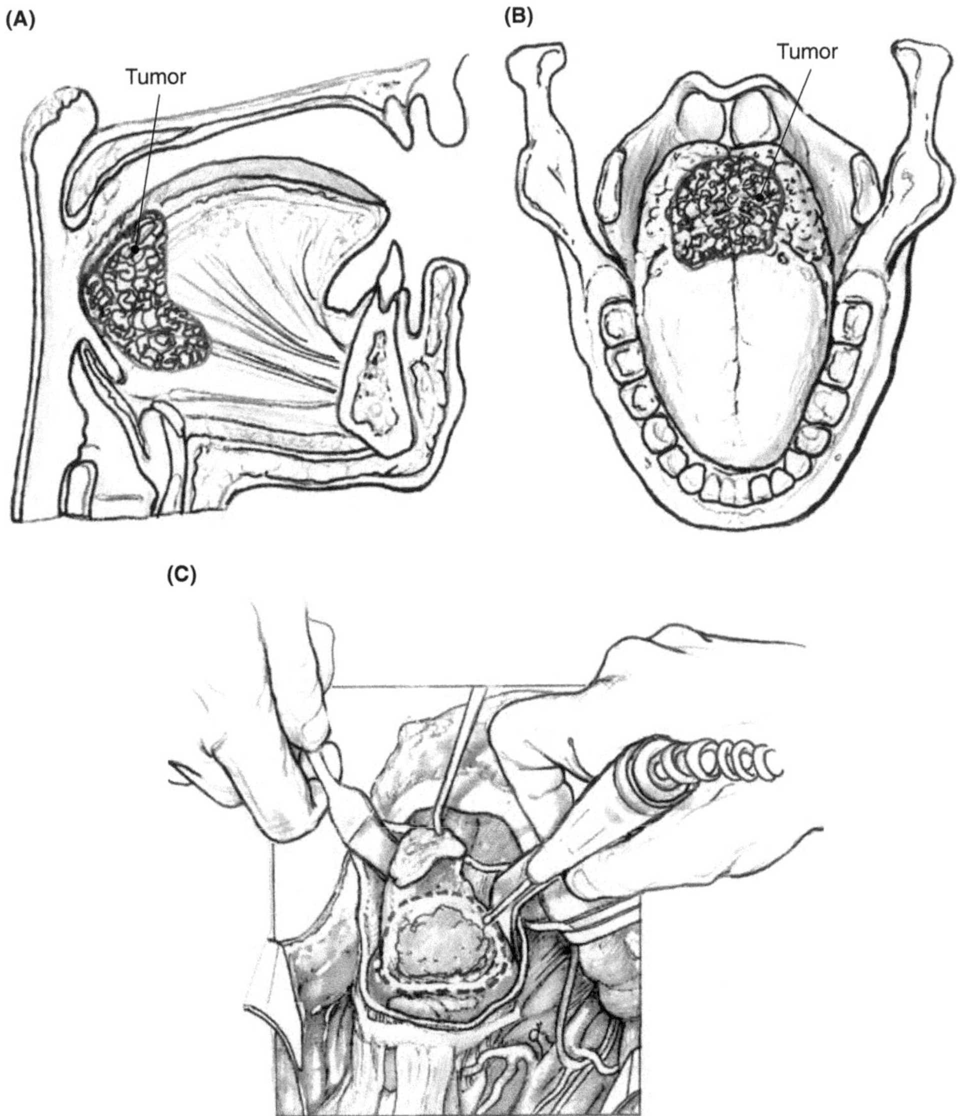

Figure 6A–E (**A**) This lateral artistic rendering demonstrates a tumor involving the total base of tongue. The anterior base of tongue is free of tumor. The vallecula is also free of tumor. Thus, only a tongue base resection is required. (**B**) Note that the lateral margins of the tongue base are intact. Thus, preservation of the hypoglossal nerves and lingual artery will be possible with preservation of mobility and vascularity to the anterior tongue. (**C**) The tumor is being excised, demonstrating preservation of the lateral neurovascular pedicle to the remaining tongue. (*Continued next page.*)

Partial Tongue Base Defects

Tongue-base defects between 25% and 75% require reconstruction with vascularized tissue in order to adequately replace lost bulk. If this bulk is not replaced, many problems can occur. For example, proper contact of the remaining tongue base with the soft palate and pharyngeal walls during deglutition and speech may not occur.

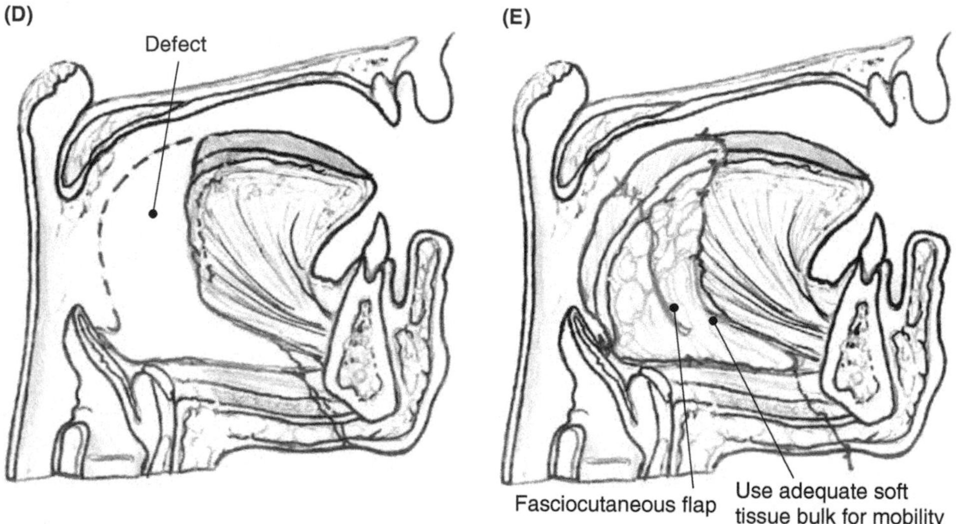

Figure 6 (**D**) Lateral view demonstrates a full thickness defect of the base of tongue. Reconstruction will require bulk to help prevent aspiration, but pliable tissue to facilitate maintenance of tongue mobility. (**E**) The radial forearm fasciocutaneous free flap has been sutured in place. Appropriate amounts of deepithelialization have been undertaken so as to provide the right amount of soft tissue bulk but maintaining mobility of the tongue.

If not reconstructed adequately, contraction of the remaining tissue may lead to significant distortion and loss of mobility of the remaining tongue. All of these factors may contribute to an increased risk of aspiration. The need for bulk must be balanced by the competing need for maximal mobility of the residual tongue. Therefore, a thinner, more pliable flap is desirable, provided it supplies sufficient bulk. For this reason, the radial forearm and ulnar forearm fasciocutaneous free flaps are preferable (Fig. 5). When more bulk is needed, a lateral arm fasciocutaneous flap is the next preference. Its use will generally cause more mobility restriction of the remaining tongue than the radial or ulnar flaps. A pedicled pectoralis major myocutaneous flap is the last option. This option is used when contraindications for a free flap are present. However, this will generally cause a greater restriction of the residual tongue mobility than a free-flap option.

Subtotal or Total Tongue Base Defects

Defects of greater than 75% of the base of tongue require greater bulk. However, the need to preserve mobility of the remaining tongue remains paramount. Therefore, the radial forearm and ulnar forearm fasciocutaneous free flaps are still the optimal selection for reconstruction if they offer enough bulk (Fig. 6). Either of these flaps may be partially de-epithelialized and rolled under itself for greater volume to fill in the tongue base defect. Generally, the volume of the flap should be greater than that of the defect to accommodate postoperative flap shrinkage (20), especially if radiation is to be administered subsequent to the reconstruction. If more bulk is needed, the lateral arm fasciocutaneous free flap is the next preference. The rectus abdominis myocutaneous free flap and latissimus dorsi flap (pedicled or free) offer

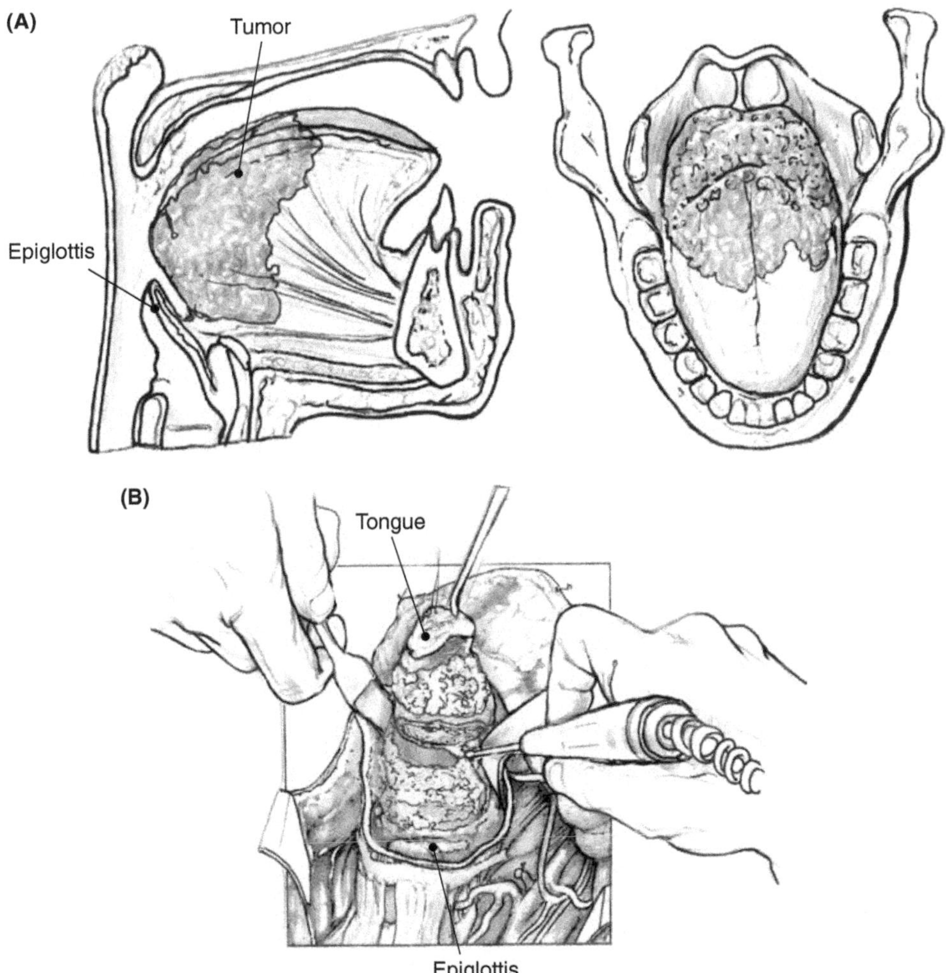

Figure 7A–D (**A**) Artist's rendering of an extensive tongue tumor that will require total glossectomy for resection. In this instance, the tumor involves significant aspects of the mobile tongue, as well as base of tongue. The lateral neurovascular pedicles will also require resection. It will not be possible to save any mobile tongue. (**B**) Removal of the whole tongue with a total glossectomy defect is demonstrated. The mandible is intact except for the mandibulotomy. The defect extends full thickness to the epiglottis. (*Continued next page.*)

even more bulk but do so at the cost of tongue mobility. When a pedicled flap is required, a latissimus dorsi flap is preferable to the pectoralis major flap due to its more pliable tissue characteristics and lesser degree of tethering.

Subtotal or Total Glossectomy Defects

In order to achieve satisfactory function of the subtotal or total glossectomy defect, the reconstruction must address two major elements: bulk and support. The reconstructive tissue must be sufficiently think to give adequate dorsal neotongue height for full contact with the soft palate and pharyngeal walls during deglutition and for good contact with the palate during articulation. Bulk also works to reduce

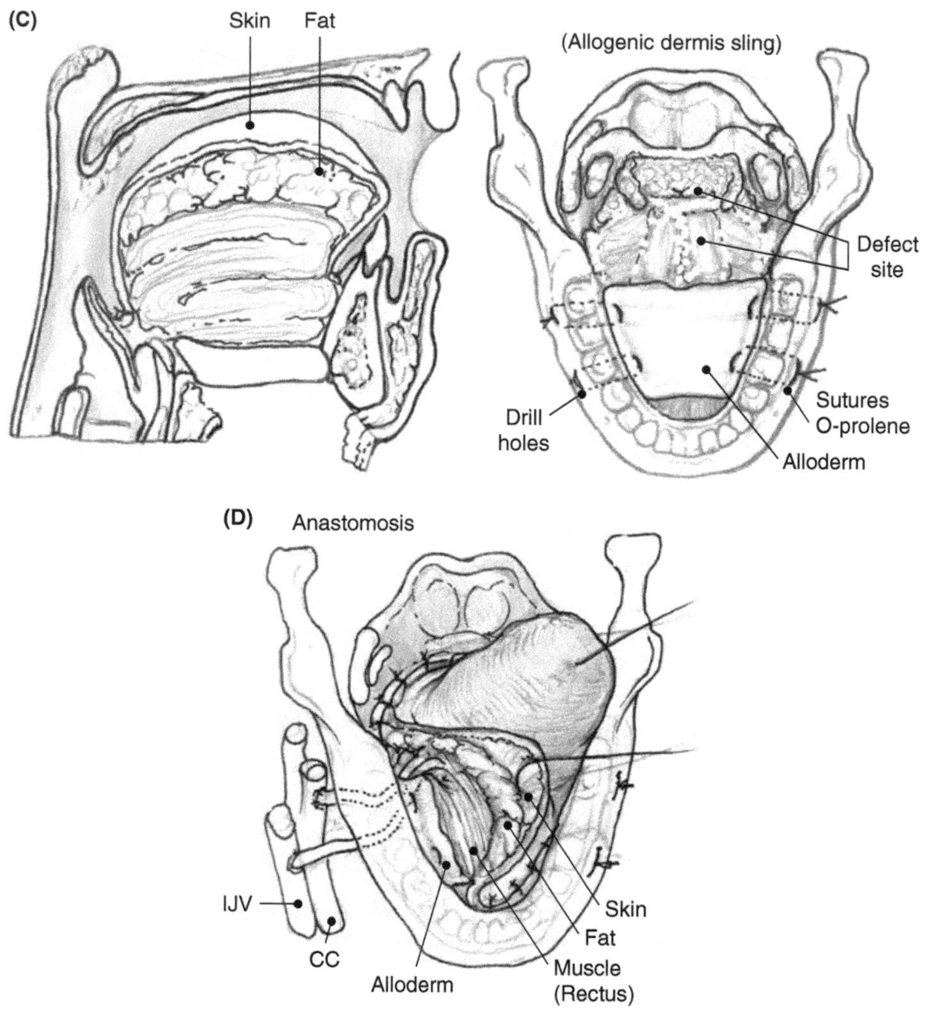

Figure 7 (C) A rectus abdominis myocutaneous free flap is used to reconstruct this defect. An allogenic dermis sling is suspended to the mandible with sutures to provide a platform on which the flap may rest. Apposition of the flap with the soft and hard palate ensures good potential for articulation. (D) Mounding of the flap is again evident with the arterial anastamosis.

aspiration by diverting secretions into the lateral gutters and yields better speech quality by decreasing resonance (21). Although, a palatal prosthesis may be worn to compensate for inadequate dorsal neotongue height, use of a prosthesis is generally discouraged because the functional loss of palatal sensation seriously impairs oral rehabilitation (22). In addition to bulk, the floor of mouth must be adequately supported in total glossectomy reconstruction. Otherwise, the floor of mouth will sag, causing effective loss of neotongue height. Ptosis of the floor of mouth may also lead to tunneling of secretions directly into the hypopharynx, increasing aspiration risk (1). For these reasons, the rectus abdominis free flap and latissimus dorsi free flap are the preferred methods of reconstruction since they offer the best bulk and support (Fig. 7). Lasting bulk is possible because both flaps contain significant vascularized fat that will not atrophy like the muscle, and both flaps are capable of motor reinnervation. This does not restore significant movement, but may partially prevent muscle atrophy. Lasting floor-of-mouth support is maintained by suturing the muscular component to the mandible to give the overlying fat and skin a firm platform (4). Some form of platform may also be fashioned with an acellular allograft dermal matrix sling. The rectus abdominis is preferred over the latissimus dorsi flap because no repositioning is necessary and a two-team approach may be used. In addition, tendinous inscriptions within the rectus abdominis muscle allow more secure suturing to the mandible (23). Unless there is a contraindication, the free latissimus dorsi flap is generally selected over the pedicled version due to the tendency of gravity to pull on the pedicle, causing ptosis and tongue tethering (24). The scapular and parascapular flap may also be used to provide good bulk and support. The parascapular flap is de-epithelialized for use as a muscular sling attached to the mandible. This supports the scapular flap, which becomes the neotongue (22). The anterolateral thigh, lateral thigh, and lateral arm fasciocutaneous flaps are also options for reconstruction. These generally do not provide the same level of bulk or support as the myocutaneous flaps. However, they do offer the advantage of potential sensory innervation. This may aid in triggering laryngeal protective mechanisms to prevent aspiration (4). Another advantage to the fasciocutaneous flaps is that they are significantly more pliable than myocutaneous flaps, although this is not as important as in partial glossectomy defects, where residual tongue mobility is an issue. If a free flap is contraindicated, a pedicled latissimus dorsi flap is preferable to the pectoralis major flap. It has a greater ease of tissue handling and less problems with tethering.

Composite oromandibular defects are discussed in detail elsewhere in this text, so reconstruction of total glossectomy defects with mandibular arch defects is briefly reviewed. The osteomusculocutaneous groin free flap, which incorporates the deep and superficial circumflex iliac vessels, has provided patients with good speech and swallowing results (25). The use of the parascapular osteomyocutaneous free flap has also been reported, with the primary limitation being the length of bone available (26). The fibula osteocutaneous flap can be used, but it requires planning and experience to ensure that perfusion to the skin pedicle is not compromised when the skin is fashioned into a neotongue.

Pedicled Myocutaneous and Muscular Flaps

The pectoralis major regional flap represented a major breakthrough in tongue reconstruction by allowing one-stage reconstruction with well-vascularized composite tissue (3). Fasciocutaneous and myocutaneous free flaps have eclipsed its utility in tongue reconstruction in most instances due to their superior tissue characteristics. However, if there is a contraindication to a free flap, or if a prior free-flap reconstruction has failed, the pectoralis flap is an option.

Anatomy and Surgical Technique

The pectoralis major myocutaneous flap is a pedicled flap, a fan-shaped muscle which derives its arterial blood supply from the pectoral branch of the thoracoacromial artery (3). The overlying skin is nourished by branches of this artery that perforate through the muscle.

The flap is designed along the medial chest to fit the glossal defect (27). The skin paddle border is incised down to the muscle, and the remaining chest wall skin is elevated to facilitate closure. After severing medial muscular attachments, the skin paddle and inferior portion of the muscle are raised as one from medial to lateral, taking care to preserve the pedicle along the lateral deep surface of the muscle. Attachments to the humerus are severed and a subcutaneous tunnel is created for the flap to travel over the clavicle into the neck. The flap is then inset and sutured into the glossectomy defect. If less bulk is desired, or if the skin flap is excessively hairy, the muscle flap can be raised alone and skin grafted. The donor site is closed primarily with suction drains.

Considerations

The most notable advantages of the pectoralis major flap are its reliability [total flap necrosis rates between 1% and 7% (27)], and the speed with which it may be harvested. The donor site should be closed primarily. The flap requires no microvascular anastamosis and is in the armamentarium of most otolaryngologists.

Disadvantages of the pectoralis flap in tongue reconstruction are multiple. The gravitational effect on the muscle and skin pedicle causes ptosis of the reconstructed area over time. This leads to poor contact with the palate and pharyngeal walls and pooling of secretions. This is exacerbated by the significant postoperative muscular atrophy of the flap. Furthermore, downward pull of the bulk of the flap causes tethering and restricted mobility of the residual tongue in partial glossectomy reconstructions. The flap itself does not have the same pliability of any of the fasciocutaneous free flaps, so residual tongue mobility is compromised. Another problem is that donor site closure causes unacceptable breast deformity in female patients. In tongue reconstruction, the flap is often excessively bulky. Occasionally, raising a muscular flap and covering it with a skin graft will eliminate some of these problems. Partial necrosis of the skin paddle and seroma or hematoma at the donor site is also frequently encountered.

Multiple studies with limited numbers have examined speech and swallowing results after pectoralis major reconstruction for base-of-tongue resection and total glossectomy (8,11,26,28–34). Although the results of these studies are somewhat mixed, most patients were able to achieve intelligible speech. In addition, most patients regained enough swallowing ability to tolerate a soft or pureed diet. Although aspiration was common, it was generally not severe enough to require discontinuation of diet or laryngectomy.

There are few direct comparative studies with other reconstructive modalities. In a study of 60 patients, pectoralis major reconstruction was compared to radial forearm free-flap reconstruction for a variety of tongue defects (33). In the study, the radial flap group had more intelligible speech, which was attributed to the greater pliability of the flap, allowing better tongue mobility. No significant difference was noted in swallowing ability. A small study comparing the pectoralis major flap to the lateral arm flap for predominantly tongue-base defects revealed inferior swallowing function in the pectoralis major group (35).

Pedicled Latissimus Dorsi Myocutaneous Flap

The pedicled latissimus dorsi myocutaneous flap is a versatile flap in the armamentarium of the head and neck surgeon, and as such has been used for many head and neck defects, including total base-of-tongue and total glossectomy defects. It may also be transferred as a free flap for tongue reconstruction, which will be discussed later in the chapter.

Anatomy and Surgical Technique

The latissimus dorsi myocutaneous flap is a composite-tissue flap with a blood supply derived from the thoracodorsal artery and vein (36). A number of perforators, most concentrated along the superior and anterior margins of the muscle, supply the overlying subcutaneous tissue and skin. The thoracodorsal nerve, whose course closely parallels the vascular pedicle, innervates the muscle.

After outlining an elliptical skin paddle that parallels the muscle fibers, an incision is made along the anterior border of the muscle (27). The thoracodorsal pedicle is located and the branch to the serratus anterior is ligated. Dissection is continued along the posterior aspect of the flap and the muscle is mobilized from the chest wall, adjacent musculature, iliac crest, vertebrae, and ribs. The tendinous insertion to the humerus is transected, as is the circumflex scapular pedicle. This allows for greater mobility and ensures that the pedicle is not kinked. A tunnel between the pectoralis major and minor is created and the pedicle is brought out through an incision inferior to the clavicle. The myocutaneous paddle is then inset along the floor of the mouth with its long axis oriented sagitally. A variation has been described in which the skin paddle is designed perpendicular to the muscle fibers (17,24). When the skin paddle is oriented sagitally in the oral cavity, the muscle fibers are oriented transversely. This allows a better dorsal projection of the flap and improved separation of the oral and pharyngeal cavities. Another skin paddle variation is the fusiform ottertail, which may provide better distal skin paddle vascularity, avoid an exteriorized vascular pedicle, and allow flap trimming after the flap is at the recipient site (36).

Considerations

The latissimus dorsi myocutaneous pedicled flap offers a significant improvement over its main alternative, the pectoralis major pedicled flap. As previously mentioned, it offers more lasting bulk that is necessary for total glossectomy reconstruction. This is due to a significant vascularized fat component, which does not atrophy like muscle (4). Flaps with significant width and at least 1.5 cm thickness have been suggested for total glossectomy reconstruction (37). The latissimus dorsi flap also gives better support to the floor of mouth than the pectoralis major flap.

A common complication of the flap is donor-site seroma, which occurred in 17 of 56 patients in one series (36). In addition, significant shoulder weakness has been noted (38). The other major drawbacks of the pedicled latissimus dorsi flap are in comparison to its free version. In the pedicled form, the pedicle may cause downward pull on the flap over time. This leads to sagging and impairment of laryngeal mobility (24). Some authors have considered the pedicled version to be unreliable compared to the free version due to concerns of external compression or pedicle kinking; in one study of latissimus dorsi flaps for subtotal/total glossectomy a failure was noted of two of three pedicled flaps whereas only 1 of 13 free flaps failed (24). However, a study of 68 pedicled latissimus dorsi flaps in head and neck reconstructions noted only one failure (36). Another drawback is that motor innervation is not possible in the pedicled version. In the free version with the perpendicular skin flap design described above, motor innervation from the hypoglossal nerve to the nerve to the thoracodorsal nerve in theory may add support to the floor of mouth by allowing flap muscle contraction in the transverse plane (17).

Although the free version is usually a better choice, the pedicled version still offers an overall good total glossectomy reconstruction if there is a contraindication to a free flap. Both methods have shown satisfactory functional results after subtotal and total glossectomy. The majority of patients are able to achieve decannulation, an oral diet, and intelligible speech (17,24,37). The major disadvantage of both is the need for repositioning and the inability to use a two-team surgical approach.

Pedicled Infrahyoid Flap

Although the authors have no personal experience with this technique, the pedicled infrahyoid flap has been described for tongue-base and total glossectomy reconstruction in 11 patients (39). This fasciomuscular flap is composed of the sternothyroid, sternohyoid, and upper omohyoid muscles, deriving its vascular supply from the superior thyroid pedicle. Voluntary movement via ansa cervicalis innervation is suggested to be a theoretical advantage for swallowing. A major disadvantage is the need for mucosal coverage of the reconstruction with a jejunal free flap or radial forearm free flap in most patients.

Fasciocutaneous Free Flaps—Radial Forearm Free Flap

Since its introduction in the 1970s, the radial forearm free flap has grown in popularity to become the workhorse of head and neck reconstruction due to its versatility, pliability, and reliability.

Anatomy and Surgical Technique

The radial forearm free flap is a fasciocutaneous flap that derives its arterial blood supply from radial artery branches running along the lateral intermuscular septum of the forearm between the brachioradialis and flexor carpi radialis (27). Nine to seventeen septocutaneous perforators supply the deep forearm fascia superficial to the muscular layer. These perforators travel to and supply the overlying skin. Due to the extensive vascularity of these perforators, the length of cutaneous territory available for harvest extends from the lower third of the upper arm to the wrist flexion crease. Proximal width extends between the humeral epicondyles, and distal width extends from the extensor pollicis longus tendon to the extensor carpi ulnaris tendon. Venous drainage includes superficial and deep systems, each of which may be used for venous flap outflow. The superficial system includes branches of the cephalic and basilic veins, while the deep system is composed of paired venae comitantes. Tendons of the brachioradialis, flexor carpi radialis, and palmaris longus can be incorporated into the flap. A vascularized segment of the lateral cortex of the distal radius can also be harvested with the flap. The medial and lateral antebrachial cutaneous nerves run in close proximity to the superficial venous system. They supply sensation to the volar forearm skin and may be harvested with the flap. Anastamosis to a sensory nerve at the recipient site (generally the lingual nerve) will provide sensory innervation.

After design of the skin paddle and tourniquet application, the radial flap is raised at the donor site starting distally, with careful attention to maintain the integrity of the intermuscular septum and vasculature therein (27). The distal radial artery and cephalic vein are ligated and transected and the superficial branches of the radial nerve are preserved. The radial artery and venae comitantes are dissected proximally. The venae comitantes can often be traced to a single vein. The antebrachial cutaneous nerves are dissected and preserved. Use of bipolar scissors will permit faster flap harvest than the scalpel (40). The tourniquet is loosened and complete hemostasis is obtained. The pedicle is then divided proximally after preparation of the recipient neck vessels as described below.

Suitable neck vessels for anastamosis at the recipient site are selected. If a neck dissection has not already been performed, an ipsilateral (or contralateral if the ipsilateral vasculature is compromised) neck exploration is performed to find suitable vessels.

The most common arterial vessels are branches of the external carotid artery. In our hands, the facial artery is the most commonly used, and the most common veins are the external jugular, internal jugular, and transverse cervical.

Microvascular anastamosis is then performed on the radial artery and on as many veins as necessary to provide adequate drainage of the flap. The forearm flap skin edges are carefully apposed to the edges of the tongue base defect. If greater bulk is desired, part of the flap may be deepithelialized and the non-epithelialized fascial portion folded under the fascioepithelial portion before suturing the epithelial edges to the edges of the recipient defect.

The donor site is closed with a circumferential pursestring stitch to minimize defect size (41). The small defect is then covered with a split-thickness skin graft of 0.015-inch thickness harvested from the lateral thigh. A petroleum impregnated gauze dressing is applied over the skin graft and the arm is bandaged and casted in 15° of extension.

Considerations

The radial forearm fasciocutaneous free flap has many characteristics that make it ideal for tongue reconstruction. It is thin and pliable, allowing good contour to the defect and maximal mobility of the residual tongue. A long vascular pedicle of 18–20 cm allows easy reach to neck vessels (12). The neurovascular anatomy is consistent and reliable. The skin is generally hairless. Cutaneous sensation is another theoretical advantage. As the donor site is located on the extremity, it allows an easy two-team approach, reducing operative time.

Disadvantages of the radial forearm free flap are minimal and mainly related to the donor site. Skin graft failure occurs in up to one-third of patients (42), usually with resultant tendon exposure. This is more likely if the paratenon layer over the tendons is not preserved when the flap is harvested. Tendon exposure may be minimized by a circumferential pursestring stitch, which leads to a smaller donor site (41). Although flap harvest leads to a significant short-term loss of function (43), this does not persist on a long-term basis despite lasting objective decreases in wrist flexion, pinch strength, and cutaneous sharp sensation (44). The potential of vascular compromise of the hand following ligation of the radial artery is a very serious potential complication. Preoperative screening with the Allen's test should prevent this complication. In the 10% of patients who fail an Allen's test another flap can be used. Experience with over 500 radial forearm flaps has demonstrated no vascular problems with the hand. Flap anastamotic failure rates are comparable to other free flaps. Reported failure rates for radial forearm free flaps used in head and neck reconstruction were 4.5% and 7.5% in series of 155 and 111 flaps respectively (45,46). In our series of over 250 flaps, the failure rate was 3.2%.

Ulnar Forearm Free Flap

On occasion, there will be circumstances where the radial forearm free flap is the reconstructive tissue of choice, but it cannot be used. In these instances, one should consider the ulnar forearm free flap. The ulnar fasciocutaneous flap and radial fasciocutaneous flap share identical tissue characteristics. If the patient fails the Allen's test with occlusion of the radial artery on the non-dominant hand, harvest of an ulnar flap on the non-dominant arm is preferred to harvest of a radial flap on the dominant arm due to the functional deficit from immobility of the dominant hand. In addition, the ulnar flap may be preferred in a hairy individual as the ulnar aspect of the forearm is less hairy than the radial aspect (42).

Anatomy and Surgical Technique

The ulnar forearm free flap is a fasciocutaneous flap which derives its arterial blood supply from branches of the ulnar artery running along the anterior medial intermuscular septum of the forearm between the flexor carpi ulnaris and flexor digitorum (20,42). Septocutaneous perforators supply the forearm fascia superficial to the muscular layer, as well as overlying skin. The length of cutaneous territory available for harvest extends 20 cm proximally from the volar wrist crease, while width varies from 10 cm proximally to 6 cm distally. Venous drainage includes superficial and deep systems. The superficial system includes branches of the basilic vein, while the deep system is composed of paired venae comitantes on either side of the ulnar artery. The medial antebrachial cutaneous nerve runs in close proximity to the basilic vein and supplies sensation to the volar forearm skin. A 10-cm pedicle may be harvested with the flap and anastamosed to a sensory nerve at the recipient site (generally the lingual nerve) to provide sensory innervation.

After design of the skin paddle and tourniquet application, the ulnar flap is raised at the donor site starting distally, with careful attention to maintenance of the vascular integrity within the thin intermuscular septum (20,42). After distal ligation, the ulnar artery and venae comitantes and basilic vein are dissected proximally. Care is taken to avoid damage to the ulnar nerve, adjacent to the ulnar artery. The medial antebrachial cutaneous nerve is dissected and preserved. Then, the tourniquet is loosened and complete hemostasis is obtained. The pedicle is then divided proximally after preparation of the recipient neck vessels as described below.

Suitable neck vessels for anastamosis at the recipient site are selected in the same manner as for the radial fascial flap. Microvascular anastamosis is then performed on the ulnar artery and the venae comitantes or superficial veins within the flap. The ulnar forearm flap skin edges are carefully apposed to the edges of the tongue-base defect. If greater bulk is desired, part of the flap may be de-epithelialized and the non-epithelialized fascial portion may be folded under the fascioepithelial portion before suturing the epithelial edges to the edges of the recipient defect.

The donor site is closed with a circumferential pursestring stitch to minimize defect size (41). The small defect is then covered with a split-thickness skin graft of 0.015-inch thickness harvested from the lateral thigh. A petroleum impregnated gauze dressing is applied over the skin graft and the arm is bandaged and casted in 15° of extension.

Considerations

The ulnar forearm free flap has essentially the same advantages for tongue reconstruction as the radial forearm free flap due to its almost identical tissue characteristics. It is thin and supple, allowing good contour to the defect and maximal mobility of the residual tongue. A long, consistent vascular pedicle of greater than 10 cm (42) allows easy reach to neck vessels, and the skin is more hairless than the radial flap. Furthermore, cutaneous sensation is possible. Because the donor site is located on the extremity, it allows an easy two-team approach, reducing operative time.

Disadvantages include donor-site morbidity similar to the radial flap. Although skin-graft failure may occur, it is much less often than with radial forearm flaps (42). In addition, the more medially based ulnar flap allows the majority of the flexor tendons to be covered when a circumferential stitch is used for closure of the donor site (41), leading to lower morbidity from skin-graft breakdown compared to the radial flap (42). The potential complication of postoperative hand necrosis, while possible, has not been reported to our knowledge. The ulnar flap is more technically difficult to harvest and anastamose than the radial flap. Although the vascular pedicle anatomy is quite reliable, the pedicle is more fragile than the radial flap and great care is required to elevate it (42). Also, the anastamosis is somewhat more challenging. The ulnar artery is typically 2.0–2.5 mm in diameter (42), compared to the 2–4 mm diameter of the radial artery (45). In addition, the venae comitantes are only 1.0–1.5 mm and do not often join, requiring two venous anastamoses and increasing operative time. However, this does not appear to cause greater flap-failure rates. In fact, in one series in which 10 ulnar flaps were used, no flap loss was reported (20), whereas in another series of 30 patients, it was reported that only two flap losses occurred, both events happening later than one week postoperatively and not likely related to the anastamosis (42). Although damage to the ulnar nerve is a concern due its proximity to the ulnar artery and multiple small perforators traveling from the artery to the nerve, no neuropraxia or other late complication related to ulnar nerve damage was noted in 30 patients (42).

Lateral Arm Free Flap

The lateral arm free flap is another excellent option for tongue reconstruction. It can be used for larger defects such as total base of tongue or total glossectomy defects in which a flap of intermediate bulk is needed.

Anatomy and Surgical Technique

The lateral arm free flap is a fasciocutaneous free flap, which derives its arterial blood supply from the posterior radial artery, a terminal branch of the profunda brachii artery (27). The artery is accompanied by paired venae comitantes, which drain the deep venous system, whereas the superficial venous system drains via the cephalic vein (47). The pedicle is located within the lateral intermuscular septum between the triceps posteriorly and the brachialis and brachioradialis anteriorly. The posterior cutaneous nerve of the arm, a branch of the radial nerve, provides cutaneous sensory innervation.

The flap is designed in an elliptical pattern with the long axis just posterior to a line from the deltoid insertion to the lateral epicondyle (27,48). Dissection is carried along the anterior margin of the skin flap to expose the septum. Dissection then proceeds along the posterior margin of the skin flap and along the fascia overlying the triceps. The posterior radial collateral artery and vein are identified within the intermuscular septum. The radial nerve is identified and carefully preserved, and the pedicle is traced proximally. The posterior cutaneous nerve of the arm is identified and skeletonized. The vascular pedicle and nerve are ligated and the flap is inset into the tongue defect after neurovascular anastamosis. Finally, the donor site is closed primarily.

Considerations

The lateral arm free flap is an excellent flap for defects, which require tissue of intermediate thickness for reconstruction, such as a total base-of-tongue defect. It is also very useful for composite defects of the base of tongue and adjacent structures: the thicker proximal paddle can reconstruct the base of tongue and the thinner distal paddle can reconstruct the adjacent structure, e.g., lateral pharyngeal wall (47). The thickness is generally between that of a radial forearm and a scapular or parascapular skin paddle (47). This flap also has the theoretical possibility of sensory innervation. A two-team approach may be used and the donor site can be closed primarily when the width of the defect is less than 7 cm. Also, there is no risk of ischemia as the posterior radial collateral artery is not necessary for upper extremity viability (47). The flap is reliable, with no failures in one series of 28 patients (35). Disadvantages include a somewhat shorter pedicle, typically 8–10 cm (12). The tissue is slightly less pliable than the radial forearm or ulnar forearm flap. In addition, vessel diameter is somewhat small: 1.0- to 2.5-mm arterial diameter and 1.0- to 3.0-mm venous diameter (35). There is significant exposure of and subsequent risk to the radial nerve. Also the flap may be hairier than a radial forearm or ulnar forearm flap.

Functional results for tongue-base reconstruction with the lateral arm are limited, but promising. In a small cohort of patients with a substantial percentage of tongue-base defects, swallowing ability was superior to another small cohort reconstructed with a pectoralis major flap (35). This flap is a good alternative to the radial forearm or ulnar forearm flap when more bulk is needed.

Scapular and Parascapular Free Flaps

The scapular and parascapular flaps are intermediate thickness fasciocutaneous flaps useful for reconstruction of total glossectomy defects.

Anatomy and Surgical Technique

The arterial supply of both flaps is based on the circumflex scapular artery (27). The artery divides into transverse and descending branches, which supply the scapular and parascapular flaps respectively. The accompanying circumflex scapular vein and its branches provide venous drainage for both flaps.

The skin paddle for either flap is designed as an ellipse over the respective arterial course of either flap (27). It is then dissected from medial to lateral over the deep fascia overlying the musculature. The pedicle is identified and branches to the teres major are ligated. Elevation of the remaining skin paddle over the muscular deep fascia is then completed. If greater pedicle length is required, the circumflex scapular pedicle may be traced back to the subscapular pedicle; this may then be transected after ligation of the thoracodorsal artery. The flap is inset into tongue base defect and vascular anastamosis is performed. If the parascapular and scapular fasciocutaneous flaps are raised simultaneously, the parascapular flap may be de-epithelialized for use as a muscular sling attached to the mandible. This provides support to the scapular flap, which becomes the neotongue (22).

The advantages of the scapular and parascapular flaps include reliable, sustained, intermediate bulk due to vascularized fat, consistent vasculature, and relatively good pliability. In addition, use of both flaps simultaneously as described above gives excellent support and bulk if needed (22). Disadvantages include the need for repositioning thus there is an inability to use a two-team approach. In addition, the positioning required for flap harvest may lead to brachial plexus injury (27).

Although, there are numerous reports on scapular or parascapular osteocutaneous flaps for repair of composite oromandibular defects involving the tongue (26), there is a paucity of literature on scapular and parascapular fasciocutaneous flaps for tongue reconstruction without associated bony reconstruction. However, in our personal experience, this flap has proven reliable for subtotal or total glossectomy reconstruction.

Anterolateral Thigh Free Flap

The anterolateral thigh flap is another intermediate-thickness, fasciocutaneous flap that is good for reconstruction of larger defects such as a subtotal or total glossectomy defect. Its volume is greater than a radial forearm or lateral arm free flap, but less than a rectus abdominis musculocutaneous flap. It is essentially equal in bulk to a lateral thigh flap (49).

Anatomy and Surgical Technique

The anterolateral thigh flap offers intermediate thickness with mobile and pliable tissue that is suitable for total glossectomy defects. A long pedicle, 8 to 20 cm, and a two-team approach make this a fast reliable flap (49). The skin paddle is large and may be designed to fit any tongue defect. The donor site is usually closed primarily. Rarely is a split thickness skin graft required, and sensory innervation of the flap is possible (49). For larger or composite defects, the flap may be combined with vastus lateralis, rectus femoris, tensor fascia lata (50), sartorius, or even iliac or fibula bone (49).

The greatest disadvantage is the variable vascular anatomy. Musculocutaneous perforators are present a significant percentage of the time. When the perforators are musculocutaneous, dissection through the vastus lateralis is necessary in order to preserve the vascular supply to the skin. The dissection is difficult due to the small size of the perforators (49) and the obliquely arranged muscle fibers (50). These small perforators tend to thrombose rapidly after congestion. Thus, salvage of a congested flap is unlikely (50). Despite this, the flap has a low failure rate: 3 of 74 in one study (50) and 2 of 38 in another study (49). Another disadvantage is that the motor nerves of the vastus lateralis may be damaged, leading to objective muscular weakness and fatigue. Subjectively, this does not lead to impairment of daily activities. Finally, if skin grafting at the donor site is required, active range of motion of the leg may be limited (51).

Lateral Thigh Free Flap

The lateral thigh flap is another fasciocutaneous flap of intermediate thickness that is suitable for reconstruction of total glossectomy defects.

Anatomy and Surgical Technique

The vascular supply of the lateral thigh flap is based on the third perforator from the profunda femoris artery (52). The perforator pierces the adductor magnus and enters the intermuscular septum between the vastus lateralis and the biceps femoris. Branches from the septum supply the overlying skin. The artery is accompanied by paired venae comitantes, which supply venous drainage for the overlying skin. These veins converge and enter the deep femoral vein. The lateral femoral cutaneous nerve supplies sensory innervation to the skin.

The skin flap is designed as an ellipse with the long axis aligned with the greater trochanter and lateral epicondyle of the femur (52). A circumferential incision is made around the flap, and the dissection is carried between the subcutaneous tissue and iliotibial tract. If sensation is desired, the lateral femoral cutaneous nerve must be traced in the subcutaneous tissue from the anterior margin of the flap prior to dissection to the iliotibial tract. The distal perforator branches are identified and traced to the third perforator, which pierces the adductor magnus. The proximal end of the adductor magnus is detached from the linea aspera of the femur, allowing exposure of the third perforator's insertion to the profunda femoris. The fourth perforator is ligated. The pedicle is transected and the paddle is sutured into the tongue defect after neurovascular anastamosis is performed.

The advantages of this flap are similar to other intermediate thickness fasciocutaneous flaps. It is a good compromise between pliability and bulk for larger reconstructions such as total glossectomy. The thicker proximal flap provides bulk, while the thinner distal flap provides contour (52). The bulk is more lasting than myocutaneous flaps due the predominance of vascularized fat, and the lateral femoral cutaneous nerve allows good innervation of the flap. Primary closure is possible. The two-team approach may be used. The flap failure rate is low, between 2% (52) and 3% (53).

The major disadvantage of the lateral thigh flap is variable vascular anatomy. The third perforator has a somewhat variable branching position from the profunda femoris artery (53). In addition, the second perforator may contribute to the arterial supply and there may be communicating vessels between the third and fourth perforators. Donor-site morbidity includes wound dehiscence (52).

Omental Free Flap

Use of the free omentum flap has been reported for head and neck reconstruction, including tongue-base, partial glossectomy, and subtotal glossectomy defects (54). Laparoscopic harvest allows significantly less morbidity than open laparotomy.

Myocutaneous and Muscular Free Flaps—Rectus Abdominis Free Flap

The rectus abdominis myocutaneous free flap is the overall best option for subtotal or total glossectomy reconstruction due to its excellent bulk and support. It has the best potential for lasting functional results.

Anatomy and Surgical Technique

The rectus abdominis free flap is based on the deep inferior epigastric artery and vein (27). The vessels travel along the undersurface of the muscle, and a number of perforating branches supply the muscle. These perforators continue through the anterior surface of the muscle to supply the overlying cutaneous layer. The rectus muscle is located between the anterior and posterior rectus sheath. The posterior sheath is made up of aponeuroses from the external and internal oblique and the transversus abdominis muscles. Below the arcuate line, the posterior sheath consists only of transversalis fascia. Thus, only fascia above the arcuate line should be harvested. The muscle is bound medially by the linea alba and laterally by the linea semilunaris. The lower six intercostal nerves supply mixed motor and sensory segmental innervation to the rectus abdominis and overlying skin.

The skin paddle is designed as an oblique ellipse from inferomedial to superolateral centered at the level of the umbilicus (27). Dissection is begun along its superior border through the skin, subcutaneous layer, and anterior rectus sheath; the inferior border is dissected in a similar manner. The lateral end of the skin paddle is raised to the linea semilunaris and the medial end is raised to the linea alba. Longitudinal incisions are performed along the anterior rectus sheath inside the linea semilunaris and linea alba to completely isolate the skin paddle aside from its anterior rectus sheath attachments. The tenth intercostal nerve is carefully identified and preserved at the lateral border of the muscle if motor innervation of the flap is planned (55). The rectus abdominis is then elevated off the posterior rectus sheath to expose the pedicle. The pedicle is followed to its origin from the external iliac artery so as to obtain maximum length. The flap is then harvested, if possible, and the anterior rectus sheath is closed primarily below the arcuate line and sewn to the posterior rectus sheath at the arcuate line. If there is any tension in the closure, a mesh or allogenic substance is used to recreate the anterior rectus sheath. The skin can always be closed primarily.

The flap is inset after microvascular anastamosis, and the tenth intercostal nerve, if harvested, is anastamosed to the hypoglossal nerve. The anterior rectus sheath and muscle are tightly sutured to the lingual aspect of the mandible and hyoid bone to create a secure oral cavity floor. The remaining deglutition muscles such as genioglossus, digastric, mylohyoid, and geniohyoid, are sutured to the muscular portion of the flap. The overlying skin paddle is sutured in place over this platform (55). The skin paddle may be designed 20% larger in length and width than the oral defect in order to allow convexity and better dorsal and posterior projection of the flap (56).

Considerations

Advantages of the rectus abdominis flap for total glossectomy reconstruction include its excellent floor-of-mouth support from the muscular sling (55), and its adequate and predictable amount of bulk due to vascularized fat in the skin paddle (56). Motor innervation aids in preventing muscular atrophy (55). It is unclear if this motor innervation also contributes to dorsal elevation in deglutition (18,55). As with most free flaps, a two-team approach is possible. The vascular anatomy is constant and reliable, and the vessels are large. Functional studies have demonstrated decent deglutition and articulation results, with a majority of patients able to achieve intelligible speech and to tolerate at least a soft diet (55,56).

Disadvantages are primarily from donor-site morbidity; furthermore, significant abdominal wall weakness, as well as ventral hernia may occur (57). Previous abdominal or vascular surgery may preclude use of this flap. Occasionally, pedicle length may be somewhat short (21).

Latissimus Dorsi Free Flap

The latissimus dorsi free flap is another good choice for total glossectomy defects. Details and considerations of this flap are discussed along with the latissimus dorsi pedicled flap in the section of this chapter in which Pedicled Myocutaneous and Muscular Free Flaps are mentioned. As a free flap, it offers the advantage of not being tethered by its pedicle. The muscle and cutaneous portions can also be positioned in a more functional way if the pedicle is mobile in the neck.

Gracilis Free Flap

The gracilis flap has been described for reconstruction of total glossectomy defects. It may be harvested as a purely muscular flap that is folded on itself longitudinally at the donor site, then skin grafted (58). Alternatively, it may be harvested as a myocutaneous flap with the muscle serving as a sling along the mandibular arch to support the cutaneous portion (59). The blood supply is based on perforators from the profunda femoris artery. Motor innervation of the flap is possible via the obturator nerve. Good swallowing function has been achieved using the gracilis for reconstruction (59).

Tensor Fascia Lata Free Flap

The tensor fascia lata fasciocutaneous flap has also been described for subtotal glossectomy reconstruction (60). The terminal branch of the lateral femoral circumflex artery provides the vascular supply. Motor innervation to the flap is possible via the superior gluteal nerve. In a clinical evaluation of five patients, speech and swallowing superior to cohorts who underwent pedicled pectoralis major myocutaneous flaps or primary closure.

Adjunctive Measures in Tongue Base and Glossectomy Reconstruction

Sensory and Motor Innervation in Tongue Reconstruction

Sensory re-innervation of the flap by cutaneous nerve anastamosis offers a theoretical potential advantage for tongue reconstruction; however, at this time, its clinical benefit is not entirely clear. Oral mucosal anesthesia has been demonstrated to be detrimental to masticatory function (61). Preservation of the superior laryngeal nerve for sensory function is critical for maximal deglutition function after tongue resection (11,29). In a study of seventeen re-innervated radial forearm free flaps used for various tongue defects, sensory fidelity was reported to be superior to the native forearm donor site and similar to normal tongue (62). Also, in another study in which eighteen radial forearm free flaps were used in oral cavity reconstruction, reinnervated flaps were shown to have sensory recovery superior to non-innervated flaps (63). Also, in an additional study of 29 patients undergoing oral cavity reconstruction with rectus and anterolateral thigh free flaps, the authors reported that these flaps provided superior function in innervated flaps. However, in a study of non-innervated flaps used for oral reconstruction, restoration of sensation in eight of eight fasciocutaneous and two or four myocutaneous flaps was achieved (64). Also, no study to our knowledge has clearly concluded that superior postoperative clinical function can be had with reinnervated flaps in oral reconstruction (65), although a significant correlation between recovery of flap sensation and both articulation and oral intake has been shown in non-innervated flaps (64). In a study of 10 ulnar free flap reconstructions of 30–100% base-of-tongue defects, there was no improvement in swallowing ability or protection of the laryngeal introitus with sensory innervation. Furthermore, the three patients described in the study who underwent neurosensory flap transfers were able to eat a regular diet long before recovery of flap sensation (20). In conclusion, free-flap sensation for tongue-base and total glossectomy defects is likely to improve deglutition and reduce aspiration, but has yet to be conclusively proven by a consensus of functional studies.

Motor function of innervated tongue reconstruction flaps is also somewhat controversial. Motor innervation of the residual tongue is clearly critical for swallowing function (4). However, the effects of flap motor reinnervation on deglutition are somewhat less clear. As noted in the previous discussion of individual flaps, motor innervation has been used for many myocutaneous or muscular free flaps in subtotal or total glossectomy reconstruction including latissimus dorsi, rectus abdominis, gracilis, and tensor fascia lata (24,55,58–60). Innervation has prevented muscular atrophy to some extent. In studies of the re-innervated muscles, electromyographic techniques revealed motor unit potentials and cineradiography showed dorsal floor-of-mouth elevation (24,55,58–60). However, the residual native deglutition musculature, rather than the flap musculature, may be responsible for much, if not all, of the movement (21,24,25). It is not clear from any of these studies if any significant voluntary or involuntary flap contraction occurs with motor innervation.

Other Procedures to Improve Swallowing Function

Various adjunctive procedures have been proposed to improve swallowing function and minimize aspiration. Laryngeal suspension, in which steel wires pull the larynx in an anterosuperior position by suspending it from the mandible (29) has been advocated by numerous authors in conjunction with total glossectomy (4,11,21,29,30). The tongue provides dynamic laryngeal support via the genioglossus to the mandible and via the styloglossus to the skull base (24). This support is lost after total glossectomy. Laryngeal suspension attempts to restore the larynx to a more physiologic position by anterosuperior traction (21). This traction attempts to position the larynx under the tongue base during deglutition, lowering the risk of aspiration. However, in the authors' experience, laryngeal suspension has not decreased aspiration risk. Furthermore, solid muscular sling reconstruction of the floor of mouth, as with a rectus abdominis or latissimus dorsi flap, should restore laryngeal position and support (37). The laryngeal support achieved with the reconstruction flap is dynamic like native laryngeal support from the tongue. With good support from the reconstructed floor of mouth, laryngeal suspension becomes unnecessary and more physiologic swallowing function is preserved.

Cricopharyngeal myotomy has also been reported (4). A lack of coordinated opening of the cricopharyngeus may occur secondary to the weak swallowing force after tongue resection, and aspiration may result. Cricopharyngeal myotomy should alleviate this in theory. However, the authors have found this procedure to be unnecessary in practice. In addition, the authors have not employed other aspiration prevention techniques such as partial laryngoplasty (4). The palatal prosthesis has been used for improvement in speech and swallowing function (21). However, an optimal tongue reconstruction should provide sufficient bulk to avoid palatal prosthesis, thereby retaining the benefit of palatal sensory innervation for oral rehabilitation (4).

CONCLUSION

The Future of Base-of-Tongue and Total Glossectomy Reconstruction

Functional tongue reconstruction has remained a challenge due to the complex motor function involved in normal deglutition and articulation. Although some current reconstruction techniques employ motor innervation, little, if any, coordinated motor function results from use of these methods. Previous studies of the canine tongue have resulted in successful autograft transplantation (66). In addition, successful microneurovascular allotransplantion of the canine hemitongue has been performed, yielding partial recovery of neuromuscular function (67). However, graft rejection represents a significant barrier to clinical application in humans at this time, because immunosuppression is generally contraindicated in cancer patients. In the future, advances in immunology or tissue engineering may lead to reconstructive methods that more closely mimic the complicated motor coordination of the tongue.

REFERENCES

1. Wells MD, Edwards AL, Luce EA. Intraoral reconstructive techniques. Clin Plast Surg 1995; 22:91–108.
2. Prince S, Bailey BM. Squamous carcinoma of the tongue: review. Br J Oral Maxillofac Surg 1999; 37:164–174.
3. Evans PH, Das Gupta AR. The use of the pectoralis major myocutaneous flap for one-stage reconstruction of the base of the tongue. J Laryngol Otol 1981; 95:809–816.
4. Urken ML, Moscoso JF, Lawson W, et al. A systematic approach to functional reconstruction of the oral cavity following partial and total glossectomy. Arch Otolaryngol Head Neck Surg 1994; 120:589–601.
5. Janfaza P, Nadol J, Galla R, et al. Surgical Anatomy of the Head and Neck. Philadelphia: Lippincott, 2000.
6. Sessions DG. Surgical resection and reconstruction for cancer of the base of the tongue. Otolaryngol Clin N Am 1983; 16:309–329.
7. Truelson JM, Pearce AN. Tongue reconstruction procedures for treatment of cancer. Aorn J 1997; 65:528, 531–534, 537.
8. Furia CL, Carrara-de Angelis E, Martins NM, et al. Video fluoroscopic evaluation after glossectomy. Arch Otolaryngol Head Neck Surg 2000; 126:378–383.
9. McConnel FM. Analysis of pressure generation and bolus transit during pharyngeal swallowing. Laryngoscope 1988; 98:71–78.
10. Hirano M, Kuroiwa Y, Tanaka S, et al. Dysphagia following various degrees of surgical resection for oral cancer. Ann Otol Rhinol Laryngol 1992; 101:138–141.
11. Weber RS, Ohlms L, Bowman J, et al. Functional results after total or near total glossectomy with laryngeal preservation. Arch Otolaryngol Head Neck Surg 1991; 117:512–515.
12. Muller C, Newlands S, Pou A. Free flap reconstructin of head and neck defects, UTMB Grand Rounds Presentation, 2002.
13. Keyserlingk JR, de Francesco J, Breach N, et al. Recent experience with reconstructive surgery following major glossectomy. Arch Otolaryngol Head Neck Surg 1989; 115: 331–338.
14. DeFries HO. Reconstruction of the tongue. Ann Otol Rhinol Laryngol 1974; 83:471–475.
15. Mikaelian DO. Reconstruction of the tongue. Laryngoscope 1984; 94:34–37.
16. Matulic Z, Barlovic M, Mikolji V, et al. Tongue reconstruction by means of the sternocleidomastoid muscle and a forhead flap. Br J Plast Surg 1978; 31:147–151.
17. Haughey BH, Fredrickson JM. The latissimus dorsi donor site. Current use in head and neck reconstruction. Arch Otolaryngol Head Neck Surg 1991; 117:1129–1134.
18. Tsue TT, Desyatnikova SS, Deleyiannis FW, et al. Comparison of cost and function in reconstruction of the posterior oral cavity and oropharynx. Free vs pedicled soft tissue transfer. Arch Otolaryngol Head Neck Surg 1997; 123:731–737.
19. McConnel FM, Pauloski BR, Logemann JA, et al. Functional results of primary closure vs flaps in oropharyngeal reconstruction: a prospective study of speech and swallowing. Arch Otolaryngol Head Neck Surg 1998; 124:625–630.
20. Salibian AH, Allison GR, Krugman ME, et al. Reconstruction of the base of the tongue with the microvascular ulnar forearm flap: a functional assessment. Plast Reconstr Surg 1995; 96:1081–1089; discussion 1090–1091.
21. Lyos AT, Evans GR, Perez D, et al. Tongue reconstruction: outcomes with the rectus abdominis flap. Plast Reconstr Surg 1999; 103:442–447; discussion 448–449.
22. Urken ML. The restoration or preservation of sensation in the oral cavity following ablative surgery. Arch Otolaryngol Head Neck Surg 1995; 121:607–612.

23. Urken ML, Turk JB, Weinberg H, et al. The rectus abdominis free flap in head and neck reconstruction. Arch Otolaryngol Head Neck Surg 1991; 117:857–866.
24. Haughey BH. Tongue reconstruction: concepts and practice. Laryngoscope 1993; 103:1132–1141.
25. Salibian AH, Allison GR, Rappaport I, et al. Total and subtotal glossectomy: function after microvascular reconstruction. Plast Reconstr Surg 1990; 85:513–524; discussion 525–526.
26. Salibian AH, Allison GR, Strelzow VV, et al. Secondary microvascular tongue reconstruction: functional results. Head Neck 1993; 15:389–397.
27. Urken ML, Cheney M, Sullivan M, et al. Atlas of regional and free flaps for head and neck reconstruction. New York: Raven Press, Ltd, 1995.
28. Robertson MS, Robinson JM, Horsfall RM. A technique of tongue reconstruction following near-total glossectomy. J Laryngol Otol 1987; 101:260–265.
29. Tiwari RM, Greven AJ, Karim AB, et al. Total glossectomy: reconstruction and rehabilitation. J Laryngol Otol 1989; 103:917–921.
30. Tiwari R, Karim AB, Greven AJ, et al. Total glossectomy with laryngeal preservation. Arch Otolaryngol Head Neck Surg 1993; 119:945–949.
31. Knuuttila H, Pukander J, Maatta T, et al. Speech articulation after subtotal glossectomy and reconstruction with a myocutaneous flap. Acta Otolaryngol 1999; 119:621–626.
32. Konstantinovic VS, Dimic ND. Articulatory function and tongue mobility after surgery followed by radiotherapy for tongue and floor of the mouth cancer patients. Br J Plast Surg 1998; 51:589–593.
33. Su WF, Hsia YJ, Chang YC, et al. Functional comparison after reconstruction with a radial forearm free flap or a pectoralis major flap for cancer of the tongue. Otolaryngol Head Neck Surg 2003; 128:412–418.
34. Furia CL, Kowalski LP, Latorre MR, et al. Speech intelligibility after glossectomy and speech rehabilitation. Arch Otolaryngol Head Neck Surg 2001; 127:877–883.
35. Civantos FJ Jr, Burkey B Lu FL, et al. Lateral arm microvascular flap in head and neck reconstruction. Arch Otolaryngol Head Neck Surg 1997; 123:830–836.
36. Hayden RE, Kirby SD, Deschler DG. Technical modifications of the latissimus dorsi pedicled flap to increase versatility and viability. Laryngoscope 2000; 110:352–357.
37. Kimata Y, Uchiyama K, Ebihara S, et al. Postoperative complications and functional results after total glossectomy with microvascular reconstruction. Plast Reconstr Surg 2000; 106:1028–1035.
38. Russell RC, Pribaz J, Zook EG, et al. Functional evaluation of latissimus dorsi donor site. Plast Reconstr Surg 1986; 78:336–344.
39. Remmert SM, Sommer KD, Majocco AM, et al. The neurovascular infrahyoid muscle flap: a new method for tongue reconstruction. Plast Reconstr Surg 1997; 99:613–618.
40. Wax MK, Winslow C, Desyatnikova S, et al. A prospective comparison of scalpel versus bipolar scissors in the elevation of radial forearm fasciocutaneous free flaps. Laryngoscope 2001; 111:568–571.
41. Winslow CP, Hansen J, Mackenzie D, et al. Pursestring closure of radial forearm fasciocutaneous donor sites. Laryngoscope 2000; 110:1815–1818.
42. Wax MK, Rosenthal EL, Winslow CP, et al. The ulnar fasciocutaneous free flap in head and neck reconstruction. Laryngoscope 2002; 112:2155–2160.
43. Skoner J, Bascom DA, Cohen JI, et al. Short-term functional donor site morbidity in radial forearm fasciocutaneous free tissue transfer. Laryngoscope. In press.
44. Brown MT, Couch ME, Huchton DM. Assessment of donor-site functional morbidity from radial forearm fasciocutaneous free flap harvest. Arch Otolaryngol Head Neck Surg 1999; 125:1371–1374.
45. Evans GR, Schusterman MA, Kroll SS, et al. The radial forearm free flap for head and neck reconstruction: a review. Am J Surg 1994; 168:446–450.
46. Vaughan ED. The radial forearm free flap in orofacial reconstruction. Personal experience in 120 consecutive cases. J Craniomaxillofac Surg 1990; 18:2–7.

47. Burkey BB, Coleman JR Jr. Current concepts in oromandibular reconstruction. Otolaryngol Clin N Am 1997; 30:607–630.
48. Wax MK, Briant TD, Mahoney JL. Lateral-arm free flap for reconstruction in the head and neck. J Otolaryngol 1996; 25:140–144.
49. Kimata Y, Uchiyama K, Ebihara S, et al. Versatility of the free anterolateral thigh flap for reconstruction of head and neck defects. Arch Otolaryngol Head Neck Surg 1997; 123:1325–1331.
50. Kimata Y, Uchiyama K, Ebihara S, et al. Anatomic variations and technical problems of the anterolateral thigh flap: a report of 74 cases. Plast Reconstr Surg 1998; 102: 1517–1523.
51. Kimata Y, Uchiyama K, Ebihara S, et al. Anterolateral thigh flap donor-site complications and morbidity. Plast Reconstr Surg 2000; 106:584–589.
52. Hayden RE, Deschler DG. Lateral thigh free flap for head and neck reconstruction. Laryngoscope 1999; 109:1490–1494.
53. Truelson JM, Leach JL. Lateral thigh flap reconstruction in the head and neck. Otolaryngol Head Neck Surg 1998; 118:203–210.
54. Nishimura T, Kanehira E, Tsukatani T, et al. Laparoscopically harvested omental flap for head and neck reconstruction. Laryngoscope 2002; 112:930–932.
55. Yamamoto Y, Sugihara T, Furuta Y, et al. Functional reconstruction of the tongue and deglutition muscles following extensive resection of tongue cancer. Plast Reconstr Surg 1998; 102:993–998; discussion 999–1000.
56. Kiyokawa K, Tai Y, Inoue Y, et al. Functional reconstruction of swallowing and articulation after total glossectomy without laryngectomy: money pouch-like reconstruction method using rectus abdominis myocutaneous flap. Plast Reconstr Surg 1999; 104: 2015–2020.
57. Sajjadian A, Deschler DG, Hayden RE. Free flap reconstruction after near-total glossectomy in the child. Otolaryngol Head Neck Surg 1999; 120:614–616.
58. Yoleri L, Mavioglu H. Total tongue reconstruction with free functional gracilis muscle transplantation: a technical note and review of the literature. Ann Plast Surg 2000; 45:181–186.
59. Yousif NJ, Dzwierzynski WW, Sanger JR, et al. The innervated gracilis musculocutaneous flap for total tongue reconstruction. Plast Reconstr Surg 1999; 104:916–921.
60. Cheng N, Shou B, Zheng M, et al. Microneurovascular transfer of the tensor fascia lata musculocutaneous flap for reconstruction of the tongue. Ann Plast Surg 1994; 33: 136–141.
61. Kapur KK, Garrett NR, Fischer E. Effects of anaesthesia of human oral tructures on masticatory performance and food particle size distribution. Arch Oral Biol 1990; 35:397–403.
62. Kuriakose MA, Loree TR, Spies A, et al. Sensate radial forearm free flaps in tongue reconstruction. Arch Otolaryngol Head Neck Surg 2001; 127:1463–1466.
63. Boyd B, Mulholland S, Gullane P, et al. Reinnervated lateral antebrachial cutaneous neurosome flaps in oral reconstruction: are we making sense? Plast Reconstr Surg 1994; 93:1350–1359; discussion 1360–1362.
64. Close LG, Truelson JM, Milledge RA, et al. Sensory recovery in noninnervated flaps used for oral cavity and oropharyngeal reconstruction. Arch Otolaryngol Head Neck Surg 1995; 121:967–972.
65. Kimata Y, Uchiyama K, Ebihara S, et al. Comparison of innervated and noninnervated free flaps in oral reconstruction. Plast Reconstr Surg 1999; 104:1307–1313.
66. Day TA, Tarr C, Zealear D, et al. Tongue replantation in an animal model. Microsurgery 2000; 20:105–108.
67. Haughey BH, Beggs JC, Bong J, et al. Microneurovascular allotransplantation of the canine tongue. Laryngoscope 1999; 109:1461–1470.

13
Hard Palate Reconstruction

J. Trad Wadsworth
Eastern Virginia Medical School, Department of Otolaryngology—Head and Neck Surgery, Norfolk, Virginia, U.S.A.

Neal Futran
Department of Otolaryngology—Head and Neck Surgery, University of Washington, Seattle, Washington, U.S.A.

INTRODUCTION

The hard palate, which comprises approximately 75% of the entire palate is a crucial component of oral cavity anatomy (1). Posteriorly, the hard palate is formed by the palatine processes of the two maxillae and the horizontal laminae of the palatine bones, and, anteriorly, by fusion with the alveolar processes of the maxillae. It is covered with thick, densely adherent, and highly glandular mucosa (1). The maxillary dentition is housed in the dense palatal alveolar bone.

The importance of the hard palate cannot be underestimated. First, and most importantly, it provides separation of the oral and nasal cavities. This not only permits differentiation in sound production but also allows breathing and chewing to occur simultaneously. It also serves as a scaffold upon which a food bolus is prepared in the oral preparatory phase of swallowing. Furthermore, coupled with the tongue, the hard palate allows for articulation of speech. Cosmetically, it aids in the support and projection of the facial soft tissues. Even subtle defects of the palate following trauma or ablative oncologic surgery can cause severe functional and cosmetic deformities. The presence of large oronasal and oromaxillary fistulae, as well as the loss of crucial tooth-bearing segments, can extensively impair phonation, oral alimentation, lip and cheek support, and midface projection (2). Thus, reconstruction of the hard palate provides one of the most challenging prospects for the head and neck reconstructive surgeon.

EVALUATION AND PLANNING

When evaluating defects of the hard palate, one must initially assess what structures are absent. Losses of bony structure, bulk, and the mucosal lining are typical findings. Furthermore, tooth-bearing segments are often lost in large oncologic resections and traumatic avulsions. Therefore, these characteristic deficiencies provide common descriptors for defect types: mucosal, anterior arch, hemipalate, subtotal, and total palatal defects. It is critical, irrespective of the defect type, to attempt to replace lost structures with similar materials.

During clinical assessment, the patient, as well as the defect, must be evaluated. The surgeon must determine whether the patient would best be served by a more rapid but less complex method of reconstruction, such as providing a mucosal lining with a skin graft and a new structure with a prosthesis, versus a potentially more elegant although time consuming procedure such as a microvascular free-tissue transfer. In any case, often the best reconstructive method for the defect may not be the preferred method for the patient, as overall health, capabilities, and desires differ among patients. Ultimately, the surgeon and the patient share the goal of restoring the patient's ability to achieve a regular diet and normal phonation, as well as acceptable cosmesis.

RECONSTRUCTIVE OPTIONS

Fortunately, surgical options for these defects are extensive, and the surgeon can tailor the reconstructive method to fit the existing defect. For example, smaller mucosal defects may respond to primary closures. However, moderate mucosal defects may require skin or acellular dermis grafts (3,4). More challenging is the resolution of large soft-tissue and bony losses.

The traditional method of reconstructing these palatal and maxillary defects is by placing a maxillofacial prosthesis to obturate the cavity, seal the palate, and provide dentition (5–7). Although the prosthesis is essential for adequate speech, swallowing, and appropriate cosmesis, such an appliance is necessarily bulky and can be cumbersome. Moreover, patients must maintain meticulous hygiene of both the prosthesis and the surgical cavity, which may be difficult for the elderly patient. Frequently, continual leakage between the nasal and oral cavities occurs, attesting to the difficulty of obtaining an adequate seal between the two cavities without causing irritation. Such leakage may further complicate the patient's speech and oral hygiene. Also, dentition must be adequate for the retention of the appliance and, as the maxillary defect increases, anchoring the device becomes problematic, and difficulties with retention and motion of the implant escalate. Thus, selecting the proper patient for this reconstructive method is imperative. Chapter 16 provides an extensive discussion on oral cavity prosthetic application and use.

Because of the reconstructive difficulties presented in this chapter, various pedicled autogenous tissues have been used to correct palatal defects. As early as 1862, von Langenbeck described the use of local palatal flaps for small defects (8).- Other authors have also advocated the use of local buccal fat, palatal, pharyngeal, and nasal septal flaps (9–11). Larger deficiencies have traditionally required more extensive reconstruction involving temporalis, forehead, and more distant tubed flaps such as the deltopectoral and upper arm flaps (12–15). Vascularized cranial bone grafts have also been used (16,17). The results of these techniques can be adequate; however, all are limited by the lack of tissue bulk, the length of vascular pedicle, and/or the need for multiple stages of reconstruction to achieve the final result.

Microvascular free-tissue transfer techniques provide a unique alternative to reconstruction of the palate and midface, and this topic will be the focus of the remainder of this chapter. Adequate amounts of bone and soft tissue can be transferred in a

(A)

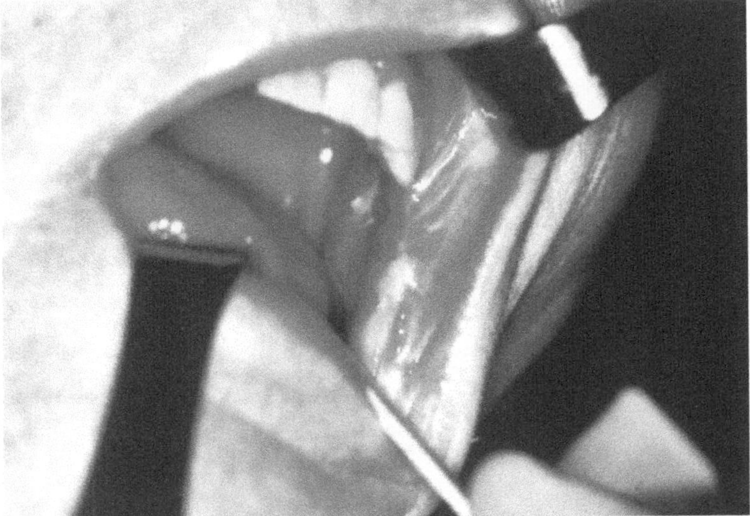

Figure 1A–F (**A**) Fifty-five-year-old female with recurrent squamous cell carcinoma of palatal and buccal mucosa. (*Continued*)

single staged procedure, thereby eliminating restrictions of pedicle length and flap geometry. Various free-tissue transfers, including myocutaneous, myofascial, and osteocutaneous flaps, can be used for reconstruction of the palate and midface. The radial forearm, latissimus dorsi, rectus abdominus, scapular, fibular, and iliac crest flaps are the most often used.

(B)

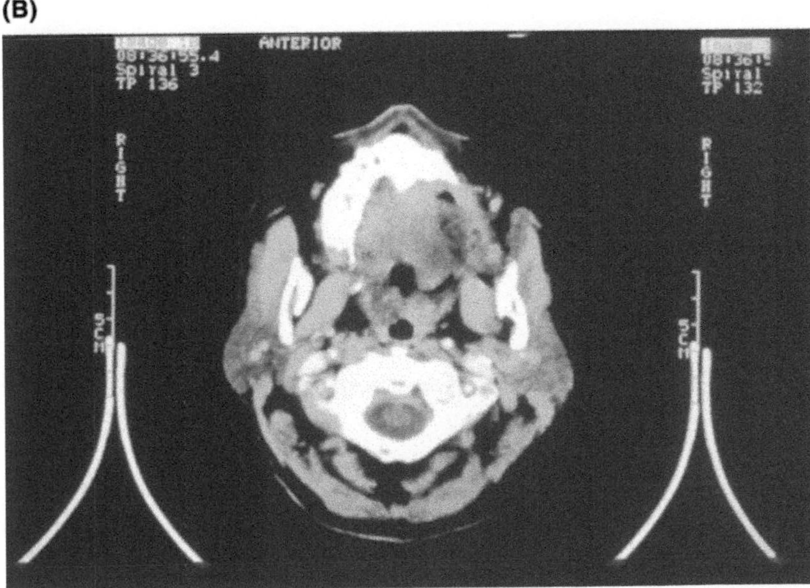

Figure 1 (**B**) CT-scan showing soft tissue infiltration. (*Continued*)

(C)

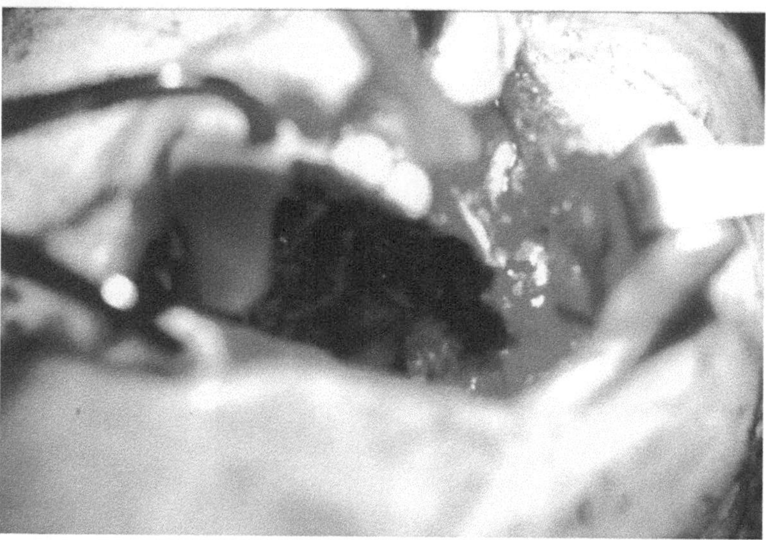

Figure 1 (C) Intra-operative view of resection cavity. *(Continued)*

Traditionally, the radial forearm free flap has been a versatile flap in head and neck reconstruction, and its application in palatal reconstruction further bolsters its utility (Fig. 1). The thin, pliable tissue characteristics of the radial forearm free flap allow the palate to be sealed and to serve as a potential surface for bearing dentures. Reports in the literature of small-case series have described the use of the radial forearm free flap to close palatal defects due to failed cleft palate repair and tumor extirpation (18,19). Cordeiro et al. (20) described the "sandwich" radial forearm osteocutaneous free flap for reconstruction of subtotal maxillectomy defects. In this report, the authors used the radial bone to recreate the maxillary arch, and the skin

(D)

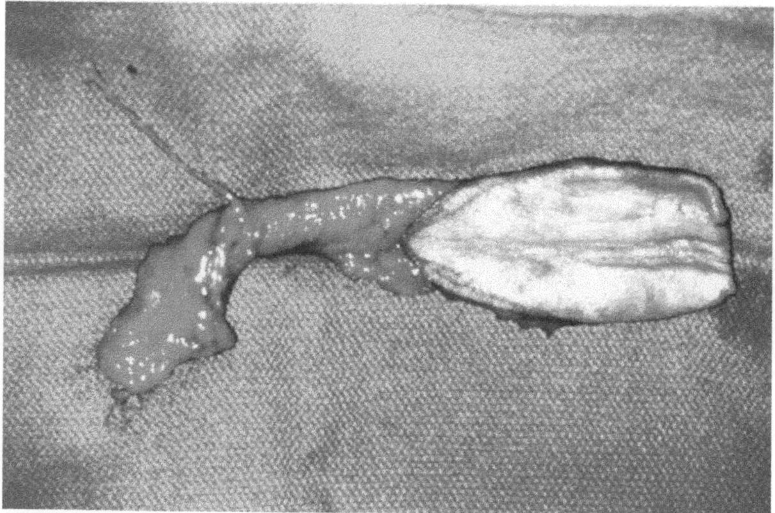

Figure 1 (D) Radial forearm free flap. *(Continued)*

(E)

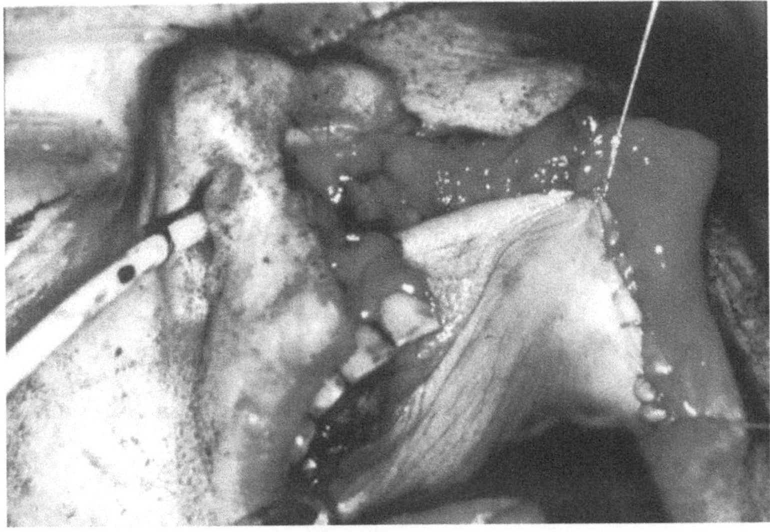

Figure 1 (E) Flap inset. (*Continued*)

paddle was folded around it, providing restoration of both the palatal and nasal linings. Theoretically, this flap could also bear osteointegrated implants. The bony component, however, is thin (3–5 mm) and is of limited length. It has excellent utility for reconstruction of the premaxilla (Fig. 2). Both the upper lip and nasal base are well supported.

Larger series of palatal and maxillary defects reconstructed with myocutaneous free flaps have been described. Shestak et al. (21,22) found that the latissimus dorsi free flap both sealed the palate and provided excellent tissue bulk in the cheek and

(F)

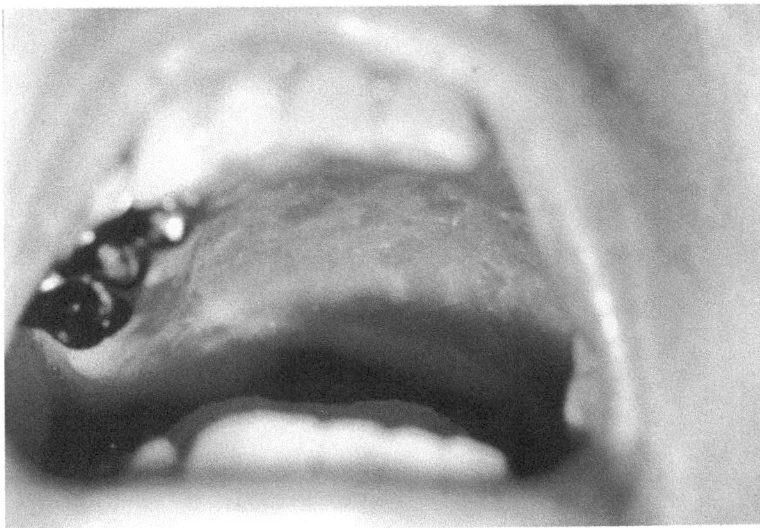

Figure 1 (F) Six-month, postoperative result.

(A)

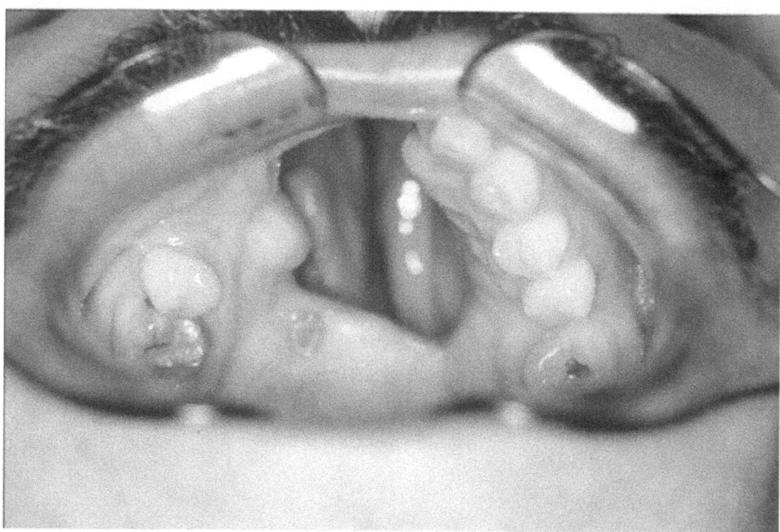

Figure 2A–E (**A**) Anterior palatal and alveolar arch defect secondary to previous gunshot wound. (*Continued*)

malar area when defects extended to these sites. Additionally, the ample pedicle length allowed microvascular anastomoses in the neck without the need for vein grafts.

Similar findings and flap attributes have been demonstrated by the use of the rectus abdominus free flap (Fig. 3). Olsen et al. (23) described 11 patients with massive sino-orbital defects who underwent reconstruction with primarily rectus abdominus free flaps. Six of the patients underwent palate reconstruction with a microvascular free-tissue transfer, and all exhibited excellent speech and deglutition.

(B)

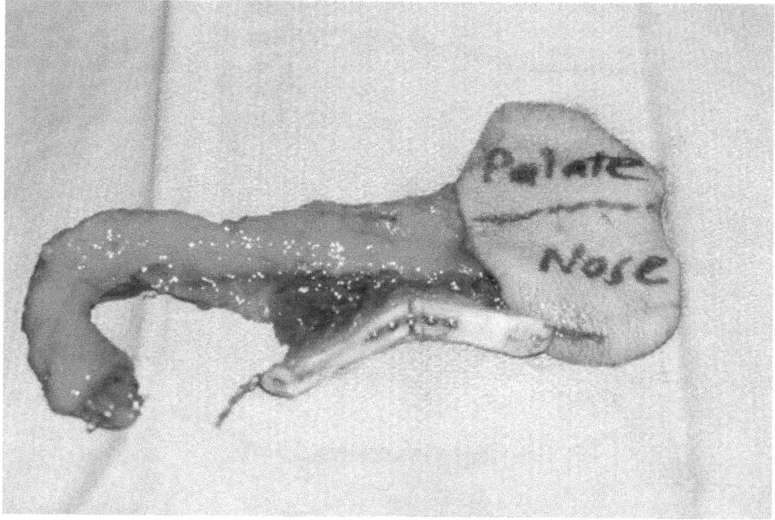

Figure 2 (**B**) Radial forearm osteocutaneous free flap with an osteotomy created to restore anterior maxillary alveolus. (*Continued*)

(C)

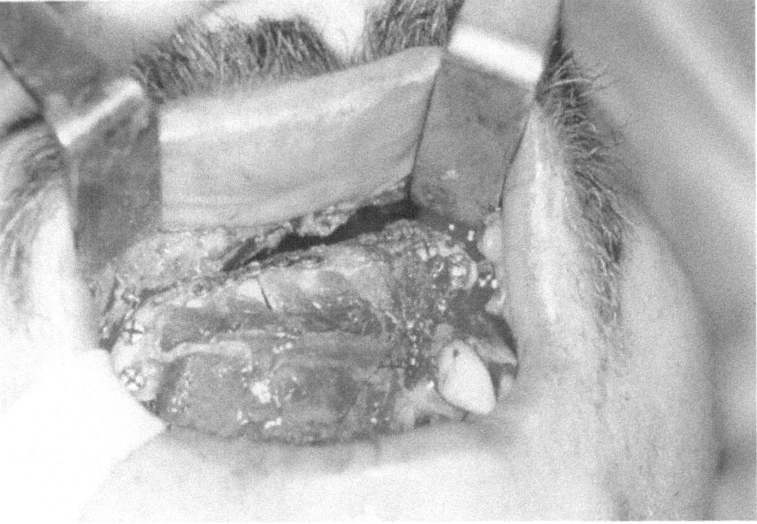

Figure 2 (**C**) Fixation of flap to residual maxilla. (*Continued*)

Some of the patients also had dental prostheses placed. Importantly, these patients also preferred living-tissue reconstruction to the problems associated with cleaning and placing a prosthesis. More recently, Browne (24) describes the successful use of the rectus abdominus free flap in a series of 12 patients, further proving the reliability of this flap in restoring both function and cosmesis to patients with these defects. These flaps are excellent for sealing the palate when adequate native teeth and/or retentive surfaces are available to support a conventional dental prosthesis and mastication.

(D)

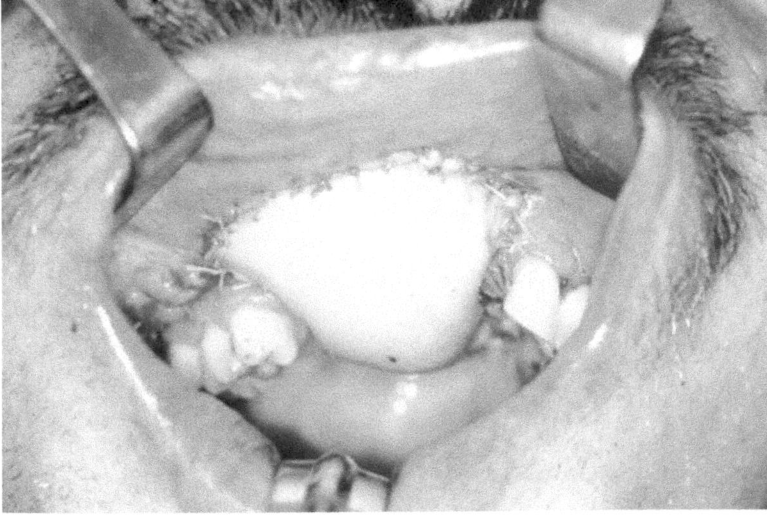

Figure 2 (**D**) Soft tissue inset. (*Continued*)

(E)

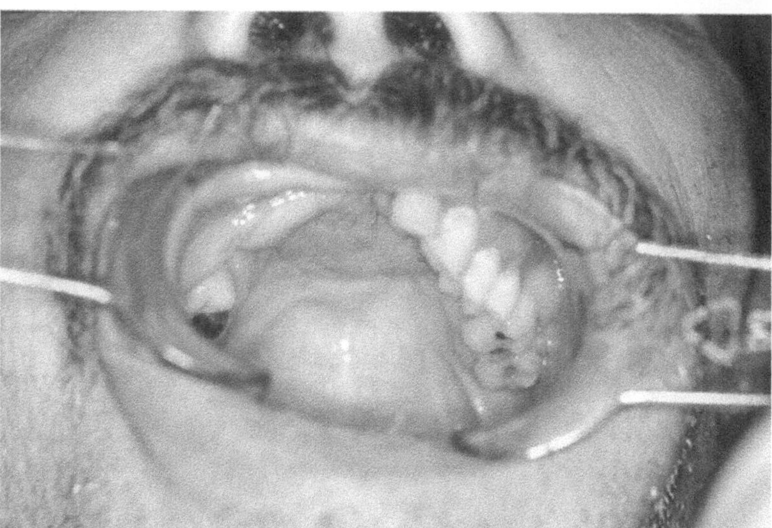

Figure 2 (E) One-year, postoperative result.

If teeth and retentive surfaces are not adequate, vascularized bone is necessary to support an implant-borne maxillary prosthesis. In this instance, the scapular osteocutaneous flap has the advantage of having a soft tissue component that can be rotated around the adequate bone stock with greater freedom than many other composite flaps (25,26). The scapular osteocutaneous flap can be particularly useful

(A)

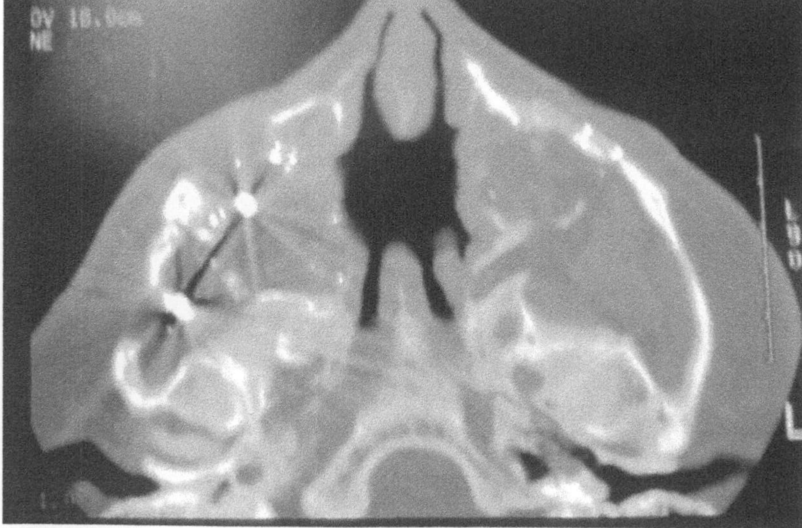

Figure 3A–F (A) Axial CT-scan of a central palatal defect created by gunshot wound which occurred 11 years previously. *(Continued)*

(B)

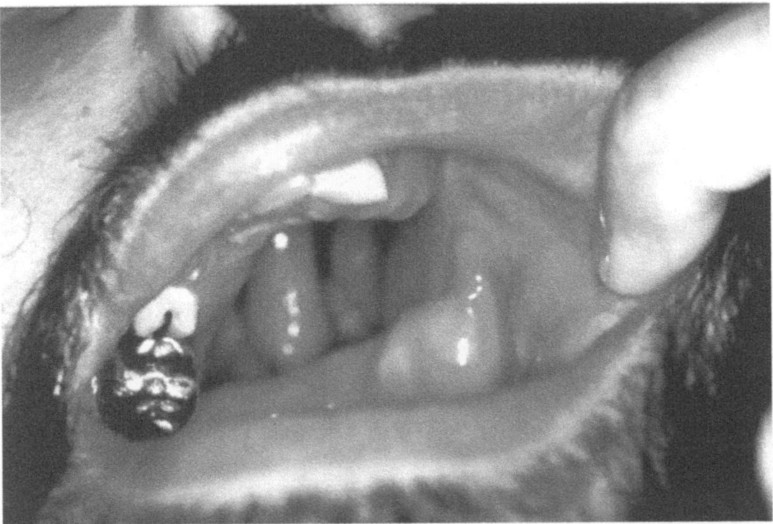

Figure 3 (**B**) Preoperative palatal defect. (*Continued*)

in larger defects in which the orbital floor, zygomatic bone, and palate all require reconstruction.

Case reports using the fibular free flap and the iliac crest free flap have emerged in the literature, as these tissue transfers have been shown to have an adequate volume of bone to support osseointegrated implants (27–30). The fibula has the advantage of a robust bone and cutaneous component with a long vascular pedicle and minimal donor site morbidity. In fact, we prefer the fibula free flap for lower maxillary defects requiring a bony reconstruction (Fig. 4).

(C)

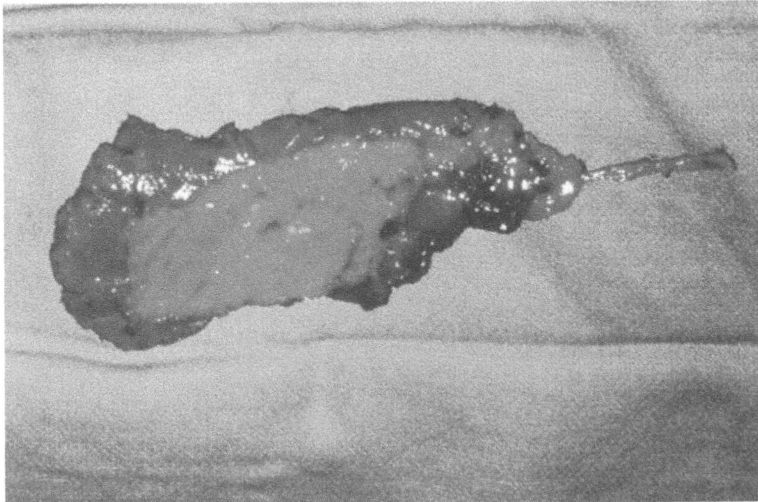

Figure 3 (**C**) Rectus abdominus myofascial free flap. (*Continued*)

(D)

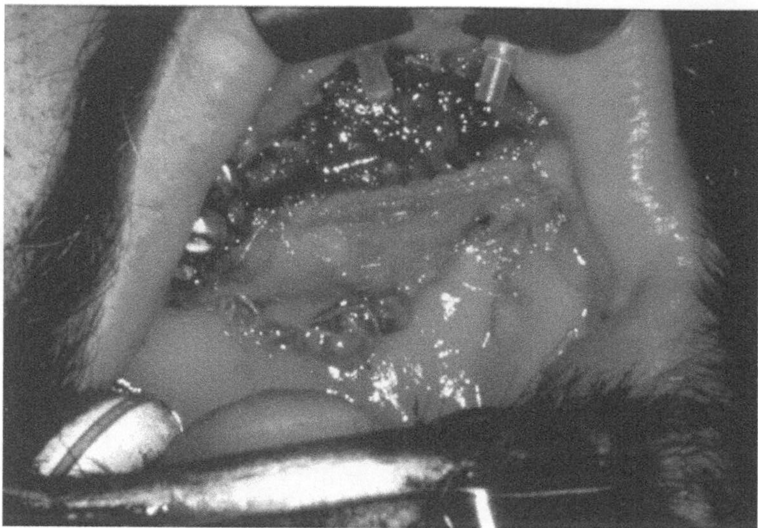

Figure 3 (**D**) Flap inset. (*Continued*)

In a series of 30 patients, described by Futran and Haller (31), all the abovementioned flaps, except the iliac crest, were used. The majority of the flaps used to reconstruct a variety of palatal defects were either rectus abdominis or fibula free flaps. Free-tissue transfer was shown to be reliable and sufficient for achieving separation of the oral and sino-nasal cavities. In addition, deglutition, speech, and an acceptable quality of life were restored for most patents.

Finally, some authors advocate the use of dual free flaps to reconstruct these complex defects (32). Although success has been reported in a small series of patients, the advantages of two separate free flaps have yet to be demonstrated.

(E)

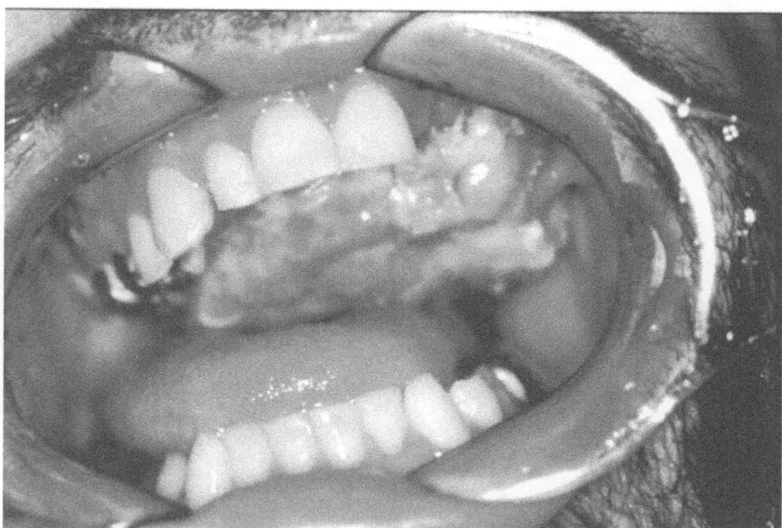

Figure 3 (**E**) Three-week, postoperative result. (*Continued*)

(F)

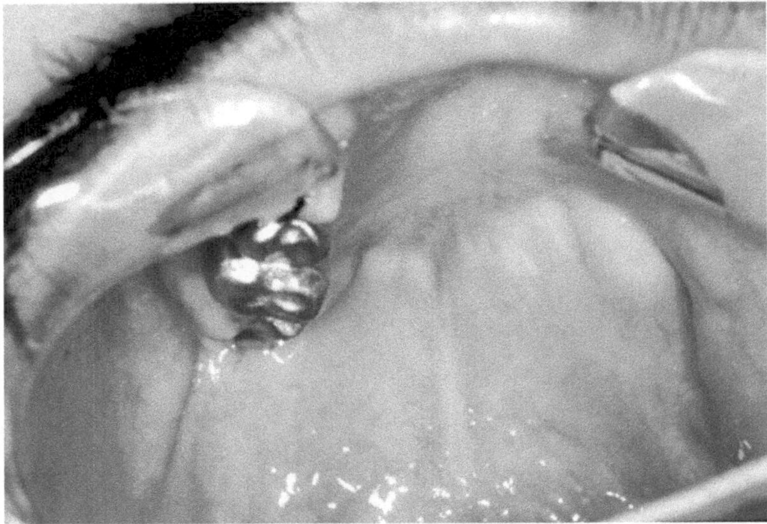

Figure 3 (F) One-year, postoperative result.

The complexity of this effort has not been shown to be more beneficial that the use of a single free flap with excellent bone stock and pliable soft tissue.

DECISION MAKING TIPS

Controversy exists in the literature concerning which flap is best to reconstruct the hard palate. Schusterman et al. (33) recommended a bone-containing free flap for

(A)

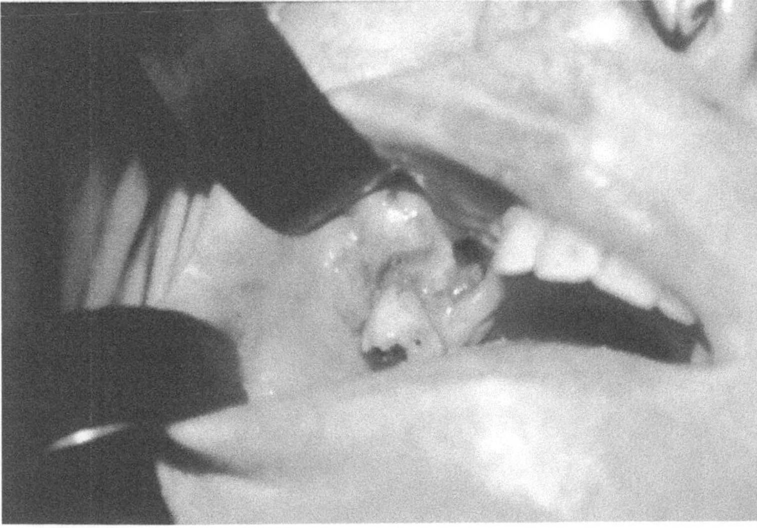

Figure 4A–L (A) Fifty-one-year-old male with recurrent adenocarcinoma of the palate status post 6800 cGy of radiation therapy. (*Continued*)

(B)

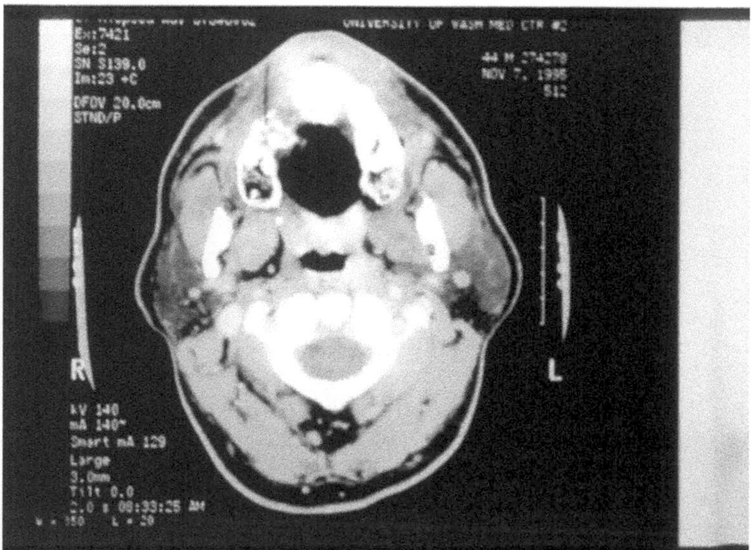

Figure 4 (**B**) CT-scan revealing bony involvement of recurrent tumor. (*Continued*)

maxillary reconstruction when bony support was needed and previous irradiation precluded the use of nonvascularized grafts. Coleman (34) suggested that the needs of the wound be matched with characteristics of the appropriate flap, including length of vascular pedicle, thickness or thinness of skin, muscle and fat, volume of soft tissue available, durability and thickness of bone, and donor-site morbidity.

Funk et al. (35) reported that the criteria for palate closure with a soft-tissue free flap includes sufficient residual dentition to retain a dental prostheses or, if

(C)

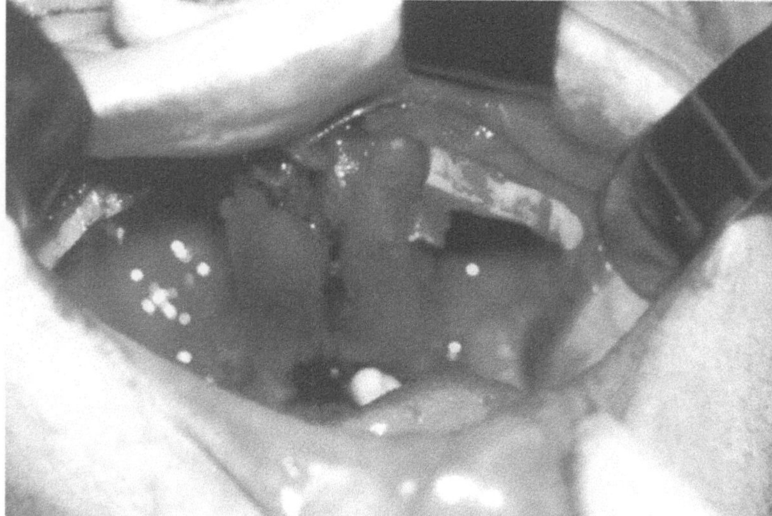

Figure 4 (**C**) Operative defect showing complete loss of hard palate. (*Continued*)

(D)

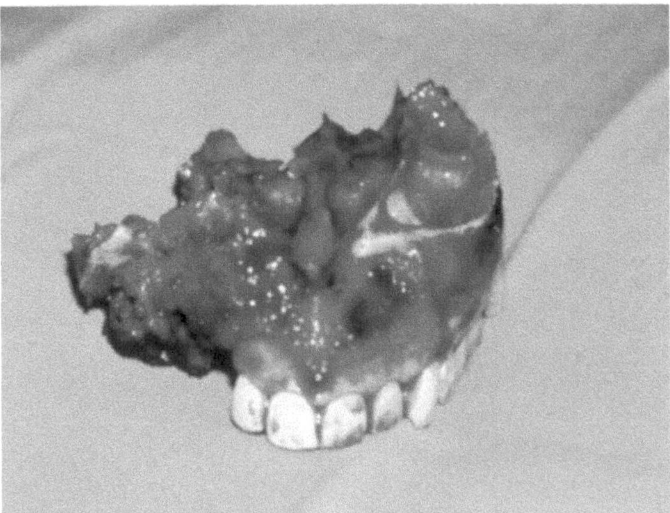

Figure 4 (**D**) Resected complete hard palate and alveolus. (*Continued*)

the anatomy of the reconstruction would allow, retention of an upper denture despite the absence of teeth. If placement of osseointegrated implants was anticipated, the scapular osteocutaneous flap was preferred. A review by Davison et al. (5) recommends free-tissue transfer closure of maxillectomy defects when substantial associated sino-orbital and/or soft-tissue defects exist. This review concludes that free-tissue transfer of vascularized bone may be ideal for reconstruction involving osteointegrated implants.

(E)

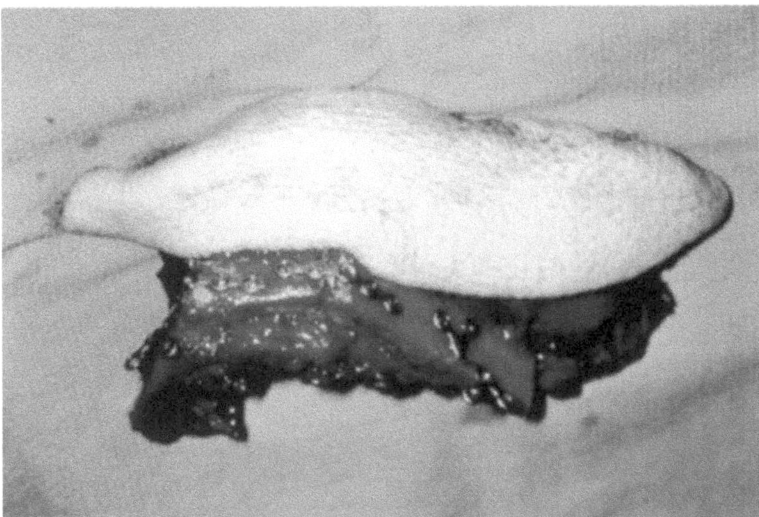

Figure 4 (**E**) Fibula osteocutaneous free flap with osteotomies to recreate the alveolar arch. (*Continued*)

(F)

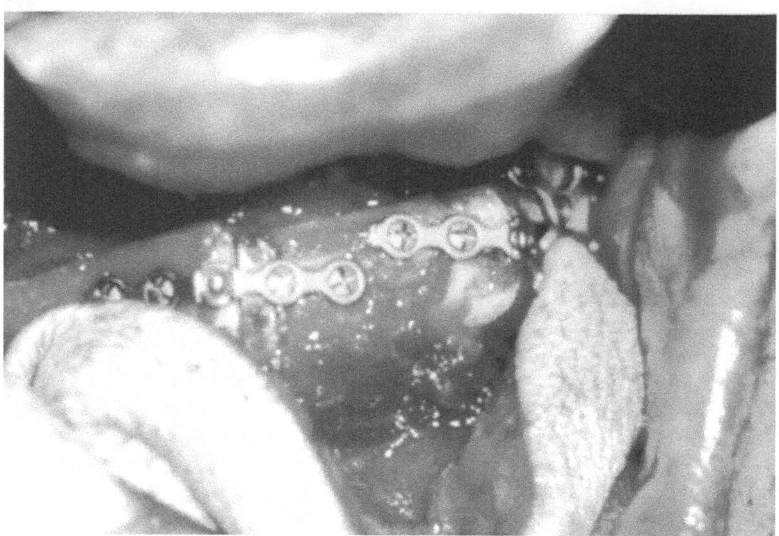

Figure 4 (F) Bony inset and fixation to residual zygomatic bone. (*Continued*)

The source of flap selection should be determined by various factors. The selection of a bone-containing free flap is largely determined by the amount, location, and quality of residual dentition and/or denture-bearing alveolar arch. In patients for whom the anterior arch is missing, the radial forearm flap provides thin, pliable tissue with minimal bulk. The incorporation of radial bone may aid in arch contour but often may not be considered suitable for placement of osseointegrated implants.

(G)

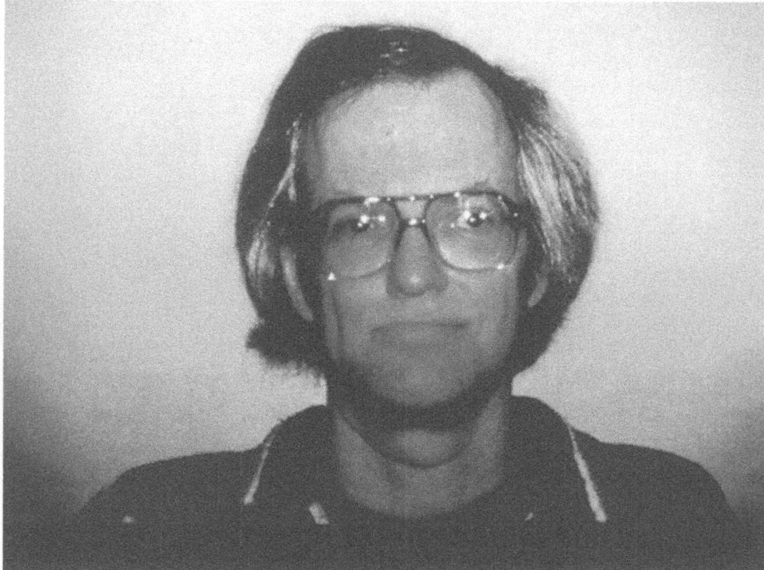

Figure 4 (G) Two-month, full face result. (*Continued*)

(H)

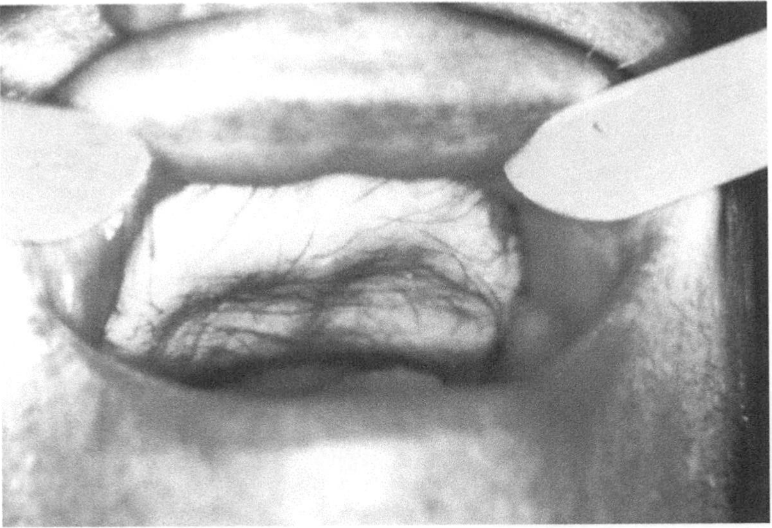

Figure 4 (**H**) Two-month, intra-oral result. (*Continued*)

In patients with hemipalatal defects, sufficient retention is usually present to support a conventional dental prosthesis so that myocutaneous free flaps can be used. Because many of these defects have associated upper midface deficits, soft tissue bulk restores these areas. In addition, cranial bone grafting can further augment the free-tissue transfer to restore the zygomatic bone and orbital floor when this is not achieved with the scapular flap.

In patients who present with total or subtotal palatectomies, little retentive surface is usually available for a conventional dental prosthesis. Therefore, these

(I)

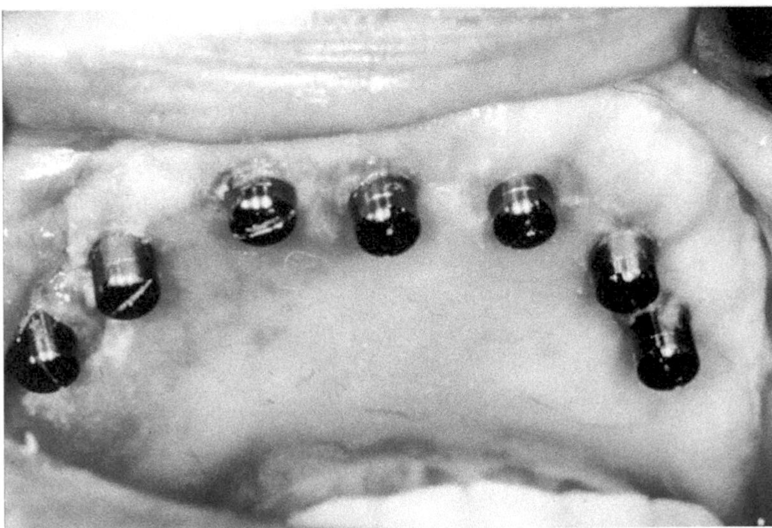

Figure 4 (**I**) Osseointegrated implants placed. (*Continued*)

(J)

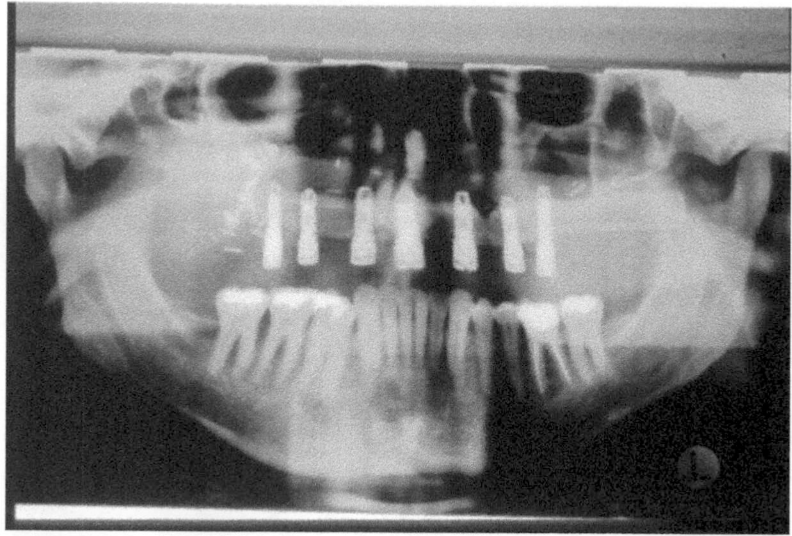

Figure 4 (J) Panorex of implants fixed into fibular bone. (*Continued*)

(K)

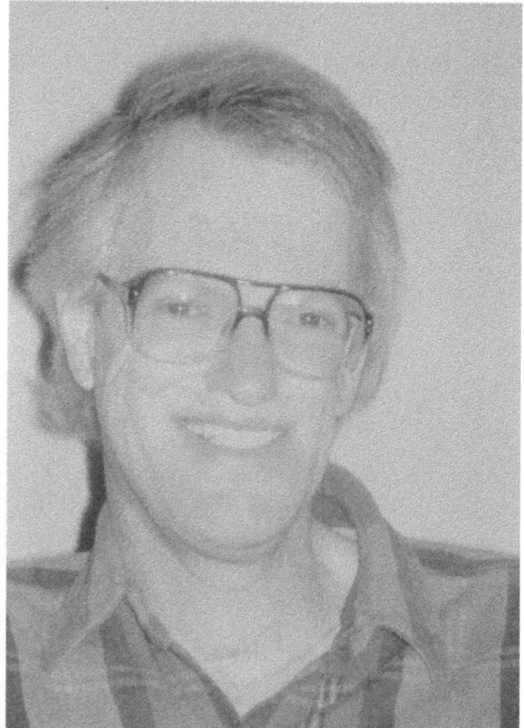

Figure 4 (K) One-year, full face result. (*Continued*)

(L)

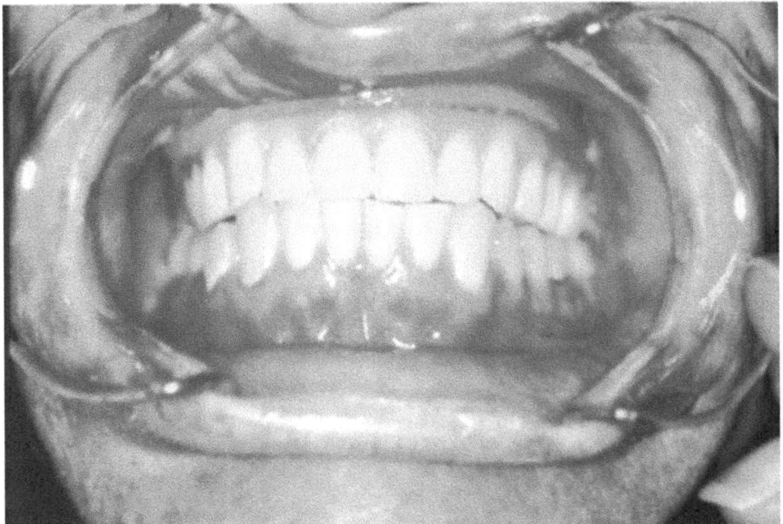

Figure 4 (L) One-year, intra-oral result with maxillary dental prosthesis in place.

patients often receive a bone-containing free flap (fibular, scapular, or iliac crest) to create the potential for implant-borne dental restoration. These are also the most complex palatal reconstructions, and may require vein grafts to achieve adequate pedicle length and geometry.

PREOPERATIVE CONSIDERATIONS

Preoperative consultation with an oral and maxillofacial surgeon as well as a maxillofacial prosthodontist should be considered for every patient for the purpose of achieving a treatment plan that leads to functional dental restoration.

The number and location of residual intact dentition and the amount of palatal bone lost dictate whether a bone-containing, free-tissue transfer or an exclusively soft-tissue, free transfer is necessary. In general, when greater than one-half of the bony palate is missing, a bone containing tissue transfer is indicated.

The patient must understand the complexity of tissue reconstruction of the palate and be motivated to follow-through with the entire prescribed treatment plan.

SPECIAL SURGICAL REQUIREMENTS

The surgeon must be very comfortable with microvascular free-tissue transfers and should be well versed in reconstructions of other areas of the head and neck, as palatal reconstruction requires complex planning and execution for satisfactory results.

The need for vein grafts should always be anticipated and prepared for, as the free-flap pedicle, after inset into the palate, may not reach the recipient vessels.

A watertight, soft-tissue seal should be created between the tissue transfer and residual maxillary structures to minimize the risk of fistulae and/or wound breakdown.

CONCLUSION

In conclusion, reconstruction of palatal defects is necessary to separate the oral cavity from the nasal and sinus cavities. Without this separation, speech is altered, and swallowing is hindered, creating a significant disability for these patients. The primary goals of reconstruction are to restore speech and to allow the patient to maintain a normal diet, although re-establishment of oral competence, midface projection, and an aesthetically acceptable appearance are also essential. Finally, functional dental restoration completes the reconstruction.

Although maxillofacial prostheses still have a role in primary reconstruction of palatal defects, free-tissue transfers have been successful and well accepted by various patients. Excellent contour and acceptable cosmesis can be achieved. In addition, the potential for dental rehabilitation with the restoration of masticatory function and normal phonation exists. The choice of free-tissue transfer should be tailored to the specific defect, denture-bearing potential of native residual tissues, and patient needs.

REFERENCES

1. Hollinshead W. Anatomy for Surgeons, The Head and Neck. Philadelphia, Pennsylvania: JB Lippincott Co., 1982:335.
2. Wells MD, Luce EA. Reconstruction of midfacial defects after surgical resection of malignancies. Clin Plast Surg 1995; 22:79–89.
3. Cho KH, Ahn HT, Park KC, Chung JH, Kim SW, Sung MW, Kim KH, Chung PH, Eun HC, Youn JI. Reconstruction of human hard-palate mucosal epithelium on de-epidermized dermis. J Dermatol Sci 2000; 22:117–124.
4. Rhee PH, Friedman CD, Ridge JA, Kusiak J. The use of processed allograft dermal matrix for intraoral resurfacing: an alternative to split-thickness skin grafts. Arch Otolaryngol Head Neck Surg 1998; 124:1201–1204.
5. Davison SP, Sherris DA, Meland NB. An algorithm for maxillectomy defect reconstruction. Laryngoscope 1998; 108:215–219.
6. Brown KE. Peripheral consideration in improving obturator retention. J Prosthet Dent 1968; 20:176–181.
7. Rahn A, Boucher L. Maxillofacial Prosthetics: Principles and Concepts. Philadelphia, Pennsylvania: WB Saunders Co., 1970.
8. Von Langenbeck B. Die Uranoplastik Mittelst Abosüng das Mucosperiostalen Guamenuberzuges. Arch Klin Chir Bd 1862; II:205–287.
9. Baumann A, Ewers R. Application of the buccal fat pad in oral reconstruction. J Oral Maxillofac Surg 2000; 58:389–392; discussion 392–393.
10. Dorrance G. The Operative Story of Cleft Palate. Philadelphia, Pennsylvania: WB Saunders Co., 1933:62–66.
11. Edgerton M, DeVito R. Reconstruction of palatal defects resulting from treatment of carcinoma of palate, antrum, or gingiva. Plast Reconstr Surg 1961; 28:306–319.
12. Kostrubala J. Repair of extensive palatal defects with skin tubes. Plast Reconstr Surg 1950; 5:512–515.
13. Colmenero C, Martorell V, Colmenero B, Sierra I. Temporalis myofascial flap for maxillofacial reconstruction. J Oral Maxillofac Surg 1991; 49:1067–1073.
14. Konno A, Togawa K, Iizuka K. Primary reconstruction after total or extended total maxillectomy for maxillary cancer. Plast Reconstr Surg 1981; 67:440–448.
15. Bakamjian VY, Poole M. Maxillo-facial and palatal reconstructions with the deltopectoral flap. Br J Plast Surg 1977; 30:17–37.

16. Ewers R. Reconstruction of the maxilla with a double musculoperiosteal flap in connection with a composite calvarial bone graft. Plast Reconstr Surg 1988; 81:431–436.
17. Choung PH, Nam IW, Kim KS. Vascularized cranial bone grafts for mandibular and maxillary reconstruction. The parietal osteofascial flap. J Craniomaxillofac Surg 1991; 19:235–242.
18. MacLeod AM, Morrison WA, McCann JJ, Thistlethwaite S, Vanderkolk CA, Ryan AD. The free radial forearm flap with and without bone for closure of large palatal fistulae. Br J Plast Surg 1987; 40:391–395.
19. Hatoko M, Harashina T, Inoue T, Tanaka I, Imai K. Reconstruction of palate with radial forearm flap; a report of 3 cases. Br J Plast Surg 1990; 43:350–354.
20. Cordeiro PG, Bacilious N, Schantz S, Spiro R. The radial forearm osteocutaneous "sandwich" free flap for reconstruction of the bilateral subtotal maxillectomy defect. Ann Plast Surg 1998; 40:397–402.
21. Shestak KC, Schusterman MA, Jones NF, Janecka IP, Sekhar LN, Johnson JT. Immediate microvascular reconstruction of combined palatal and midfacial defects. Am J Surg 1988; 156:252–255.
22. Shestak KC, Schusterman MA, Jones NF, Johnson JT. Immediate microvascular reconstruction of combined palatal and midfacial defects using soft tissue only. Microsurgery 1988; 9:128–131.
23. Olsen KD, Meland NB, Ebersold MJ, Bartley GB, Garrity JA. Extensive defects of the sino-orbital region. Results with microvascular reconstruction. Arch Otolaryngol Head Neck Surg 1992; 118:828–833; discussion 859–860.
24. Browne JD, Burke AJ. Benefits of routine maxillectomy and orbital reconstruction with the rectus abdominis free flap. Otolaryngol Head Neck Surg 1999; 121:203–209.
25. Swartz WM, Banis JC, Newton ED, Ramasastry SS, Jones NF, Acland R. The osteocutaneous scapular flap for mandibular and maxillary reconstruction. Plast Reconstr Surg 1986; 77:530–545.
26. Granick MS, Ramasastry SS, Newton ED, Solomon MP, Hanna DC, Kaltman S. Reconstruction of complex maxillectomy defects with the scapular-free flap. Head Neck 1990; 12:377–385.
27. Sadove RC, Powell LA. Simultaneous maxillary and mandibular reconstruction with one free osteocutaneous flap. Plast Reconstr Surg 1993; 92:141–146.
28. Nakayama B, Matsuura H, Ishihara O, Hasegawa H, Mataga I, Torii S. Functional reconstruction of a bilateral maxillectomy defect using a fibula osteocutaneous flap with osseointegrated implants. Plast Reconstr Surg 1995; 96:1201–1204.
29. Anthony JP, Foster RD, Sharma AB, Kearns GJ, Hoffman WY, Pogrel MA. Reconstruction of a complex midfacial defect with the folded fibular free flap and osseointegrated implants. Ann Plast Surg 1996; 37:204–210.
30. Brown JS. Deep circumflex iliac artery free flap with internal oblique muscle as a new method of immediate reconstruction of maxillectomy defect. Head Neck 1996; 18:412–421.
31. Futran ND, Haller JR. Considerations for free-flap reconstruction of the hard palate. Arch Otolaryngol Head Neck Surg 1999; 125:665–669.
32. Freije JE, Campbell BH, Yousif NJ, Matloub HS. Reconstruction after infrastructure maxillectomy using dual free flaps. Laryngoscope 1997; 107:694–697.
33. Schusterman MA, Reece GP, Miller MJ. Osseous free flaps for orbit and midface reconstruction. Am J Surg 1993; 166:341–345.
34. Coleman JJ III. Osseous reconstruction of the midface and orbits. Clin Plast Surg 1994; 21:113–124.
35. Funk GF, Laurenzo JF, Valentino J, McCulloch TM, Frodel JL, Hoffman HT. Free-tissue transfer reconstruction of midfacial and cranio-orbito-facial defects. Arch Otolaryngol Head Neck Surg 1995; 121:293–303.

14
Reconstruction of the Soft Palate and Velopharyngeal Complex

Craig W. Senders
Department of Otolaryngology, University of California—Davis Medical Center, Sacramento, California, U.S.A.

INTRODUCTION

The treatment of velopharyngeal dysfunction is challenging due to the complex anatomy of the velopharyngeal sphincter, which is responsible for separating the nasal cavity from the mouth during speech and swallowing. The velopharyngeal sphincter is comprised of three muscles: the levator veli palatini, the uvularis, and the superior constrictor muscle. The first two muscles are palatal muscles. The levator veli palatini elevates the palate, and the uvularis, located centrally, creates a bulge on the nasopharyngeal surface of the soft palate, aiding in sphincter closure (Fig. 1) (1). Typically, the levator veli palatini muscle is the major contributor to sphincter closure. The third muscle, the superior constrictor muscle, contributes to closure laterally and posteriorly and effects a coronal pattern to velopharyngeal closure (Fig. 2) (2,3).

The symptoms of velopharyngeal dysfunction include difficulty swallowing, regurgitation of liquids, and alterations in speech (4). Most patients learn to adapt to swallowing problems but often require surgical or prosthetic help with speech problems. Typically, these patients have hypernasal resonance with escape of air through the nose (5,6). This can be seen easily using a laryngeal mirror placed below the nostrils during the production of sounds that would not be expected to cause air to pass through the nose. In the English language, velopharyngeal closure is expected during all sounds except "M," "N," and "NG." For all other sounds, nasal emission would be abnormal.

The evaluation of velopharyngeal dysfunction optimally includes a speech pathology evaluation. The surgeon's evaluation for inappropriate velopharyngeal emission should start with simple repetitive phrases like "ba ba ba ba" or "to ta to ta." The evaluation should progress to two syllable words without "N's," "M's," or "NG's" such as "blackboard," "tabletop," or "shirttail." It is important to use sentences that do not include nasal sounds like "Black cats are fast," "Tall trees grow fast," and "Red shorts are bright." Moreover, the use of sentences can uncover velopharyngeal dysfunction, which is only present during connected speech (5). To aid in

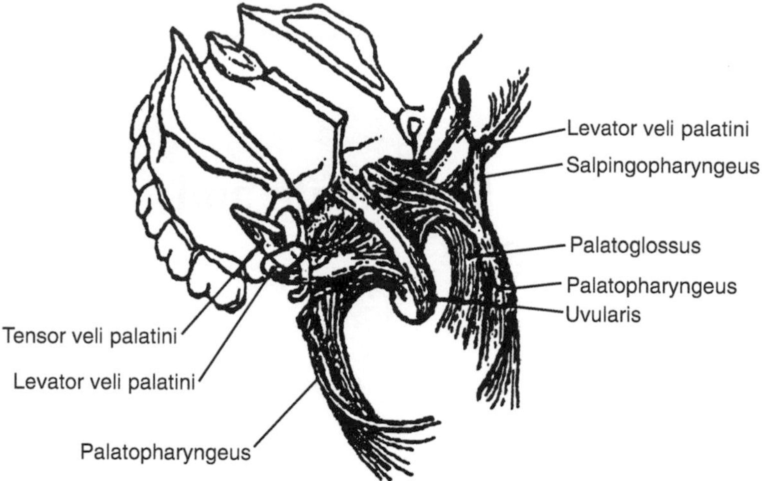

Figure 1 Anatomy of the velopharyngeal sphincter. *Source*: From Ref. 1.

the decision to treat prosthetically or surgically, one should assess nasal escape, hypernasal resonance, and intelligibility during single task and connected speech.

EVALUATION AND PLANNING

The most common cause of velopharyngeal dysfunction is a patient with a post-repair cleft palate or a child with a submucous cleft palate. The most common cause

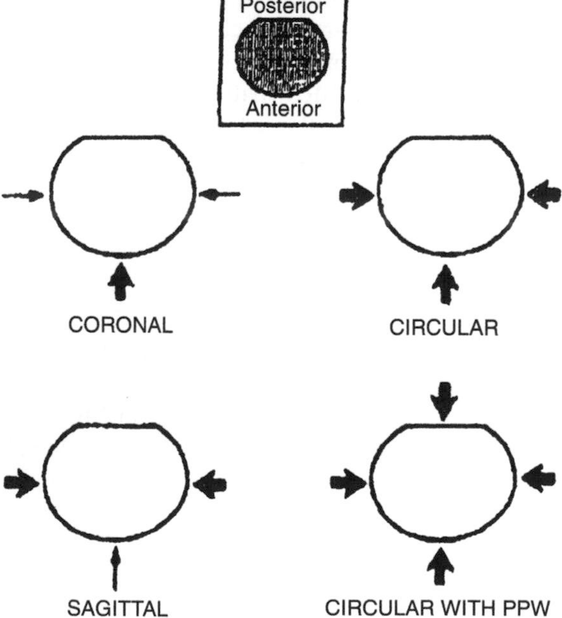

Figure 2 Patterns of closure of the velopharyngeal sphincter. (*Bold arrows indicate most motion*) The coronal pattern is the most common. *Source*: From Ref. 3.

of velopharengeal dysfunction in the head and neck surgeons' practice is typically post-head-and-neck cancer surgery or due to a cerebral-vascular accident. The superior constrictor muscle and the muscles of the soft palate, except for the tensor veli palatini muscle, are innervated by the tenth cranial nerve (1). The tensor veli palatini muscle, which opens the eustachian tube, is innervated by the fifth cranial nerve. A tumor resection that required the sacrifice of the tenth cranial nerve on one side would be expected to cause ipselateral velopharyngeal dysfunction in addition to vocal cord paralysis and dysphagia. If, after a period of time, the patient failed to adapt, surgical or prosthetic intervention would be appropriate.

Head neck cancer which involves the velum directly, would be the most common scenario presented to the head and neck surgeon. Typically, patients who have partial resections of their oral pharynx and palate do better than one might expect with their speech post-operatively. As would be expected, the larger the resection of the palate and surrounding tissues, the worse the outcome (7). Resections of the soft palate that also involve the tongue not only create problems with velopharyngeal competence, but also interfere with articulation and swallowing, and intelligibility is greatly reduced. For this reason, major reconstructive efforts are typically left until after the patient has healed and recovered from primary surgery. However, at the time of the primary surgery, every effort should be made to reduce the size of the velopharyngeal defect, or if possible, to close it primarily (Fig. 3) (8–10).

After surgery, patients are allowed to heal; evaluation of velopharyngeal function is most meaningful three or more months following the surgery. At this time, a full assessment of the velopharyngeal dysfunction is made and a flexible nasopharyngoscopy is performed. The classification schemes for velopharyngeal function are based upon the contributions of the muscles which aid in velopharyngeal closure (Fig. 2) (3). However, from the surgeon's standpoint, the defect which is left during maximum velopharyngeal closure is what directs the surgical or prosthetic therapy. A pharyngeal flap or a dynamic pharyngoplasty can be tailored to close the defect observed during maximal velopharyngeal function. Defect-directed therapy offers patients the best results with the least morbidity (Fig. 4) (3).

RECONSTRUCTIVE OPTIONS

Prosthetic Therapy

In many patients, prosthetic management is appropriate for the velopharyngeal dysfunction. Because it is not permanent, it can be started within a month after surgery and modified as needed as the patient heals. Prosthetic management is appropriate in patients who are poor surgical candidates, patients who are already using a palatal prosthesis to obturate the hard palate, patients with sleep apnea, and in patients in whom more than three-fourths of the soft palate has been removed. Patients who use dentures already have an advantage over other patients as the prosthetic device can be incorporated into the dentures. Additionally, some patients will prefer prosthetic management over surgical management. An advantage of prosthetic management is that the device can be removed at bedtime to allow easier breathing. The device can also be modified as many times as necessary to optimize speech results.

For many patients, retention of a large prosthesis is problematic. Retention can be improved with the use of implants with or with out magnets to serve as anchors. Another technique to improve retention is allowing the prosthesis to cover a large area of sensate mucosa in the oral cavity, because the insensate nature of a prosthesis

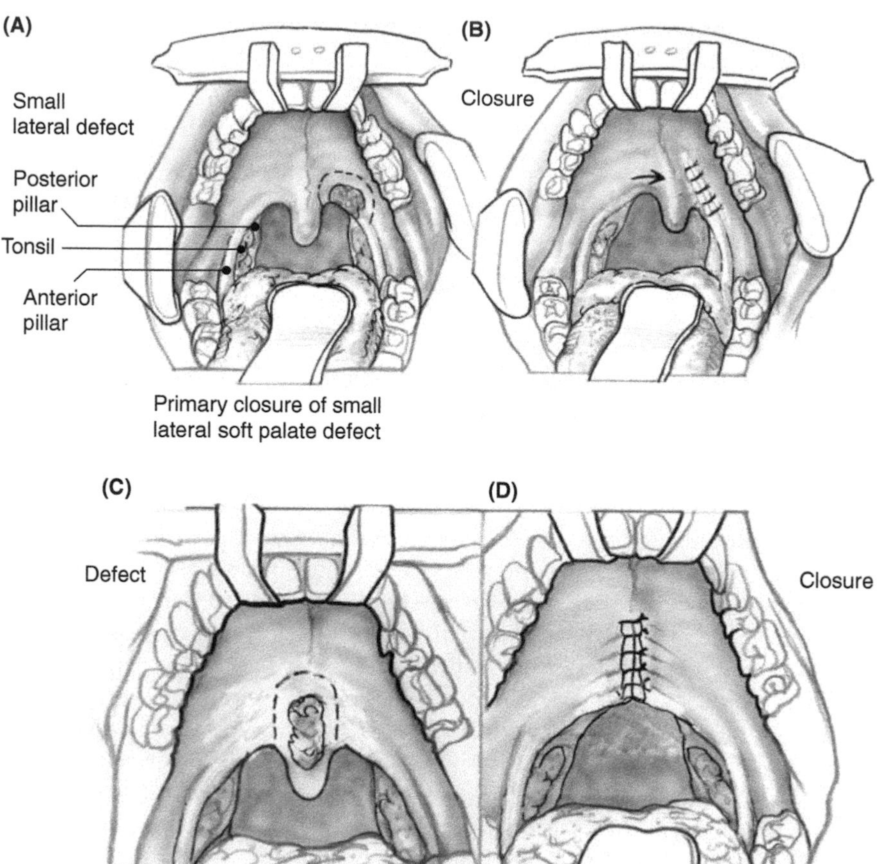

Figure 3 Examples of primary closure: (**A**) A primary carcinoma of the soft palate. (**B**) With small defects, primary closure is the best option. (**C**) A primary carcinoma involving the uvula. (**D**) An attempt at primary closure is appropriate.

negatively affects articulation, which is often already hampered in patients who have undergone a cancer resection (8).

The Dynamic Pharyngoplasty

The dynamic pharyngoplasty is becoming the most popular technique for the treatment of velopharyngeal dysfunction in cleft patients (11). It is ideal for a patient with mild neurological dysfunction in that it reduces the nasopharyngeal opening that must be closed to allow velopharyngeal competence (12,13). The best results are observed in patients who have retained some neurological function, such as a patient with a unilateral neurological defect, possibly due to resection of the tenth cranial nerve. In this situation, a unilateral dynamic pharyngoplasty can be used to close the velopharynx unilaterally.

A common pitfall of this surgery is to create a new sphincter at a height insufficient for velopharyngeal function (14). At nasopharyngoscopy, the level of maximal closure should be determined. The level of the new sphincter always needs to be as high as the inferior margin of the adenoids and often higher. If there is a significant adenoid pad, an adenoidectomy should be preformed two to three months prior to

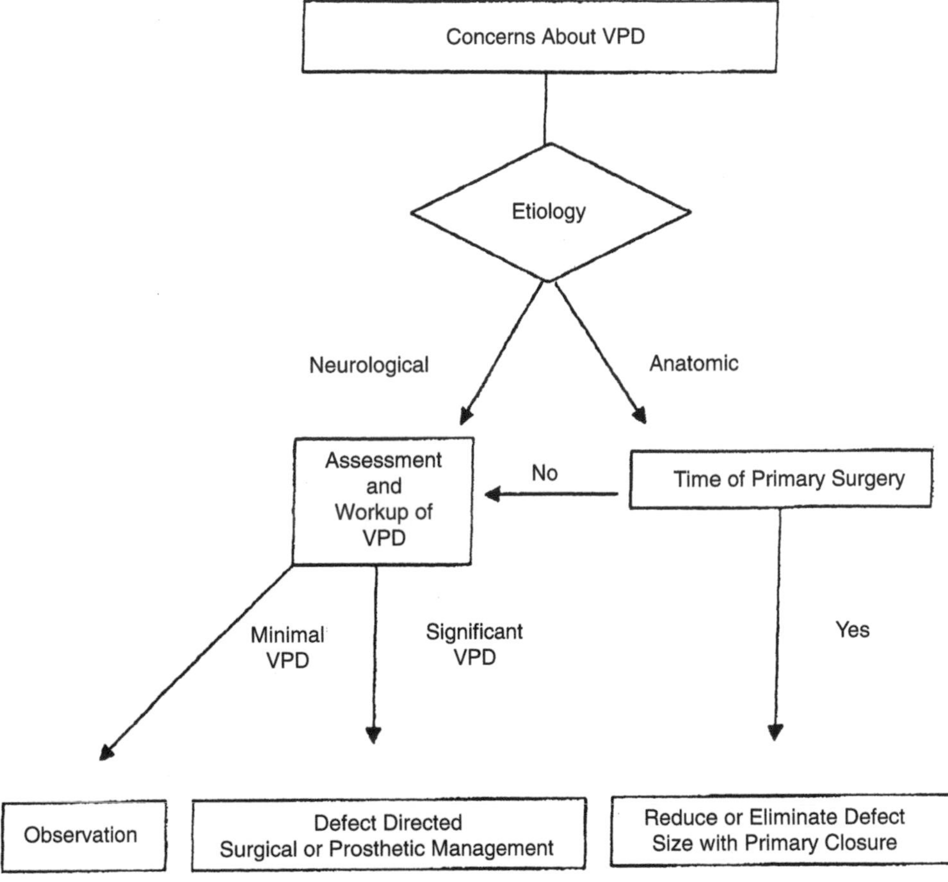

Figure 4 Treatment algorithm for VPD (velopharyngeal dysfunction).

the definitive surgery. Removal of the adenoids preoperatively will allow creation of the neosphincter at a higher level. The tonsils should typically be removed with the adenoids, unless they are diminutive.

For the dynamic pharyngoplasty, a Dingman mouth gag is typically utilized and the surgical bed is typically injected with 1% lidocaine and 1:100,000 epinephrine. All patients should be visually evaluated for an aberrant internal carotid artery. If pulsations are observed, care is taken to not damage this vessel.

A superiorly based lateral pharyngeal flap is created by making an incision just anterior and parallel to the posterior tonsillar pillar that extends inferiorly to the level of the tongue (Fig. 5). This incision involves mucosa, palatoglossus muscle and the superior constrictor muscle. The posterior margin of the incision is made at or just before the junction of the posterior and lateral pharyngeal walls. The flap width should be one to two centimeters. The anterior incision extends superiorly to the apex of the tonsillar fossa. The posterior incision extends to the desired height of the to-be-created neosphincter. At the desired height, the incision makes a right angle turn and passes across the nasopharynx from one side to the other. The mucosa and superior constrictor muscle are cut and the alar fascia is exposed.

The lateral pharyngeal flap is then sewn in place in the nasopharynx using long lasting absorbable suture. The surgeon can fine-tune the amount of medialization of the soft palate by how far he pulls the lateral flap across the midline.

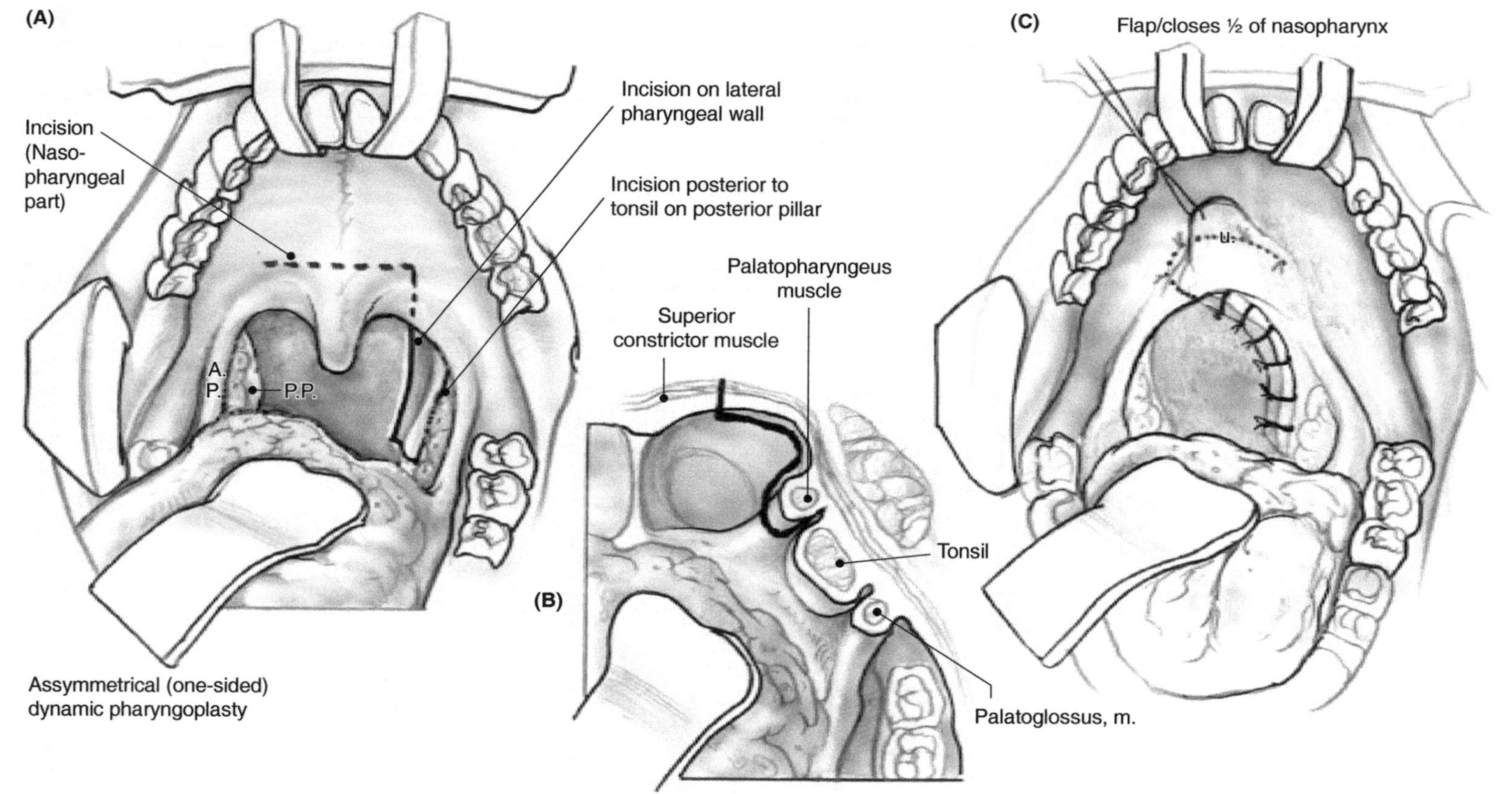

Figure 5 Unilateral dynamic pharyngoplasty: (**A**) Incisions. (**B**) Cross-section showing lateral flap incisions. (**C**) Flap sewn in place at the level of maximal velopharyngeal closure.

The patient should be given pre- and post-operative antibiotics and monitored with a pulse oximeter. The patient should be discharged when able to drink fluids well. Speech therapy should start one-month post-operatively, with a full evaluation six-months post-operatively.

Asymmetrical Pharyngeal Flap

The asymmetrical pharyngeal flap is ideal in a patient that has an anatomical defect of the soft palate. If the defect is too large (greater than three-fourths of the soft palate) it is difficult to create a port that a patient is able to breathe through and also close during speech or swallowing. Pharyngeal flaps have a tendency to cause long-term post-operative snoring and in some patients sleep apnea (15–17). The larger the flap the greater the tendency toward this outcome. Therefore, in patients that have minimal velopharyngeal motion, an almost totally occlusive flap would likely lead to sleep apnea and should be avoided.

Pharyngeal flaps can also be combined with radial forearm free flaps (10,18–20). This combination has been described for total soft palate reconstruction (19,20). In patients with little or no velopharyngeal function remaining, these combined flaps would have to almost totally occlude the nasopharynx. This would be an appropriate treatment for a patient who was already tracheotomy dependent. In the authors experience, patients with minimal residual palate are best managed prosthetically if they are not tracheotomy dependent.

To create asymmetrical pharyngeal flap, a Dingman mouth gag is typically utilized and the surgical bed is injected with 1% lidocaine and 1:100,000 epinephrine. The posterior pharyngeal wall should be carefully evaluated for pulsations, as this may indicate an aberrant internal carotid artery. If pulsations are seen within the planned pharyngeal flap harvest area, prosthetic management should be considered.

The pharyngeal flap is elevated first (Fig. 6). The width of the pharyngeal flap should be 25% wider than the intended defect that it is to close. The flap, which contains the superior constrictor muscle, is raised in the fascial plane known as the alar fascia. To determine the correct plane, one can identify the mobility of the constrictor muscles in relation to the paraspinous muscles. The length of the pharyngeal flap should be generous enough to easily close the defect, keeping in mind that the longer the flap the greater the chances of hypopharyngeal narrowing and post-operative sleep apnea. Inferiorly the flap should come to a point to help identify the midline of the pharyngeal flap later. The flap is raised superiorly as far as is practical and to the level of maximum sphincter function. A right angle scissor can extend the lateral incision superiorly and also separate attachments to the paraspinous muscles and ligaments.

A pocket is then created in the soft palate to receive the pharyngeal flap. This pocket should extend as far, as is practical to allow a large adhesive area between the pharyngeal flap and the soft palate. Laterally, it is often more practical to back elevate a mucosal and muscle flap which will then overlap the pharyngeal flap. With the asymmetrical pharyngeal flap, the goal is to not leave a lateral pharyngeal port as is commonly done in the typical patient that has velopharyngeal dysfunction with a cleft. Rather here, the goal is to close the side of the nasopharynx with the soft palate defect thereby, allowing the opposite side to work as the velopharyngeal sphincter. In order to accomplish this the pharyngeal incision must communicate with the palatal incision. Laterally, the flap is sewn in place with absorbable sutures at the maximum depth of the pocket as well as on the margins of the pocket.

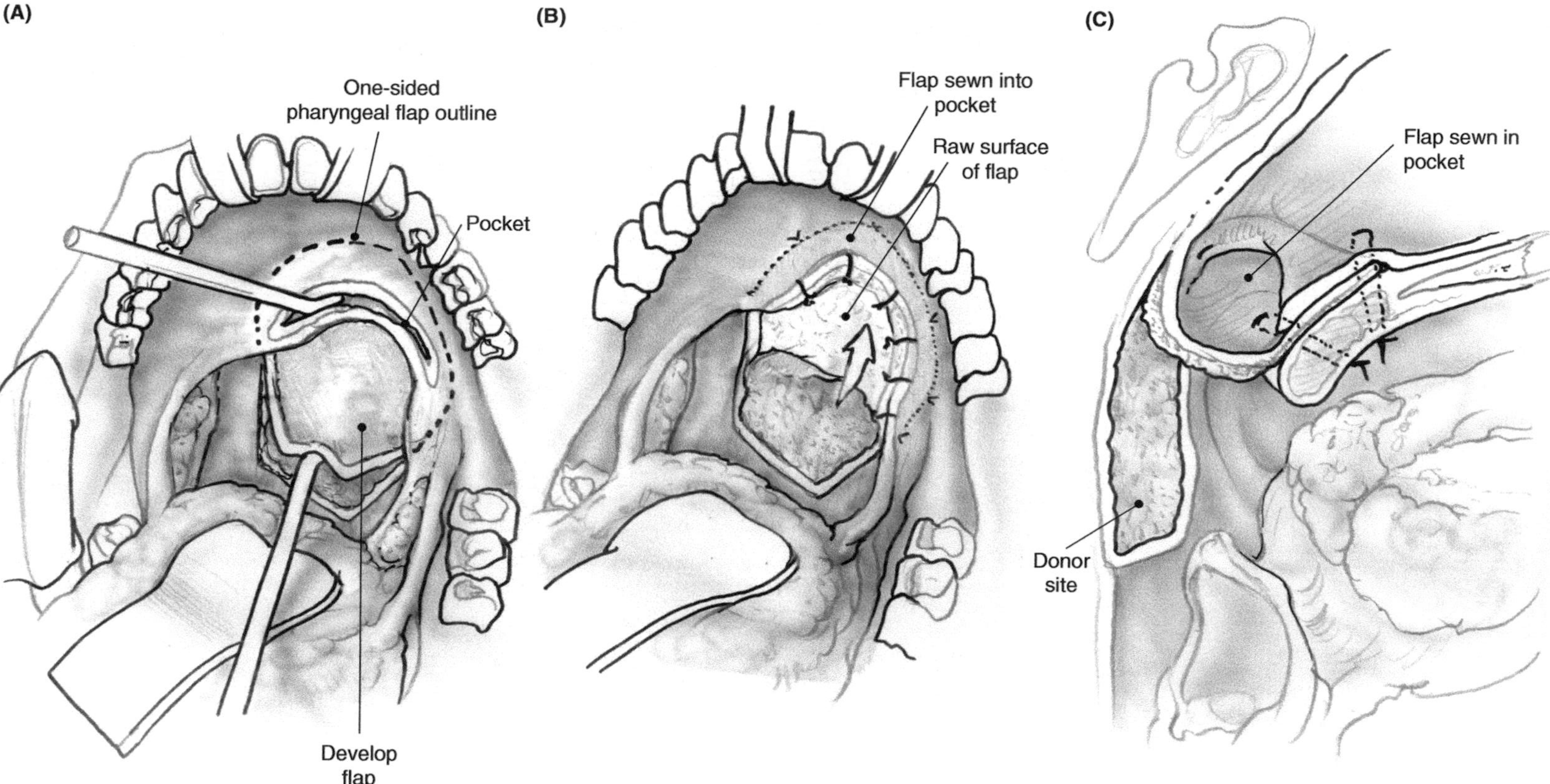

Figure 6 Asymmetrical pharyngeal flap: (**A**) A symptomatic defect of the soft palate. (**B**) Flap sewn in place. (**C**) Cross-sectional view showing flap sewn in place. *Note*: There is not a lateral port on the side closed with the pharyngeal flap.

The patient is maintained on pre- and post-operative antibiotics and monitored with a pulse oximeter. The patient should begin speech therapy one-month post-operatively. After appropriate speech therapy, a full speech evaluation should be made six-months post-operatively.

CONCLUSION

The reconstruction of soft palate defects should be individualized. Small defects can be repaired at the time of tumor resection. Otherwise the palatal defect should be partially closed and the patient fully evaluated two to three months later. By determining the defect in velopharyngeal closure, prosthetic or surgical management is customized.

REFERENCES

1. Sykes J, Senders C. Pathologic anatomy of cleft lip and palate. Biol Basis Facial Plast Surg 1993; 5:57–71.
2. Croft CB, Shprintzen RJ, Rakoff SJ. Patterns of velopharyngeal valving in normal and cleft palate subjects: a multi-view videofluoroscopic and nasendoscopic study. Laryngoscope 1981; 91:265–271.
3. Gray S, Pinborough-Zimmerman J. Diagnosis and treatment of velopharyngeal incompetence. Facial Plast Surg Clin N Am 1996; 4:405–412.
4. Crockett DM, Bumsted RM, Van Demark DR. Experience with surgical management of velopharyngeal incompetence. Otolaryngol Head Neck Surg 1988; 99:1–9.
5. Senders C, Bernstein L. Cleft lip and palate: Orolaryngology. Philadelphia: Lippencott-Raven, 1997.
6. Trost-Cardamone JE. Coming to terms with vpi: a response to loney and bloem. Cleft Palate J 1989; 26:68–70.
7. Pauloski BR, Logemann JA, Colangelo LA, Rademaker AW, McConnel FM, Heiser MA, Cardinale S, Shedd D, Stein D, Beery Q, et al. Surgical variables affecting speech in treated patients with oral and oropharyngeal cancer. Laryngoscope. 1998; 108: 908–916.
8. Gillespie MB, Eisele DW. The uvulopalatal flap for reconstruction of the soft palate. Laryngoscope 2000; 110:612–615.
9. Zohar Y, Buler N, Shvilli Y, Sabo R. Reconstruction of the soft palate by uvulopalatal flap. Laryngoscope 1998; 108:47–50.
10. Lacombe V, Blackwell KE. Radial forearm free flap for soft palate reconstruction. Arch Facial Plast Surg 1999; 1:130–132.
11. Sloan GM. Posterior pharyngeal flap and sphincter pharyngoplasty: the state of the art. Cleft Palate Craniofac J 2000; 37:112–122.
12. Jackson IT. Sphincter pharyngoplasty. Clin Plast Surg 1985; 12:711–717.
13. Moss AL, Pigott RW, Albery EH. Hynes pharyngoplasty revisited. Plast Reconstr Surg 1987; 79:346–355.
14. Riski JE, Serafin D, Riefkohl R, Georgiade GS, Georgiade NG. A rationale for modifying the site of insertion of the orticochea pharyngoplasty. Plast Reconstr Surg 1984; 73:882–894.
15. Morris HL, Bardach J, Jones D, Christiansen JL, Gray SD. Clinical results of pharyngeal flap surgery: The iowa experience. Plast Reconstr Surg 1995; 95:652–662.
16. Senders CW, Fung M. Factors influencing palatoplasty and pharyngeal flap surgery. Arch Otolaryngol Head Neck Surg 1991; 117:542–545.

17. Wells MD, Vu TA, Luce EA. Incidence and sequelae of nocturnal respiratory obstruction following posterior pharyngeal flap operation. Ann Plast Surg 1999; 43:252–257.
18. Townend J. Combined radial forearm and pharyngeal flaps for soft palate reconstruction. Br J Oral Maxillofac Surg 1998; 36:156–157.
19. Brown JS, Zuydam AC, Jones DC, Rogers SN, Vaughan ED. Functional outcome in soft palate reconstruction using a radial forearm free flap in conjunction with a superiorly based pharyngeal flap. Head Neck 1997; 19:524–534.
20. Penfold CN, Brown AE, Lavery KM, Venn PJ. Combined radial forearm and pharyngeal flap for soft palate reconstruction. Br J Oral Maxillofac Surg 1996; 34:322–324.

15
Cleft Lip and Palate

Jonathan M. Sykes
Facial Plastic and Reconstructive Surgery, University of California—Davis Medical Center, Sacramento, California, U.S.A.

Travis T. Tollefson
Facial Plastic and Reconstructive Surgery, Department of Otolaryngology—Head and Neck Surgery, University of California—Davis Medical Center, Sacramento, California, U.S.A.

INTRODUCTION

Clefts of the lip and palate are complex congenital deformities that have significant physical and psychological effects. Successful management of these deformities requires a team approach in order to diagnose and treat the problems associated with clefting.

An interdisciplinary cleft team should include a speech therapist, social worker, pediatrician, geneticist, orthodontist, oral surgeon, otologist, audiologist, and cleft surgeon (1). Most patients with clefting have significant dental, speech, and audiologic issues that require attention. It is also important to address psychosocial and genetic concerns of the patient and family. Although care of the cleft patient is inherently complex, successful treatment is extremely rewarding.

This chapter will outline the epidemiology, embryology, pathophysiology, and classification of cleft deformities. Specific repairs for treatment of unilateral and bilateral cleft lip and palate defects will be discussed.

Epidemiology

The overall incidence of clefting of the lip and/or palate is approximately 1 in every 750 live births in the United States. The distribution of cleft disorders includes: isolated cleft palate, 30%; and cleft lip with or without cleft palate, 70% (isolated cleft lip 20%, cleft lip and palate 50%). Cleft lip with or without cleft palate is unilateral in 80% of patients. The highest incidence of cleft lip with or without cleft palate is seen in Native Americans (3.6 per 1000 live births) and Asians (2.1 per 1000 live births). African Americans have the lowest incidence (0.3 per 1000 live births) compared to Caucasians (1 per 1000 live births). Isolated cleft palate is genetically distinct from cleft lip with or without cleft palate and exhibits no racial predilection with an overall incidence of 1 per 1000 live births. Isolated cleft palate is twice as common in females, whereas cleft lip with or without palate is more frequently seen in males.

Although, an isolated cleft palate is most commonly non-syndromic, many syndromes have been associated with cleft palate. These include Stickler's syndrome which is an autosomal dominant disorder associated with progressive myopia, hearing loss, arthropathy, and Pierre Robin sequence (cleft palate, microgenia, and relative macroglossia (Fig. 1). Van Der Woude syndrome (autosomal dominant associated with lip pits), Goldenhar's syndrome (autosomal dominant, hemifacial

(A)

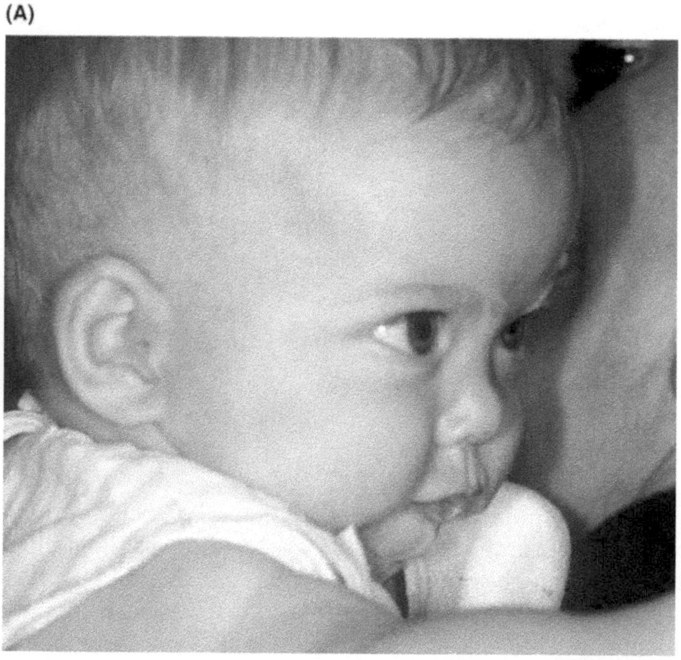

(B)

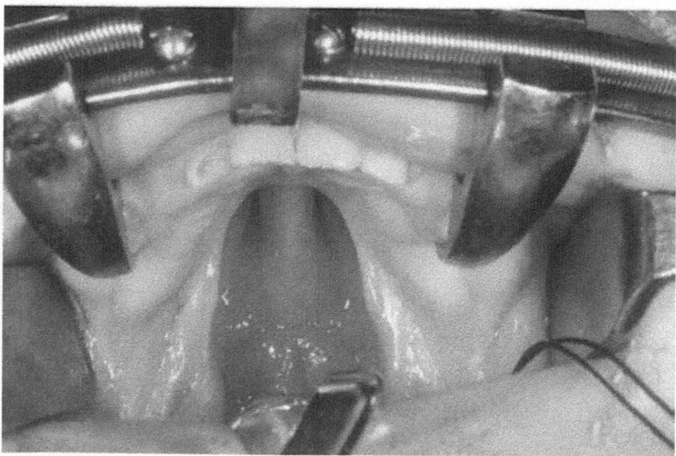

Figure 1 (**A**) Lateral view of a child with Pierre Robin sequence (micrognathia, relative macroglossia, and a U-shape cleft palate). (**B**) Intraoral view of U-shaped cleft palate.

microsomia, ocular dermoid or coloboma, kidney, and vertebral anomalies, and auricular deformities), oro-facial-digital syndrome (x-linked, with mandibular hypoplasia, tongue and palate clefting), and Treacher-Collins (autosomal dominant, lower lid colobomas, downward slanting palpebral fissures, hypoplastic zygomatic arches, and low-set ears) are other examples of syndromic cleft palate disorders. Velo-cardio-facial syndrome is autosomal dominant with variable expression of ventriculoseptal defect, right aortic arch, malar flattening, and nasal or auricular deformities. An aberrant internal carotid artery should be of particular interest when considering pharyngeal flap surgery in a patient with velo-cardio-facial syndrome (2).

Embryology

The lip and palate normally develop during the embryonic period (the first 12-weeks of intrauterine life). The midportion of the face develops anterior to the forebrain by the differentiation of the broad midline frontonasal prominence. The primary palate begins to form at approximately four- to five-weeks gestation and forms the initial separation between the oral and nasal cavities. The primary palate, or median palatine process, is formed by the fusion of the paired median nasal prominence (MNP). The paired MNP fuse during the sixth week and form the premaxilla, consisting of the hard palate anterior to the incisive foramen, the central maxillary alveolar arch, and associated lateral and central incisors (3,4).

The fused MNPs develop into the philtrum of the upper lip, columella, and nasal tip. The lateral elements of the upper lip (from the philtral column laterally) are derived from the paired maxillary processes. The cheek, maxilla, zygoma, and secondary palate are also formed from the maxillary processes. Therefore, the upper lip is formed from both the median nasal and maxillary processes (5).

Development of the primary palate is embryologically distinct from that of the secondary palate. The incisive foreman divides the palate into primary (anterior to the incisive foramen) and secondary palate (posterior to the incisive foramen). The secondary palate begins developing at approximately eight-weeks of gestation. Formation of the secondary palate occurs by inferior and medial growth and migration of the palatal shelves (the medial projections of the maxillary processes). As the palatal shelves displace inferiorly (similar to a drawbridge), the developing nasal cavities expand laterally and inferiorly.

The normal sequence of palatal formation begins when the palatal shelves and nasal septum contact each other, and proceeds in an anterior-to-posterior direction beginning at the incisive foramen. Palatal closure first occurs at the incisive foramen at approximately eight-weeks of gestation and is usually completed through the uvula by 12 weeks. The paired palatal shelves are initially separated by the developing tongue. Growth of the mandible with associated anterior movement of the tongue allows the palatal shelves to migrate inferiorly and assume a more horizontal orientation. If fetal development and migration of the mandible does not proceed normally, the paired palatal shelves cannot migrate inferiorly and medially. Lack of contact of these shelves creates palatal clefting. This malformation can result in the Pierre Robin sequence (U-shaped cleft palate, micrognathia, and relative macroglossia) (2). The degree of clefting of the secondary palate is related to many factors including interruption of the fusion process. Therefore, the palatal abnormality can range from a complete cleft of the secondary palate to a bifid uvula and/or submucous soft palate cleft (6).

EVALUATION AND PLANNING

Cleft Lip and Palate Classification

Many classification systems have been suggested for cleft lip and palate. Interruption of the normal embryologic development of the lip and palate results in different severities of clefting. The upper lip and primary palate develops between four- and eight-weeks of gestation. Disruption of this development can cause clefts of the upper lip and alveolus (primary palate). Cleft lips may be unilateral or bilateral, and maybe complete or incomplete. The upper lip clefting may be isolated, may be associated with clefts of the alveolus and palate, or may be associated with other malformations (syndromic clefts). Clefting of the upper lip, with or without associated palatal clefting, is caused by failure of the MNPs to make contact with the lateral nasal process and the maxillary process during embryogenesis. Interruption of this embryologic process creates maldevelopment of some or all of the upper lip, the central maxillary arch, the anterior portion of the palate, and the base of the nose and nasal tip.

The degree of clefting of the upper lip, alveolus, and nose is related to the amount of the embryologic insult to the upper lip. The lip deformity ranges from a minor malformation of the normal development of the lip to a complete interruption of all layers of the lip and base of the nose. A microform cleft of the upper lip is a minor malformation of normal lip development caused by dehiscence of the orbicularis oris muscle with no overt clefting of the epidermis of the upper lip (Fig. 2). A more significant interruption of the upper lip development is referred to as an incomplete cleft lip (Fig. 3). An incomplete unilateral cleft lip involves a through-and-through defect of skin, muscle, and mucosa of the lower aspect of the lip, but does not extend superiorly through the entire height of the lip. A complete unilateral cleft lip occurs when the defect involves all tissue layers of the upper lip and extends through the entire height of the lip and floor of the nose (Fig. 4). A cleft of the alveolus is almost always associated with complete unilateral cleft lip.

A bilateral cleft lip occurs with disruption of lip development on both sides. In the incomplete bilateral cleft lip, there is usually some skeletal continuity between the lateral maxillary processes and the central premaxilla. For this reason, there is often little or no protrusion of the premaxilla in incomplete bilateral cleft lips. In the

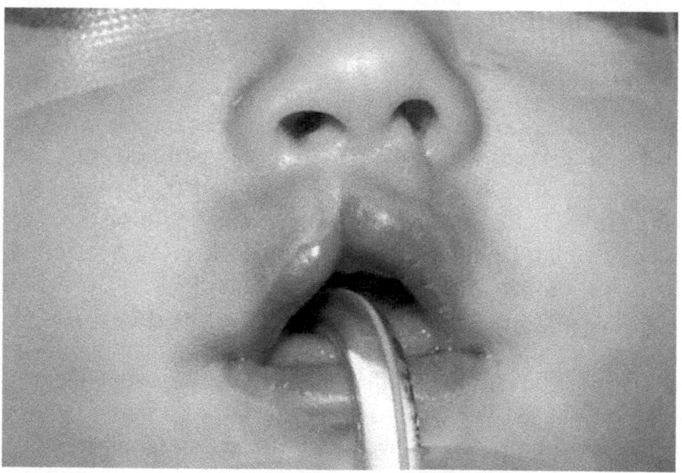

Figure 2 A six-month-old child with a microform cleft lip.

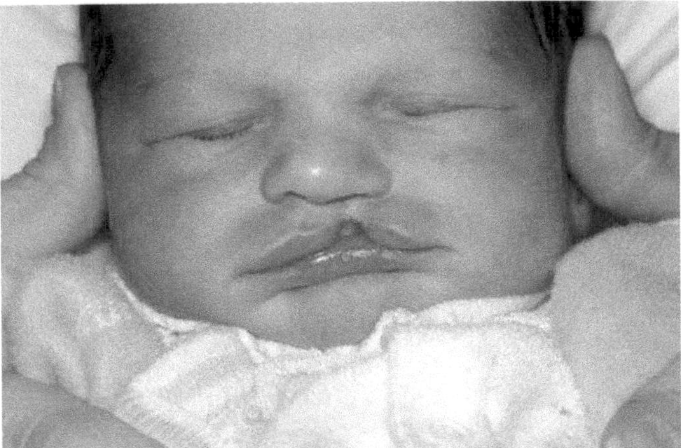

Figure 3 A three-month-old child with an incomplete cleft lip.

complete bilateral cleft lip deformity, the central premaxilla is totally detached from each lateral maxillary process. This may result in a "locked out" premaxilla (Fig. 5).

Either unilateral or bilateral cleft lip deformities may be isolated or associated with alveolar or palatal clefting. The bilateral cleft lip deformity is more likely than the unilateral cleft lip deformity to be associated with secondary palate clefting because a greater interruption of lip development is required to create a bilateral cleft lip deformity.

Secondary Palate

The secondary palate is composed of the horizontal plate of the maxilla and palatine bone. In normal development between weeks eight and twelve embryologically, the secondary palate closes in the anterior-to-posterior direction. Interruption of the normal fusion of the secondary palate causes various degrees of palatal clefting. Clefts of the secondary palate can be variable in expression, depending upon the

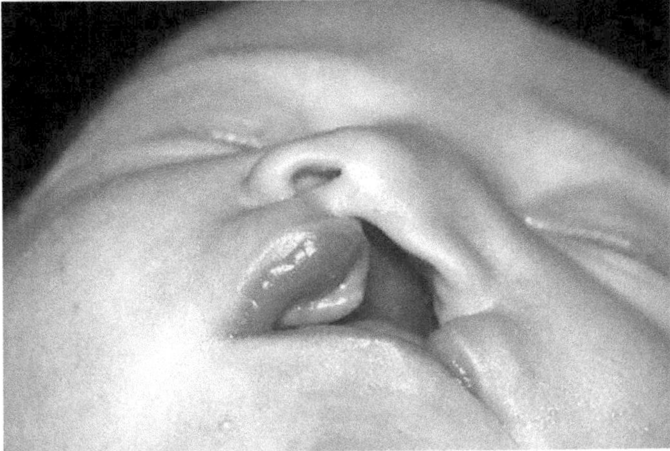

Figure 4 A base view of a three-month-old child with complete left cleft of the lip and palate.

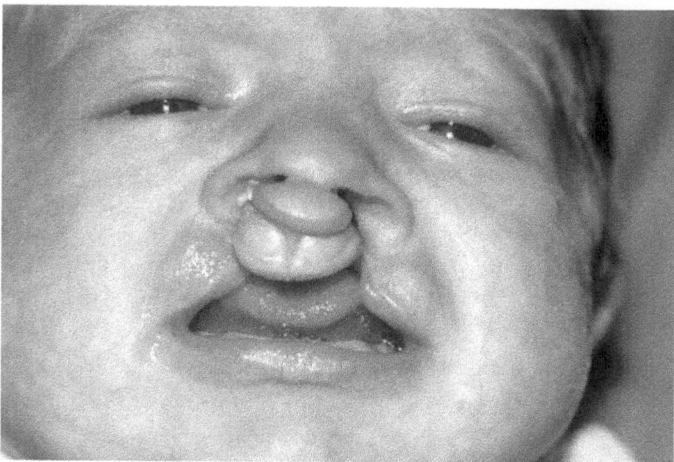

Figure 5 Three-month-old child with symmetrical complete bilateral cleft lip and cleft palate. Note the anterior protrusion of the premaxilla and prolabium associated with very poor projection of the nasal tip and short collumella.

timing and degree of interruption of palatal development. The most common condition and the smallest expression of soft palate clefting is the bifid uvula. This common deformity occurs when there is a lack of normal fusion of the uvula. A submucous cleft of the soft palate occurs when there is dehiscence of the muscles of the soft palate. In this condition, the palatal mucosa is intact but there is incomplete development of the underlying palatal musculature. A submucous cleft palate often requires speech therapy and sometimes requires surgical repair. Full-thickness clefting of the soft palate can manifest with either an incomplete (Fig. 6) or complete secondary palatal cleft (Fig. 7). Complete clefting of the secondary palate may result from total interruption of the normal formation of the palate posterior to the incisive foramen, while incomplete secondary clefts include the range of soft palate clefts that do not extend into the secondary hard palate (7).

A complete cleft of the lip and palate includes a cleft of the secondary palate with a complete cleft lip and may be unilateral or bilateral. The complete unilateral

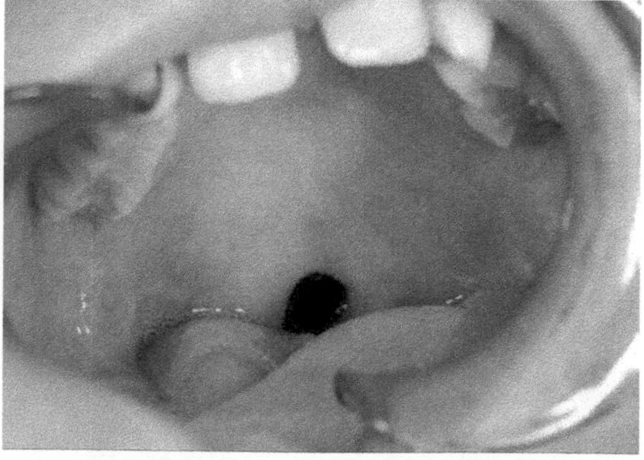

Figure 6 Intraoral photograph of an incomplete secondary palate cleft.

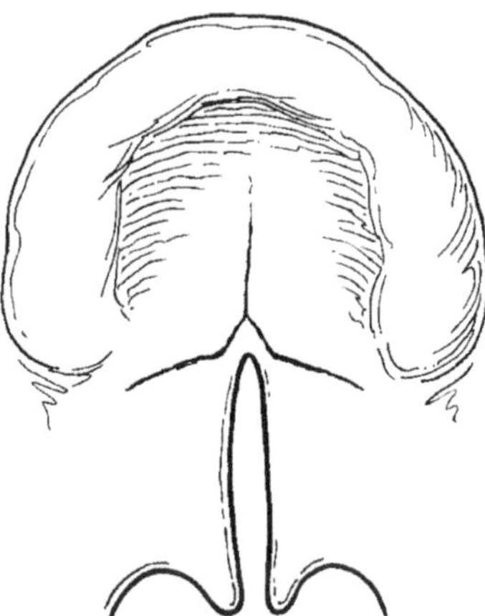

Figure 7 Schematic diagram of cleft of the soft palate. *Source*: From Ref. 6.

cleft lip and palate usually involves attachment of the vomer to the maxillary palatal shelf of the non-cleft side (Fig. 8). Complete bilateral clefts of the lip and palate usually have the central vomer and premaxilla detached from the two lateral palatal shelves (Fig. 9). In all cases, clefting of the lip and palate is variable in expression and typically follows known embryologic patterns.

Timing of Cleft Repair

The decision to repair a cleft lip or palate deformity is based the severity of the deformity, consideration of speech development, facial growth, psychological effect on the child, and family, and safety of anesthesia. The timing of repair of various cleft deformities is outlined in Table 1 (8). In patients with palatal clefting with or without clefts of the lip, tympanostomy tube placement is performed at age three-to-six months. This surgery is performed at an early age to minimize the likelihood of chronic ear

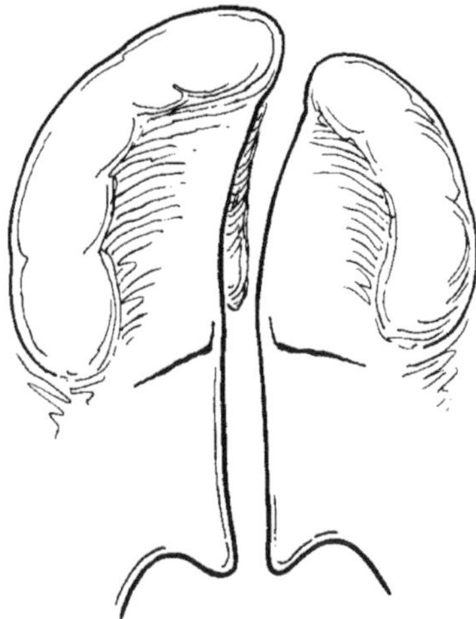

Figure 8 Schematic diagram of a complete unilateral cleft of the hard and soft palate. *Source*: From Ref. 6.

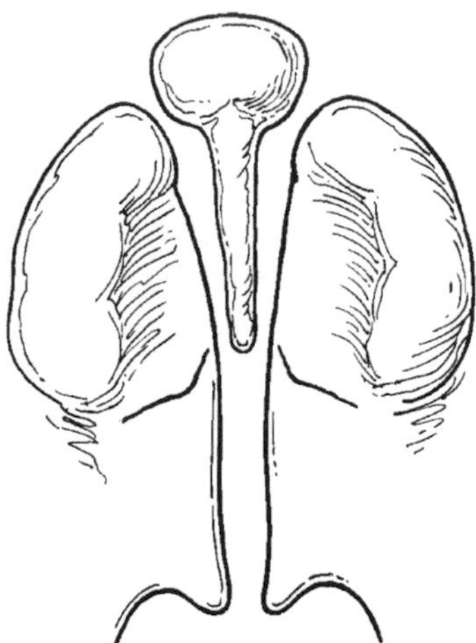

Figure 9 Schematic diagram of a complete bilateral cleft palate. *Source*: From Ref. 6.

disease and conductive hearing loss by aerating the middle ear. In patients with cleft lip and palate, the tympanostomy tube is placed simultaneous to the cleft lip repair. In these patients, surgery is performed at approximately three months of age and includes cleft lip repair, cleft tip rhinoplasty, and tympanostomy tube placement. Most surgeons follow the "rule of 10s" to determine eligibility for the initial cleft lip repair. The child should be more than 10 weeks old, over 10 pounds, and have a hemaglobin count of >10 g. Cleft palate repair is performed prior to the initial development of speech. This is usually performed at nine to fifteen months of age. Long acting tympanostomy tubes are placed at the time of palatoplasty.

The cleft and craniofacial team closely monitors the speech development after cleft palate repair with emphasis beginning at two years of age. Velopharygeal dysfunction (VPD) should be evaluated with nasopharyngoscopy and video fluoroscopy. If the degree of VPD is significant, speech therapy is undertaken at approximately three years of age. If aggressive speech therapy is unsatisfactory, surgical correction of VPD should be performed between four and six years of age.

Table 1 Timing and Management of Cleft Lip and Palate

Procedure	Age
Cleft lip repair	3 mo
Tip rhinoplasty	
Tympanostomy tubes	
Palatoplasty	9–18 mo
T-tube placement	
Speech evaluation	3–4 yr
Velopharyngeal dysfunction	4–6 yr
Workup and surgery (if necessary)	
Alveolar bone grafting	9–11 yr
Definitive cleft nasal reconstruction	12–18 yr
Orthognathic surgery (if necessary)	At mandibular growth completion (>16 yr)

Further surgical treatments for cleft deformities include alveolar bone grafting at ages 9 to 11 years, internal and external nasal reconstruction (cleft septorhinoplasty) at ages 12–18 years and orthognathic surgery after growth of the facial skeleton is complete. The need for these interventions is related to the initial deformity as well as the growth and development of the patient.

The Unilateral Cleft Lip Deformity—Pathologic Anatomy

A unilateral cleft of the upper lip can involve alterations in all layers of the lip including skin, muscle, mucosa, and underlying skeletal framework. The external appearance of the defect is determined by the extent of the underlying muscular and skeletal deformity. Subcutaneous (microform) cleft lip involves partial or total clefting of the upper lip musculature. Partial (incomplete) cleft lip involves skin, muscle, and mucosa, but may spare the underlying skeletal structures. Complete unilateral lip deformities involve all tissue layers.

The principle muscle of the lips is the orbicularis oris (Fig. 10). The fibers of this muscle encircle the oral orifice within the substance of the lips (9). The orbicularis oris muscle consists of a superficial and a deep layer. This muscle is not a true sphincter, with the superficial and deep components arising as separate muscles from the modiolus at each oral commissure (10).

In the unilateral cleft lip deformity, there is discontinuity of the orbicularis oris muscle in the region of the cleft (Fig. 11). The muscles of the unilateral cleft lip have two distinct differences when compared with normally developed lip musculature. First, the muscles are hypoplastic in the region of the cleft. Second, the muscles cannot cross the cleft gap and are prevented from attaching to their normal sites and find substitute insertions. Although, it is obvious that no muscle crosses the cleft gap in complete lip clefting, the skin bridge in incomplete clefts has also been found to contain no functional musculature. Muscle dissections by Fara et al. (11) on stillborn babies with incomplete clefts confirm that the muscles in unilateral cleft lips are more hypoplastic on the medial side than on the lateral side of the cleft. Additionally, these dissections reveal that the upper lip muscles in incomplete clefts did not cross the cleft gap unless the skin bridge was at least one-third of the height of the lip.

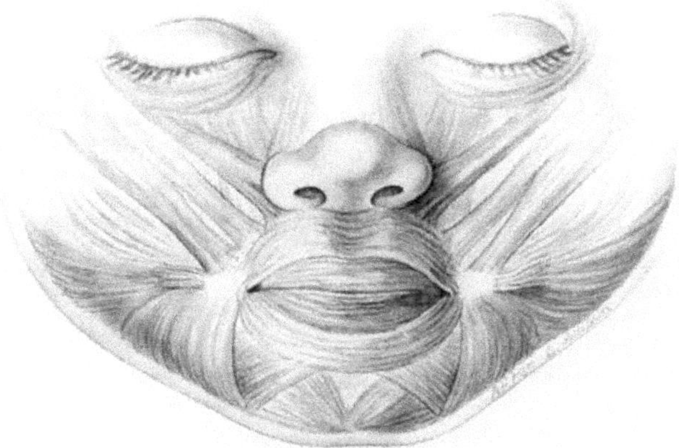

Figure 10 Normal architecture of the orbicularis oris muscles as they relate to the other facial musculature. *Source*: From Ref. 6.

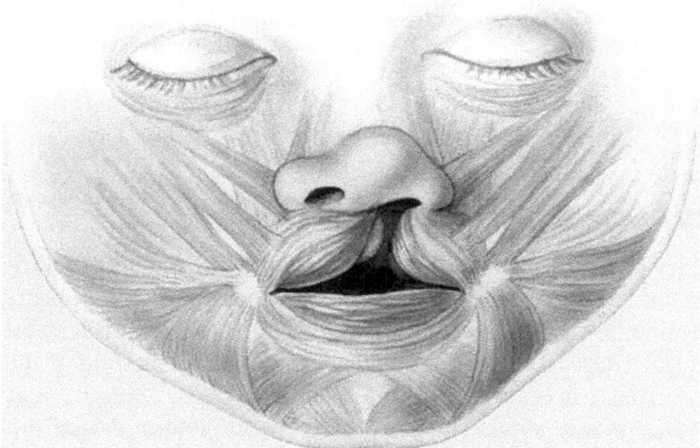

Figure 11 Diagram of the orbicularis oris musculature in the unilateral complete cleft lip deformity. The orbicularis oris muscles inserts along the cleft margin, alar base, and collumella. *Source*: From Ref. 6.

Even if the orbicularis oris muscle is present in the skin bridging the incomplete cleft, the orientation of the musculature is abnormal.

The major vascular supply to the lips and nose arises from the facial artery, which is a branch of the external carotid artery. The facial artery gives a rise to the superior and inferior labial arteries at each oral commissure. The paired superior labial arteries anastomose in the midline of the upper lip and the two inferior labial arteries similarly anastomose in the lower lip. In the unilateral cleft lip deformity, the aberrant vascular supply parallels the findings of the unilateral cleft lip musculature. As with the musculature, the blood supply on the lateral aspect of the cleft is better developed than is the vasculature on the medial side. In the incomplete cleft lip deformity, a terminal branch of the superior labial artery crosses the epithelial skin bridge.

RECONSTRUCTIVE OPTIONS

Unilateral Cleft Lip Repair

The first documented unilateral cleft lip repair was performed in the Tang Dynasty in China in approximately 390 AD. Many techniques have been described over the years for repair of the unilateral cleft lip deformity. Ambroise Par repaired the unilateral cleft by freshening the cleft edges and skewering the two sides of the cleft with a long needle (12). The needle was then wrapped with thread in a figure eight fashion. Thompson (14) described modifications of straight-line closures for repair of the unilateral cleft lip deformity. All straight-line techniques closed the cleft defect adequately, but often resulted in vertical scar contracture and notching of the upper lip.

Wide, complete, unilateral cleft lips are also difficult to repair by the straight-line method. In the mid 20th century, various geometric closure techniques were proposed for repairing the unilateral cleft lip. Geometrical techniques, such as modified Z-plasties, quadrangular flaps, and triangular flaps, were designed to decrease the amount of lip shortening that occurred with cleft lip repair and to improve orbicularis oris muscle realignment and function (13,15,16). The triangular flap designed by Tennison (13) and the quadrangular flap of Le Mesurier (12) are reliable, consistent methods for decreasing vertical lip contraction in the unilateral cleft lip repair. Geometric cleft lip repair techniques provide a reproducible method to repair the lip. Exact measurements can be made with calipers to ensure reliable tension-free closure of the lip. The basic disadvantage of geometric designs is that the incisions always violate the curved philtral column on the non-cleft side, creating a scar that crosses boundaries of known anatomical subunits. In addition, geometric repairs require exacting presurgical measurement and lack flexibility during surgical applications.

Rotation–Advancement Repair of the Unilateral Cleft Lip Deformity

The rotation-advancement flap technique for repair of the unilateral cleft lip deformity was introduced by Ralph Millard (17) in 1957. This incorporated aspects of multiple previously described repairs. This method maximizes flexibility for the surgery while minimizing the amount of normal lip tissue discarded. This method is the most commonly used technique today for unilateral cleft lip repair. The advantages and disadvantages of the Millard rotation advancement flap technique are shown in Table 2 (18).

The primary goals of unilateral cleft lip repair are to reconstruct normal lip anatomy and to restore lip function. Other goals include closure of the nasal floor, correction of nasal tip asymmetry, and narrowing of the alveolar cleft (18). The rotation-advancement flap technique designs two major full-thickness flaps that can be approximated to repair the cleft without notching of the lip. This design allows reconstitution and reorientation of the orbicularis oris muscles.

The main advantage of the rotation-advancement flap technique is its flexibility in application. This procedure allows continuous modifications during the design, incision, and execution of the repair. Another advantage is that the incisions are designed to place the eventual scar in the new philtral column. In contrast, most geometric flap designs violate the philtral subunit.

Measurement and Flap Design

The important reference points of the rotation-advancement flap technique are summarized in Table 3 and Figure 12. Some of these points are anatomical points, whereas the other points are "measured." Several measurements may be used to maximize flap design and eventual lip aesthetics. The ultimate objective of these

Table 2 Millard Rotation-Advancement Cleft Lip Repair

Disadvantages	Advantages
Requires experienced surgeon	Flexible
Possible excessive tension	Minimal tissue discarded
Extensive undermining required	Good nasal access
Vertical scar contracture	Camouflaged suture line
Tendency to small nostril	

Table 3 Millard Rotation-Advancement Reference Points

Non-cleft side (NCS)	Cleft side (CS)
1. Center (low point) of Cupid's bow	7. Commissure (CS)
2. Peak of Cupid's bow—(lateral NCS)	8. Peak of Cupid's bow
3. Peak of Cupid's bow—(medial NCS)	9. Medial tip of advancement flap
4. Alar base	10. Midpoint of alar base
5. Columellar base	11. Lateral alar base
6. Commissure—(NCS)	x. Back-cut point

measurements is to ensure that the length of the rotation flap (3 to 5 + X) equals the length of the advancement flap (8,9) (Table 4).

Incision of skin with a #15C blade creates two major full thickness flaps: A (rotation) and B (advancement) raised in a supraperiosteal plane. One minor skin flap, the collumellar flap (C flap) is elevated in a subcutaneous plane and used for nasal floor closure. The perialar incision (cleft side) creates a full thickness alar flap

(A)

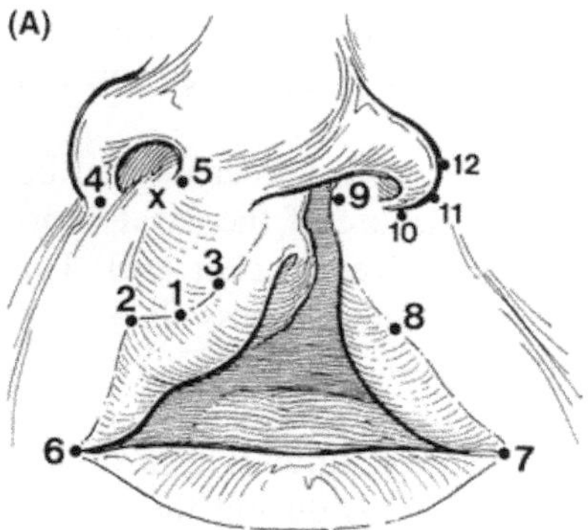

(B)

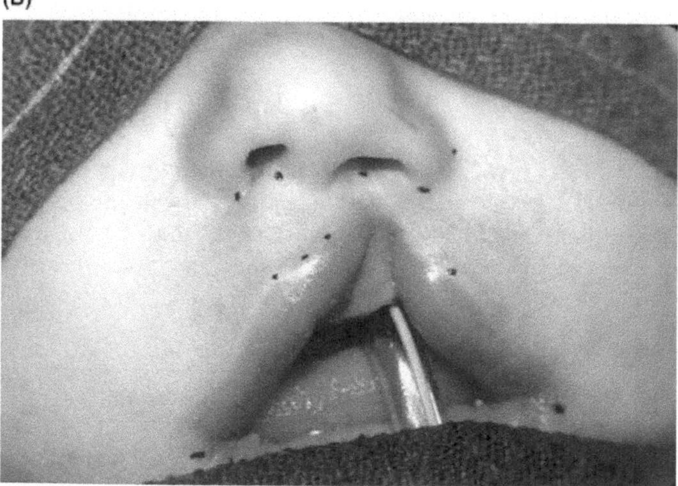

Figure 12A–D (**A**) Schematic diagram of the reference points associated with Millard rotation advancement unilateral cleft repair. (**B**) The reference points marked on a three-month-old patient with incomplete cleft lip. (*Continued*)

(C)

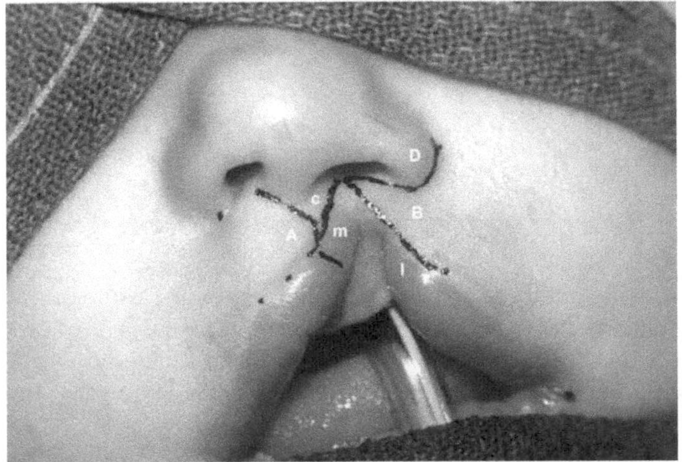

(D)

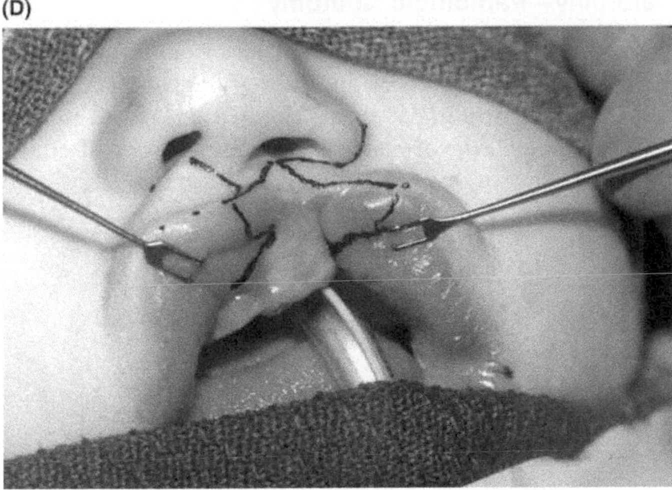

Figure 12 (**C**) Flap design on the same patient. (**D**) View of the M (*medial mucosal*) and L (*lateral mucosal*) flaps.

(D flap). Mucosal flaps are incised with a #11 blade and include the M (medial mucosal), and L (lateral mucosal) flaps (Table 5). After incising and dissecting these lip flaps, dissection and reapproximation of the orbicularis oris muscle is performed. This closure maximizes lip function while minimizing tension across the eventual lip

Table 4 Flap Design Measurements

Reference points	Range (mm)
1 to 2 = 1 to 3	2–4
2 to 6 = 8 to 7	20
2 to 4 = 8 to 10	9–11
3 to 5 + X = 8 to 9	

Table 5 Flaps

Skin flaps	Mucosal flaps
A—Rotation flap	M—Medial mucosal flap
B—Advancement flap	L—Lateral mucosal flap
D—Alar rim–(cleft side)	
C—Columellar base soft tissue (non-cleft side)	

wound. The Millard rotation-advancement lip repair also allows active closure of the nasal floor and nasal tip rhinoplasty (Fig. 13). Complete access to the nasal tip can be obtained through the standard perialar and cleft margin incisions, without creating additional nasal incisions. This allows for improved symmetry of the nasal tip and relative equalization of the alar base.

The Bilateral Cleft Lip Deformity—Pathologic Anatomy

Although, the central segment of the bilateral cleft lip deformity is an entity which has no correlate in the unilateral deformity, the configuration of the two lateral segments of the bilateral cleft lip deformity are similar to the lateral segment of the unilateral deformity. In normal development, the orbicularis oris muscle grows laterally to medially into the mid-portion of the lip or prolabium. Therefore, the amount of

(A)

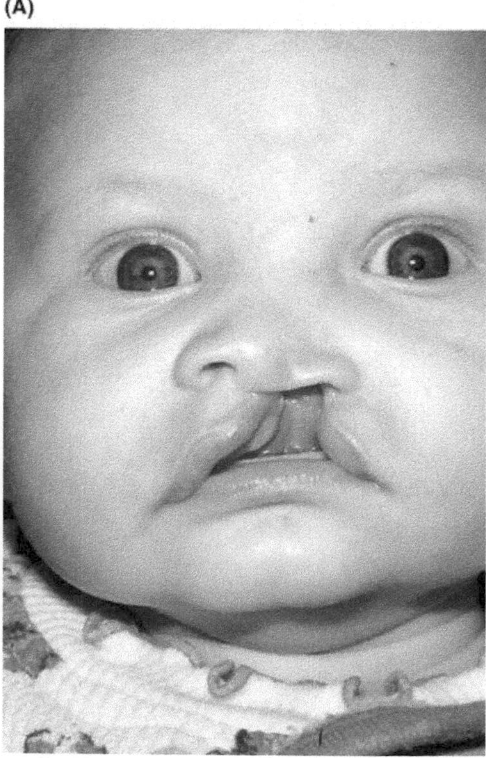

Figure 13 (A) A three-month-old patient with complete left cleft lip and palate. (*Continued*)

(B)

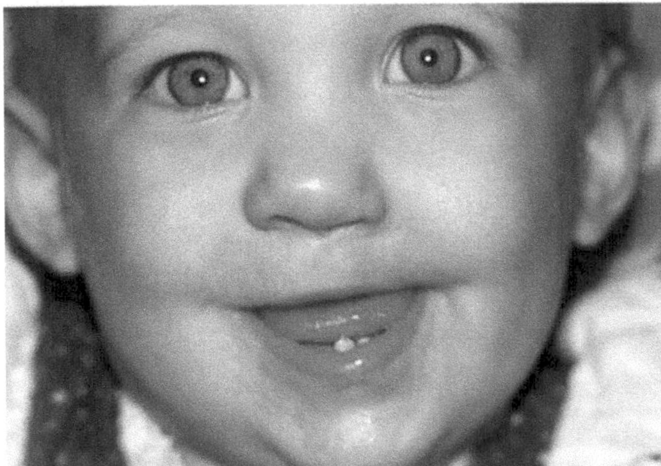

Figure 13 (**B**) A 10-month-old after Millard rotation advancement unilateral cleft lip repair performed at three months of age.

muscle present in the prolabium depends on the extent of the cleft deformity. Incomplete bilateral clefts generally have a diminished amount of misdirected muscle fibers present, whereas complete bilateral clefts have no muscle present in the prolabium. In the incomplete bilateral cleft lip, there is usually some skeletal continuity and very little protrusion of the premaxilla and prolabium. The premaxilla in complete bilateral cleft lips usually protrudes more than it does in the incomplete deformity; therefore, the columella of the nose is usually shorter in the complete bilateral cleft lip deformity than in the incomplete bilateral deformity. Most bilateral cleft lip deformities tend to be symmetrical. This advantage allows the cleft surgeon to create a bilaterally symmetrical lip via a single-staged operation, in contrast to the unilateral cleft lip repair, in which the surgeon attempts to match the abnormal cleft side to the normal, or non-cleft side.

The arterial network and musculature of the lateral elements of the complete bilateral cleft lip parallels that of the lateral segment in the unilateral deformity. The abnormal insertion of the cleft lip musculature follows the margin of the cleft (Fig. 14) (19,20). The arterial supply in bilateral cleft lips is characterized by an aberrant course of the superior labial artery. This artery runs superiorly along the edge of the cleft and anastomoses with the angular and lateral nasal arteries. This abnormal course is similar to that in the lateral segment of the unilateral deformity. In the bilateral complete cleft lip deformity, the prolabial segment receives its blood supply from the septum, columella, and premaxilla.

Bilateral Cleft Lip Repair

The extent of deformity and the philosophy of the operating surgeon can influence the timing and technique for repair of the bilateral cleft lip deformity. The repair can be performed after presurgical orthopedics or lip adhesion, both defined to narrow the cleft gap and to better align the center segments. Definitive bilateral lip repair can be performed in a single stage or carried out in two separate surgical

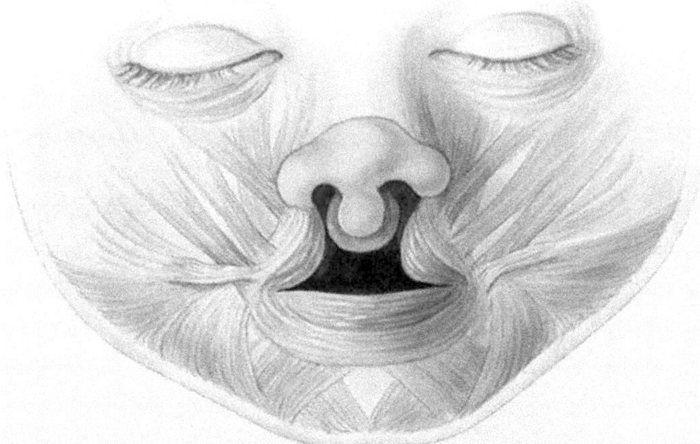

Figure 14 Schematic diagram illustrating abnormal insertion of the orbicularis musculature in the bilateral cleft lip deformity. *Source*: From Ref. 6.

procedures. Bilateral cleft lip adhesion may be indicated in patients with a wide complete bilateral cleft lip, alveolus, and secondary palate (21). This procedure converts a complete bilateral cleft lip deformity to an incomplete deformity, and allows the repair to be performed under more favorable conditions with reduced tension. Bilateral cleft lip adhesion exerts an orthopedic force on the premaxilla, which inhibits forward growth of the premaxilla and results in an improved position in relation to the lateral lip segments.

Several factors should be considered when deciding between a single-stage versus a two-staged lip repair. The two-staged technique can allow improved vascularity to the central prolabial segment and the capability to apply the techniques of the Millard rotation advancement repair to each side of the bilateral repair (22). However, the two-staged repair has two significant disadvantages: (i) it tends to create asymmetry of the lip as the first side lip closure has rapid growth of the lip after supplying vascularity to the repaired lip—this asymmetry is difficult to correct; (ii) it does not allow muscle to be advanced to cross the central prolabial segment, and can produce a secondary deformity from this lack of muscle.

The single staged bilateral cleft repair, as described by Millard in 1977, is designed to produce an intact lip with scars mimicking the philtral columns. This technique maximizes symmetry of the lip and is designed to reorient the orbicularis oris from each lateral lip segment across the central prolabial segment. This reoriented lip musculature improves lip aesthetics and decreases tension across the two vertical lip incisions (23).

Palatoplasty

The goals of cleft palatoplasty are to allow the patient to develop normal speech development and to prevent nasal regurgitation by closure of the congenital oral nasal fistula. Successful palatal cleft repair requires adherence to several important surgical principles including an atraumatic technique to minimize injury to flap vessels, adequate flap mobilization to minimize wound tension, two-layered closure of

Table 6 Principles of Palatoplasty

Minimize wound tension
Tissue preserving "atraumatic" technique
Two-layer closure (oral and nasal layers) over hard palate
Three-layer closure (oral, muscle, nasal layers) of soft palate
Recreation of soft-palate muscular sling

the oral and nasal mucosa to prevent post-operative fistula formation, and recreation of the soft palate muscular sling to maximize velopharyngeal function and speech (Table 6) (24).

The specific technique used to repair palatal clefts is based on the surgeon's experience and the cleft type. In all cases, an atraumatic "no touch" technique should be used to minimize injury to the palatal wound edges and to maximize blood supply to the periphery of the palatal flaps. Monopolar cautery should be avoided. It is important to recreate the velopharyngeal muscular sling to minimize the chance of post-operative velopharyngeal dysfunction. If the above-mentioned principles are followed, post-operative fistulae are rare and the incidence of velopharyngeal dysfunction can be minimized.

Timing of Cleft Palate Repair

The timing of repair of cleft deformities is outlined in Table 1. Other interventions for the cleft patients (including orthodontic therapy, alveolar bone grafting, cleft nasal reconstruction, and orthognathic surgery) are related to the degree of the original deformity and the growth of the face. It can be noted that in cleft patients who do not undergo palatoplasty at a young age, midfacial growth is normal (25). Ross (26) has noted that midfacial growth disturbance is most related to the type of cleft palate repair and the timing of palatoplasty. The decision to perform palatoplasty at approximately one-year-of-age is made to improve speech and with the knowledge that facial growth may be altered.

von Langenbeck Palatoplasty

Closure of clefts of the hard palate by elevation of bipedicled mucoperiosteal flaps was first reported in the early 19th century by Dieffenbach (27), Warren (28,29), and von Langenbeck (30). This method involves incisions along the cleft margin (medial) and adjacent to the alveolar ridge (lateral). Undermining the bipedicled flaps in the subperiosteal plane allows flap release and advancement. The bipedicled flaps can be approximated in a "drawbridge" fashion to achieve closure of the hard-palate cleft.

The von Langenbeck repair (bipedicled flap palatoplasty) employs several important principles of palatoplasty (Fig. 15). Most importantly, the use of a two-layered closure (oral and nasal layers) decreases the incidence of post-surgical fistula when compared to the fistula rate of closure of only the oral layer. The use of a two-layered closure prevents fistula formation if there is slight wound breakdown of either the oral or the nasal layer because the second layer remains intact. The other important principle in the bipedicle flap technique is to achieve adequate flap mobilization to minimize tension across the wound edges.

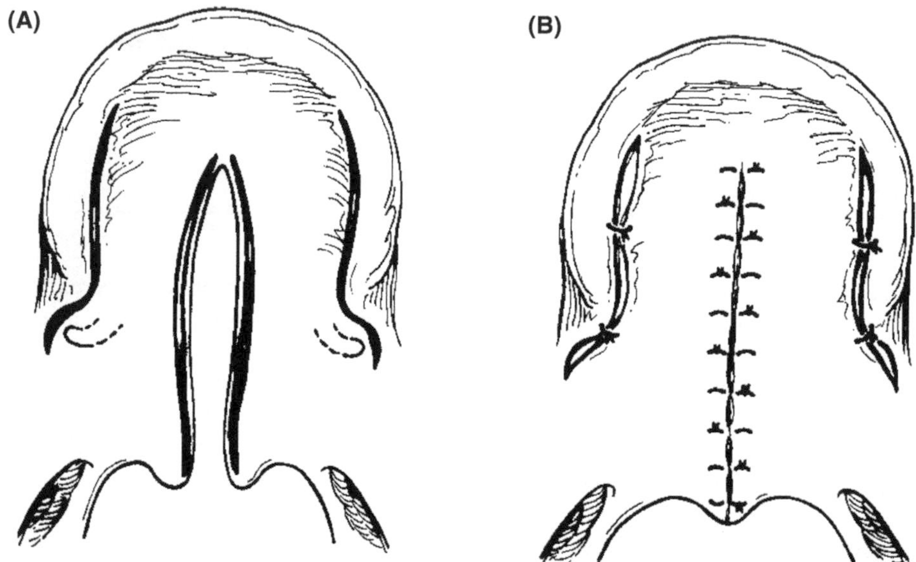

Figure 15 (**A**) The von Langenbeck palatoplasty. Two bipedicled flaps supplied by the greater palatine and incisive arteries are shown. (**B**) Schematic diagram showing closure after the von Langenbeck palatoplasty procedure.

The major disadvantage of the von Langenbeck palatoplasty is not allowing visualization of the vascular pedicle of the palatal flaps. The greater palatine vascular pedicle is located approximately one centimetre medial to the upper second molar tooth. Identification of this pedicle allows greater flap mobilization and can decrease wound tension in wide palatal clefts. For this reason, most surgeons connect the medial and lateral cleft incisions anteriorly, thereby converting the bipedicled flaps to posteriorly based unipedicled flaps. These three-flap (incomplete clefts) and two-flap (complete clefts) repairs allow increased visualization of the vascular pedicle, increased flap mobilization, and decreased wound tension.

Three-Flap Palatoplasty

Clefts of the secondary palate (the entire soft palate and the hard palate posterior to the incisive foramen) can be repaired using the three-flap palatoplasty. The medial and lateral incisions are identical to those used in the von Langenbeck (bipedicled flap) technique. The lateral incisions are made adjacent to the tooth crowns and carried around the maxillary tuberosity. The medial cleft margin and lateral incisions are joined anteriorly by oblique incisions that connect at the level of the canine teeth laterally. This converts the bipedicle flaps to posteriorly based unipedicled mucoperiosteal flaps (Fig. 16).

The posteriorly based unipedicle flaps are elevated in a submucoperiosteal plane and contain the greater palatine vessels. Dissection is carried posterior to the greater palatine neurvascular pedicle (space of Ernst) to further mobilize the flaps and minimize tension. Meticulous release of the malaligned soft palatal musculature is performed. After the nasal mucosa is elevated, complete closure of the nasal layer is accomplished prior to muscle closure. This allows repositioning of the velopharyngeal muscular sling from an oblique to a more physiologic transverse orientation.

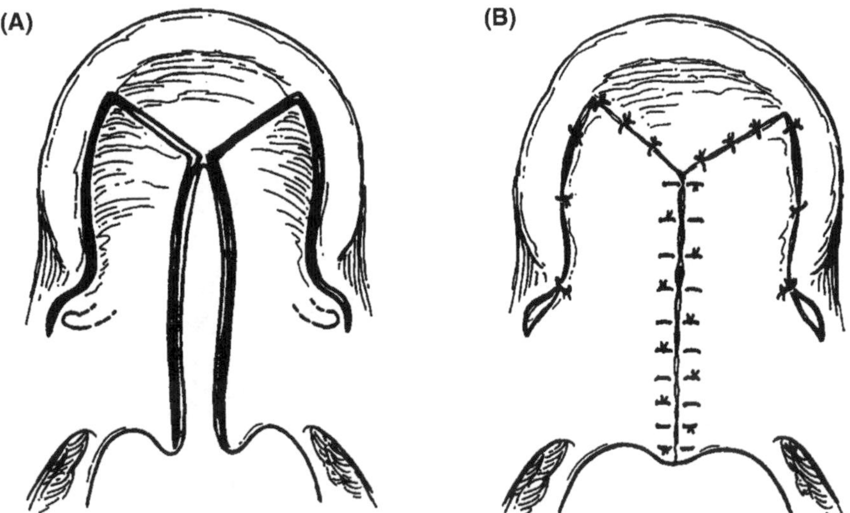

Figure 16 (**A**) The three-flap palatoplasty incisions are illustrated. (**B**) Schematic diagram after closure of the nasal and oral layer of the three-flap palatoplasty for repair of the complete secondary cleft palate deformity.

After closure of the nasal layer and the posterior muscular layer, the oral layer is closed in a single layer approximating the medial cleft margin incisions. At least one "tacking" suture is used to coapt the oral and nasal layers and to prevent dead-space and hematoma formation.

Two-Flap Palatoplasty

Complete palatal clefts (primary and secondary palate) are best repaired with the two-flap palatoplasty technique. The exact technique used for unilateral versus bilateral complete clefts is slightly different. In the complete unilateral cleft palate, the medial cleft margin incisions are carried anteriorly almost to the alveolar cleft. These medial incisions are joined to two curved lateral incisions, creating two posteriorly based palatal flaps.

The principles of elevation are the same as in other cleft palate techniques. Subperiosteal flap elevation with an atraumatic technique is performed to expose and isolate the neurovascular pedicles (Fig. 17). After flap elevation, the palate is again repaired in layers, beginning with the nasal layer. The soft-palate musculature is again closed with interrupted sutures, decreasing the tension across the palatal wound. Closure of the oral palatal mucosa followed by a coapting suture is then performed. In complete clefts, the entire cleft with exception of the anterior alveolar cleft is thus closed.

Furlow Palatoplasty

In 1978, Leonard Furlow (31,32) first described the double-reversing Z-plasty, or Furlow palatoplasty. This technique is usually used to repair a submucous cleft or a cleft of the soft palate only. The procedure involves the creation and closure of

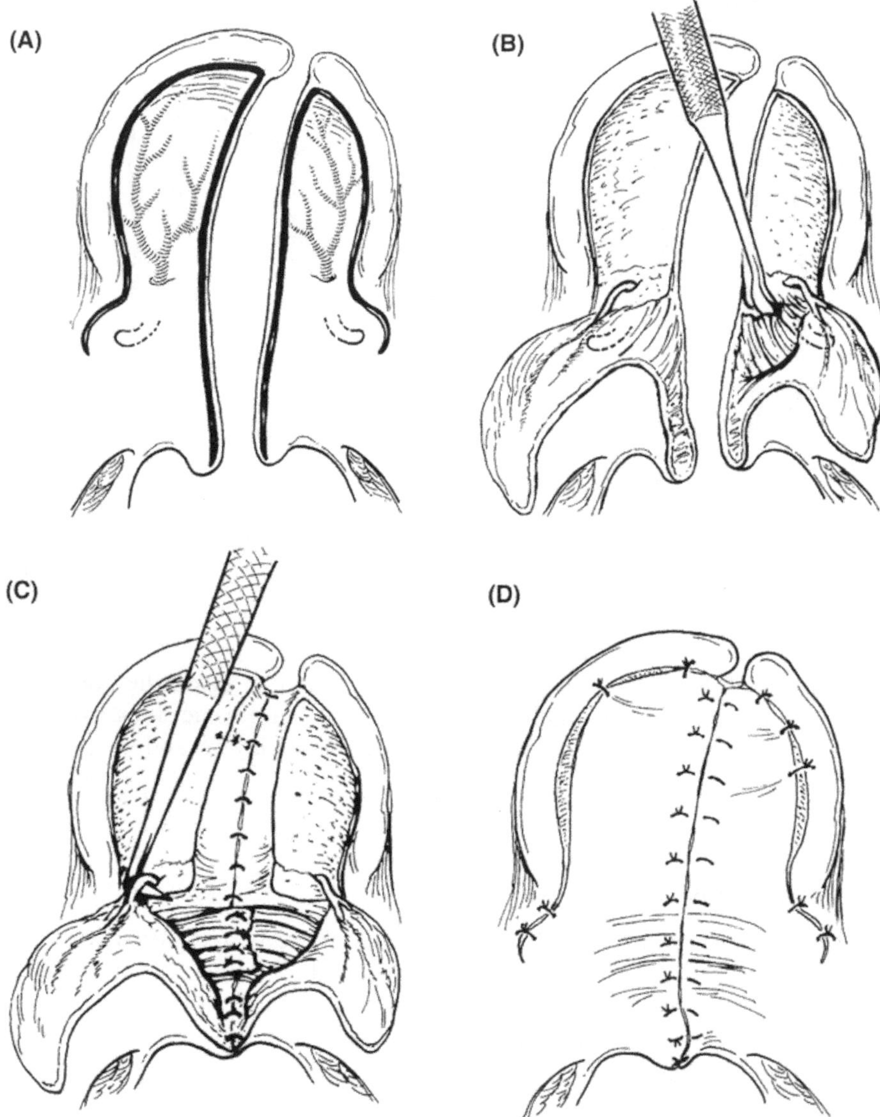

Figure 17 (A) Diagram of the repair of a complete unilateral cleft palate deformity with the incisions for a two-flap palatoplasty marked. (B) Elevation of the flaps of the subperiosteal plane dissecting out the greater palatine arteries bilaterally. (C) Dissection posterior to the greater palatine arteries in the space of Ernst. Note that the nasal mucosa and soft palate musculature have been closed in the oral flaps await closure. (D) Repair of the oral musculature in a complete unilateral cleft lip deformity.

two opposing Z-plasties of the oral and nasal mucosa. The repair is designed to recreate the muscular sling of the soft palate and to lengthen the palate.

The medial limbs of the double-reversing Z-plasty technique are made at the margin of the soft-palate cleft. A full-thickness incision is made through the palate in the midline to create a soft palate cleft if a submucous cleft of the soft palate, without through-and-through clefting is being repaired. On one side, an incision is made extending from the cleft margin obliquely toward the hamulus laterally (Fig. 18).

Dissection is carried on this side deep to the soft palatal musculature. This posteriorly based oral mucosal flap contains both oral mucosa and soft-palate muscle. On the opposite side, an incision is made in the oral mucosa from the uvula to the ipsilateral hamulus. This triangular oral mucosal flap does not contain soft palate musculature.

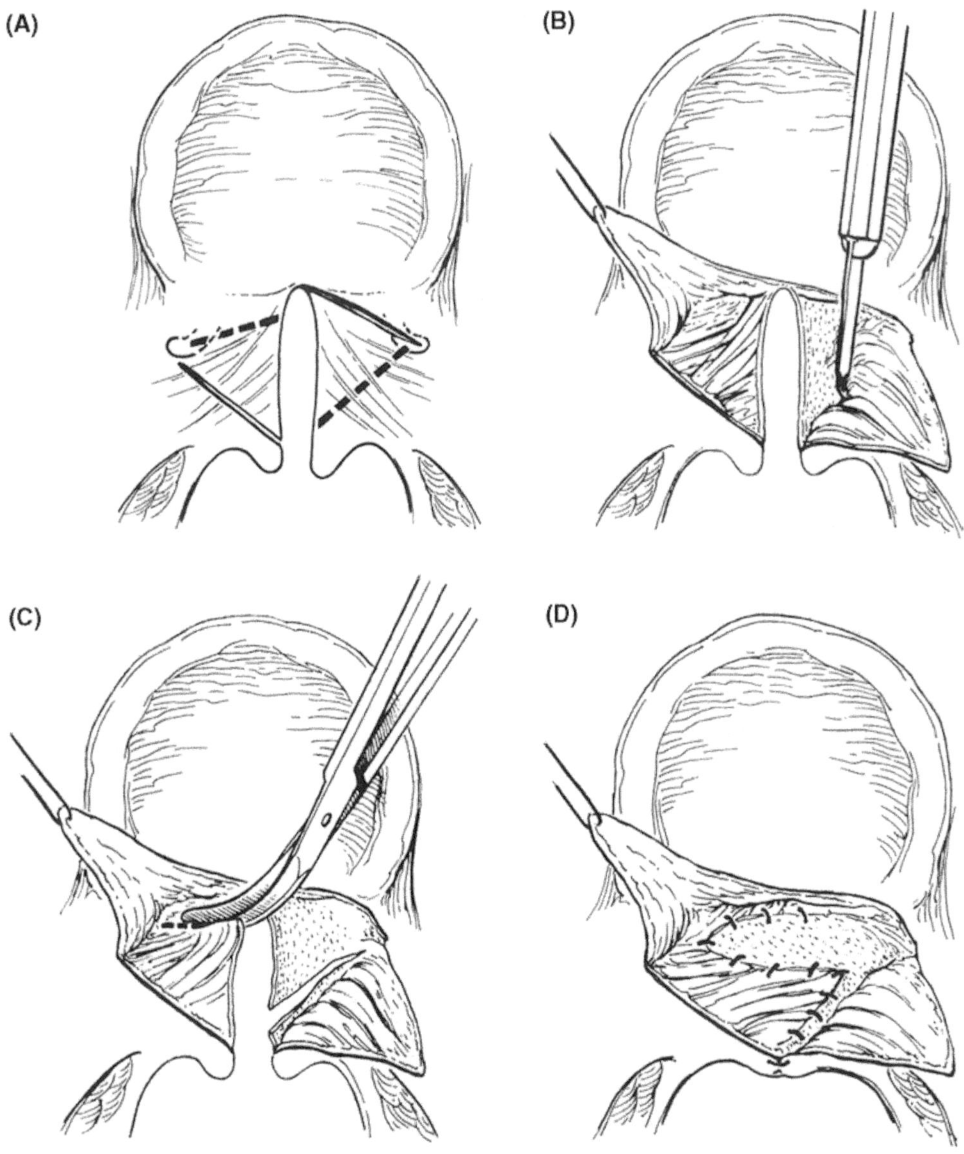

Figure 18A–E (**A**) Diagram of a Furlow palatoplasty (double reversing Z-plasty). Note that the dotted lines (----) indicate the nasal incisions and the straight lines (——) indicate the oral incisions. (**B**) Elevation of the oral flaps bilaterally. Note that the patient's left flap is elevated below the musculature, so that the oral flap contains both oral mucosa and palatal musculature. The right flap contains only oral mucosa. (**C**) Incision of the flaps with curved scissors on the nasal side. (**D**) Closure of the nasal mucosal and palatal musculature. (*Continued*)

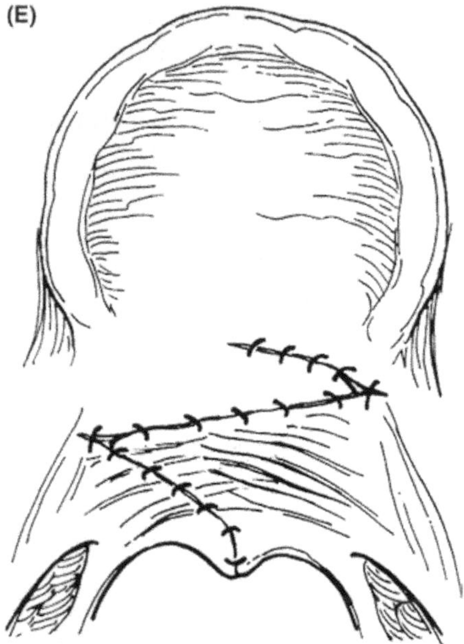

Figure 18 (E) After closure of the oral mucosa.

Mirror-image incisions (to the oral mucosal incisions) are then made to create two triangular-shaped nasal flaps on the nasal side. The anatomy of the soft palate musculature is important in dissection, elevation, and transposition of the oral and nasal flaps. The levator veli palatini muscles are located immediately adjacent to the nasal (not the oral) mucosa, elevation of these muscles from the nasal mucosa is often difficult (Fig. 19). It is important that the muscular sling of the soft palate be reoriented to a horizontal direction during closure of the Z-plasty flaps. For this reason, the soft-palate musculature must be based posteriorly within the flaps. Right-handed surgeons can more easily perform the difficult dissection of the soft-palate musculature from the nasal mucosa on the patient's left or contralateral side; left-handed surgeons should design the incisions in the mirror image.

Transposition of all four flaps is accomplished after dissection of both oral and nasal flaps. The nasal flaps are first transposed and reapproximated. The soft-palate muscular sling is then reoriented and closed with 4–0 braided absorbable suture. The oral flaps are then re-approximated. A post-operative fistula is usually prevented in

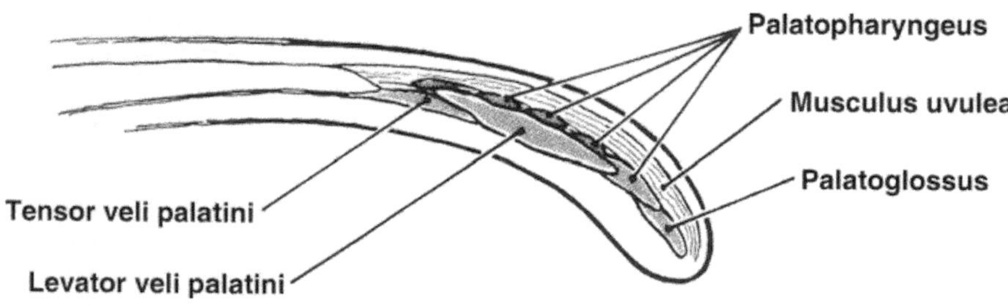

Figure 19 Sagittal view of the soft palate showing that the palatal musculature is closer to the nasal mucosa than it is to the oral mucosa.

Table 7 Preferred Palatoplasty Techniques

Cleft type	Technique
Complete unilateral	Two-flap
Complete bilateral	Two-flap (with vomerian flaps)
Secondary palate	
Complete	Three-flap
Incomplete	
Soft palate	(Furlow) double-reversing Z-plasty
Submucous	(Furlow) double-reversing Z-plasty

that the oral and nasal suture lines do not overlie one another. This technique both lengthens the palate and recreates the velopharyngeal muscular sling.

Preferred Techniques

Certain palatoplasty techniques are most suitable for specific cleft palate classifications. A summary of preferred surgical techniques for repair of cleft palate is listed in Table 7 (24). They include two-flap palatoplasty for complete unilateral and bilateral clefts, three-flap palatoplasty for incomplete clefts, and double-reversing Z-plasty (Furlow's technique) for submucous clefts and incomplete secondary palate clefts (soft palate).

CONCLUSION

Management of patients with cleft lip and palate should include a multi-disciplinary team approach to initially assess feeding and growth, as well as evaluate for other abnormalities. Further evaluation will address the development of speech and hearing. Surgical repair of cleft lip and palate deformities is a challenging, but rewarding experience.

REFERENCES

1. Koepp-Baker H. The craniofacial team. In: Bzoch K, ed. Communicative Disorders Related to Cleft Lip and Palate. Boston: Little, Brow, 1979.
2. Gorlin R, Pindborg J, Cohen M. Syndromes of the head and neck. New York: McGraw-Hill, 1976.
3. Enlow D. Facial growth 3rd ed. Philadelphia: WB Saunders, 1990:316–334.
4. McCarthy J. Plastic surgery, cleft lip and palate and craniofacial anomalies. Philadelphia: WB Saunders, 1990:2515–2552.
5. Gaare JD, Langman J. Fusion of nasal swellings in the mouse embryo: surface coat and initial contact. Am J Anat 1977; 150:461–475.
6. Sykes J, Senders C. Pathologic anatomy of cleft lip, palate, and nasal deformities. In: Meyers A, ed. Biological Basis of Facial Plastic Surgery. New York: Thieme Medical Publishers, 1993.
7. Stark RB. The pathogenesis of harelip and cleft palate. Plast Reconstr Surg 1954; 13: 20–39.

8. Sykes J, Senders C. Cleft palate, Practical pediatric otolaryngology. Philadelphia: Lippincott-Raven Publishers, 1999.
9. Barkitt A, Lightoller G. The facial musculature of the Australian aboriginal. J Anat 1928:33–57.
10. Latham RA, Deaton TG. The structural basis of the philtrum and the contour of the vermilion border: a study of the musculature of the upper lip. J Anat 1976; 121:151–160.
11. Fara M, Chlumska A, Hrivnakova J. Musculis orbicularis oris in incomplete hare-lip. Acta Chir Plast (Prague) 1965; 7:125–132.
12. LeMesurier A. Method of cutting and suturing lip in complete unilateral cleft lip. Plast Reconstr Surg 1949; 4:1.
13. Tennison CW. The repair of the unilateral cleft lip by the stencil method. Plast Reconstr Surg 1952; 9:115–120.
14. Thompson J. An artistic and mathematically accurate method of repairing the defect in cases of harelip. Surg Gynecol Obstet 1912:498–505.
15. Skoog T. A design for the repair of unilateral cleft lips. Am J Surg 1958; 95(2):233–236.
16. Randall P. A triangular flap operation for the primary repair of unilateral clefts of the lip. Plast Reconstr Surg 1959; 331:95.
17. Millard JDR. A primary camouflage of the unilateral hare-look. Transactions of the First International Congress of Plastic Surgery, Stockholm, Sweden, 1957.
18. Ness JA, Sykes JM. Basics of Millard rotation-advancement technique for repair of the unilateral cleft lip deformity. Facial Plast Surg 1993; 9:167–176.
19. Lee, FC. Orbicularis oris muscle in double harelip. Arch Surg 1946; 53:409.
20. Mullen T. The developmental anatomy and surgical significance of the orbicularis oris. West J Surg 1932; 40:134–141.
21. Seibert RW. Lip adhesion. Facial Plast Surg 1993; 9:188–194.
22. Millard D. Adaptation of rotation-advancement principle in bilateral cleft lip. Trans Int Soc Plast Surg 1960; 2:50.
23. Schultz L. Bilateral cleft lips. Plast Reconstr Surg 1946; 1:338.
24. Sykes J, Senders C. Cleft palate. Plast Reconstr Surg 1999; 49:809.
25. Innis C. Some preliminary observations on unrepaired harelips and cleft palates in adult members of the Dusan tribes of North Borneo. Br J Plast Surg 1962:173.
26. Ross R. Treatment variables affecting facial growth in complete unilateral cleft lip and palate. Cleft Palate J 1987; 24(1):5–77.
27. Dieffebach J. Beitrage zur Gaumennath. Lit Ann Heilk 1828; 10:322.
28. Warren J. On an operation for the cure of natural fissures of the soft palate. Am J Med Sci 1828; 3:1.
29. Warren J. Operations for fissures of the soft and hard palate (palatoplastie). N Engl Q J Med Surg 1843; 1:538.
30. von Langenbeck B. Operation der angebornen totalen Spaltung des harten Gaumens nach einer neuer Methode, Dtsch Kin, 1861:321.
31. Furlow L Jr. Double reversing Z-plasty for cleft palate. In: Millard JDR, ed. Cleft Craft, Alveolar and Palatal Deformities. Boston: Little, Brown, 1980:519.
32. Furlow L Jr. Cleft palate repair by double opposing Z-plasty. Plast Reconstr Surg. 1986; 78(6):724–738.

16
Dental and Prosthetic Reconstruction of the Oral Cavity

Betsy K. Davis
Department of Oral and Maxillofacial Surgery, Medical University of South Carolina, Charleston, South Carolina, U.S.A.

Eleni Roumanas
Department of Biomaterials, Advanced Prosthodontics, and Hospital Dentistry, UCLA School of Dentistry, Los Angeles, California, U.S.A.

INTRODUCTION

This chapter presents treatment guidelines regarding the rehabilitation of head and neck cancer patients. Resection of head and neck tumors often results in severe facial disfigurement and functional disabilities which affect speech, deglutition, control of saliva, and mastication (1,2). Rehabilitation is an essential part of cancer treatment. Rehabilitative efforts involve multiple treatment modalities involving multidisciplinary teamwork. Members of the team include head and neck surgeons, radiation therapists, medical oncologists, facial reconstructive surgeons, maxillofacial prosthodontists, speech and swallowing therapists, physical therapists, and nutritionists. Today, treatment for head and neck cancers involve surgery, radiation therapy, chemotherapy, or some combination thereof. Superior rehabilitation efforts rely on close coordination and communication among the resection surgeon, reconstructive surgeon, and maxillofacial prosthodontist (3–5).

Optimal results for head and neck cancer patients are achieved when all members of the treatment team consult with the patient preoperatively. Patients should be referred to the maxillofacial prosthodontist as early as possible to determine the status of the oral cavity and dentition. Prosthetic rehabilitative efforts can be reviewed with the patient and this is an ideal time to obtain impressions, maxillomandibular records, and photographs. For either surgical or prosthetic reconstruction, pre-operative impressions and photographs serve as a guide in the reconstruction of the defect. Advances in prosthetic reconstruction often complement the cosmesis and function of flap reconstruction. Because many head and neck cancers involve such cosmetic and functional anatomic structures as the ear, nose, palate, and orbit, it is essential that the resection surgeon, reconstructive surgeon, and maxillofacial prosthodontist discuss surgical and prosthetic reconstructive options prior to definitive procedures. For either treatment modality, it is important that patients have realistic expectations of surgical and/or prosthetic reconstruction (3,4,6).

EVALUATION AND PLANNING

Proper communication between the resection and reconstructive teams is essential for post-treatment outcomes. Surgeons should be familiar with the universal numbering system of teeth (Fig. 1). This universal system numbers teeth sequentially in the adult from 1 to 32, starting with the right maxillary third molar, going to the left maxillary third molar, continuing with the opposing left mandibular third molar, and finishing with the right mandibular third molar (4).

As a general rule, edentulous patients are more difficult to rehabilitate than dentate patients. The surrounding oral anatomy plays a greater role in prosthesis support and retention. For the maxilla, the tuberosity, alveolar ridge, and hard palate are the major support areas for a prosthesis in the edentulous arch; whereas, for the mandible, the alveolar ridge, buccal shelf, and retromolar pad are the major support areas. Preservation and/or reconstruction of these structures are critical for the support and retention of the prosthesis (Figs. 2 and 3) (4).

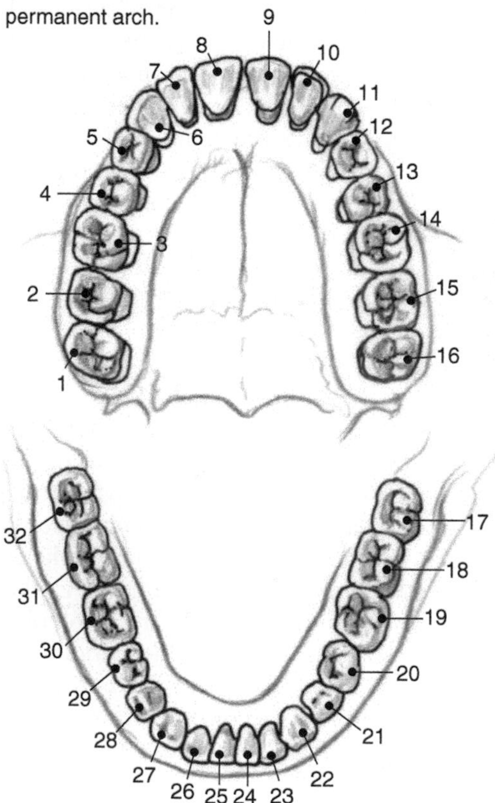

Figure 1 Universal numbering system is the acceptable method of tooth identification.

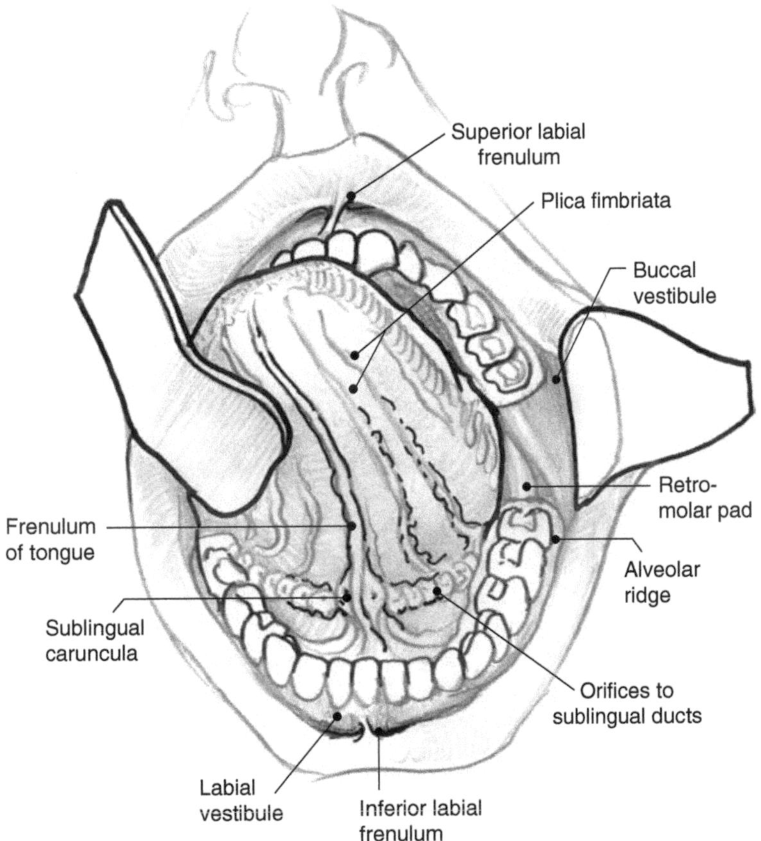

Figure 2 Anatomical structures which need consideration.

During the head and neck examination, the surgeon should identify acute or chronic pathologic conditions related to the dentition or supporting structures such as gross caries, poor oral hygiene, plaque, periodontal disease, or tissue irritation from poorly fitting prostheses. Next, referral to the maxillofacial prosthodontist can confirm any preexisting acute or chronic oral pathologic condition with appropriate radiographs such as a panoramic, periapical, bitewing, or occlusal films. The panoramic radiograph may be particularly of diagnostic value to the surgeon, because it confirms bony invasion of the maxilla or mandible by tumor. Impressions, maxillomandibular records, or photographs can be obtained at this initial visit as well (4).

RECONSTRUCTION OPTIONS

Chemotherapy/Radiation Therapy (Tables 1 and 2)

Patients receiving chemotherapy are at an increased risk of oral infection. Side effects of treatment include mucositis, xerostomia, oral bleeding, petechiae, ecchymosis, and nutritional deficiencies. The goal of the dental examination prior to treatment is to identify susceptible areas of infection and provide appropriate treatment of either restorative procedures and/or extractions (4,7).

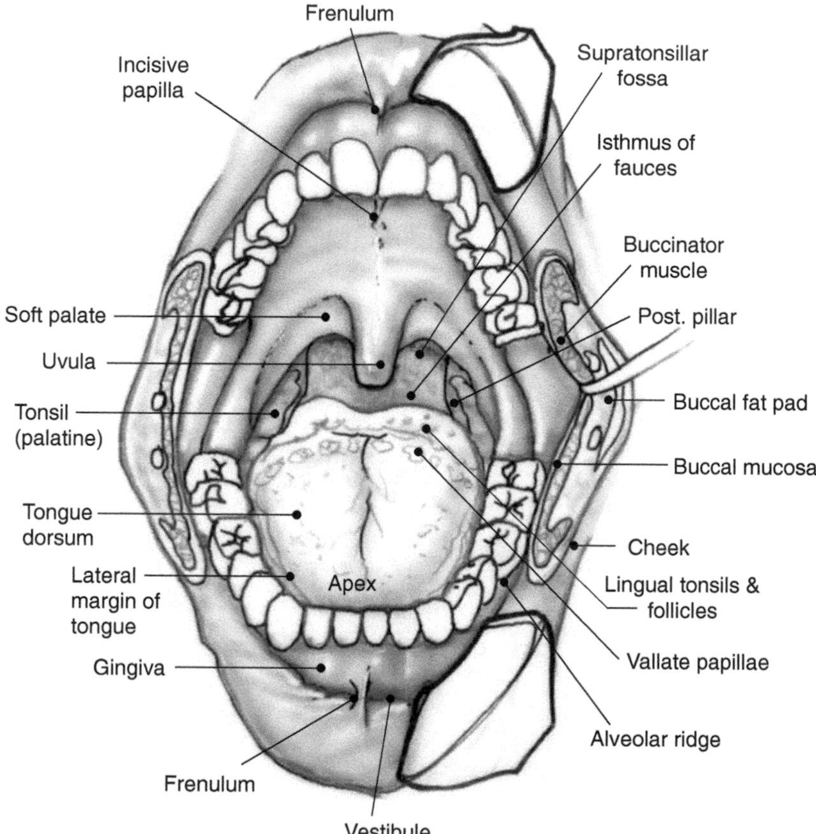

Figure 3 Anatomical structures which need consideration for maxillary rehabilitation.

On the other hand, patients receiving radiation therapy involving the salivary glands experience xerostomia, increased risk of dental caries, trismus, fibrosis, loss of taste, and increased risk of osteoradionecrosis. The severity of the morbidity correlates to the radiation dose, volume of tissue treated, and age of the patient. Goals of the dental examination are to identify any teeth requiring extraction or restoration, evaluate hygiene compliance of the patient, schedule needed treatment such as dental cleanings and scaling, and fabricate fluoride carriers. Pre-radiation dental extractions should be scheduled as soon as possible, because of the required ten-day to three-week healing period which must precede radiation therapy. Close communication with the radiation therapist is essential to identify any stents that may be needed, including a tongue depressing stent or a shielding stent (4,8).

Table 1 Treatment Considerations During Chemotherapy

Dental treatment	Oral side effects
Identify risk of oral infection	Mucositis
Restorative treatment	Petechiae
Extractions	Ecchymosis
	Nutrition deficiency

Table 2 Treatment Considerations During Radiation Therapy

Dental treatment	Oral side effects
Pre-XRT extractions	Xerostomia
Fluoride carriers	Dental caries
Stents	Trismus/Fibrosis
Mouth opening exercises	Mucositis/Candidiasis
	Loss of taste
	Increased risk of ORN

Maxillary Defects: Hard Palate (Table 3)

Maxillary defects are rehabilitated quite effectively prosthetically (9). Surgical closure of maxillary oncologic defects may not be indicated after resection due to the inability to monitor for recurrence of the neoplasm. Also, surgical reconstruction of large defects often fails to effectively reproduce palatal contour, which adversely affects bolus control and speech, and bulky flaps may prevent placement of an intraoral prosthesis. Most patients with maxillary defects can be restored to near-normal appearance and function with prostheses. Rehabilitation of maxillary defects can be immediate and straightforward, with predictable results. Resection of maxillary tumors involving the palate may result in nasal drainage into the oral cavity and impaired mastication and speech, which can be minimized with prosthetic obturation. Moreover, after rehabilitation, most patients with maxillary resections may lead relatively normal lives with little facial disfigurement (Figs. 4 and 5) (3,9).

At the time of surgical resection, an immediate surgical obturator can be wired or screwed into place to support the packing (Figs. 6 and 7). The obturator will provide separation from the oral cavity and sinus cavity, allowing the patient to eat and drink by mouth and to speak. In addition, several modifications can be performed surgically to enhance the prosthetic prognosis. Retention of as much of the maxilla, in particular, the premaxilla, if oncologically sound, enhances the stability and support for the obturator prosthesis. Patients who have a tapering arch form will benefit greatly from the retention of the premaxilla. Preservation of the cuspid eminence, if oncologically sound, aids in the stability and support of the prosthesis and minimizes collapse or contraction of the cheek into the large maxillectomy defect. Retention of key teeth, particularly the cuspid tooth, increases the retention and support of the prosthesis. Transalveolar resection cuts should be made as distant as feasible from the tooth adjacent to the resection to ensure an adequate amount of

Table 3 Treatment Considerations for Hard Palate Defects

Surgical modifications	Obturators
Retain as much as hard palate as possible, particularly premaxilla	Surgical
Retain key teeth (cuspid),	Interim
Consider implants	Definitive
Skin graft cheek flap	
Remove inferior turbinate	Troubleshooting
Remove medial wall of maxillary sinus	Nasal leakage
Cover medial aspect with palatal mucosa	Hypernasal speech

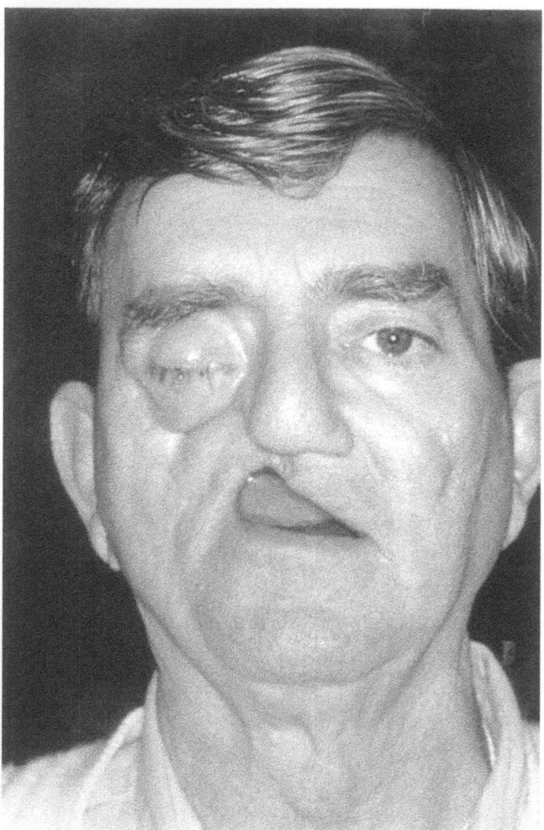

Figure 4 Patient who experienced maxillectomy and postoperative radiation therapy without an obturator. Note severe facial disfigurement.

bone around the tooth adjacent to the defect. Teeth in the path of resection should be extracted, and the cut made through the posterior portion of the extraction socket, increasing the clinical usefulness of the tooth adjacent to the maxillary defect and aiding in retention of more bony support (Fig. 8) (3,4,9).

The most difficult patient to obturate effectively is the edentulous maxillectomy patient (Fig. 9). Endosseous implants have dramatically improved the retention, stability, and support of the obturator (Figs. 10 and 11). However, implants alone do not provide adequate support and retention of the obturator prosthesis. Implants function predictably only when the defect has been designed to facilitate support, retention, and stability for the obturator prosthesis. The use of implants in the residual premaxilla provides the best retention of the obturator prosthesis, because the anterior maxillary segment is situated opposite to the most retentive portion of the defect, located along the posterior lateral wall (1,3,4,9). Roumanas et al. reported an 82.6% success rate of implants in non-irradiated bone sites and a 63.6% success rate in irradiated bone (10). Implants in the anterior maxilla had an accelerated rate of bone loss, which was 2.6 times greater than bone loss from implants in the posterior maxilla. Occlusal loading and delivery of excessive lateral torquing forces appear to be the cause of the patterns of bone loss with resultant failures (1,10).

Finally, proper preparation of the defect itself is as important as maximal preservation of palatal hard structures is. Lining the reflected cheek tissue with a

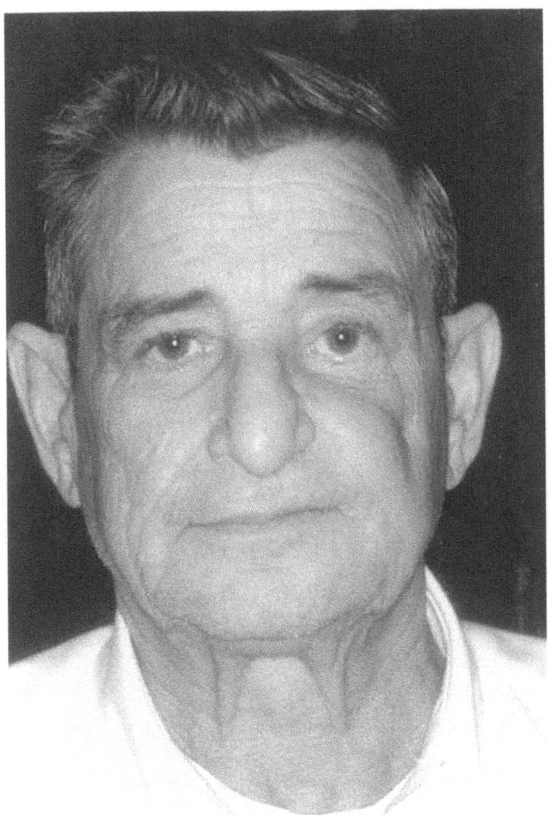

Figure 5 Patient who experienced maxillectomy and postoperative radiation therapy with an obturator. Note minimum facial disfigurement.

split-thickness skin graft improves the tolerance and retention of the obturator prosthesis because the keratinized surface is a more effective denture-bearing and supportive surface than is respiratory mucosa or poorly keratinized squamous epithelium (Fig. 12). The skin graft increases flexibility of the cheek flap and limits its contracture after surgery, thereby allowing the prosthodontist to achieve near-normal facial contour by displacing the cheek on the resected side with the obturator prosthesis. The scar band at the skin graft-mucosal junction creates a lateral undercut superiorly. Engagement of the scar band superiorly and inferiorly enhances support, retention, and stability of the prosthesis (Fig. 13) (3–5,9).

The inferior turbinate and medial wall of the maxillary sinus in partial palatectomies should be removed to prevent interference with obturation of the maxillary defect by the prosthesis. The exception is when the defect is small enough to be covered completely by conventional denture prosthesis. In that situation those structures can be retained. Otherwise, with larger defects, it is best to remove these structures (3–5,9).

During surgical resection, it is advantageous to cover the medial aspect of the resection with palatal mucosa (Fig. 14). The medial margin of the defect is one of the axes around which the obturator prosthesis rotates during function. If allowed to granulate and epithelialize spontaneously, the medial aspect will be lined with

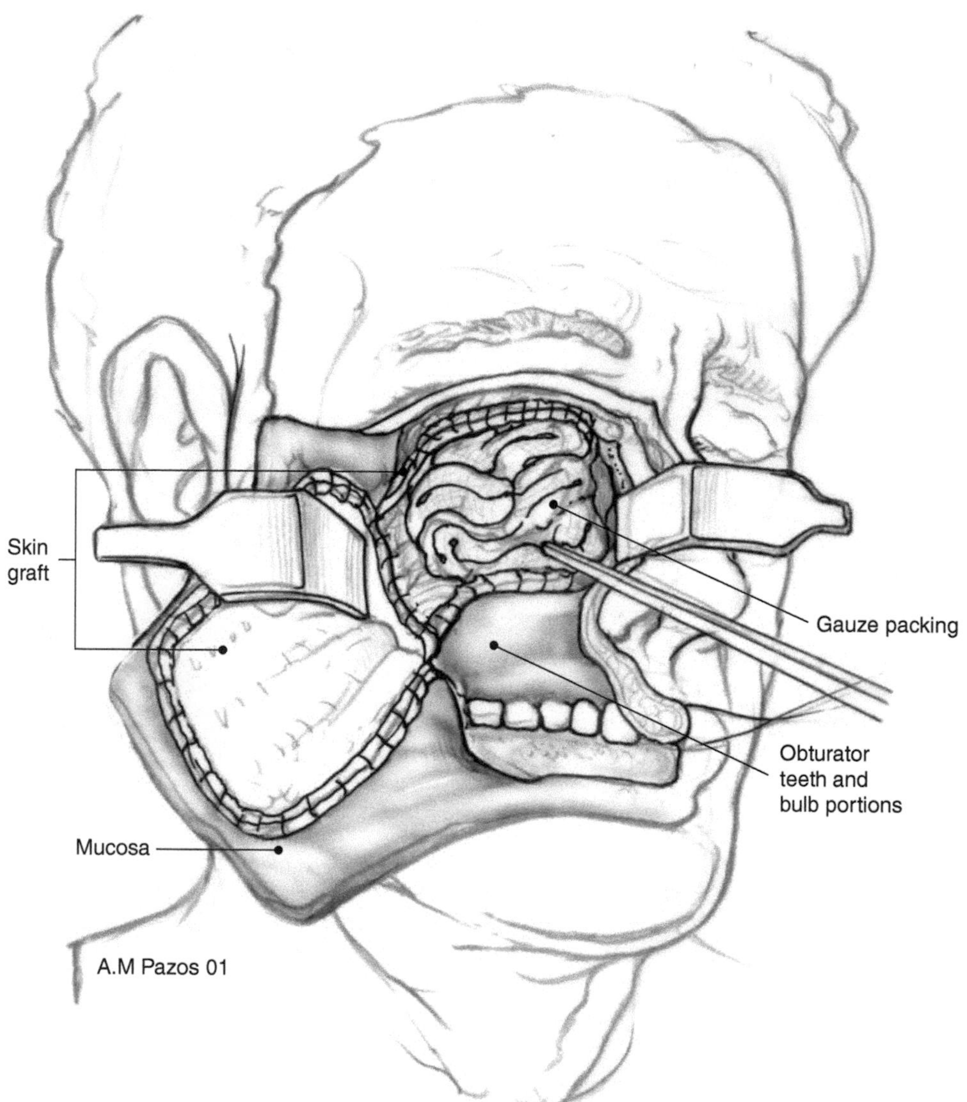

Figure 6 An immediate surgical obturator is wired in at the time of the resection surgery and helps to retain the packing.

respiratory mucosa or poorly keratinized squamous epithelium, which is an inferior denture-bearing surface. If the medial margin of the defect is covered with keratinized mucosa, the prosthesis may engage this surface, facilitating lateral stability of the prosthesis (Fig. 15) (3–5,9).

Maxillary Defects: Soft Palate (Table 4)

Velopharyngeal anatomic defects require a team approach among the speech pathologist, maxillofacial prosthodontist, and surgeon. Large defects of the soft palate are frequently best restored prosthetically. Pharyngeal flaps or free flaps are not effective in restoring velopharyngeal closure in this highly dynamic region, especially if the

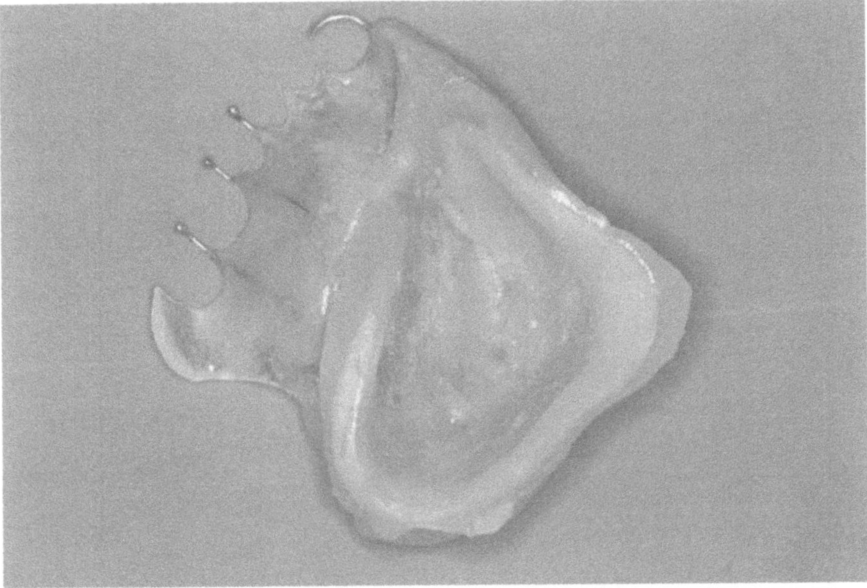

Figure 7 The immediate surgical obturator is relined at the time of unpacking.

defect is large. Functional velopharyngeal closure is difficult to achieve with surgical reconstruction; therefore, the patient's speech becomes hypernasal or hyponasal. When half or more of the soft palate is involved with the tumor or when there is a large midline, soft-palate defect and prosthetic rehabilitation is planned, the entire

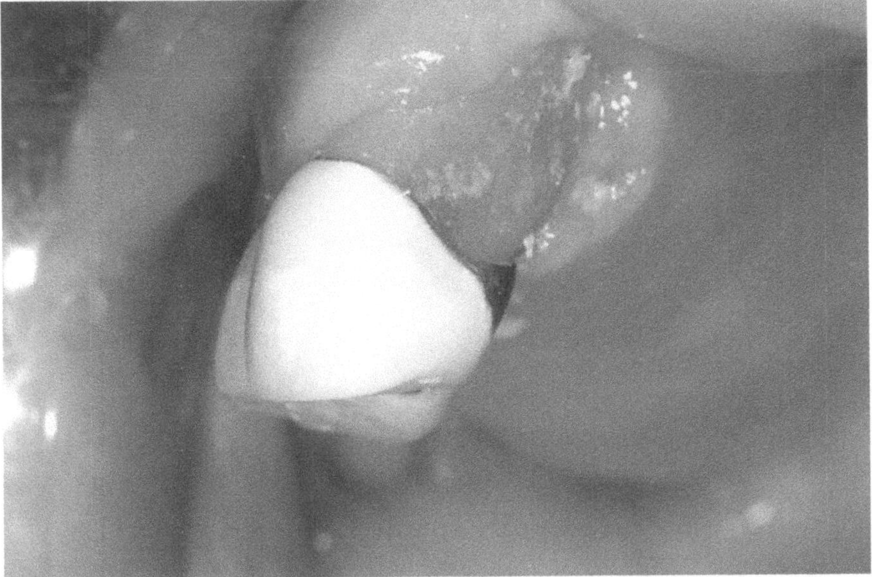

Figure 8 Transalveolar cuts should be made through the extraction socket. In this situation, the cut was made between the teeth. Note the lack of bone support around the abutment tooth.

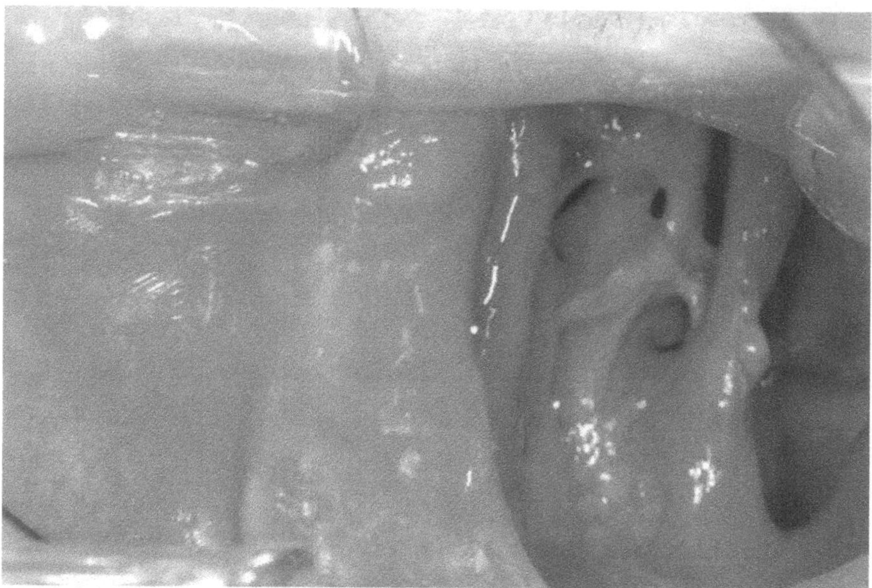

Figure 9 Placement of dental implants in the alveolar ridge will greatly improve the prosthetic prognosis in the edentulous maxilla.

soft palate should be removed. Retaining a band of residual soft palate that lacks innervation and/or the capability of normal elevation hinders prosthetic reconstruction by blocking access to the area of greatest motion of the residual lateral and posterior pharyngeal walls. The edentulous patient is the exception to this rule

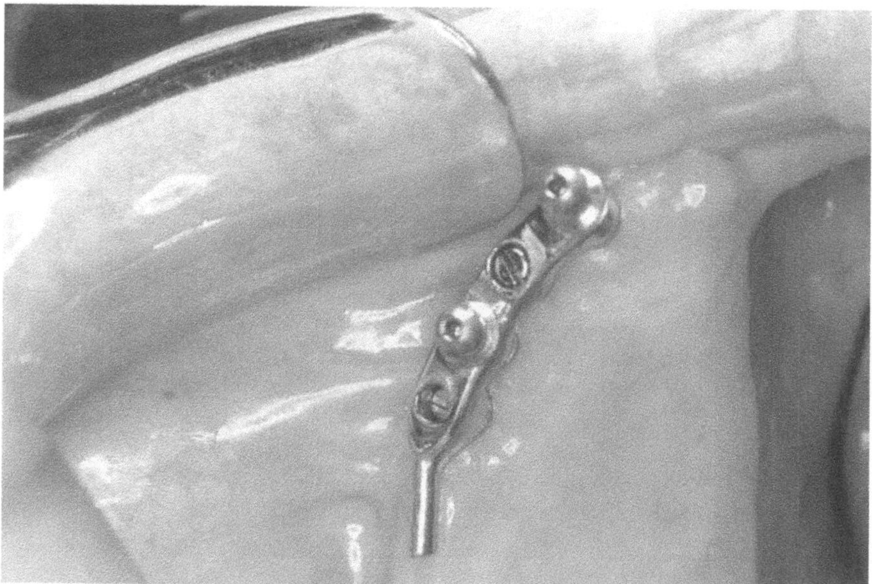

Figure 10 Placement of dental implants provides a mechanical means of retention for the obturator.

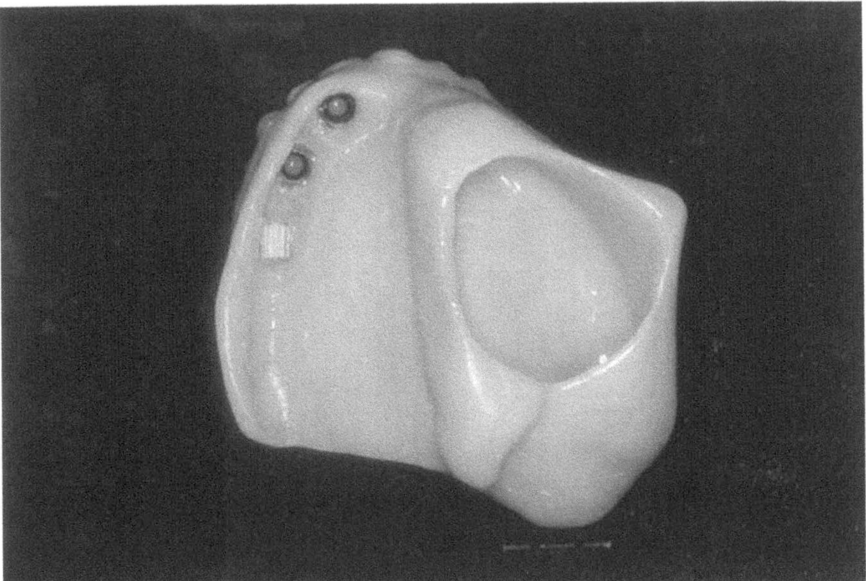

Figure 11 Implant housing mechanism in the obturator.

in that a distal band of residual soft palate may be advantageous for retention of the prosthesis (3–5,11).

When unilateral defects of the lateral and posterior pharyngeal wall are reconstructed surgically, the resulting lack of lateral pharyngeal wall movement of the

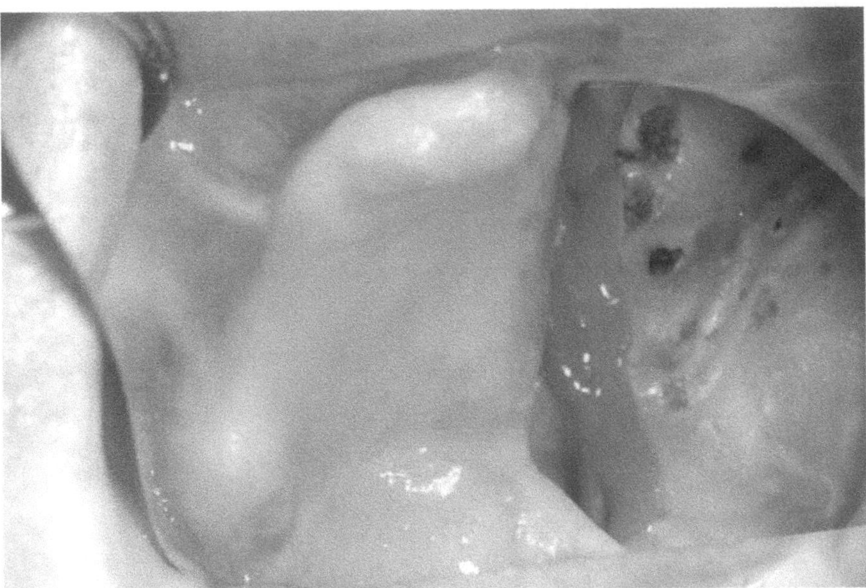

Figure 12 Lining the reflected cheek tissue with a split-thickness skin graft improves the tolerance and retention of the obturator prosthesis. The resulting scar band improves obturator retention.

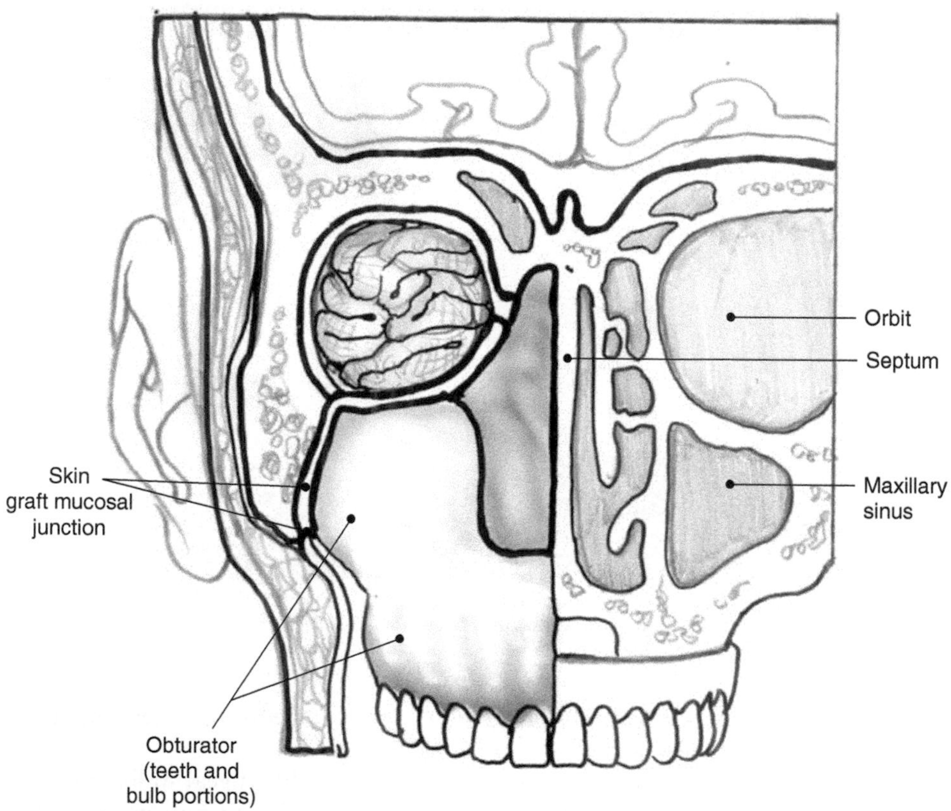

Figure 13 Engagement of the scar band superiorly and inferiorly enhances support, retention, and stability of the prosthesis.

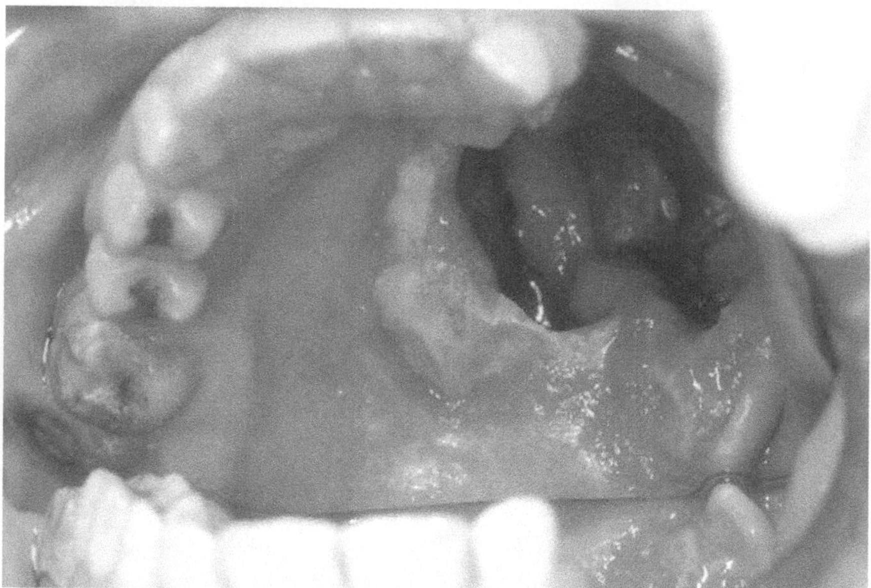

Figure 14 In this situation, the exposed bone is an inferior denture-bearing surface. The medial aspect of the resection should be lined with palatal mucosa.

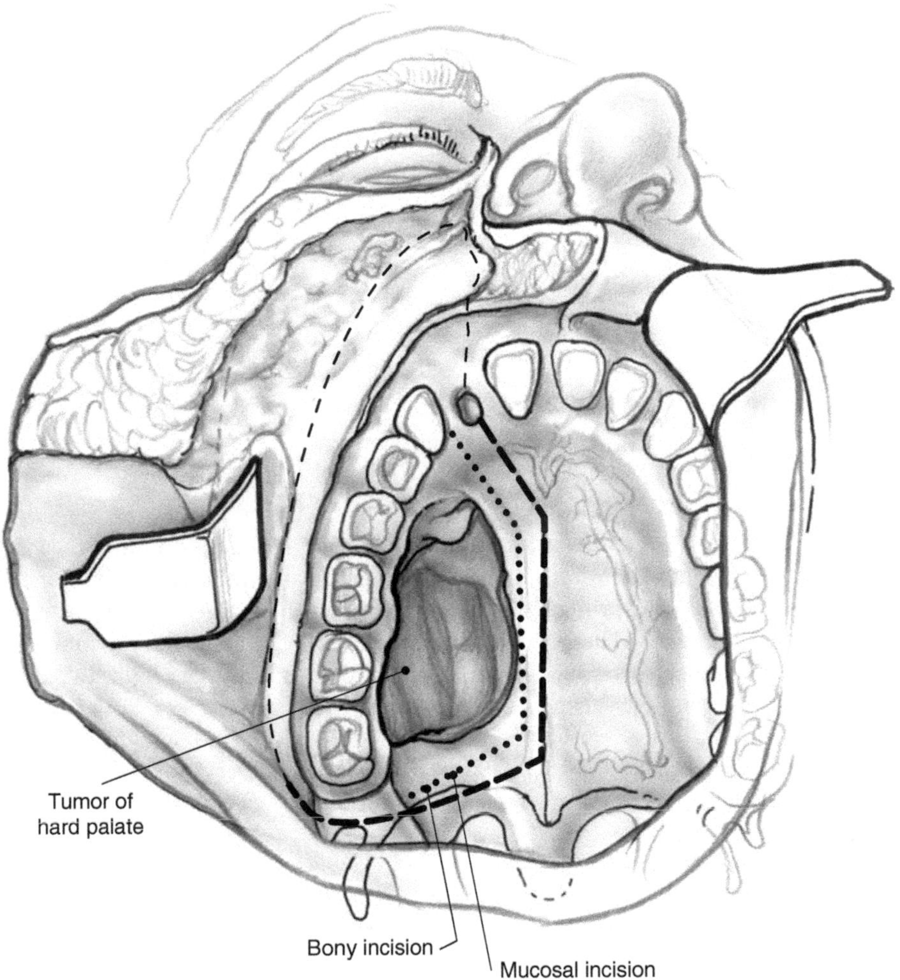

Figure 15 Lining the medial resection with palatal mucosa facilitates lateral stability of the prosthesis. This can be achieved by sparing more mucosa than bone.

reconstructed area mandates the use of a speech appliance which interacts with the normal functioning velopharyngeal complex on the opposite site, if normal levels of speech and swallowing are restored (3–5,11).

Mandible/Tongue Defects (Table 5)

Resection defects or tumors of the mandible, tongue, and adjacent structures are much more difficult to rehabilitate than maxillary defects. Resections of this type result in dysfunctions of speech, deglutition, and salivary control, and are often accompanied by severe facial disfigurement (Fig. 16) (12). Surgical advancements of microvascular free flaps and endosseous implants have greatly improved the reconstructive and rehabilitative results (1,3,12,13). Although restoration of tongue-mandibular defects is primarily a surgical responsibility, it requires the careful coordination of the resection surgeon, reconstructive surgeon, and maxillofacial prosthodontist. The development of

Table 4 Treatment Considerations for Soft Palate/Pharyngeal Wall Defects

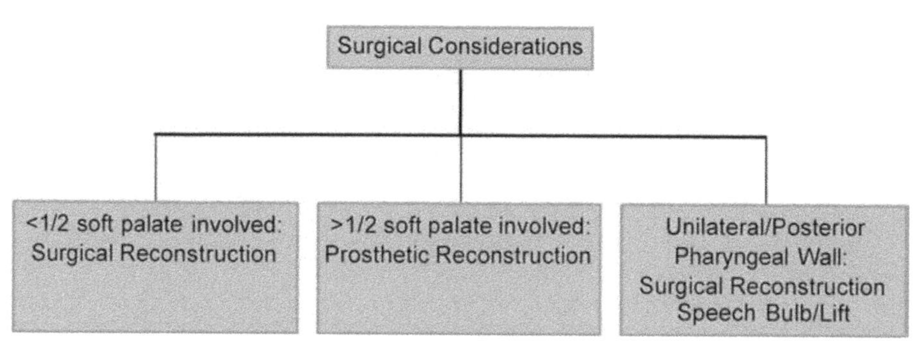

microvascular free flaps has greatly improved the patient's post-resection function with some patients approaching preresection levels of speech and swallowing. Previously, oral defects that were closed primarily with tongue flaps (Figs. 17 and 18) are now being restored with free flaps. These flaps restore tissue bulk, preserve tongue mobility and function, and enhance speech and swallowing. With loss of tongue bulk, the ability to manipulate the bolus is severely compromised. Free flaps restore bulk needed for bolus manipulation and speech articulation. Palatal speech and swallowing aids can be used as a supplement for these patients under the supervision of a speech and swallowing therapist and may be effective in improving speech articulation and swallowing in selective patients (3,5).

The maxillofacial prosthodontist can fabricate surgical stents that can be used as a guide during surgical reconstruction to ensure reestablishment of normal maxillomandibular skeletal relationship (13,14). In the past, mandibular defects, which were not reconstructed, resulted in severe deviation of the mandible with resulting abnormal maxillomandibular relationships. The use of free flaps to replace the resected mandible and soft tissue has eliminated much of the mandibular deviation. Today, reconstruction of mandibular defects with microvascular free flaps can result in near-normal articulation of teeth on the non-resected side. If the patient is not a candidate for surgical reconstruction, a course of mandibular guidance therapy can be used to help prevent mandibular deviation. Reconstruction of a buccal and lingual vestibule with free flaps or skin grafts enhance6s the prosthetic prognosis (1,3,5).

Table 5 Treatment Considerations for Mandible/Tongue Defects

Mandible defects	Tongue defects
Reconstruct surgically	Reconstruct surgically
Consider reconstructive stent (helps to maintain maxillomandibular relationship and pre-resection occlusion)	Consider palatal speech/swallowing appliance
Parallel mandible to maxilla	Palatal augmentation appliance
Consider placement of implants and/or maintenance of dentiion	

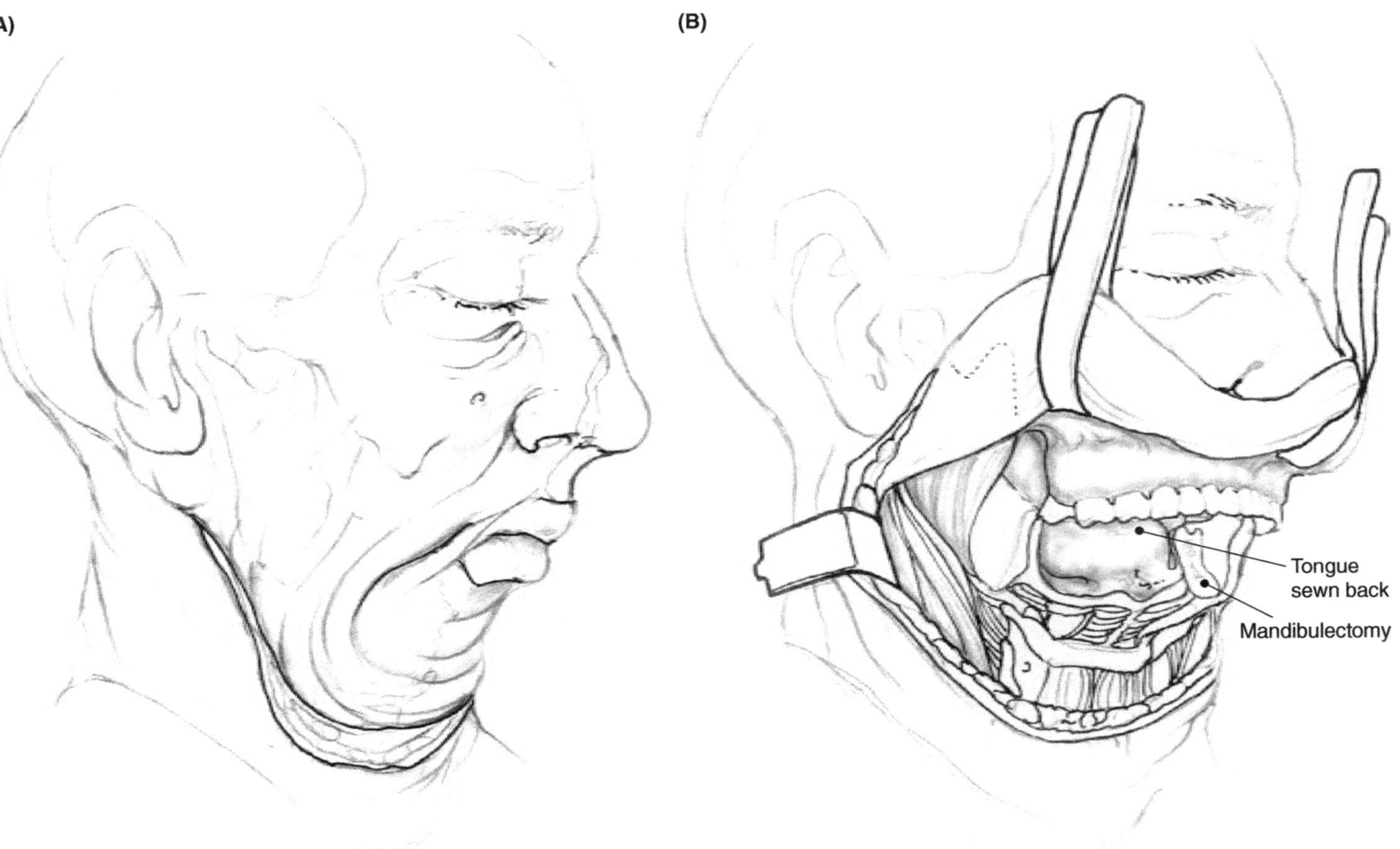

Figure 16 Resection of the anterior mandible results in severe dysfunctions of speech, deglutition, and salivary control.

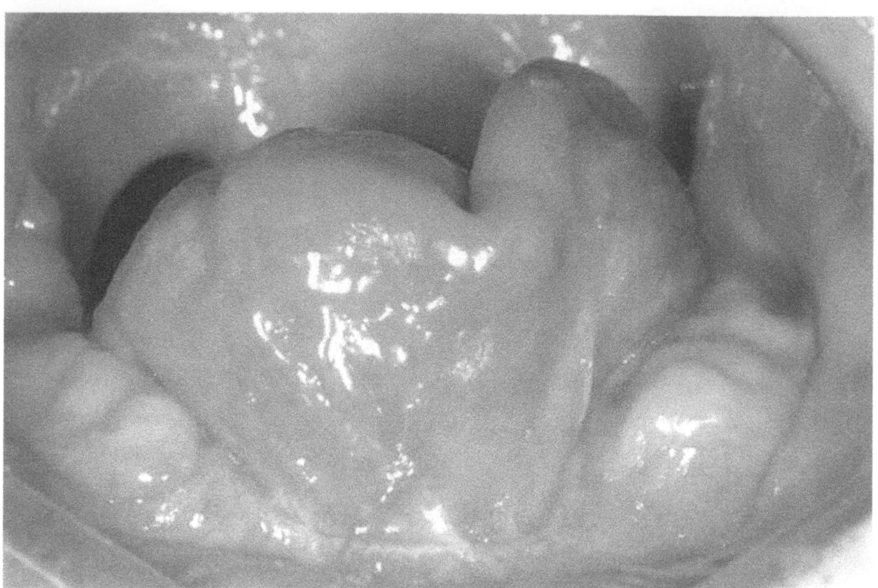

Figure 17 Tongue defects should not be closed primarily, limiting tongue mobility.

Endosseous implants can be used to retain the resection prosthesis. Whether considering reconstructed or native mandible, a general rule for implant placement is to have 10 mm of vertical bone with 6 mm of horizontal bone width available to ensure predictable results (Fig. 19). Roumanas et al. reported greater than 90% success for implants placed in fibula free flaps (15). If implants are planned, a surgical guide dictating the number and position of implants should be fabricated by the

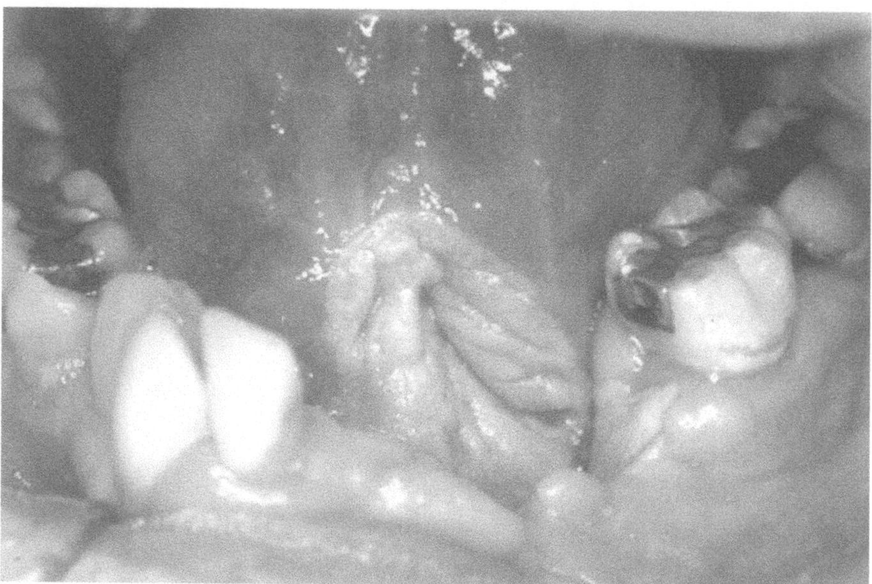

Figure 18 The defect should be lined with skin, which increases tongue mobility.

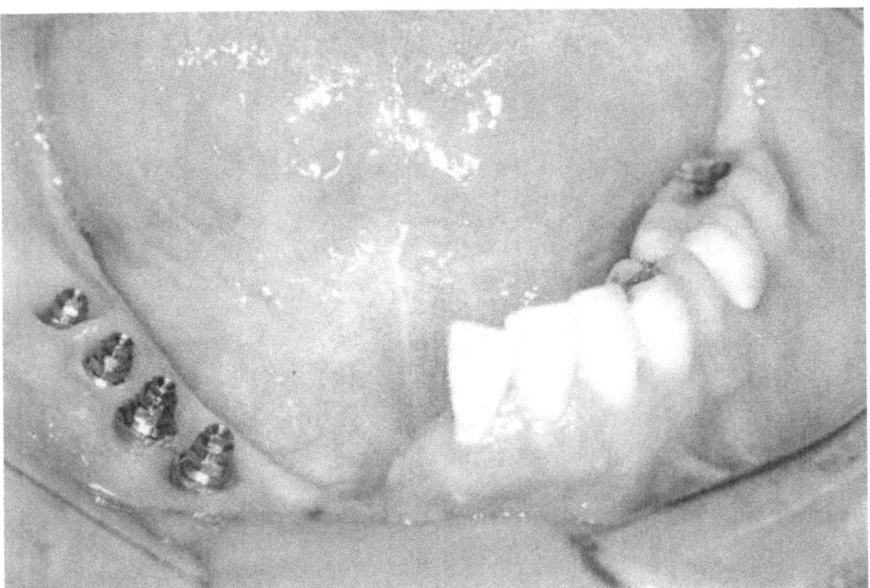

Figure 19 Implants placed in free-tissue transfer aid in the retention of the resection prosthesis.

maxillofacial prosthodontist to ensure proper positioning and angulation of implants during surgical placement.

Lateral mandibular defects in dentate patients who have undergone reconstruction with either free flaps or bone grafts need special consideration before implant placement. The use of implants on the reconstructed side is justified only if motor and sensory innervation of the adjacent soft tissue is intact. When the lingual and hypoglossal nerves are sacrificed, the patient cannot detect and therefore cannot manipulate the bolus on the resected side. Hence, masticatory efficiency is only improved when the motor and sensory innervation is intact. Conventional removable partial dentures designed to support the lip and improve aesthetics are sufficient for the needs of these patients (3–5).

Complex Midface Defects

Perhaps, the most difficult defects to rehabilitate are midfacial defects due to loss of extensive portions of the face, nose, upper lip, orbital contents, and often, the oral cavity (Fig. 20). When these tumors extend into the oral cavity resulting in resection of the maxilla or mandible, mastication, swallowing, saliva control, and speech articulation are adversely affected. The resulting facial disfigurement can create severe psychological problems for the patient. Many of these patients can be rehabilitated with a combination of surgical and prosthetic modalities (3,5,15).

A maxillectomy defect with an orbital exenteration is particularly challenging. If portions of the maxilla are involved, it is usually preferable to reconstruct the palatal portion prosthetically. The use of an immediate surgical obturator greatly aids the speech and deglutition in the post-operative period. There are a number of advantages of prosthetic reconstruction and rehabilitation which include: the

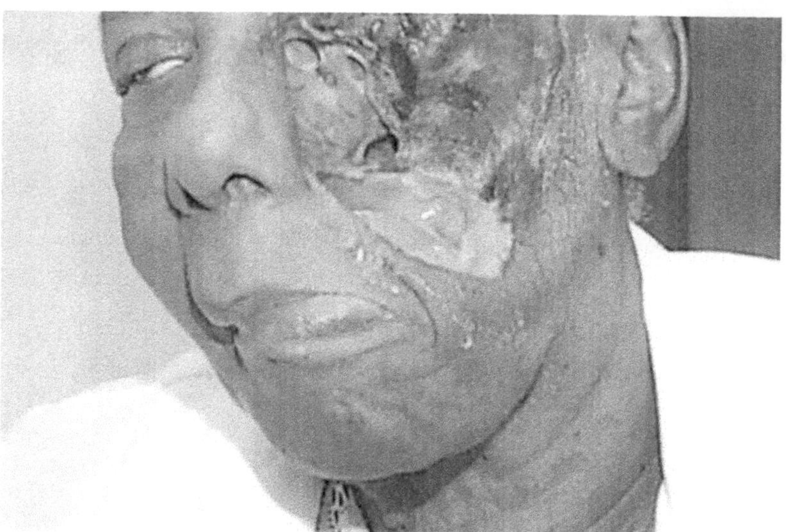

Figure 20 An example of a midface defect in which functions of swallowing, speaking, and cosmesis are severely compromised.

cavity can be monitored; speech and swallowing can be fine-tuned to ensure tongue contact with the palate; and velopharyngeal insufficiency can be minimized in those patients who have had soft palate resections. The prosthesis can also serve as tooth replacement and provide projection for the upper lip and anterolateral midface (3,5,16).

Separating the oral portion from the orbital portion with a free-tissue transfer is a desirable modification that can be performed at the time of surgical resection (17). If the orbital floor or palatal defect is extensive, a scapular osteocutaneous flap can be used, providing a more stable palatal reconstruction. Also, this may prevent the gravitational inferior displacement that often occurs with soft tissue flap reconstruction. Most large lateral facial defects are best restored surgically.

The most difficult problem for large midfacial defects from a prosthetic standpoint is providing retention, stability, and support for the prosthesis, which is accomplished using prostheses retained by implants and yields a result that has greater patient acceptance (1). Implants, however, cannot compensate for proper defect preparation; therefore, at the surgical resection, key teeth should be salvaged and all exposed tissue surfaces that can be usefully engaged by the prosthesis should be lined with skin grafts. The choice of prosthetic or surgical reconstruction of intraoral defects is dependent on the etiology, anatomic structures involved, and size of the defect. In most situations, small defects are more amenable to surgical reconstructions, whereas, larger defects are better restored prosthetically. The surgical site can be closed either primarily or with flap reconstruction. Raw surfaces can be lined with a split-thickness skin graft. Mucosal flaps are useful to close small medial defects and nasolabial flaps are useful for anterolateral defects (1,3,5,16).

Decision Making Tips

Radiation Therapy: Need dental evaluation for pre-radiation extractions, fabrication of fluoride carriers, radiation stents, and mouth opening exercises.

Chemotherapy: Dental evaluation to identify risk of infections and possible restorative treatment and/or extractions.

Hard Palate Defects: Need obturator and design defect so it has retentive qualities.

Soft Palate: If $< 1/2$ of soft palate involved, perform surgical reconstruction; otherwise, prosthetic reconstruction.

Mandible/Tongue Defects: Reconstruct surgically, place special emphasis on maxillomandibular relationship and consider placement of implants.

CONCLUSION

Superior rehabilitation is achieved only when there is close communication among members of the treatment team. Consideration of prosthetic design at the time of surgical resection and reconstruction greatly improves patients' functional outcomes. Thereby, allowing patients the ability to be able to speak, swallow, and masticate more effectively.

REFERENCES

1. Beumer J III, Roumanas E, Nishimura R. Advances in osseointegrated implants for dental and facial rehabilitation following major head and neck surgery. Semin Surg Oncol 1995; 11:200–207.
2. Ross B. The clinician and the head and neck cancer patient psychodynamic interactions. In: Beumer J III, Curtis T, Firtell D, eds. Maxillofacial Rehabilitation Prosthodontic and Surgical Considerations. St. Louis: Mosby, 1979:5–6.
3. Davis BK, Roumanas ED, Nishimura RD. Prosthetic-surgical collaborations in the rehabilitation of patients with head and neck defects. Otolaryngol Clin N Am 1997; 30:631–645.
4. Martin J, Lemon J, Chambers M. Surgical techniques to enhance prosthetic rehabilitation-oral and dental oncologic principles. In: Bailey B, ed. Head & Neck Surgery-Otolaryngology. Lippincott-Raven: Philadelphia, 1998:1855–1865.
5. Martin JW, Lemon JC, King GE. Maxillofacial restoration after tumor ablation. Clin Plast Surg 1994; 21:87–96.
6. Ordway D. The crisis of cancer: challenge to change. J Prosthet Dent 1977; 37:184–189.
7. Klokkevold P. Cancer chemotherapy: oral manifestations complications and management. In: Beumer JI, Curtis T, Marunick M, eds. Maxillofacial Rehabiliation: Prosthodontic and Surgical Considerations. St. Louis: Ishijaku Euro America, 1996:25–42.
8. Kramer D. The radiation therapy patient treatment planning and posttreatment care. In: Taylor T, ed. Clinical Maxillofacial Prosthetics. Chicago: Quintessence Publishing Company, 2000:37–52.
9. Curtis T, Beumer J III. Restoration of acquired hard palate defects: etiology disability and rehabilitation. In: Beumer III J, Curtis T, Marunick M, eds. Maxillofacial Rehabilitation: Prosthodontic and Surgical Considerations. St. Louis: Ishijaku Euro America, 1996:225–226, 233–240.
10. Roumanas ED, Nishimura RD, Davis BK, Beumer J III. Clinical evaluation of implants retaining edentulous maxillary obturator prostheses. J Prosthet Dent 1997; 77:184–190.
11. Curtis T, Beumer J III. Speech velopharyngeal function and restoration of soft palate defects. In: Beumer JI, Curtis T, Marunick M, eds. Maxillofacial Rehabilitation: Prosthodontic and Surgical Considerations. St. Louis: Ishijaku Euro America, 1996: 285–330.

12. Beumer J III, Marunick M, Curtis T. Acquired defects of the mandible: etiology treatment and rehabilitation. In: Beumer J III, Curtis T, Marunick M, eds. Maxillofacial Rehabilitation: Prosthodontic and Surgical Considerations. St. Louis, Ishijaku Euro America, 1996:113–224.
13. Markowitz BL, Calcaterra TC. Preoperative assessment and surgical planning for patients undergoing immediate composite reconstruction of oromandibular defects. Clin Plast Surg 1994; 21:9–14.
14. Markowitz BL, Roumanas E, Calcaterra T. Surgical stents for composite mandible reconstruction. Plast Reconstr Surg 1995; 96:194–198; discussion 199–200.
15. Roumanas ED, Markowitz BL, Lorant JA, Calcaterra TC, Jones NF, Beumer J III. Reconstructed mandibular defects: fibula free flaps and osseointegrated implants. Plast Reconstr Surg 1997; 99:356–365.
16. Beumer J III, Marunick M, Roumanas E, Nishimura R. Restoration of facial defects: etiology disability and rehabilitation. In: Beumer JI, Curtis T, Marunick M, eds. Maxillofacial Rehabilitation: Prosthodontic and Surgical Considerations. St. Louis: Ishijaku Euro America, 1996.
17. Hochman M. Reconstruction of midfacial and anterior skull-base defects. Otolaryngol Clin N Am 1995; 28:1269–1277.

17
Mandibular Reconstruction

Deepak Gurushanthaiah
Department of Head and Neck Surgery, Oakland Medical Center, Oakland, California, U.S.A.

Jeffrey R. Haller
Rocky Mountain Allergy Center, Missoula, Montana, U.S.A.

INTRODUCTION

The mandible is an important structure for function, esthetics, and quality of life. Etiologies for mandibular defects include ablative cancer surgery, trauma, osteoradionecrosis, and infection. Repair of these defects remains a challenge for the head and neck reconstructive surgeon. Ideally, reconstruction would provide a solid arch to articulate with the upper jaw to restore preoperative occlusion and cosmesis, maintain oral competence to allow fluent, intelligible speech and a normal swallow, and allow for dental rehabilitation with functional mastication. These goals can be met for most mandibular defects.

Many different techniques have been described throughout the years. Some of the more common ones include alloplastic implants, autogenous bone grafts, and reconstruction plates. The use of vascularized tissue and bone, increased graft survival rates and improved outcomes. Pedicled osteomyocutaneous flaps were pioneered by Conley in the 1970s (1). The limitations of these were overcome with the use of free flaps over the last twenty years and have essentially become the gold standard with most mandibular reconstruction, particularly anterior and large defects.

EVALUATION AND PLANNING

The optimal technique for reconstruction continues to be debated. Several issues need to be addressed including the patient's desires and expectations, the medical stability of the patient, compliance, adjunctive radiation therapy, and oral contamination of the recipient bed.

Medical problems such as peripheral vascular disease, coronary artery disease, obesity, and even psychosocial/psychiatric issues play a significant role in the ultimate choice of reconstruction. Lengthy operations may not be tolerated by these individuals and a less complex procedure may be chosen. Imaging studies should be obtained as appropriate for the nature of the disease that is being treated.

There are often two anatomic issues to address in mandibular reconstruction. Universally, a bony defect is present. In addition, there often exists a soft tissue component that needs attention. This varies with the extent of resection but undoubtedly influences the ultimate reconstruction method. Hence, the reconstructive surgeon needs a wide variety of techniques available in their armamentarium. Foster et al. (2) showed that mandibular reconstruction with vascularized bone grafts versus non-vascularized bone grafts had a higher incidence of bony union, required fewer operations to achieve bony union, and had better success with dental implants. All of these factors applied to lateral mandibular defects as well. No one method deals with all the factors affecting each patient with a mandibular defect. One option that should always be considered is no reconstruction of the mandible. Komisar (3) concluded that mandibular continuity did not enhance the functional rehabilitation in the majority of patients he studied with oropharyngeal malignancies.

Another consideration with mandibular reconstruction is sensory reinnervation of the soft tissue surrounding and included in the defect which is reconstructed. The improvements over the last decade have made this feasible. Sensory branches of various free flaps have been identified and anastomosed to the lingual nerve stump when soft tissue flaps are used. Interposition and nerve grafts have also been used to bridge the gap of inferior alveolar nerve and mental nerve to regain sensation of the lower lip and help prevent drooling and improve poor oral function (4).

RECONSTRUCTIVE OPTIONS

Non-Vascularized Grafts

From a historical perspective, materials such as wax and paraffin have been injected beneath the skin and molded to create an esthetically acceptable cosmetic appearance. The foreign body reaction to these materials was worse than the ultimate cosmetic outcome. Implants such as pins, trays, and plates made of various materials including silastic, polyurethane-reinforced Dacron mesh, stainless steel, vitallium, and titanium have been used. Millard used a medullary K-wire beneath a notched rib graft cortex to accommodate bending for an anterior defect. Other sources include ilium, clavicle, and fibula. High failure rates led to abandonment of these techniques. Barring plates and screws which are now widely used in mandibular reconstruction other alloplastic implants have fallen out of favor because of decreased stability and higher rates of infection and extrusion.

Free Bone Grafts

Autogenous bone grafts have been in use since the 1900s. They provide an isogenic material that allows the transplantation of viable osteoblasts and osteoprogenitor cells that continue to lay down new bone in a recipient bed. Hence, they have been noted to be resistant to extrusion.

The healing of bone grafts relies on tissue regeneration rather than simple repair with scar formation. The most widely accepted theory for graft incorporation is Axhausen's "two-phase" theory (5). Bone formed in the graft initially arises from cells that remain after reconstruction that proliferate and form new osteoid that is laid out in the framework of the graft. The first phase is approximately four weeks and determines the ultimate size of the bone graft. A sufficient number of osteoblastic cells must survive and be viable in order to provide bulk. In the second phase, there is no new bone growth but phase I bone is replaced. Pluripotential host cells are transformed into osteoblastic cells that remodel phase I bone and organize the graft. This is thought to be mediated by bone morphogenic protein which induces host fibroblasts to grow into the graft. Urist (6) has shown high concentrations of BMP in cortical bone. Phase II starts at about two weeks, peaks at six weeks, and wanes around six months. If the host tissue cannot support the second phase of osteogenesis because of hypovascularity and hypocellularity, delayed resorption of the graft will occur, often resulting in its total loss.

There are four types of autogenous free bone grafts: corticocancellous blocks, cancellous bone, cortical bone, and particulate bone/cancellous marrow. Corticocancellous bone has given mixed results because of late resorption in the center causing fractures secondary to decreased phase I bone formation and difficulty with vascularization of the transplant from the thick plate separating the cancellous bone from the hosts tissues. Osteoblasts that do survive die before they can be reperfused. Cancellous bone gets enough phase I bone formation and adequate phase II bone formation when the defect is small and has surrounding bone and periosteum. With larger defects and no periosteum, cancellous bone on its own does not provide enough rigidity and you get diminished phase II bone production and late graft resorption. Particulate bone/cancellous marrow has by far the best osteogenic potential with sufficient viable osteoblasts and mesenchymal cells for both phases of osteogenesis. The particulate nature of the bone and increased surface area allows for rapid revascularization. However, you have no structural integrity and need some support. Alloplastic or allogenic cribs or trays that are biocompatible and/or resorbable have been developed for this purpose. Our approach with this technique is to use reconstruction bars for stabilization and pack cortical bone around the plate. Homologous bone (freeze drying methods) exhibits little immunogenicity and the lack of any viable cellular component leads to its eventual resorption. Allogenic mandible, rib, and ilium have all been used. Metal mesh trays can be used in combination with corticocancellous bone chips or particulate bone. It is fenestrated to allow vascular and cellular ingrowth. This is effective when using an external approach for secondary reconstruction and avoiding oral contamination. The allogenic bone cribs have replaced these because they are essentially biodegradable.

Reconstruction with particulate bone has met with varied success. In the pre-free flap era, Lawson et al. (7) noted a failure rate of 54% for primary reconstruction using titanium hollow screw reconstruction plates (THORPs) with particulate cancellous bone. This improved to a 90% success rate when reconstruction was delayed. The high failure rate was attributed primarily to the inability of the graft to tolerate oral contamination. Hence, it is infection and extrusion that are problems plaguing this technique. Higher success rates were noted when reconstruction was not done primarily.

Additional bone substitutes for mandibular reconstruction include a variety of autogenous free bone grafts, irradiated or cryopreserved mandible, and alloplastic materials. The overall success rate for these in immediate reconstruction has been less than ideal (8–10). They do not provide the integration that occurs when using vascularized bone flaps.

Reconstructive Bars/Plates

Some form of rigid fixation is necessary for mandibular reconstruction to secure the remaining bone fragments and any grafts, which are used to provide adequate

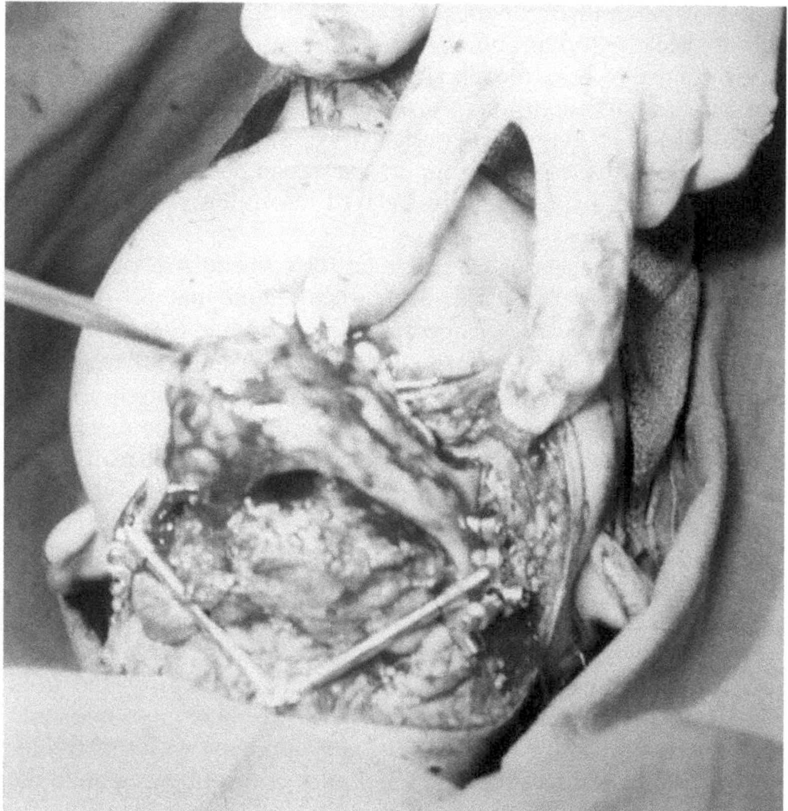

Figure 1 Interlocking bridging device prior to reconstruction.

healing and maintain mandible position. The type of rigid fixation used can vary but the technique should remain constant. Whichever plate is decided upon, it should be contoured before the resection to bridge the defect with an adequate amount of fixation on either side of it. Usually, two-point fixation on each side of the defect is minimal. This is essential to maintain proper occlusion. Occasionally, MMF is necessary before the resection to ensure the occlusal relationship. If the tumor is in the way and does not allow adequate plate contouring, an interlocking bridging device can be used to maintain occlusion while resection and reconstruction is performed (Fig. 1). Sometimes, this is not even possible and a plate must be designed by visualization alone. It should also be mentioned that some reconstructive surgeons prefer to use mini-plates for the mandible rather than the larger, more bulky plates and bars that are used prevalently.

Reconstruction bars/plates have undergone a constant evolution over the last several decades since their inception. Their continued improvement in design and composition has established a niche in mandible reconstruction. They can be used alone or with local flaps and both pedicled and free musculocutaneous, fasciocutaneous, or osteomusculocutaneous flaps. Their role and in what combination is determined anatomically by factors such as location and size of the defect. Again, medical stability of the patient can dictate what type of reconstructive technique is used. In patients with a short life expectancy, a plate alone may occasionally be used understanding that it is temporary and over time will be met with complications. It should be understood that using a plate alone in reconstruction of the mandible is rarely considered to be an ideal method.

The THORP was the first design with screws that locked to the plate, so essentially worked as an internal external fixator. It decreased screw loosening if there was bone loss at the plate bone interface. This tended to be a problem with earlier plates. The THORP plate did see good success rates early on, but it had its own problems. The plate was extremely thick and had sharp edges. This led to difficulty bending the plate to achieve appropriate contour and also resulted in increased soft tissue extrusion rates. Since that time, plates have evolved to be a lower profile, more rounded contour, and more malleable locking plates which are proving to be more effective and result in less complications.

Benoist (11) reported an unsatisfactory experience with failure rates as high as 80%. Contrary to this report, Raveh et al. (12) in a series using the titanium-coated hollow screw and reconstruction plate with a pedicled myocutaneous flap showed success in 100% of his patients. Gullane and Holmes (13) reported similar success with a different reconstruction bar. They attributed the success to the use of a vascularized myocutaneous flap. Blackwell (14) looked at 15 patients reconstructed with the THORP plate combined with soft tissue free flaps for lateral mandibular defects and found the overall failure rate to be 40% with a minimum one year follow-up.

Reconstruction bars provide reasonable reliability for mandibular reconstruction when combined with well-vascularized soft tissue. It offers an expedient method suitable for patients of poor health not able to tolerate lengthy operations. Additionally, reconstruction bars may work well for lateral mandibular defects of the body and ramus if the patient does not wish to pursue dental implantation. Anterior defects treated with a plate and no bone undoubtedly will end up with soft tissue erosion and plate exposure (Fig. 2). The aesthetic outcome is also extremely unsatisfactory when comparing the results with vascularized bone combined with a reconstruction plate.

The general feeling is that reconstruction plates alone should only be used as a temporary repair of any defect. Given time, they will extrude or even fracture. When placing a reconstruction bar with an osseous free flap, the soft tissue will heal to the bone and the bone will absorb the associated forces so there is less chance for extrusion. For this reason, some surgeons elect to secure these bone flaps with mini-plates. The senior author elects to use the low profile, locking 2.0 reconstruction plate to keep hardware to a minimum.

Vascularized Grafts

Vascularized bone allows for healing despite compromised recipient beds such as irradiated bone and soft tissue. Hoffman et al. (15) showed histological evidence that vascularized bone flaps healed with bone continuity similar to that of a fracture. This is in contrast to non-vascularized bone, which heals by resorption of old bone and deposition of new bone, "creeping substition". Remodeling takes place in non-vascularized bone with marked bone resorption and loss of cortex.

Pedicled Osteomyocutaneous Flaps

Pedicled osteomyocutaneous flaps were introduced in the 1970s as a means for mandible reconstruction and were the first attempts to bring vascularized bone to the defect. Prior to this era, soft tissue pedicled flaps were used to cover defects and allow healing to occur. A secondary reconstruction with bone was performed at a later date. This was successful as long as oral contamination was avoided. With

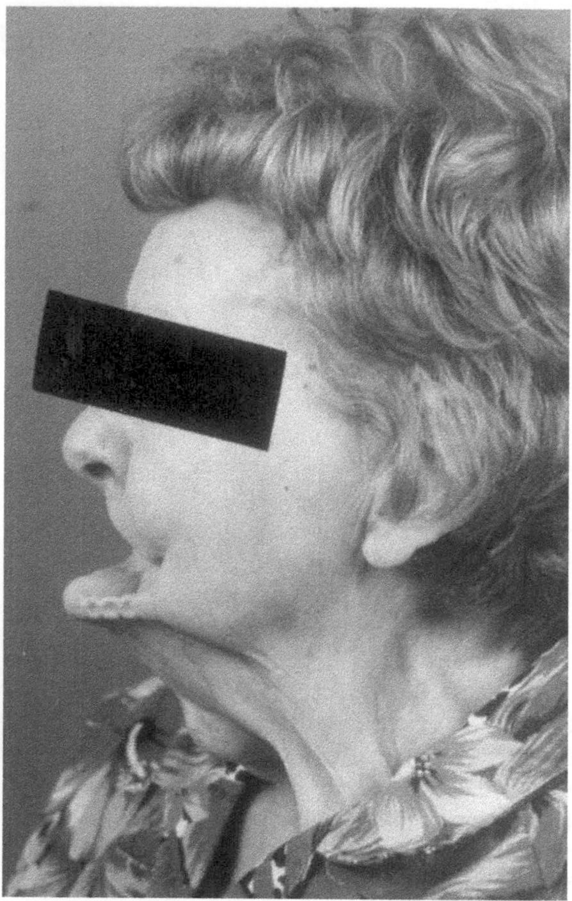

Figure 2 Reconstruction plate alone used for anterior defect showing signs of erosion.

the advent of newer techniques these have fallen out of favor but will be mentioned for historical significance. The osteocutaneous flaps that have been used include sternocleidomastoid muscle with medial clavicle, trapezius muscle with scapula, pectoralis major muscle with rib, lateral trapezius with acromial end of clavicle, temporalis muscle with temporoparietal bone, and deltopectoral flap with acromial end of clavicle. Krespi et al. (16) included rhomboids with the trapezius muscle, theoretically lengthening the segment of scapula that would remain viable. Limited bone length, questionable bone stock for dental implantation, limited arc of rotation and flap mobility, poor survival of cutaneous components, variable success rates, high donor-site morbidity, and random or collateral vascular supply to the osseous component has made these methods less attractive today.

Free Flaps

Technological advancement, improved post-operative care, and refinement in microsurgical technique over the last 20 years has led to an increase in the use of vascularized free bone grafts for reconstruction of mandibles. As a result, they have become the gold standard in mandible reconstruction against which other methods are compared. Urken et al. (17) recently reviewed his experience with microvascular tissue transfer in oromandibular reconstruction and cited a 96% success rate in 210 cases over 11 years. Most experienced microvascular surgeons would match this value with success rates in excess of 90%.

Microvascular free flaps allow long-term reliability and stability along with the ability to osseointegrate for dental rehabilitation in one primary stage (18). Evolution of flaps has made neurosensory innervation possible over the last decade. Numerous studies over the last decade have shown success using various methods of anastomoses. Urken's (17) review described 49 patients who underwent nerve grafts to restore sensation to the lower lip by bridging the gap between the inferior alveolar nerve and the mental nerve following hemimandibulectomy. This undoubtedly helps with oral competence thereby facilitating speech and swallowing. Vascularized bone is resistant to infection, resorption, and extrusion. It heals similar to bone in a fracture with rigid fixation securing the segments. Bone grafts heal more indirectly and they still require rigid fixation of mandibular defects.

In addition, for anterior mandibular defects, no other reconstruction methods have the ability of vascularized free bone flaps for providing a solid arch necessary to restore form and function. Therefore, when suitable for specific patients, reconstruction with vascularized bone is the preferred method of mandibular reconstruction. During the past decade, a variety of donor sites for vascular bone flaps and soft tissue have evolved. Ideally, the bone must provide adequate length, width, and height to span the defect and accommodate endosteal implants and withstand the forces of mastication. They may need an adequate soft tissue component to fill any large defects created from extirpation for good form and function. There is not a single flap that works well for all defects; hence, we will discuss a variety of flaps emphasizing their advantages and disadvantages (Table 2). Eight different sites have been employed using this technique: scapula, fibula, ilium, radius, humerus, ulna, metatarsus, and rib. Most centers today use one the first three flaps because of their versatility and reliability. The senior author finds the fibula to be the most useful, versatile, and reliable in regards to harvesting technique and application and is the flap of choice at our institution for mandibular reconstruction.

Table 1 Evaluation and Planning

- I. Patient factors
    - A. Patient's desires/expectations
    - B. Medical condition
        - 1. Peripheral vascular disease
        - 2. Coronary artery disease
        - 3. Obesity
    - C. Compliance
    - D. Psychosocial
- II. Defect factors
    - A. Location
        - 1. Anterior
        - 2. Lateral
        - 3. Posterior
    - B. Size
    - C. Soft tissue defect
    - D. Oral contamination
- III. Associated treatment
    - A. Radiation therapy

Table 2 Free Flaps and Their Characteristics

	Scapula	Fibula	Ilium	Forearm
Soft tissue availability	+++	++	++	+++
Two team approach	+	+++	++	+++
Donor site morbidity	++	+++	++	±
Soft tissue mobility	+++	++	+	+++
Sensate potential	−	+++	−	+++
Ossepotegration	±	++	+++	−

Rating scale from (−) to (+++). (−) indicates least favorable and (+++) indicates most favorable.

When designing a bone graft for use in mandibular reconstruction there are several important points to keep in mind for an optimal outcome. There should be complete bone contact at each end of the defect and at all osteotomy sites. The periosteum should be left intact on the bone graft during the harvest and while making osteotomies. The vascular pedicle must be protected. Finally, some form of rigid fixation should be used to provide a framework to stabilize the bone segments between the cut ends of the mandible and between osteotomy sites. The senior author now incorporates small 2.0 mm locking reconstruction plates with his fibula free flap reconstructions because with 100% bone contact as described above large, heavy plates are not needed for strength. Our method of reconstruction involves bridging the proposed resection area with a plate of sufficient length to allow 2–4 fixation points on either side of the defect. This allows for appropriate occlusion to be maintained by ensuring proper mandibular alignment. Once the mandibular segment is resected, a template is fashioned using silastic blocks (Fig. 3A). First, it is cut to the length of the defect. Osteotomies are simulated by removing wedge blocks until the natural contour of the mandible is achieved. The bone graft is then sculpted to match the template (Fig. 3B). Care is taken to preserve periosteum laterally and obtain 100% bone to bone contact. This will allow for the best healing. Fixation is then applied to the graft.

Scapula: The scapula osteocutaneous free flap is attractive for use in composite defects of the head and neck necessitating a large soft tissue component. Based on the subscapular artery, this system of flaps can include the lateral scapula and overriding skin as well as latissimus dorsi and serratus anterior muscles (19). The vascular anatomy allows the bone to be positioned independently of the skin paddle. The bone is corticocancellous and can provide from 10 cm to 14 cm of length. When facial reanimation is desired, the latissimus dorsi muscle may be reinnervated.

The biggest disadvantage to this flap is the positioning difficulty during the operation. It requires the patient to be in a lateral decubitus position and makes a two-team approach difficult. Cross-sectional area of the flap can be limited on a case-to-case basis making osseointegration questionable. Also, sensory reinnervation has not been described.

Fibula: First described by Taylor et al. (20) in 1974 for reconstruction of long bone defects, the fibula free flap has become a workhorse in mandible reconstruction. Hidalgo (21) described its use for mandibular reconstruction in 1988. Its blood supply originates from the peroneal artery via endosteal and periosteal branches. Excellent segmental periosteal blood supply allows the fibula to be osteotomized as many times as necessary to recreate the natural contour of the mandible. Up to 25 cm of bone can be procured with this flap making it the only flap available for total mandible

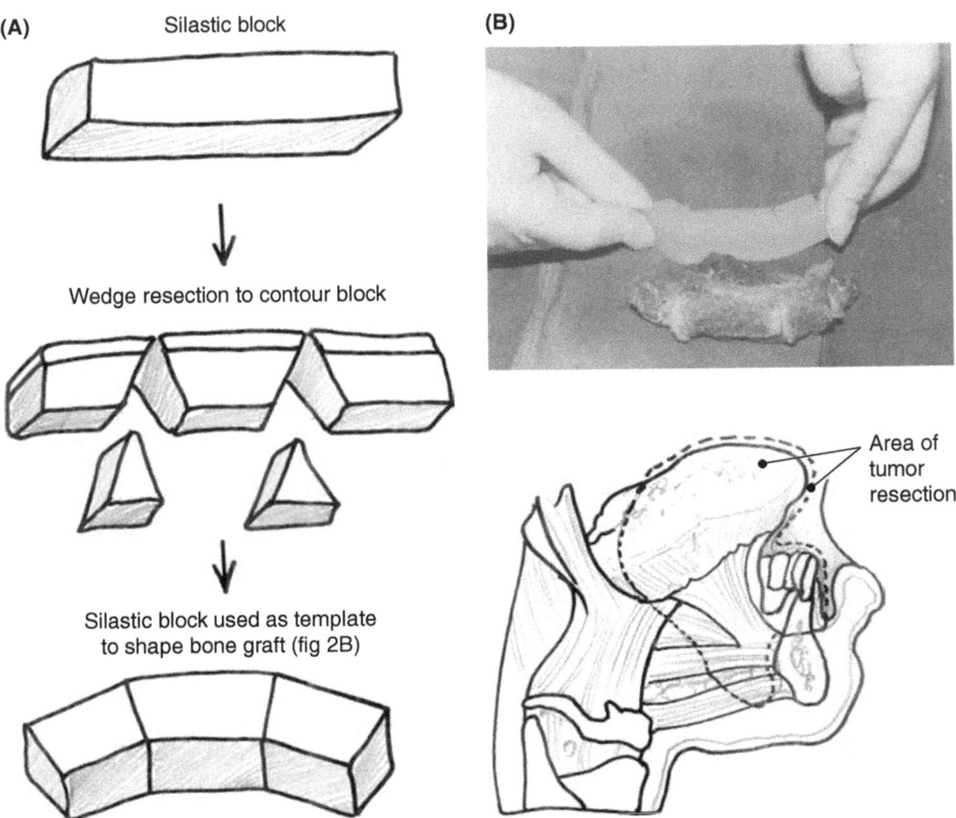

Figure 3 (**A**) Illustration of technique used to create silastic template for bone graft. (**B**) Fibula free flap with osteotomies performed to match contour of silastic template.

reconstruction. The location provides an easy two-team approach making it more attractive. It works well for implantation and dental restoration. Frodel et al. (22) showed adequate bone stock in a cadaver study comparing four different flaps: fibula, scapula, ilium, and radius. Hayden described the lateral cutaneous nerve to the calf as a sensory nerve to the skin paddle and the sural communicating nerve to bridge the inferior alveolar nerve defect allowing a sensate osteocutaneous flap.

The major disadvantage to this flap in the past has been an unreliable skin paddle with variable septocutaneous perforators. Incorporating a cuff of soleus muscle or dissecting cutaneous perforators through the soleus muscle has basically eliminated most of these concerns.

Ilium: The large amount of bone available and the natural contour of the ilium make it a popular replacement for the resected mandible. The vascular supply to this flap is based on the deep circumflex iliac artery. A major advancement of this flap was the identification of the ascending branch of the DCIA as the dominant supply to the internal oblique muscle. Urken et al. (23,24) modified this flap for mandibular reconstruction and obtained excellent results with it. A total of 14–16 cm of bone can be procured, a moderate soft tissue component, and it has sufficient height for osseointegration. Hence, this has become a popular flap for composite defects. The use of iliac crest is indicated opposed to fibula in patients with significant peripheral vascular disease, history of vein stripping or varicosity, prior leg trauma, or those with signs of venous or arterial insufficiency.

Limitations of this flap include the poor pliability of the overlying skin and the overall bulk of the flap that can add difficulty while insetting the flap. Also, the dissection involved in harvesting this flap involves dividing most of the lower abdominal muscles making donor site morbidity an issue.

Radius: The radial forearm fasciocutaneous flap has been widely used in head and neck reconstruction because it is thin and pliable, two ideal qualities for oral reconstruction. The underlying radius can be included in this graft to create an osteocutaneous flap. A total of 10–12 cm and 40% circumference of the bone can be harvested. In addition, a cutaneous sensory nerve to the skin paddle has been isolated and good results have been demonstrated with reinnervation. For these reasons, there are reconstructive surgeons who state that this flap should be considered among the "first line" choices for oromandibular reconstruction (25).

There are several major disadvantages to using this bone flap. The limited bone width and length is not enough for osseointegration or structural strength for mastication. Pathological fractures of the remaining radius have been reported in up to 25% of the patients. Grip, pinch, and range of motion were significantly reduced in the affected hand when fractures occurred. Bowers et al. (26) published results from a cadaveric study of fresh frozen radii showing that plating the segmental defect created in the radius with a dynamic compression plate increased the strength in torsion and four point bending when compared to one that was not plated. These findings may renew interest in this flap.

Ulna: The ulnar flap receives its vascular supply from the ulnar artery. It is similar to the radius in the amount of bone available and quality of skin component hence, it has the same disadvantages. The antebrachial cutaneous nerve can be anastomosed to a recipient nerve in the head and neck for a sensate flap. Limited experience exists with this flap in the head and neck.

Humerus: The humerus is based on the profunda brachii artery. It's soft tissue component is the lateral arm flap which is used as a fasciocutaneous flap on its own. Ten centimeters of length and 1/6 the diameter of bone can be procured using this flap. It also has the advantage of sensory supply via the posterior cutaneous nerve. Additionally, the donor site can usually be closed primarily. Disadvantages include a short vascular pedicle and smaller lumen diameter that the other two arm flaps. Again, the quantity of bone is usually insufficient and hence, it has seen limited use in head and neck reconstruction.

Metatarsus: The metatarsus osteocutaneous flap is supplied by the dorsalis pedis artery and is based on the second metatarsal bone. It has been used to reconstruct anterior floor of mouth mandibular composite defects. The skin is thin and receives sensory input from the superficial peroneal nerve. The pliability of the skin is a major advantage of this flap (27).

Disadvantages of metatarsus include difficulty in flap elevation and limited amounts of bone and skin. The average length of the second metatarsal bone is 7–8 cm and only approximately 10 cm of skin can be procured. Atherosclerotic disease can narrow vessel lumen diameter. The donor-site morbidity rate can be significant, including poor healing of the skin graft over the paratenons, repeated breakdowns from local trauma, and loss of sensation to the dorsum of the foot (27).

Rib: In addition to its use as a pedicled flap rib has also been described as a free vascularized graft. McKee (28) used it clinically as a free flap for mandibular reconstruction in 1974. The rib can be harvested anteriorly or posteriorly and is based on the intercostal vessels. It can be transferred with latissimus dorsi or serratus anterior muscles for added soft tissue (29,30).

The major disadvantage to using this flap is the limited amount of bone available. It is soft bone and is not amenable to osseointegration. In addition, the vascular pedicle is short and, there is a risk of pneumothorax during harvesting (31). For these reasons, other donor sites are usually preferred before rib is used.

LOCATION OF MANDIBULAR DEFECTS

Anterior Defects

Cosmesis obviously takes on a large part in planning of operative intervention. Leaving an anterior defect of the mandible undoubtedly gives a poor cosmetic outcome resulting in the unsightly "Andy Gump" deformity. In addition, speech and swallowing will be less than optimal because of the poor articulation of the maxilla and mandible as well as the lips. Restoring the anterior arch resuspends the soft tissues of the oral cavity. Reconstruction bars can be bent to provide the natural shape of the mandible and vascularized bone can be fixed to these plates (Fig. 4). Bone

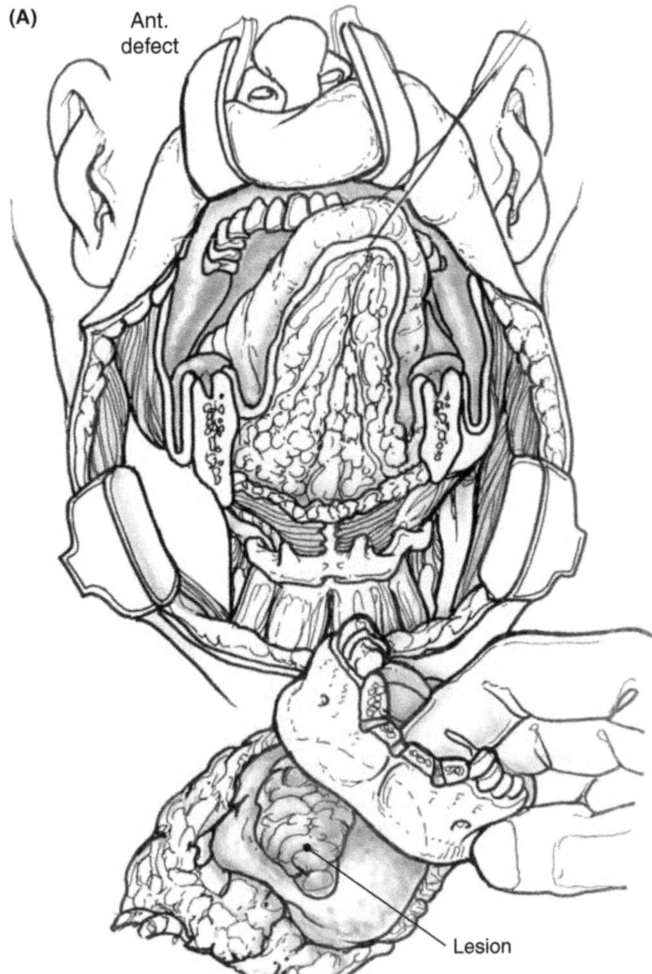

Figure 4A–C Vascularized bone fixed to reconstruction bar in mandibular defect. (*Continued*)

(B)

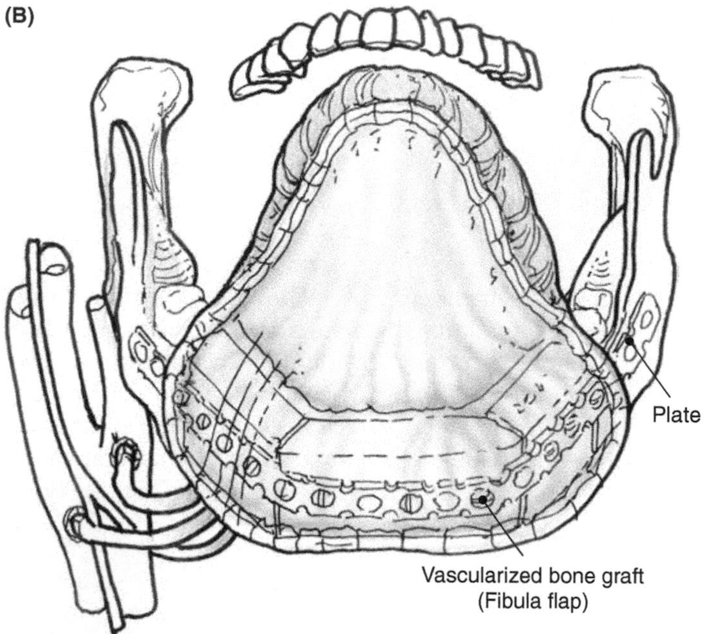

Figure 4 (*Continued*)

reconstruction is the only reliable method for anterior defects. While a free bone graft may be used for small defects without soft tissue loss or an irradiated bed, free flaps are generally the first choice. Particulate or cortical bone can be used and will give good structural support but does not have the bone stock necessary to facilitate dental implants. The most ideal reconstruction of medium to large bony defects of the anterior mandible is vascularized bone graft. We prefer to use the fibula flap because of its versatility but both the iliac and scapula free flaps can be used with excellent results.

Lateral Defects

Although most reconstructive surgeons would agree that an osseous free flap is ideal for anterior defects, the treatment of lateral mandibular defects remains a controversial topic in mandibular reconstruction. Several options exist and the argument is that vascularized bone may not always be necessary. In fact, as mentioned previously, no reconstruction is always an option. The obvious disadvantage to this is in cosmesis since all patients will suffer from a mandibular swing to the resected side on mouth opening. Komisar (3) compared composite resection patients with and without reconstruction and found decreased masticatory function in the reconstructed patients. He suggests that restoration of mandibular continuity does not enhance the functional rehabilitation of the majority of patients with oropharyngeal malignancy. It appeared to limit mandibular motion and hence the scarring and decreased range of motion observed in this group of patients may have contributed to a greater number tolerating only a liquid diet. Non-reconstructed patients could open their mouths to a larger degree along a deviated plane of motion. All resections were of lateral or anterolateral origin. This data is older now and is likely influenced

(C)

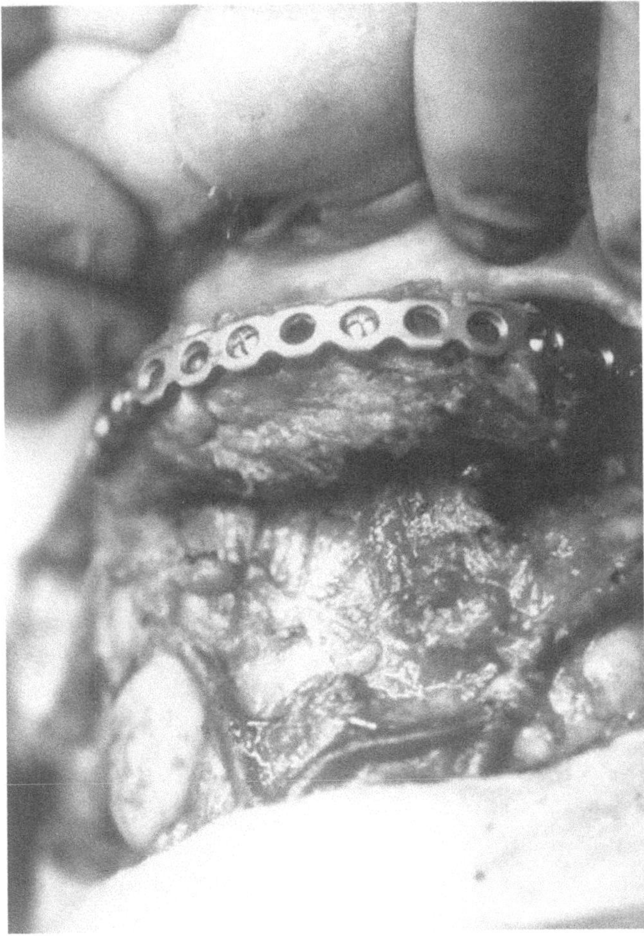

Figure 4 (*Continued*)

by the fact that reconstruction was performed using non-vascularized bone grafts and outcomes were assessed subjectively by patients. Newer studies such as Curtis et al. (32) looked at objective measures including bite force assessed at the first molar and incisal edge, a measure of tongue and cheek function, and patient reports of food they could eat and found that reconstructed patients have better overall function than non-reconstructed patients.

Smaller lateral defects with healthy vascularized tissue, no oral contamination, a non-irradiated bed, and with minimal soft tissue defect many still allow for free bone grafts. This may require secondary reconstruction, especially in oncologic and trauma surgery where it may be difficult to keep oral contamination low. Using a plate alone is an option with small lateral defects. As mentioned before, this would increase complications of soft tissue erosion and potential plate fracture. The plate flap technique without bony reconstruction has been shown to be effective in these smaller defects. Blackwell et al. (33) revisited the topic of plate and flap for lateral defects and showed a 93% success rate. He found the use of newer, better-designed plates decreased the

(A)

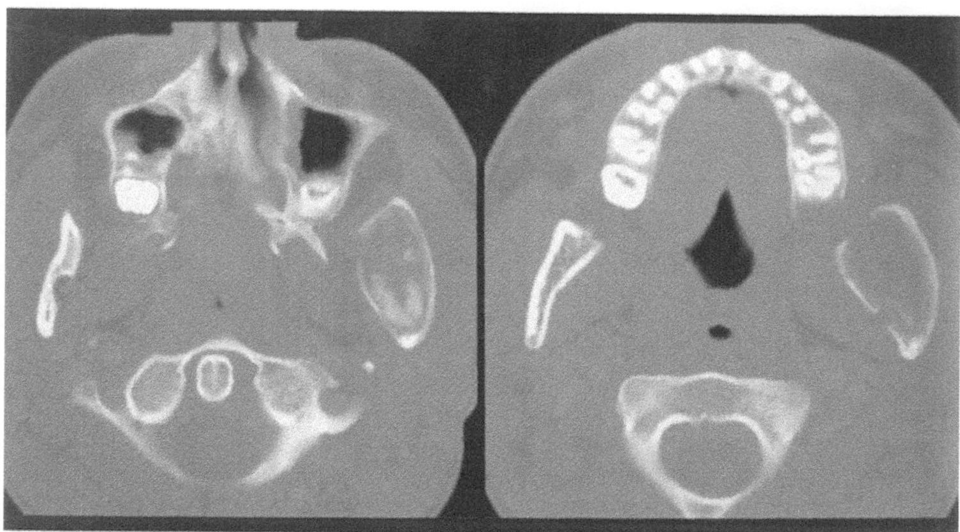

(B)

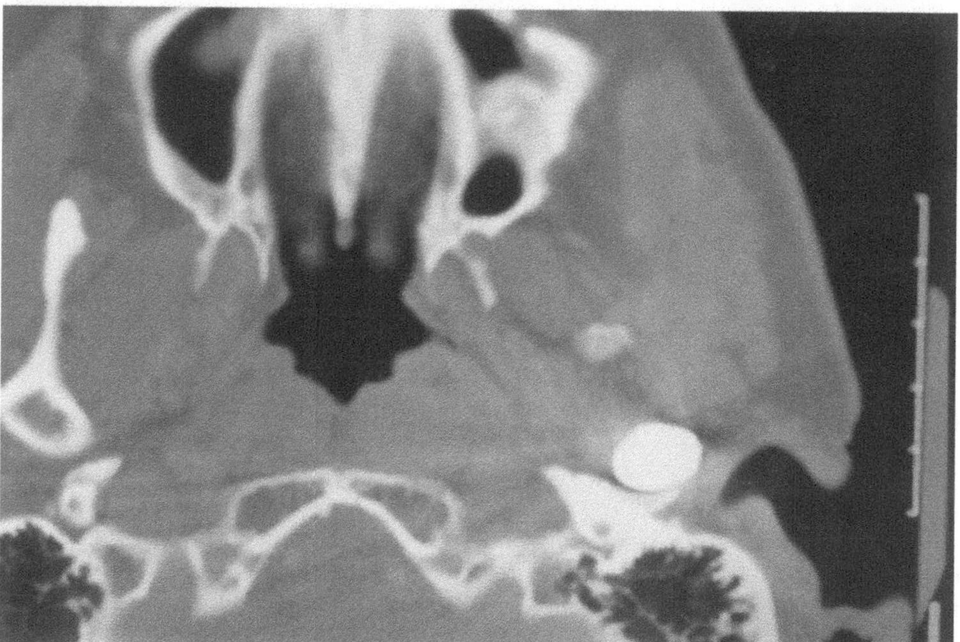

Figure 5A–H (**A**) Preoperative axial CT scan demonstrating left mandibular ameloblastoma. (**B**) Post-operative axial CT scan showing fibula free flap in glenoid fossa. (*Continued*)

incidence of plate exposure. This was in contrast to his original paper showing a 29% incidence of hardware related reconstructive failures and is now using this technique for small lateral mandibular defects (14).

Areas which would be problematic to use this type of reconstruction include larger defects of bone and large volume defects medial to the mandible resection.

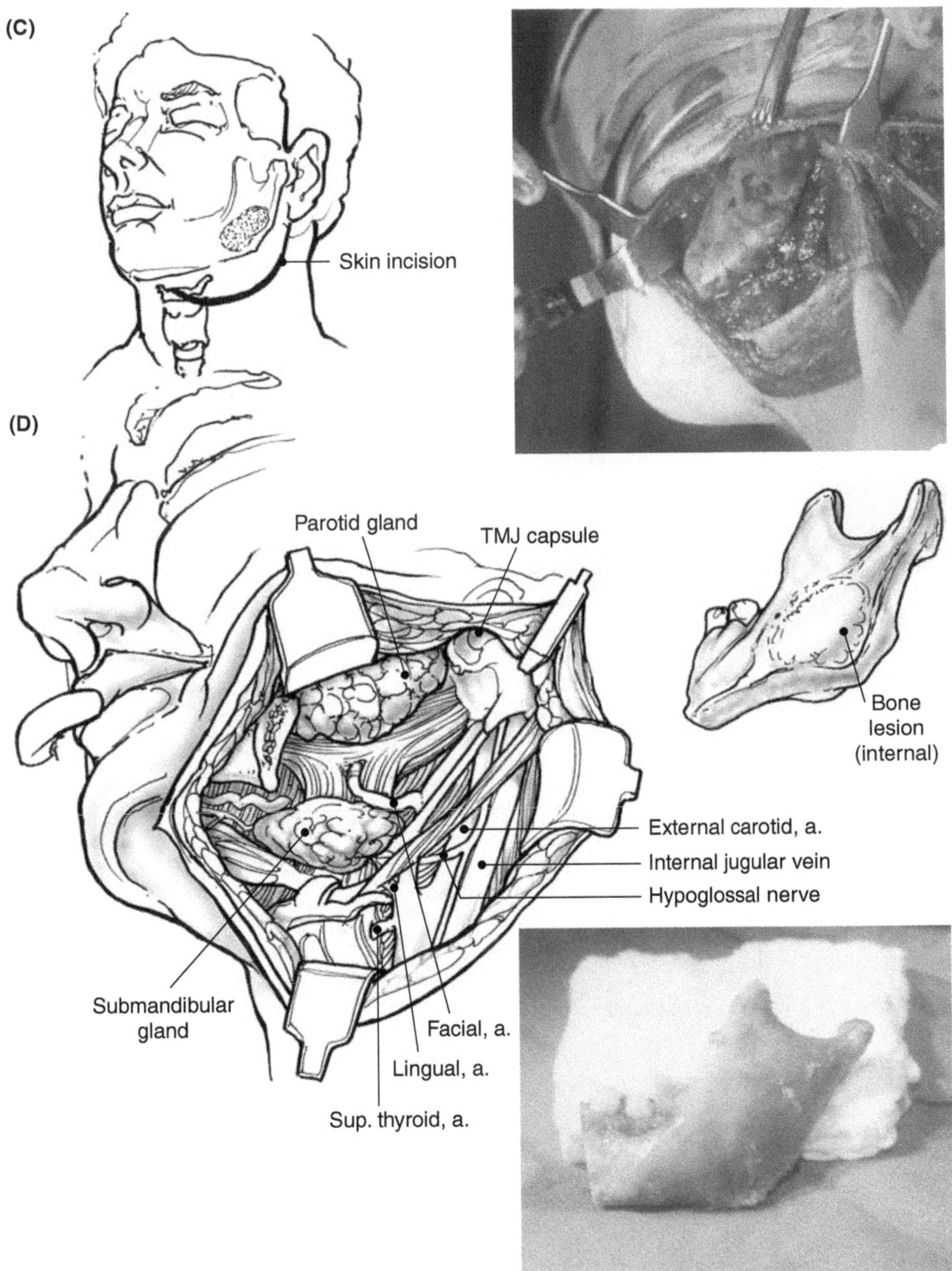

Figure 5 (**C** and **D**) Intraoperative view of mandible and resected specimen. (*Continued*)

This can lead to contraction of tissues inwards against a rigid plate hence, erosion of skin, mucosa and even flap is more likely to occur. It is in these circumstances where the patient would be best served with vascularized bone grafts. Also, if segmental resection includes any tooth-bearing mandible, the patient would be best served with vascularized bone to allow dental implantation.

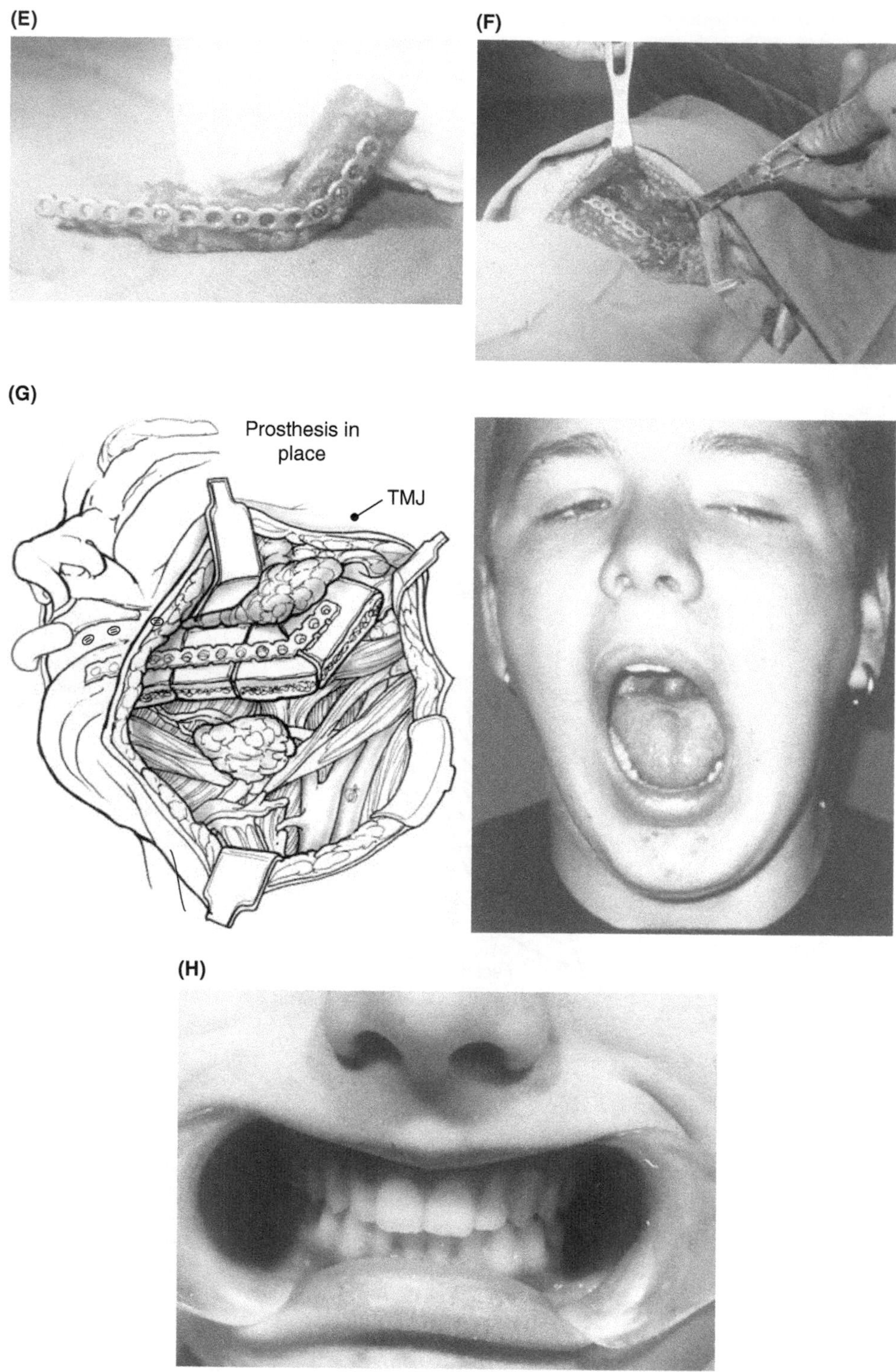

Figure 5 (**E**) Fibula free flap contoured and affixed to recontruction plate. (**F**) Inset free flap in defect. (**G** and **H**) Post-operative photographs showing jaw opening with greater that 4.5 cm incisor to incisor distance and excellent occlusion.

Posterior Defects (Condylar)

Four methods have been advocated for condylar/posterior defect. One can incompletely reconstruct the mandibular ramus so it does not extend to the glenoid fossa. This relies on the contralateral joint for alignment and motion. By not entering the joint, there is thought to be a decreased chance of fibrosis and therefore, it doesn't decrease jaw motion. Prosthetic condyles which are part of the reconstruction plate have been used alone or with a free flap. Too much pressure is created in the joint and these patients develop pain over time secondary to wear. Also, erosion through the glenoid can occur with displacement into the middle cranial fossa. This is no longer food and drug administration (FDA) approved in the United States. However, it could be used temporarily while awaiting permanent reconstruction. Mounting the resected condyle on the end of a flap with a miniplate has been described. Costochondral grafts can also be used in a similar fashion. The problem here is that resorption of the graft tends to occur in the glenoid fossa. Of course, vascularized free flaps into the glenoid fossa provide a method to maintain mandibular height and TMJ motion. We believe that the best results are achieved by placing vascularized bone directly into the glenoid fossa and have good success rates using this technique. Figure 5 illustrates a patient reconstructed using this technique. Soft tissue flaps are used in these posterior condylar defects as an acceptable alternative for those patients who have poor general health, poor tumor prognosis, or who are not good surgical candidates for a complex surgical procedure (34).

CONCLUSION

Mandibular reconstruction continues to challenge the head and neck surgeon. Figure 6 provides an algorithm to consider when determining the best method for reconstruction of the mandible. Although, no method meets all the requirements, free tissue transfer techniques allow us to more consistently and reliably meet the

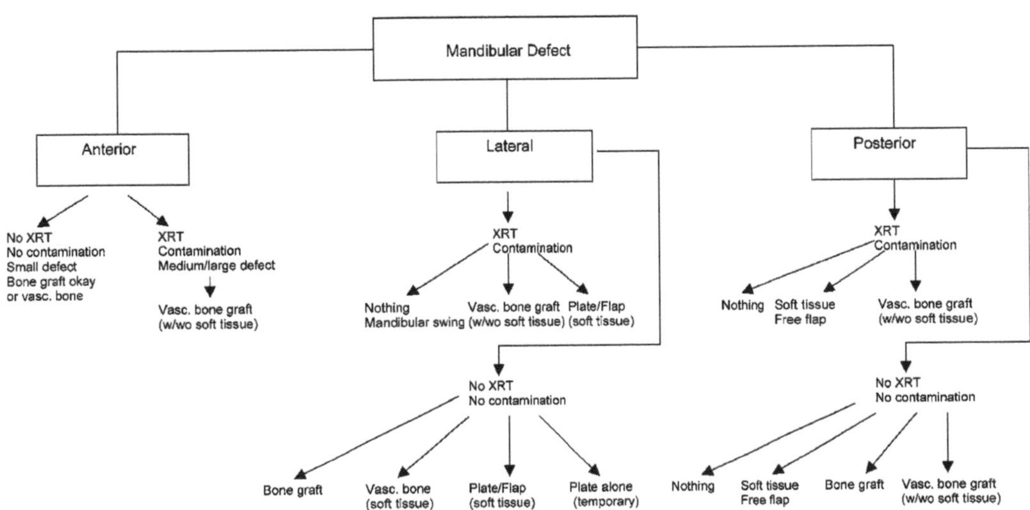

Figure 6 Algorithm for mandibular reconstruction based on location.

needs of the patient. Each donor site has specific advantages and disadvantages. There must be adequate bone and soft tissue to reconstruct the particular defect. The status of the patient will always play a role in reconstruction selection. If suitable, we believe mandibular reconstruction with vascularized bone provides optimal function and cosmesis. Successful reconstruction requires thoughtful selection of a donor site tailored to each patient's needs. We have passed the era when successful oromandibular reconstruction is judged by survival of the flap or graft. With flap survival rates exceeding 95%, the focus is now on function and aesthetics. Objective means to measure functional deficits and postoperative results are available and need to be instituted into meaningful comparative studies (35).

REFERENCES

1. Conley J. Use of composite flaps containing bone for major repairs in the head and neck. Plast Reconstr Surg 1972; 49(5):522–526.
2. Foster RD, Anthony JP, Sharma A, Pogrel MA. Vascularized bone flaps versus nonvascularized bone grafts for mandibular reconstruction: an outcome analysis of primary bony union and endosseous implant success. Head and Neck 1999; 21:66–71.
3. Komisar A. The functional result of mandibular reconstruction. Laryngoscope 1990; 100:364–374.
4. Shibahara T, Noma H, Takasaki Y, Nomura T. Repair of the inferior alveolar nerve with forearm cutaneous nerve graft after ablative surgery of the mandible. J Oral and Maxillofacial Surgery 2000; 58:714–717.
5. Axhausen W. The osteogenetic phases of regeneration of bone, a historical and experimental study. J Bone Joint Surg Am 1956; 38-A:593.
6. Urist MR. The substratum for bone morphogenesis. Dev Biol 1970; 4(suppl):125.
7. Lawson W, Boek S, Loscalzo L, et al. Experience with immediate and delayed mandibular reconstruction. Laryngoscope 1982; 92:5–10.
8. Hamaker RC. Irradiated autogenous mandibular grafts in primary reconstructions. Laryngoscope 1981; 91:1031–1051.
9. Leipzig B, Cummings CW. The current status of mandibular reconstruction using autogenous frozen mandibular grafts. Head Neck Surg 1984; 6:992–996.
10. Schmoper RR. Mandibular reconstruction using a special plate: animal experiments and clinical experience. J Maxillofacial Surg 1983; 11:99–106.
11. Benoist M. Experience with 220 cases of mandibular reconstruction. J Maxillofacial Surg 1978; 6:40–49.
12. Raveh V, Stitch H, Sutter F. The use of titanium-coated hollow screw and reconstruction plate system in bridging of lower jaw defects. J Oral Maxillofacial Surg 1984; 42:281–286.
13. Gullane PJ, Holmes H. Mandibular reconstruction-new concept. Arch Otol Head Neck Surg 1976; 112:714–719.
14. Blackwell KE, Buchbinder D, Urken ML. Lateral mandibular reconstruction using soft-tissue free flaps and plates. Arch Otolaryngol Head Neck Surg 1996; 122:672–678.
15. Hoffman HT, Harrison N, Sullivan MJ, et al. Mandible reconstruction with vascularized bone grafts. Arch Otolaryngol Head Neck Surg 1991; 117:917–925.
16. Krespi YP, Oppenheimer W, Flanzer JM. The rhombotrapezius myocutaneous flaps. Arch Otol Head Neck Surg 1988; 114:734–738.
17. Urken ML, Buchbinder D, Costantino PD, Sinha U, Okay D, Lawson W, Biller HF. Oromandibular reconstruction using microvascular composite flaps. Arch Otol Head Neck Surg 1998; 124:46–55.

18. Urken ML, Buchbinder D, Vickery C, Weinberg J, Sheiner A, Biller HF. Primary placement of osseointegrated implants in microvascular mandibular reconstruction. Otol Head Neck Surg 1989; 101:56–73.
19. Aviv JE, Urken ML, Buchbinder D, Vickery C, Weinberg H, Biller HF. The combined latissimus dorsi-scapular free flap in head and neck reconstruction. Arch Otol Head Neck Surg 1991; 117:1242–1250.
20. Taylor GI, Miller GH, Ham FJ. The free vascularized bone graft. Clinical extension of microvascular techniques. Plast Reconstr Surg 1975:533–539.
21. Hidalgo DA. Fibular free flap. A new method of mandibular reconstruction. Plast Reconstr Surg 1989; 84:71–77.
22. O'Leary MJ, Martin PJ, Hayden RE. The neurocutaneous free fibula flap in mandibular reconstruction. Otolaryngol Clinica N Am 1994; 27(6):1081–1096.
23. Urken ML, Vickery C, Weinberg H, et al. The internal oblique-iliac crest osseomyocutaneous microvascular free flap in head and neck reconstruction. J Reconst Microsurg 1989; 5:203–214.
24. Urken ML, Vickery C, Weinberg H, et al. The internal oblique-iliac crest osseomyocutaneous free flap in oromandibular reconstruction: report of 20 cases. Arch Otol Head Neck Surg 1989; 115:339–349.
25. Thoma A, Khadaroo R, Grigenas O, Archibald S, Jackson S, Young JEM, Veltri K. Oromandibular reconstruction with the radial-forearm osteocutaneous flap: Experience with 60 consecutive cases. Plast Reconst Surg 1999; 104:368–378.
26. Bowers KW, Edmonds JL, Girod DA, Jayaraman G, Chua CP, Toby EB. Osteocutaneous radial forearm free flaps. J Bone Joint Surg 2000; 82-A(5):694–704.
27. McLeod AM, Robinson DW. Reconstruction of defects involving the mandible and floor of mouth by free osteocutaneous flaps derived from the foot. Br J Plast Surg 1982; 35: 239–246.
28. McKee BM. Microvascular bone transplantation. Clin Plast Surg 1978; 5:283–292.
29. Schmidt D, Robson M. One stage composite reconstruction using latissimus myocutaneous free flap. Am J Surg 1982; 144:470–472.
30. Maruzanma V, Urita V, Ohnishi K. Rib-latissimus dorsi osteomyocutaneous flap in reconstruction of a mandibular defect. Br J Plast Surg 1985; 38:234–237.
31. Serafin D, Ricfbohl R, Thomas I, et al. Vascularized rib periosteal and osteocutaneous reconstruction of the maxilla and mandible: an assessment. Plast Reconst Surg 1980; 66:718–721.
32. Curtis DA, Plesh O, Miller AJ, Curtis TA, Sharma A, Schweitzer R, Hilsinger RL, Schour L, Singer M. A comparison of masticatory function in patients with or without reconstruction of the mandible. Head and Neck 1997; 19:287–296.
33. Blackwell KE, Lacombe V. The bridging lateral mandibular reconstruction plate revisited. Archives Otolaryngol Head Neck Surg 1999; 125:988–993.
34. Kroll SS, Robb GL, Miller MJ, Reese GP, Evans GRD. Reconstruction of posterior mandibular defects with soft tissue using the rectus abdominis free flap. Br J Plast Surg 1998; 51:503–507.

18
Composite Defects of the Oromandibular Complex

Douglas A. Girod
Department of Otolaryngology—Head and Neck Surgery, University of Kansas School of Medicine, Kansas City, Kansas, U.S.A.

Terance T. Tsue
Medical Research Service, Veterans Affairs Medical Center, Kansas City, Missouri, and Department of Otolaryngology—Head and Neck Surgery, University of Kansas School of Medicine, Kansas City, Kansas, U.S.A.

INTRODUCTION

The oral cavity presents tremendous complexity of both form and function. Located in a highly visible location, it plays a key role in aesthetics, oral competence, articulation, mastication, deglutition, taste, oral hygiene, respiration and airway protection. Thus any alteration in the structure of the oral cavity can impact significantly on daily activities and social interaction.

Surgical resection of tumors of the oral cavity, alone or in combination with radiotherapy remains a mainstay of current management. The consequence of therapy invariably results in some degree of dysfunction and adversely affects the patients' quality of life. Due to the complex anatomical structures comprising the oral cavity, the larger the soft tissue defect the greater the impact on function. The resulting dysfunction is magnified considerably when a portion of the mandibular arch is resected along with the soft tissues creating a composite defect. While the options for therapy and the overall cure rates have changed very little over the last 15 to 20 years, there has been considerable progress in the reconstruction of the oral cavity.

An increased awareness of the importance of soft tissue mobility and sensation for oral cavity function, and mandibular continuity for cosmesis and potential dental rehabilitation has fueled significant advancements in reconstructive techniques. The result has been a movement away from loco-regional reconstructive options toward more complex microvascular techniques for the management of these highly complicated defects.

RELEVANT ANATOMY

The anatomy and physiology of the oral cavity has been discussed in detail earlier in this text (chapters 2 and 3). When contemplating the management of large composite defects of the oromandibular complex it is useful to divide the oral cavity into three major regions: anterior, lateral and posterior. Each of these three regions has specific anatomical and functional issues, each of which must be considered for planning of a successful reconstruction. While it may not be possible to specifically address all aspects of the anatomy and function with the reconstructive approach chosen, the recognition of these issues will allow for maximal benefit despite the necessary compromises. Obviously, all defects do not fall conveniently into artificial divisions and may involve two or even all three of these regions. Regardless, the issues remain the same and should be considered appropriately.

Anterior Defects. Composite defects of the anterior oromandibular complex pose the single greatest challenge in head and neck reconstruction due to the tremendous cosmetic and functional importance of this region. Comprising the entire lower 1/3 of the face, symmetry and projection are critical aesthetic components that are largely determined by the anterior mandibular arch and the lower lip. Sensation and tension of the lower lip dictates oral competence (to avoid drooling) while movement of the lip facilitates the articulation of speech. In addition to providing projection of the chin, the mandibular arch is necessary for mastication, a contact point for the tongue for articulation and as an anchor for the musculature for the lower 1/3 of the face, the upper neck, the tongue and the hyoid-laryngeal complex. The anterior tongue is one of the most intricately mobile structures in the human body. Its' role in mastication, deglutition, articulation and taste cannot be over-stated.

It is this remarkable high density of aesthetic and functional components coming together in the midline of the anterior oromandibular complex that makes aggressive and thoughtful reconstruction of this region so challenging, yet absolutely necessary.

Lateral Defects. The cheek skin, muscle and buccal mucosa provide the lateral wall to the oral cavity. It is of obvious facial aesthetic importance and provides lateral tension to keep the food bolus between the teeth for mastication. The lateral mandible supports dentition, maintains mandibular position and serves as an anchor for the mylohyoid musculature. The lateral floor of mouth and lateral tongue are most needed for successful mastication and mobility. Overall, lateral defects of the oromandibular complex are less debilitating and better tolerated than anterior defects. This makes a successful and functional reconstruction a readily achievable goal in most instances.

Posterior Defects. Lesions involving the posterior oromandibular complex are often not confined to the oral cavity. Direct extension into the palate, nasopharynx, oropharynx, hypopharynx and tongue base are common and must be anticipated. The additional involvement of these structures can have a significant impact on both speech and swallowing. The reconstructive approach must place a high priority on these additional soft tissue components to achieve overall success.

EVALUATION AND PLANNING

The evaluation of the head and neck surgery patient has been extensively covered in chapter 6. Several specific issues, however, relate to composite defects of the oromandibular complex. The majority of these defects will consist of two primary layers of tissue requiring reconstruction – bone and either mucosa or skin. The largest and most difficult defects to manage involve all three layers of tissue – mucosa, bone and skin.

It is the reconstructive surgeons mandate to determine the impact of the anticipated defect and the relative import of the soft tissue and bony deficits. The different components of the deficit will have varying degrees of impact on cosmesis and function, which dictates the priorities for the planned reconstruction. As might be predicted – the larger the defect, the fewer the reconstructive options.

Soft Tissue Aspects. In most settings it will be the degree of soft tissue loss that will determine the long-term functional outcome for any given patient. The cheek, lip, floor of mouth and soft palate all consist of very thin and mobile tissues. Replacement of these structures with heavy, bulky and relatively immobile tissues will usually restrict the mobility of the remaining tissues and thus impair function further.

The exception to this rule is when the soft tissue loss will result in an inadequate amount of remaining mobile tissues to produce function. In this setting, replacement of lost tissues using tissues of increased bulk and relative immobility can serve to provide a solid foundation for the patient to work with during rehabilitation. This is the case for extensive lower lip and large oral tongue deficits.

Mandibular defects. Reconstruction of the mandible is the primary focus of chapter 17 and has been extensively discussed. This chapter will review reconstruction of the mandible in the context of larger combined composite defects. The location, amount and length of mandibular loss should play a key role in dictating the reconstructive approach for a patient. It is important to remember that not all portions of the mandible are equally important. Whereas posterior or lateral defects may potentially be managed with a reconstruction plate alone, anterior defects will rarely if ever, be successfully managed with a plate over the long term.

Sensory and motor nerve deficits. The impact of the loss of nerve function from resection of cranial nerve branches has been previously discussed in chapter 3. This loss must be anticipated and, whenever possible, the reconstruction plan should include the use of sensate tissues and interposition nerve grafts to facilitate rehabilitation.

While none of the pedicled flaps have the potential for reinnervation by surgical means, there are several options for sensate free flaps including the radial forearm, lateral arm, lateral thigh, dorsalis pedis, ulnar forearm and the fibula osteocutaneous free flap (1–6).

The loss of the inferior alveolar nerve with resection of the mandible is unavoidable other than for a marginal mandibulectomy or limited midline defects. Loss of sensation to the lip is less debilitating than the loss of lingual nerve function but still produces an additional handicap to be dealt with during rehabilitation. The use of cable nerve grafts from the posterior inferior alveolar nerve stump to the mental nerve should be planned whenever possible. The loss of the facial or hypoglossal motor nerves also requires cable nerve grafting provided there is adequate terminal muscle mass remaining for function. The primary sources for donor nerve grafts include the greater auricular nerve, cervical supraclavicular sensory nerves, sural nerve and medial or lateral antebracheal cutaneous nerves from the forearm (harvested during forearm flap elevation).

Cutaneous Defects. The direct involvement of facial skin by a neoplasm of the oral cavity significantly complicates the reconstruction of the oromandibular complex. It is absolutely critical that this eventuality be anticipated and the reconstructive plan prepare for the management of this problem. Most commonly involved are the cheek and neck skin via buccal or submandibular spread although direct involvement from erosion of the lateral mandibular cortex also occurs. Smaller cutaneous defects may be managed with local tissue rearrangement techniques allowing the reconstruction to focus on the intraoral reconstruction. Larger skin and through and through defects will require a more aggressive reconstructive approach. Anterior lesions of the oral cavity may directly involve the lower lip, resulting in a most challenging reconstruction from a functional and cosmetic perspective (7–12).

Rehabilitation. The patient's long-term motivation and capacity for physical and dental rehabilitation should be assessed and contribute to the reconstruction decision-making process. Not all patients are motivated to achieve a full return of function. Others lack the necessary resources to achieve full rehabilitation – especially dental rehabilitation.

The importance of dental rehabilitation for cosmesis, mastication and diet is reviewed in chapter 16. While soft tissue mobility and sensation are still more important for function, only aggressive dental rehabilitation will make near normal function a possibility. The native mandible will support endoseous dental implants for many people although patients with edentulous status of prolonged duration may lack sufficient mandibular bone stock as a result of bone resorption. The donor options for free flap reconstruction of the mandible have been examined for the suitability for dental implantation with the most consistent to least consistent for the support of dental implants being the iliac crest, the fibula, the scapula and the radius bone (13,14). If the patient is anticipated to be capable of this level of endoseous implant rehabilitation then the bony reconstruction should be planned appropriately (13,15,16).

RECONSTRUCTIVE OPTIONS FOR THE OROMANDIBULAR COMPLEX

The use of skin grafting, acellular dermis (Alloderm, Lifecell Corp, Branchburg, New Jersey) and local tissue transfer, have been discussed in detail in previous chapters. These techniques have application for limited intraoral soft tissue defects or occasionally with soft tissue defects associated with a marginal mandibulectomy but will rarely be adequate to manage a composite defect of the oromandibular complex. These large two and three layer composite defects will necessitate a more aggressive reconstructive approach.

The options for the management of two and three layer composite defects of the oromandibular complex are outlined in Table 1.

Regional Tissue Transfer

Prior to the establishment of microvascular free tissue transfer as a reliable and superior reconstruction technique for the oral cavity, several regional flaps were developed to provide reconstructive options. The anterior oral cavity however, posed particular difficulty for most of these flaps given the arc of rotation required by a pedicled flap to reach the midline floor of mouth or alveolar ridge. Both the forehead flap and the deltopectoral flap are unable to reliably reach the midline oral cavity for staged reconstructions. The superiorly-based sternocleidomastoid flap and the

Table 1 Reconstructive Options for the Oromandibular Complex

Two Layer Defects (bone plus mucosa or skin)
Pectoralis Major Myocutaneous Flap + reconstruction plate
Radial Forearm Fasciocutaneous Flap + Reconstruction Plate
Osteocutaneous Radial Forearm Flap
Osteocutaneous Fibula Flap
Osteocutaneous Scapula Flap
Osteocutaneous Iliac Crest + Radial Forearm Fasciocutaneous Flap
Three Layer Defects (bone plus mucosa and skin)
Radial Forearm Fasciocutaneous Flap + Reconstruction Plate
Osteocutaneous Radial Forearm Flap
Osteocutaneous Scapula Flap
Combination of Multiple Flaps
Free Flap + Pectoralis Major Myocutaneous Flap
Radial Forearm Fasciocutaneous Flap + Osteocutaneous Fibula, Scapula or Iliac crest Flap

trapezius myocutaneous flap in its various forms have similar limited rotation restricting their reach to the midline. Only the pectoralis major myocutaneous pedicled flap (PMMF) has found a long-term place in reconstructive options for the oral cavity.

Pectoralis Major Myocutaneous Pedicled Flap (PMMF) Combined With a Reconstruction Plate

The PMMF has been a workhorse in head and neck reconstruction since it was popularized by Ariyan in the 1970s (17–24). The PMMF has immediate proximity to the neck, is well vascularized, found outside the usual neck radiation ports, quickly dissected and tremendously versatile. For these reasons, it remains a reliable tool in the reconstructive surgeon's armamentarium (22,23). While bone (rib) has been raised with this flap (25), it has limited vascular supply from the muscular perforating vessels to the periosteum, thus limiting its reliability. The PMMF can be raised with or without skin and subcutaneous fat depending on the purpose for the flap.

For anterior defects of the oromandibular complex, the loss of bone will result in a severe retracted "Andy Gump" deformity if only a soft tissue reconstruction is completed (Fig. 1). Therefore, the primary setting where the PMMF will be a useful option for an anterior defect is when a marginal mandibulectomy has been performed leaving adequate anterior mandible intact. The chest skin elevated with the PMMF can be used to repair the anterior floor of mouth, alveolar ridge and anterior tongue if necessary.

Lateral and posterior oromandibular composite two layer defects involving mandible and mucosa can be successfully managed with a PMMF alone. The cutaneous portion of the flap is used to repair the soft tissue defect including the buccal mucosa, alveolar ridge, floor of mouth, tongue, palate and pharynx. The skin paddle of the PMMF is fairly bulky and is not readily contoured to recreate the soft palate and tends to decrease tongue mobility. The loss of the mandibular body, angle and/or ramus will disrupt mandibular continuity and cause shifting of the mandible to

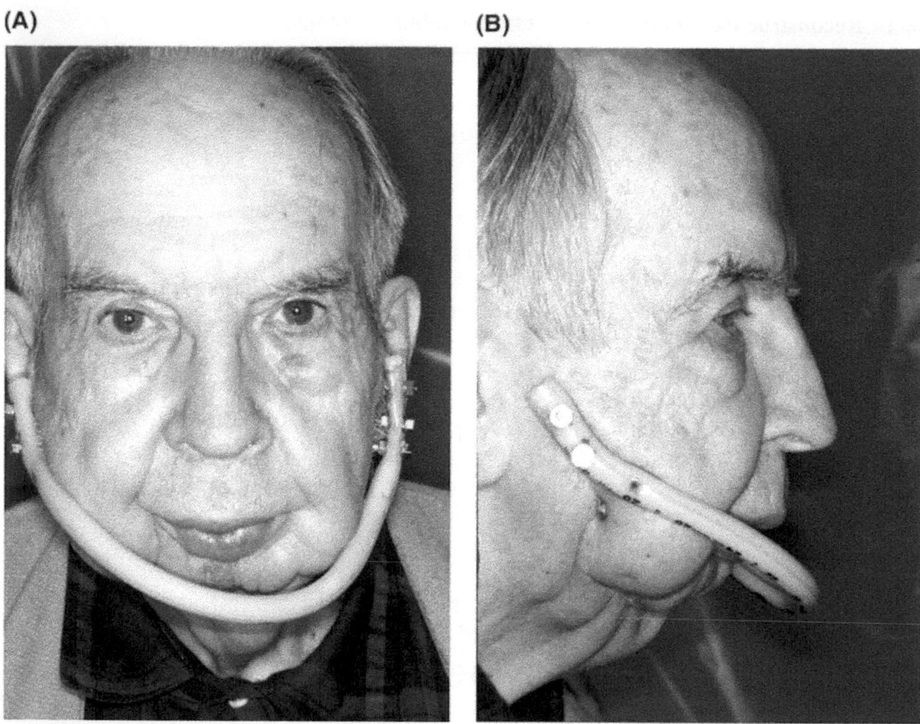

Figure 1 Patient with an anterior mandibular defect resulting in an "Andy Gump" deformity. An external fixator holds the remaining mandible in proper anatomic position.

the side of defect secondary to unopposed muscular forces. Soft tissue mobility will usually be better than with primary closure as, however, the malocclusion and cosmetic deformity resulting from the shift of the mandible will persist. To avoid this problem the PMMF can be combined with a bridging locking reconstruction plate to maintain mandibular continuity.

Reconstruction plates have undergone significant evolution over the last 15 years. Titanium has been established as the most biocompatible metal for plate implants. The introduction and subsequent modification of the locking screw plate has provided increased stability in the form of an "implantable external fixator" which is ideal for use in place of or as an adjunct to bone reconstruction (26–29). The evolution of this technology has been toward smaller lower profile plates and screws ranging from the original 4 mm hollow screw titanium hollow screw reconstruction plate (THORP) system (Synthes North America, seen in Figs. 2A, 3D, 4C, 5C, and 7C) to the 2.4 mm single locking screw system (as seen in Figs. 6C, 8A, and 11C) and the most recent 2.0 mm locking screw system (as seen in Fig. 3A). The 2.0 mm system however, does not provide adequate stability for use without bone grafting. Currently, for reconstruction of the mandible with a plate alone, the authors prefer the 2.4 mm locking screw plates and screws. This plate offers the needed stability yet is much easier to work with compare to the older hollow screw (THORP) plates.

While the use of a bridging reconstruction plate to replace a portion of the mandible may be a more expedient technique than osteocutaneous reconstruction, especially for the patient with a low likelihood of long-term survival, the risk of plate complications remains high (28,30–32). This is especially true for defects of the anterior mandibular arch. Therefore, this approach is most successful for smaller lateral and posterior defects of the oromandibular complex (33). To minimize the risk of complications, most surgeons would now prefer to proceed with primary bone and soft tissue reconstruction if possible, even in the poor prognosis patient.

Technique

PMMF Harvest. The PMMF relies on the pectoral branch of the thoracoacromial artery for vascular supply to the flap. This artery emerges deep to the mid clavicle and runs between the pectoralis major muscle and its deep fascia toward the inferior insertion of the muscle on approximately the sixth rib and the aponeurosis of the external oblique muscle. The initial planning and mapping of the flap is critical for success.

The most cephalad reach of the flap into the oral cavity from the clavicle (the point of rotation) must be measured. This is most effectively done by unfolding a surgical sponge and securing one end to the mid clavicle with one hand and laying the sponge out over the anticipated course of the flap in the neck to the furthest point of the defect subsequently leaving the one end of the sponge fixed at the clavicle, the other end of the sponge can then be rotated to the chest to demonstrate the inferior most extent of skin paddle required. This should be performed without contaminating the chest surgical field from the neck.

The skin paddle should be outlined on the chest centered at the midpoint between the sternum and the nipple. The skin is excised in a superior to inferiorly oriented fusiform shape to facilitate primary closure of the chest wound (Fig. 2B). The superior incision is directed in a curvilinear fashion to the anterior axillary line so as to preserve the vascular supply for a potential future deltopectoral flap.

Dissection is carried out around the skin paddle down to the fascia of the pectoralis muscle where it is tacked with absorbable sutures to minimize shearing forces during dissection and rotation. The surrounding chest skin is then elevated off the pectoralis muscle in all directions in a subfascial plane–again preserving the vascular supply to a deltopectoral flap over the upper chest for future considerations. The PM muscle insertions are then released from the ribs inferiorly taking care to cauterize perforating vessels emerging from the intercostal muscles. As elevation proceeds superiorly, care is taken to elevate the deep fascia with the muscle to protect the pectoral branch of the thoracoacromial artery. The vascular pedicle will become visible under the fascia and will be noted to pass more medially as it is traced superiorly. The superior extent of the dissection is the clavicle. The motor nerves to the pectoralis will be identified and divided during muscle elevation. Next, the medial and lateral attachments of the pectoralis muscle are divided from inferiorly to superiorly. The medial attachment is divided 1–2 cm from the medial intercostal notch to avoid the perforating vessels from the internal mammary arteries. There will be an additional vascular pedicle divided laterally as the humeral head of the muscle is divided. Preservation of this lateral pedicle will severely limit the arc of rotation of the flap. The muscle is divided superiorly all the way to the clavicle to maximize rotation. Care must be taken at this point not to damage the vascular supply to the muscle as it runs more medially.

A tunnel is then elevated on top of the muscle in a subcutaneous plane over the clavicle and into the neck. This passageway should measure at least four finger breadths in width to allow the passage of the muscle over the clavicle and into the neck without constriction. The muscle is then folded on itself from an inferior to

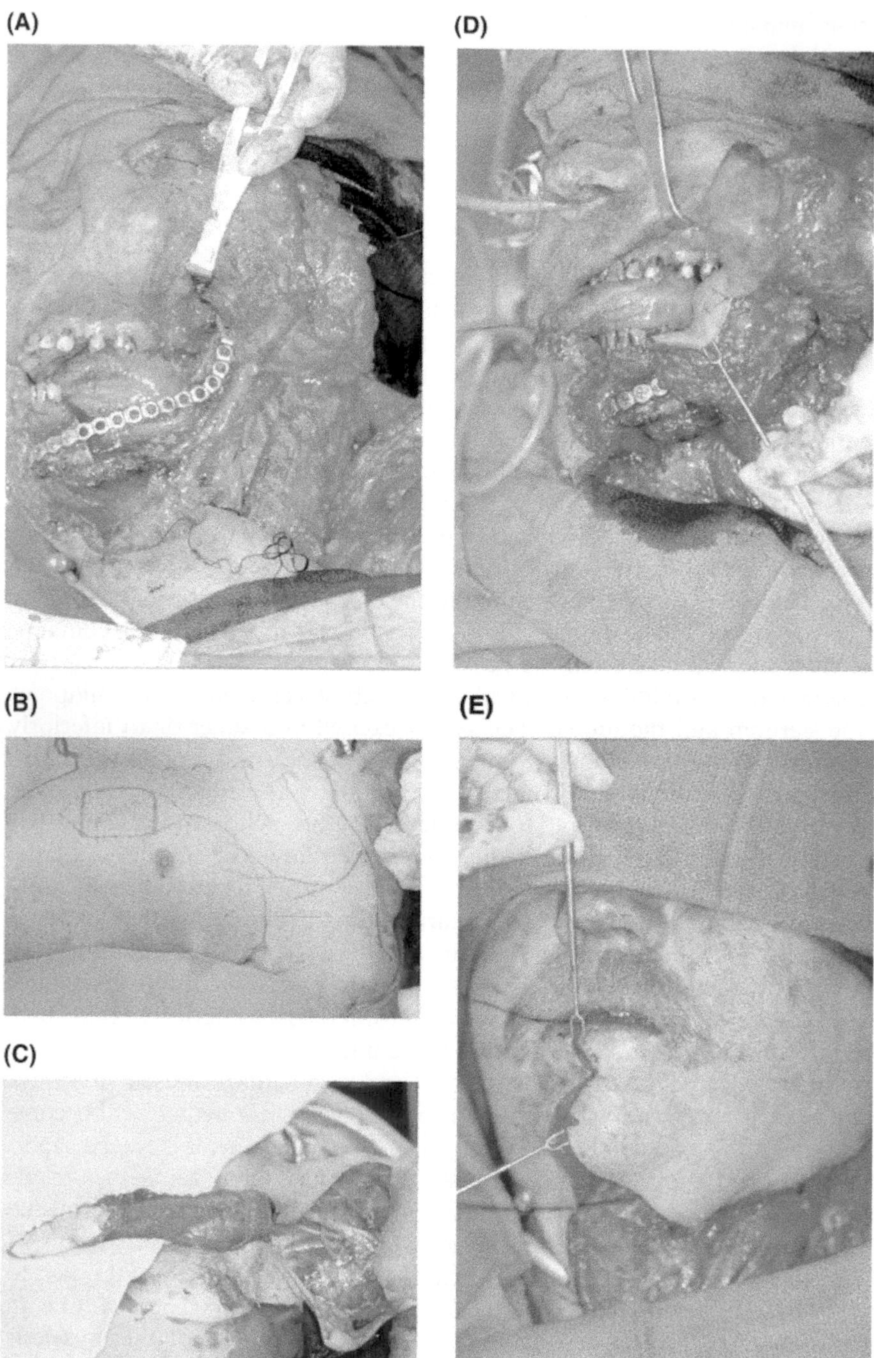

Figure 2 Reconstruction of an oral cavity defect using a reconstruction plate and a pectoralis major myocutaneous pedicled flap. (**A**) Oral cavity and mandibular defect with reconstruction plate spanning the bone defect. (**B**) Skin paddle for the PM flap is outlined on the chest along with the incision to the anterior axillary line which preserves a future deltopectoral flap. (**C**) Harvested PM muscle with skin paddle based on the clavicular head of the muscle containing the vascular pedicle. (**D**) PM flap rotated into the neck with the cutaneous paddle relining the oral cavity defect. The PM muscle is suspended to the plate for support. (**E**) Closure of the lip spit incision after reconstruction.

superior direction and the distal muscle with the attached skin paddle is carefully passed though the tunnel and into the neck (Fig. 2C). It is critical that the skin not suffer extreme shearing forces from the muscle and the muscle is not twisted which can kink the vascular pedicle as it passes over the clavicle.

If the sternocleidomastoid muscle remains intact in the ipsilateral neck it should be removed to make room for the bulk of the PMMF. Once in the neck, the PMMF is rotated into place and the skin paddle tacked into position. For anterior oral cavity defects, the inferior-most chest skin will be placed in the most anterior portion of the defect. For posterior defects the most distal reach for the skin paddle will be the palate or nasopharynx.

The reconstruction plate will usually be formed, fitted and pre-drilled prior to resection and then removed to allow tumor ablation (see next section). To maximize exposure, the reconstruction is initiated with the soft tissue repair and the PMMF inset prior to the reapplication of the plate. The skin paddle is used to fill the defect using absorbable interrupted sutures to create a water-tight closure (Fig. 2D). The muscular pedicle of the PMMF is routed under the plate to avoid compression of the vascular pedicle by the plate resulting is distal flap ischemia. Once the plate is fitted, care should be taken to extensively support the PM muscle to the plate and surrounding soft tissues tissues. This reduces the chance of tension ischemia of the skin paddle, separation of the flap-mucosal repair and the likelihood of the soft tissue pulling away from the plate.

The muscle should then be spread out across the neck to cover the great vessels and provide an even distribution of the bulk. The neck incision should ideally be closed in an airtight fashion with the adequate placement of suction drains. In some patients however, the bulk of the PM muscle will not allow closure without constricting the muscle and therefore the vascular pedicle. In this setting it is preferable to leave a portion of the incision open and place a meshed split thickness skin graft over the exposed muscle.

Reconstruction Plate Application

Whenever possible the reconstruction plate should be fitted and secured prior to the resection of the mandible. Malleable templates are available which are easily conformed to the native mandible. The appropriate length plate can then be bent to match the template form. Placement of the plate at the appropriate height of the mandible is important. If the patient will have good dentition in the remaining mandible the plate must be placed below the tooth roots to avoid damage from the bicortical screws. The plate should be high enough however, so that the neoalveolus height matches the remaining alveolus. Along the anterior midline mandible the bone projects several millimeters beyond the level of the teeth at the mentum. Placement of the plate at this level will result in an over projection of the neomandible and increase the chance for plate complications as well as being cosmetically sub-optimal

For anterior defects in the edentulous patient, the tendency toward over projection can be compensated for by "setting back" the plate one hole on each side of the jaw. This effectively narrows the arch and somewhat under projects the mandible but reduces the stresses on the covering soft tissues and may reduce the likelihood of plate exposure. In the dentulous patient, this can be managed by drilling off the bone at the lower edge of the mandible in the midline to allow placement of the plate at the appropriate level without distortion of the dental occlusal relationships of the remaining teeth.

If the presence of tumor on the lateral aspect of the mandible prevents the pre-bending of the plate prior to resection, several approaches are available. After resection the plate can be molded free-hand using a template to estimate the desired size and shape of the neomandible (Figs. 3A and B). If adequate dentition remains the mandible can be put into mandibulo-maxillary fixation to maintain occlusal relationships prior to fitting the plate. Alternatively, a "fixed bridge" device (Synthes, Paoli, Pennsylvania) may be placed prior to resection, removed for resection, and then replaced to ensure the remaining mandible segments are in appropriate anatomical orientation to each other before the plate is designed and bent free-hand (Figs. 3C and D). In some instances, the fix-bridge device can be left in place during the mandibulectomy, reducing the steps involved with plate bending. Lastly, computed tomography images of the mandible can be sent to commercial providers to fabricate a plastic model of the patient's own mandible preoperatively. This allows the fashioning of the plate to the model, which is then transferred to the patient. The cost of this approach may be prohibitive.

Advantages. The PMMF is handily located immediately adjacent to the neck, is supplied by a predictable robust vascular pedicle, lies outside the usual neck radia-

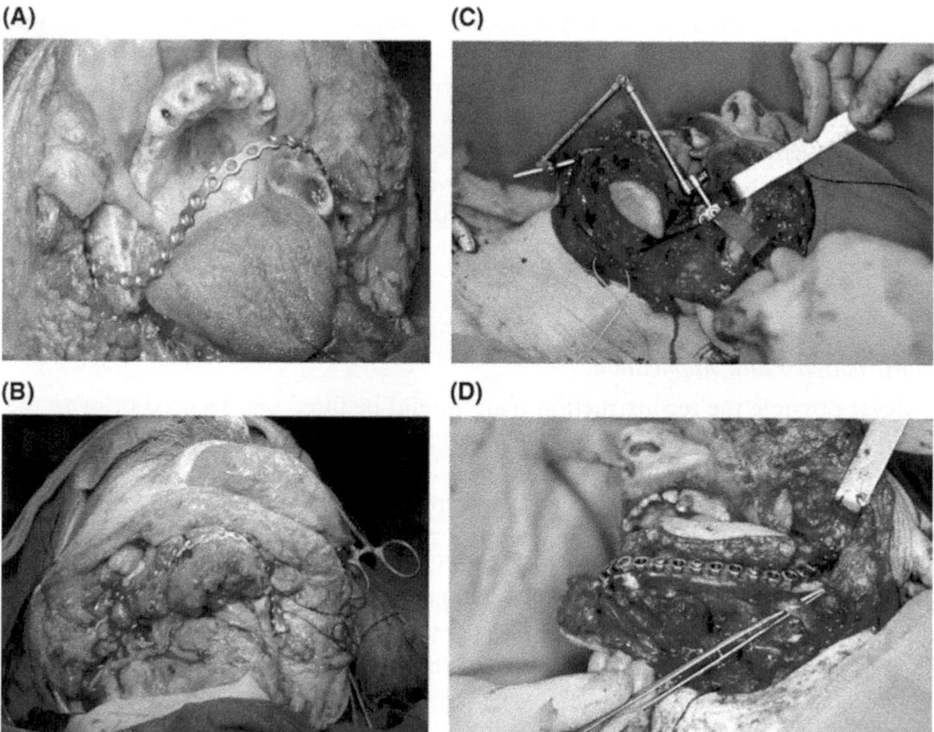

Figure 3 Formation of a plate for mandibular reconstruction when the lateral cortex of the mandible is involved by tumor precluding the pre-bending of the plate prior to resection. (**A**) Reconstruction plate bent free-hand to replaced the resected mandible. This patient is edentulous and thus occlusion is less of an issue. (**B**) Free tissue transfer bone secured to the plate for mandibular reconstruction. (**C**) An intra-operative fixed bridge device secures the position of the non-resected mandible, which allows a plate to be bent and secured after the resection and maintain occlusal relationships. (**D**) Plate and free tissue bone graft in place after removal of the fixed bridge device.

tion field, can be quickly dissected and remains tremendously versatile. The muscle rotated with the skin for vascular supply can also be used for tongue bulk and great vessel coverage. Mandibular continuity and therefore overall form and anatomical relationships are maintained with the use of a reconstruction plate. The added time required to apply a reconstruction plate to the mandible is modest and requires only minimal additional training for the surgeon. The long-term biocompatibility of the newer titanium plates has been proven to be safe and reliable.

Disadvantages. As a pedicled flap, the PMMF has restrictions in arc of rotation and distal reach. The skin paddle is usually very thick and fatty providing more bulk than may be ideal. In addition, partial necrosis of the distal skin paddle can be seen, bone cannot be reliably transferred with the muscle, and wound healing can be delayed. A post-operative orocutaneous fistula incidence of up to 30% can be anticipated (34–36); however, most fistulas will heal readily given the good vascularity of the pecturalis major (PM) muscle even in the post-radiation setting. The donor site morbidity consists of chest deformity and scar, and some upper extremity weakness from muscle loss.

The primary issues with the use of a reconstruction plate and PMMF relate to potential plate complications and the inability to achieve any degree of dental rehabilitation. For posterior and lateral mandibular defects, this approach can be successful in many instances. Plate fracture, mobility or exposure still occur up to 40% of the time in the first year following surgery necessitating additional surgery (32,33,37). Plate reconstruction of the anterior mandibular arch is even less reliable given the extreme muscular and gravitational forces experienced in this location.

Distant Tissue Transfer

The multitude of free tissue transfer options for the reconstruction of the oral cavity has been extensively described in earlier chapters of this text. Experience over the last 15 to 20 years has proven that reconstruction of the oral cavity and pharynx with free tissue transfer techniques has resulted in shorter hospital stays (36,38) fewer post-operative complications including infection and fistula rate and comparable or lower overall cost (36,38–40) when compared with pedicled flap reconstruction. Functional outcome measures are discussed in detail later in this text under a separate chapter. While these measures are difficult to obtain given the diversity of patient populations and clinical experience some studies (38) have confirmed the superiority of free tissue transfer over pedicled flap reconstruction.

This discussion will focus on those options most useful in the reconstruction of composite defects of the oromandibular complex. Excellent options exist for bony reconstruction of the mandible, sensate soft tissue reconstruction of the oral cavity and muscle bulk as needed for tongue reconstruction. Unfortunately, not all these features are ideally available in any one defined flap. Therefore it is the reconstructive surgeons mandate to prioritize the various tissue requirements of the reconstruction and then select the appropriate flap for a given patient.

Fasciocutaneous Radial Forearm Free Flap Combined with a Reconstruction Plate

The radial forearm free flap (RFFF) described by Yang (1978) is an ideal source for thin pliable skin that can be successfully transferred in a sensate fashion to the oral cavity (2,4,6,41–46). Large amounts of skin are available for transfer and the ease of harvest, the long vascular pedicle and the ability to harvest the flap simultaneous to ongoing work in the neck have made this the new workhorse for head and neck reconstruction. There is less bulk, more available skin, limitless options for positioning and sensate capacity when compared to the PMMF, making the RFFF the preferred choice of most surgeons in this setting.

Other fasciocutaneous options include the ulnar forearm free flap, the lateral arm flap and the lateral thigh flap. Each of these flaps has advantages and disadvantages but lack the versatility and pedicle length of the RFFF.

Following resection of the mandible with an extensive loss of soft tissue, the defect can be managed with a reconstruction plate to re-establish mandibular continuity and facial contour and a fasciocutaneous RFFF for soft tissue reconstruction (Fig. 4). This approach can be successful for both two and three layer defects. As discussed previously, the use of a reconstruction plate to replace mandible, span a defect and maintain continuity carries a risk of delayed complications, especially for anterior defects (Fig. 5). The use of vascularized bone flaps should at least be considered when planning the reconstruction approach.

The fasciocutaneous RFFF is the most commonly utilized free flap to provide the soft tissue reconstruction over a reconstruction plate. All the advantages of this flap described above hold true in this setting. The reliability and versatility of the RFFF remain unequaled in oral cavity reconstruction.

Technique

The harvest of the RFFF has been described elsewhere in this text so will not be repeated. In most instances, it will be desirable to have a sensate flap so care must be taken to identify and harvest the medial and lateral antebrachial cutaneous nerves along with the flap. Maximal pedicle length is obtained to allow easy reach from the midline anterior oral cavity to the great vessels in the neck.

Prior to flap inset, care should be taken to smooth all cut edges of bone along the mandibulectomy to minimize the risk of delayed bone exposure. Nerve grafting should occur fairly early in the flap insertion process while exposure is maximized. If the lingual nerve has not been sacrificed during the resection, leaving a stump for grafting, an end-to-side anastomosis can be performed by making a partial incision of an intact lingual nerve. Other potential recipient nerves include the inferior alveolar nerve, the greater auricular nerve and cervical sensory nerves.

On inset, significant contouring of the flap is possible to recreate the gingivolabial sulcus and anterior floor of mouth using buried tacking sutures from flap fascia to periosteum or the reconstruction plate. Care must be exercised not to excessively tighten down the flap as post-operative flap edema can result in venous congestion and pedicle thrombosis if adequate laxity for expansion is not provided. The flap can be thinned and recontoured at a later date in a staged fashion if desired.

Advantages. The RFFF can be transferred with a greater than 95% success rate making this a highly reliable option (47–50). The improved vascularity and versatility of the long vascular pedicle when compared to a PMMF result in a post-operative fistula rate of less than 5% (36,38). The thin skin with limited subcutaneous fat maintains better tongue mobility than the bulk of the PMMF. The recovery of sensation through nerve grafting improves oral function in the long-term. Reduced operative time and potential donor site morbidity compared to osteocutaneous flap reconstruction. The RFFF combined with a reconstruction plate allows

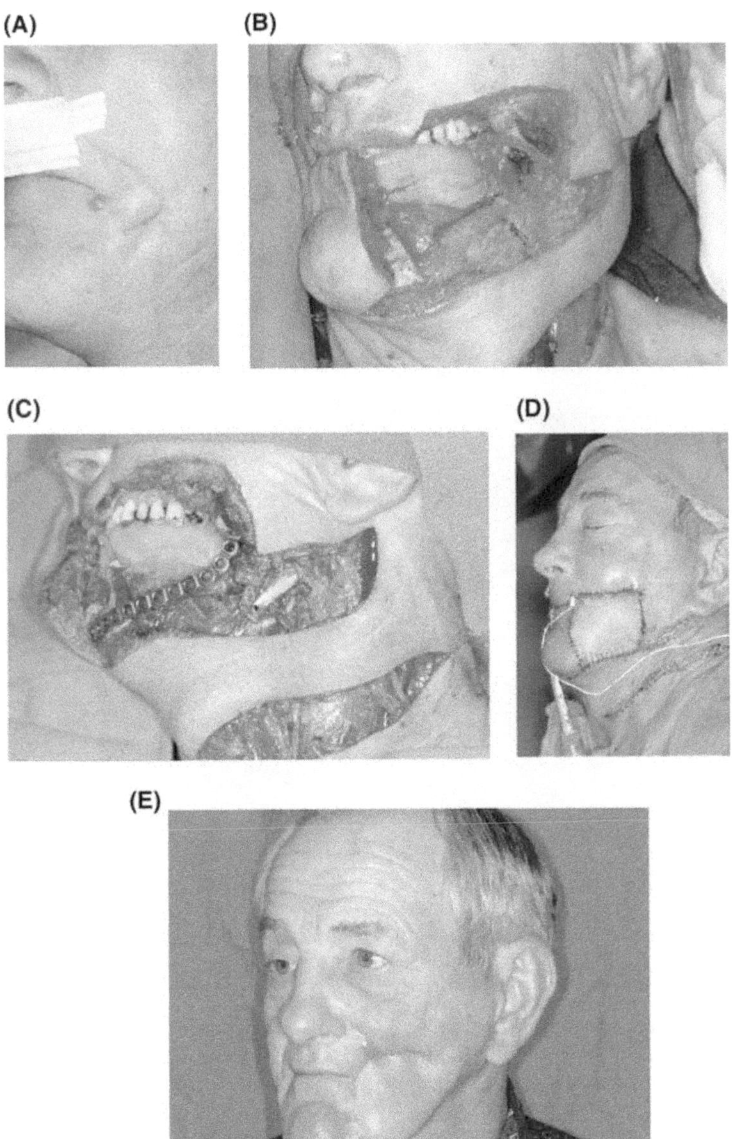

Figure 4A–E Reconstruction of a full thickness buccal composite defect with a reconstruction plate and a fasciocutaneous RFFF. (**A**) Recurrent buccal carcinoma involving skin with prior radiation therapy. (**B**) Complete through and through buccal defect following resection. (**C**) Reconstruction plate placed to span the bone defect. (**D**) Closure of the soft tissue defect with a fasciocutaneous RFFF. The mid portion of the flap is de-epithelialized to allow the skin paddle to fold onto itself and thus line the buccal defect and the cheek defect. (**E**) Six month follow-up appearance.

for a concentrated focus on the soft tissue reconstruction using the highest quality transferable skin available.

Disadvantages. Increased operative time and additional expertise, equipment requirements and close post-operative monitoring are required for the successful performance of microvascular free tissue transfer. Although hospital length of stay

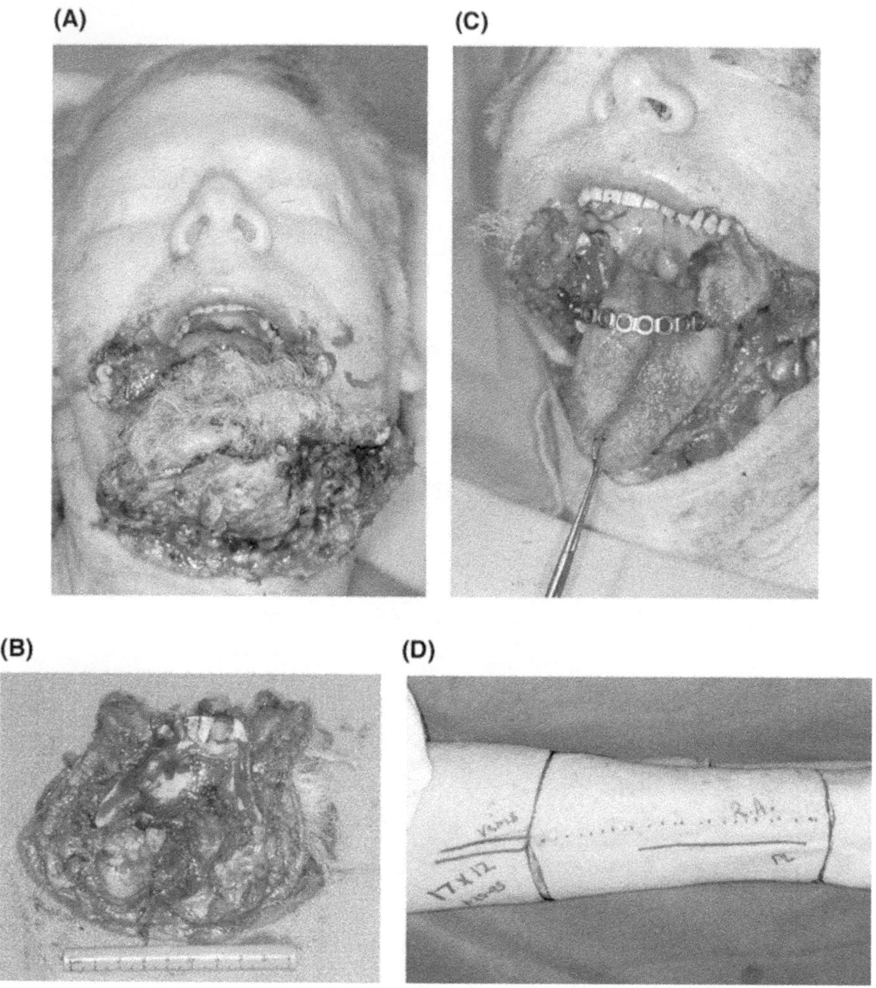

Figure 5A–H Resection and reconstruction of a large T4N3M0 squamous cell carcinoma of the lower lip using a reconstruction plate and fasciocutaneous RFFF. (**A**) Lower lip carcinoma involving the entire lower lip, portions of the upper lip, the chin, mandible, and gingiva with a large necrotic submental lymph node. (**B**) Composite resection specimen. (**C**) Oral cavity, lip and neck defect with a reconstruction plate in position. (**D**) Outline of a large cutaneous paddle for the radial forearm free flap (RFFF). (*Continued*)

is reduced, overall costs are about comparable to PMMF reconstruction given the additional operative costs for free tissue transfer (36,38). There is no potential for dental rehabilitation in the absence of bone reconstruction. As with the PMMF and reconstruction plate there remains a high probability of plate exposure or failure even in the short term, particularly for anterior defects (Fig. 5H) (32,37).

Osteocutaneous Fibula Free Flap

The osteocutaneous fibula free flap has become the mainstay for mandibular reconstruction at most institutions. The fibula is touted as the "the most donateable bone in the body" with up to 25 cm of bone available for harvest and usually has adequate

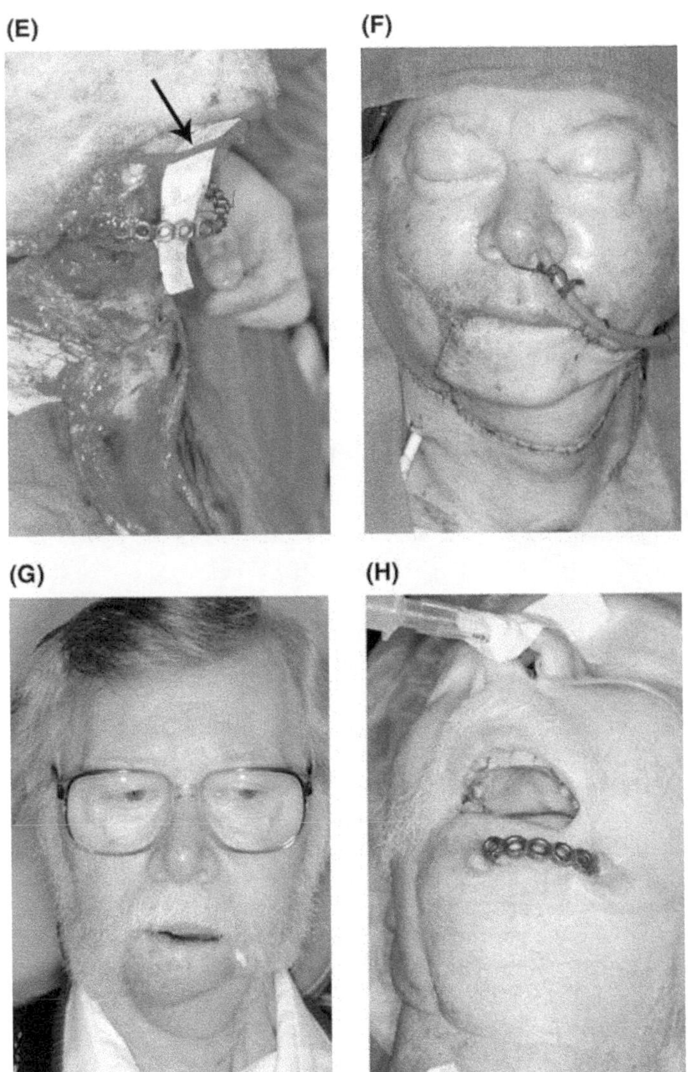

Figure 5 (**E**) Palmaris longus tendon secured to the maxilla bilaterally to suspend the skin of the RFFF to create a new lower lip. (**F**) Closure of the defect using the large fasciocutaneous RFFF. (**G**) One month postoperative appearance, eating a soft diet and preparing for radiation therapy. (**H**) One year postoperative appearance with the exposure of the reconstruction plate at the anterior mandibular arch.

bone stock to support dental implantation. With such lengths of bone available the entire mandible may be reconstructed with vascularized bone if required. Multiple osteotomies may be performed to shape the fibula to reconstruct the anterior arch, body, angle and/or ramus of the mandible as long as the fibular periosteum is not disrupted (Fig. 6). The vascular angiosome of the fibula flap is based on the deep peroneal artery which takes off from the bifurcation of the popliteal artery with the posterior tibial artery just below the knee. The cutaneous portion of the flap is supported by septocutaneous or musculocutaneous perforating vessels passing along the posterior crural septum and/or through flexor hallucis longus, tibialis posterior,

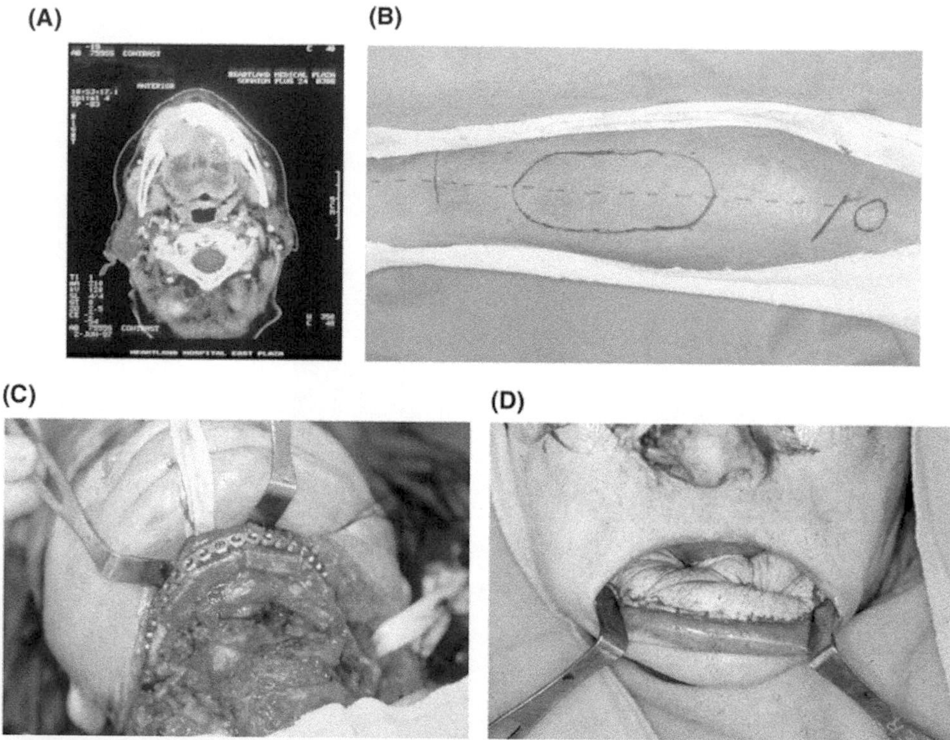

Figure 6 Reconstruction of the anterior oral cavity and mandibular arch with a fibula osteocutaneous free flap. (**A**) CT scan of the neck showing mandible erosion from direct tumor extension of an anterior floor of mouth carcinoma. (**B**) Outline of the cutaneous paddle for the fibula osteocutaneous free flap. (**C**) Facial degloving approach reconstruction of the anterior mandibular arch with a reconstruction plate securing the fibula bone graft. The fibula has undergone two osteotomies preserving the periosteum, to allow reformation of the rounded arch. (**D**) Intra oral soft tissue reconstruction is accomplished with the cutaneous paddle of the flap from the lateral leg.

or soleus muscles to supply the subcutaneous tissues (51,52). These perforating vessels can be quite variable in location and quantity effecting the placement and reliability of the skin paddle. The skin of the lower lateral leg is thin and pliable with large amounts of skin available if needed. The skin may be transferred in a sensate fashion using the lateral sural cutaneous nerve, which is a branch of the common peroneal nerve. With smaller skin paddles the donor defect may be closed primarily, with larger defects, a split thickness skin graft is utilized. In one study, there are fewer donor site complications with skin graft closure when compared to primary closure (53).

Technique

The harvest technique for the fibula osteocutaneous free flap has been described in detail in chapter 17 and will not be repeated here. However, when reconstructing major defects of the oral cavity, the necessary placement of the flap may make vascular pedicle length an issue. The pedicle length of the fibula as harvested is quite short (4 cm or less). This will usually need to be lengthened by elevating the periosteum off the proximal fibula graft and resecting proximal bone. In most cases, this sacrifice of bone is not an issue as adequate bone will remain for mandibular repair. If a complete or near-complete mandibular reconstruction is needed, vein grafting from the neck to the flap pedicle may be necessary.

For repair of anterior oromandibular defects the arch of the mandible will need to be reconstructed. The authors have found that locking screw reconstruction plates work well to maintain the position of the remaining mandible and provide a framework to secure the bone grafts during healing (Fig. 6C). More recently available low profile small (2.0 mm) plates provide adequate support yet should be less likely to result in later plate exposure (Fig. 3A).

The skin paddle of the fibula flap is thin and pliable and can be contoured to recreate the structures of the oral cavity or replace external skin for two layer defects (Fig. 6D). For larger three layer defects the mid portion of the skin paddle can be de-epithelialized, keeping the subcutaneous fascia intact. This allows the skin to be folded onto itself and utilized to reconstruct both internal and external defects. In most instances, however, there is inadequate skin and questionable cutaneous vascular supply to allow for extensive soft tissue reconstruction.

If a sensate flap is indicated the sural cutaneous nerve should be harvested with the skin paddle and anastomosed to an appropriate recipient nerve in the oral cavity or neck (54).

Advantages. The distant location of the lower extremity from the oral cavity makes simultaneous harvest with the head and neck procedure straightforward. The available length of bone and adequate bone stock for dental implantation make the fibula an optimal bone for mandibular reconstruction. The skin of the lower extremity is thin and pliable and may be transferred in a sensate fashion.

Disadvantages. The primary disadvantage of the fibula flap is the limitations of the skin paddle. Adequate skin is not available for larger soft tissue defects or most 3-layer defects requiring a second flap for soft tissue repair. The somewhat unreliable nature of the presence and location of the cutaneous perforator vascular supply require that an alternative option be available on every case (although infrequently utilized). The limited rotational mobility of the skin paddle relative to the bone also limits soft tissue reconstruction is some settings. If dental implants are not planned, the fibula bone results in a very broad and rounded neomandible, which is quite difficult to fit for a tissue-borne prosthesis.

The long-term morbidity of fibula harvest includes some sensory deficit to the lower extremity and potential joint instability (53,55). The use of a walking aid for several months is not unusual and physical therapy may be required for achievement of maximal rehabilitation.

Osteocutaneous RFFF

The RFFF has also been described as an osteocutaneous flap (OCRFFF) with harvest of a portion of the radius bone based on perforators in the intermuscular septum passing to the periosteum (5,56,57). This significantly broadened the applicability of the forearm flap in reconstructive surgery. While seemingly the best of options with tremendous soft tissue characteristics and an option for bone harvest, the widespread acceptance of the OCRFFF has been limited by two significant issues.

First is the amount and quality of bone stock available for harvest. The length of radius bone that can be safely harvested without unacceptable forearm dysfunction is limited to 10–12 cm. The insertions of the pronator teres muscle proximally and the brachioradialis tendon distally define the relative limits of bone harvest. To avoid compromise of the integrity of the radius bone, the thickness of the bone harvested is recommended to be limited to 40% of the circumference of the radius by most authors (58,59). This is generally does not provide adequate bone stock to support endosseous dental implants (13,14).

The second and more problematic issue is that of donor site morbidity. Removing a segment of bone from the radius significantly weakens the bone, especially to torsional forces. This has resulted in a post-operative pathologic radius fracture rate of up to 66% with an average of 23% (60–63). This weakening of the donor radius bone has prompted some to recommend the OCRFFF be abandoned for the other osteocutaneous flap options (59).

Despite the limitations of bone availability with the OCRFFF, it has been used successfully for oromandibular reconstruction with fewer complications than the fasciocutaneous RFFF with plate reconstruction (37,59,64,65) (Fig. 7). For limited mandibular defects, the radius bone is very adequate and can easily bear a tissue-borne prosthesis (denture). As previously mentioned, the bone of the OCRFFF is usually not sufficient for the support of dental implants. Unfortunately, many patients do no have the financial means for dental implantation which is frequently not covered by many third-party payers. In this setting, the radius bone provides a superior contour for the support of a tissue-borne prosthesis when compared to either the fibula or scapula bone.

If the segmental mandibular defect is 5 cm or less the OCRFFF can be effectively utilized to equal or exceed the bone stock of the fibula in a given patient. The radius bone graft is harvested to provide a length of bone just longer than twice that of the defect. A central segment of the radius is then excised allowing the bone to be folded onto itself to create a full tube of bone (Fig. 8). This should allow dental implantation in most patients.

The OCRFFF offers the highest quality soft tissue available for oral cavity reconstruction and adequate bone for limited mandibular defects. With a modification of the harvest technique to include the prophylactic internal fixation of the radius bone, the donor site morbidity can now be successfully minimized (65,66). With the risk of pathological fracture of the radius eliminated, the OCRFFF offers a very useful technique with tremendous versatility for reconstruction of the oromandibular complex.

Prophylactic Internal Fixation of the Radius Bone

The impact of harvesting 50% circumference of the radius for OCRFFF on bone strength has been shown to significantly reduced radius strength by 82% for torsional forces and 76% for 4-point bending forces (66,67). Harvest of the same bone graft (8 cm long and 50% of the circumference of the radius) followed by prophylactic internal fixation of the radius bone using an orthopedic reconstruction plate resulted in a reduction of radius bone strength by only 30% for torsional forces and 26% for 4-point bending forces.

This significant improvement in bone strength after graft harvest, using a reliable and proven orthopedic surgical technique, has successfully prevented the problem of pathologic fracture of the radius bone in the clinical setting. No clinically significant radius fractures were reported in 52 patients utilizing this method of OCRFFF harvest (65). Additionally, grip strength and wrist range of motion was not impaired by harvest of this flap on long-term follow-up.

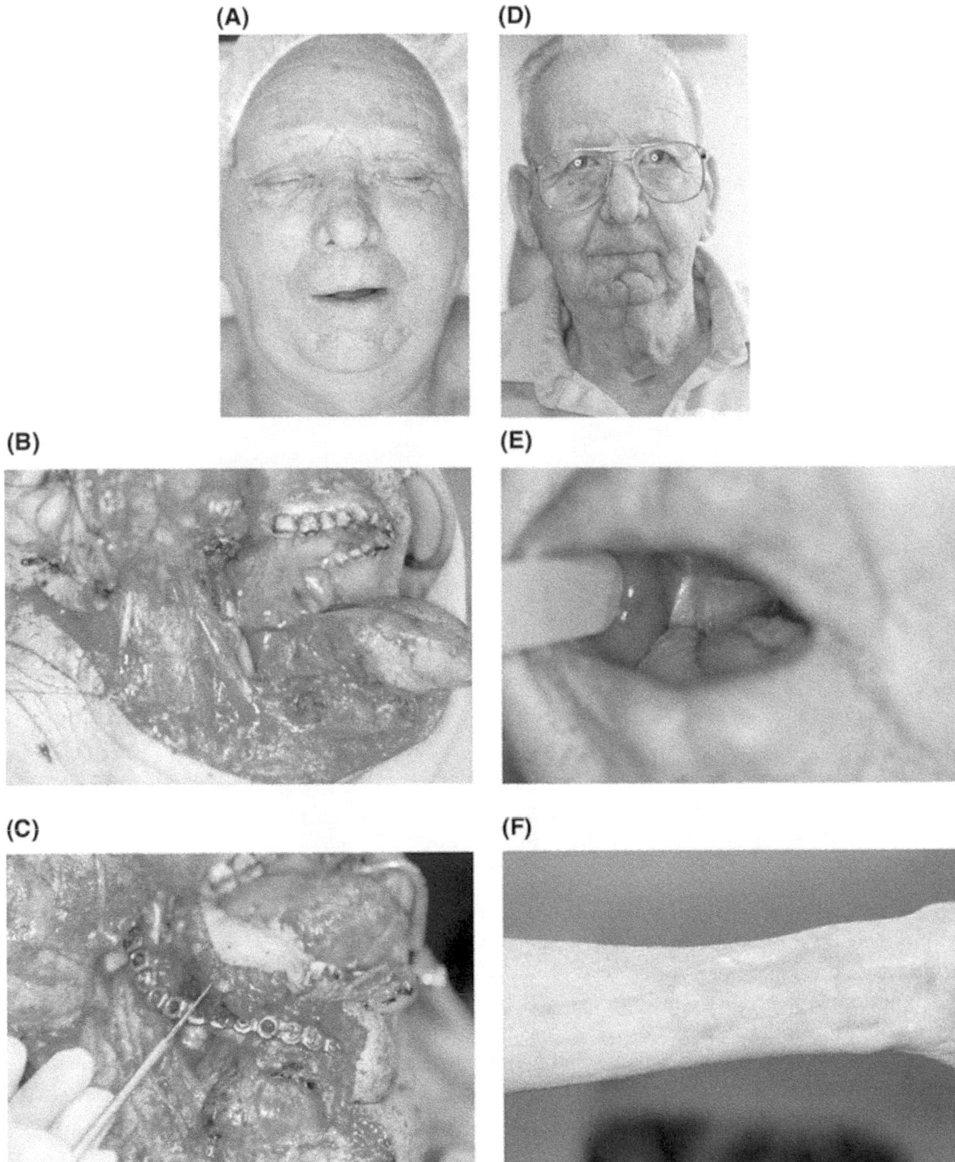

Figure 7 Reconstruction of a posteriolateral oral cavity and pharyngeal defect with an osteocutaneous radial forearm free flap (OCRFFF). (**A**) Pre operative frontal view of patient prior to surgery. (**B**) Defect of the angle and lateral body of the mandible, posterior floor of the mouth, posteriolateraloral tongue, base of the tongue, soft palate and lateral pharyngeal wall. (**C**) Reconstruction plate securing the radius bone graft in place with the forearm skin repairing the extensive soft tissue defect in a sensate fashion. (**D**) Postoperative appearance three months after radiation therapy. Patient is eating a normal diet. (**E**) Intraoral appearance of reconstructed alveolar ridge and soft palate after radiation therapy. (**F**) Long –term appearance of the forearm after harvest of the OCRFFF.

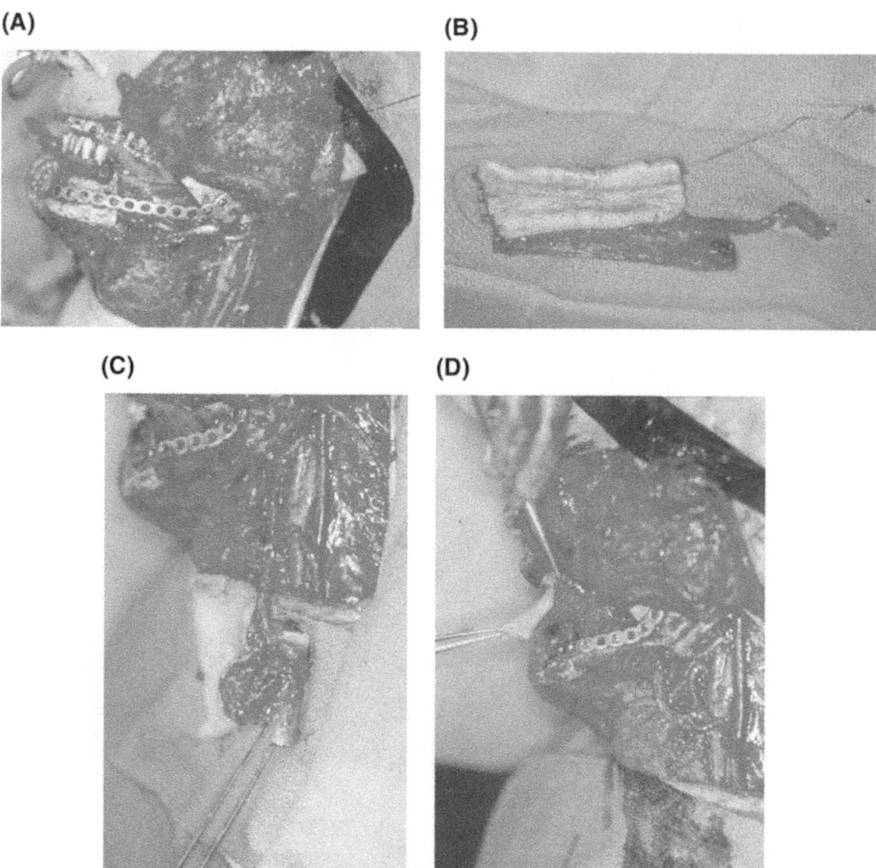

Figure 8 Reconstruction of a lateral oral cavity composite defect from recurrent buccal carcinoma with a "double barreled" OCRFFF. (**A**) Lateral defect of the mandible, floor of the mouth and buccal mucosa after resection with a reconstruction plate spanning the defect and maintaining occlusal relationships. (**B**) Harvested OCRFFF with 11 cm of radius bone harvested for reconstruction. (**C**) OCRFFF in the neck after microvascular anastomosis has been completed. The radius bone has had a 1cm segment removed in the mid portion allowing the bone to be folded onto itself to create a full tube of bone graft. This improves the quality of bone to allow dental implantation. (**D**) Inset of the flap to reconstruct the mandibular and soft tissue deficits.

OCRFF Modified Harvest Technique

The method for the harvest of the OCRFFF is very similar to that for a fasciocutaneous RFFF with a few specific modifications (65,68) (Fig. 9). Skin paddle design is more proximal (2cm from the wrist crease) and with an ulnar bias. This ensures adequate skin coverage of the plated radius bone to avoid the potential risk of plate exposure. The skin paddle is then elevated in a subfascial plane until it is based on the intermuscular septum between the brachioradialis and the flexor carpi radialis muscles and tendons.

The flexor digitorum superficialis muscle must then be released from the radius to allow visualization of the flexor pollicis longus muscle. This muscle belly must be split over the volar surface of the radius bone and the periosteum incised longitudinally with a scalpel to outline the length of bone needed for harvest. This

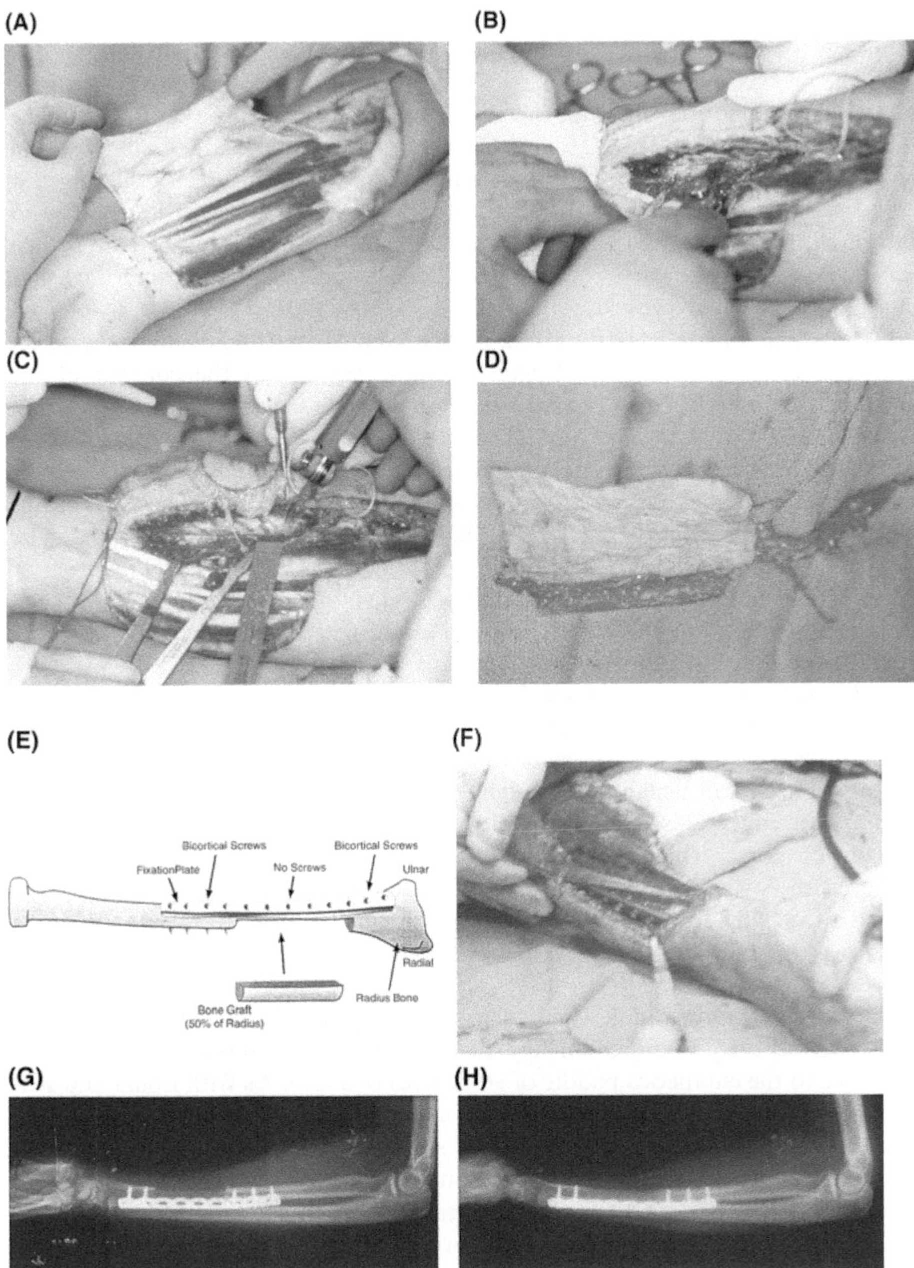

Figure 9 Technique for harvest and internal fixation of the radius bone for the OCRFFF. (**A**) The skin paddle of the flap is harvested with a proximal and ulnar bias to allow adequate remaining to cover the internal fixation plate. (**B**) The oscillating saw is used to make a horizontal cut through the radius bone to remove 50% of the circumference of the bone as a graft. (**C**) The proximal and distal vertical cuts are made at a bevel with a metal ruler placed in the horizontal cut to prevent past-cutting. (**D**) Harvested OCRFFF with skin, radius bone, vascular pedicle and two cutaneous nerves. (**E**) Diagram of plate fixation technique for the radius bone. At a minimum three screws are placed proximal and two screws distally. (**F**) Plate fixation completed after flap harvest. (**G**) Lateral forearm radiograph two months post op showing plate and screw position and graft defect. (**H**) Lateral forearm radiograph six weeks post op showing significant bone healing of the graft defect.

is designed to include 50% of the circumference of the radius and the length desired. The bone graft length is limited by the insertions of the brachioradialis tendon distally and the pronator teres muscle proximally. The pronator muscle can be partially taken down to extend the length of the graft available but must be reattached. The distal cut must be made at least 2.5 cm from the radial styloid to allow later fixation of the radius. The bone is then split in the longitudinal plane with an oscillating saw at its mid-portion. Proximal and distal cuts are made on a bevel with care taken to avoid past-cutting which can further weaken the bone. The dorsal periosteum is then incised to allow complete mobilization of the bone graft based on the intermuscular septum and the vascular pedicle.

The dorsolateral aspect of the radius is exposed proximal and distal to the defect and an appropriately sized reconstruction plate is bent to fit the contour of the radial aspect of the bone. Most recently, titanium low contact dynamic compression plates have been the fixation device of choice. The wrist extensors are retracted and at least two bicortical screws are placed distal to the defect. Proximally, the supinator muscle is visualized and care taken to avoid the interosseus nerve, which passes through the supinator. If a long bone graft has been harvested, the supinator can be elevated in the subperiosteal plane and the plate placed beneath it. Three to four bicortical screws are placed proximal to the defect. No screws are placed into the remaining radius bone of the defect to avoid additional stress points in the bone. The final plated donor site is shown in Figure 9G.

Additional measures are taken during the soft tissue closure of the forearm donor site. The flexor pollicis longus muscle is sutured over the remaining radius bone to provide coverage of the plate. The released edge of the flexor digitorum superficialis muscle can usually be brought over the flexor carpi radialis tendon to the radial skin edge. This provides additional coverage of the radius donor site and tendon coverage, which aids in skin graft take. A meshed split thickness skin graft is used to cover the remaining cutaneous defect and the arm immobilized in an ulnar gutter splint for seven days. Once the splint is removed, the donor site is covered for protection during healing but full activity with the donor arm and wrist is encouraged.

The harvested radius bone is vascularized via perforating vessels found in the intermuscular septum. The septum has adequate length to allow rotation of the bone relative to the cutaneous paddle of 90 degrees or more. As with fibula and scapula flaps, osteotomies may be performed to allow conformation of the graft to the defect if the periosteum is maintained. When securing the radius bone in the defect the exposed marrow portion of the bone should face away from the reconstruction plate (lingually). This allows significant bone remodeling to produce additional bone formation to close the marrow space with cortical bone over time.

The radius bone at the graft donor site also undergoes significant bone remodeling and reconstitution over a five to six-month-period (Figs. 9G and 9H) (65).

Advantages. The ease of harvest of abundant thin pliable sensate skin of the forearm is ideal for oral cavity reconstruction. There is significant independent mobility of the fasciocutaneous paddle relative to the bone graft, which facilitates soft tissue reconstruction. The long vascular pedicle of the RFFF provides unequaled versatility for flap placement. The 50% thickness of radius bone harvested with the OCRFFF provides long-term durability and stability for mandibular reconstruction and forms a relatively thin neo-alveolar ridge, which can be fitted with a tissue-born prosthesis (denture). The OCRFFF can be rapidly harvested concurrently with the head and neck resection. The donor site morbidity of this flap harvest is significantly less than that of the fibula, scapula and iliac crest free flaps if the radius bone is managed with prophylactic fixation.

Disadvantages. There is an additional step to the operation of performing prophylactic internal fixation of the radius bone although the time required is still less than that for the harvest of a scapula flap or a second flap. The harvested portion of the radius bone is usually inadequate for the support of dental implants unless the mandible defect is less than 5 cm in length as mentioned above.

Scapula Osteocutaneous Free Flap

The osteocutaneous scapula free flap remains one of the most versatile flaps available for harvest in the human body (69–75). The subscapular arterial system offers tremendous amounts of skin, the latissmus dorsi and serratus anterior muscles and scapular bone for harvest, all supplied by one major vascular pedicle, which has both favorable length and caliber. These different tissue components each have a separate vascular branching supply allowing for almost limitless degrees of orientation in relation to each other and the recipient bed. The skin of the upper lateral back is usually quite thick with considerable subcutaneous fat resulting in significant soft tissue bulk, which can be used to advantage in some reconstructive situations. This bulk will reliably remain on a long-term basis without atrophy. The skin, which can be harvested alone as a fasciocutaneous flap, can also be separated into scapular and parascapular skin paddles based on the transverse and descending branches of the circumflex scapular artery, respectively (71,72,76). Unfortunately, there has been no corresponding segmental nervous supply to the skin of the region, which precludes the harvest of skin as a sensate flap. Recently, however, dorsal cutaneous rami of the T1 or T2 spinal nerves have been described, which may allow for sensate transfer of scapular cutaneous paddles (1).

A total of 10–14 cm of bone is available for harvest from the lateral border of the scapula for mandibular reconstruction supplied by the periosteal branch of the circumflex scapular artery. The separation of the bony and fasciocutaneous components of the flap resulting from unique vascular supplies can be as much as 4 cm, allowing for significant versatility in hard and soft tissue orientation during reconstruction. Osteotomies may be safely performed for mandibular contouring as long as the periosteum is preserved. The harvested scapular bone has a thick border along the free edge of the scapula but transitions quickly to thin bone 1–2 cm medial to the edge. The resulting limited bone stock may not be adequate for the support of endosteal dental implants (13,14).

The scapular osteocutaneous flap remains an optimal choice for the reconstruction of the oromandibular complex when the surgeon is faced with large complex defects, especially those involving a large surface area or with three-layer composite defects involving both the oral cavity and external soft tissues.

For extremely large defects, some surgeons have employed the scapular "mega flap" which includes scapular bone and extensive skin as described above, but also the latissmus dorsi muscle and or the serratus anterior muscle for additional bulk and coverage (77,78). The muscles are based on the thoracodorsal artery and vein which branch off the subscapular vessels and therefore can be harvested on the same vascular pedicle requiring only one arterial and venous anastomoses. The mega flap offers significant mobilization of the various tissue components relative to each other as a result of the branching vascular supply providing great reconstructive versatility for the largest of defects.

Technique

The harvest of the scapula osteocutaneous free flap has been described in detail elsewhere in this text. The patient must be placed on a bean bag mattress on the operating room table to allow the intraoperative change of position from supine for the head and neck ablation or recipient site preparation to the lateral decubitus position for the harvest of the scapula flap. The patient is usually returned to the supine position for flap inset and head and neck closure prior to returning to the lateral decubitus position for closure of the donor site defect. The entire upper extremity and hemi-back must be prepped into the surgical field prior to placement in the supine position at the outset of the procedure.

Planning of the flap requires careful consideration of the defect location and size of the intraoral and external soft tissue deficits. The two skin paddles are designed in a "V" shape (Fig. 10) with the base of the "V" oriented over the medial aspect of the triangular space which is bounded by the teres major and minor muscles and long head of the triceps muscle at the lateral border of the scapula. The skin paddles are separated the by de-epithelialization of an intervening portion of skin and then folding the paddles on themselves when an external defect is to be reconstructed. When deciding which shoulder to utilize as the donor site and how large to design the scapular and parascapular skin paddles one must take into account the final configuration of the inset skin in relation to the vascular pedicle. It is advisable to map out the transverse and descending cutaneous branches of the circumflex scapular artery using doppler ultrasonography prior to the design of the fasciocutaneous paddles.

When harvesting the bone of the lateral border of the scapula a cuff of muscle should be preserved to ensure periosteal integrity. The superior limit of bone harvest is 1–2 cm below the glenoid fossa to ensure stability of the joint. The vascularity of the tip of the scapula may be questionable, especially after multiple osteotomies. This can be improved by also harvesting the angular branch of the thoracodorsal artery as part of the pedicle, which also supplies the scapula tip.

Reconstruction of the mandible is performed similar to other osteocutaneous flaps by using a low profile reconstruction plate to retain mandible remnant orientation and provide a framework for securing the bone grafts. The thick edge (lateral border) of the scapula is positioned superiorly to provide an alveolar ridge and facilitate the possible placement of endosteal dental implants.

The skin paddles are inset following reconstruction of the mandible. The bulky nature of the skin paddles precludes extensive contouring on inset and may require future revision to achieve the final desired product (79). The bulk may desirable for reconstructing large tongue, cheek, chin, and lip defects. Portions of the skin paddle may be completely de-epithelialized for use as a source of additional buried soft tissue bulk.

The cutaneous portion of the flap should be designed to allow primary closure of the donor site. This can be achieved even with the harvest of large amounts of skin. It is important to reattach the divided edge of the teres major muscle to holes drilled in the cut edge the scapula or the infraspinatus fascia to maximize post-operative function of the shoulder. Shoulder immobilization for five to seven days should be followed by physical therapy for shoulder mobility.

Advantages. The multiple tissue components transferable on the subscapular vascular pedicle, which has good length and caliber allows for very complex reconstructions. A large amount of skin may be harvested with additional bulk available.

The donor site can usually be closed primarily, avoiding the need for a skin graft. Up to 14 cm of bone is available for mandible reconstruction.

Disadvantages. The necessity to reposition the patient several times during the operation usually precludes simultaneous ablation and flap harvest, which adds significant length to the procedure. There is no reported opportunity for the restoration of cutaneous sensation to the flap due to the lack of cutaneous nerves. The bone of the scapula is often inadequate to support endosseous dental implant rehabilitation.

Long-term shoulder dysfunction can result from the harvest of the scapula osteocutaneous flap with winging of the scapula, decreased range of motion and chronic pain. These problems can usually be minimized with careful technique and aggressive physical therapy.

MULTIPLE FLAPS FOR THE RECONSTRUCTION OF OROMANDIBULAR DEFECTS

The approach of choosing the best source available for each of the required tissue components of a given defect (bone, skin, muscle) will often lead to the consideration of multiple flaps for one patient (80,81). For very large two-layer defects and many three-layer defects there may be inadequate tissue available with most single flap options requiring either a compromise of the reconstruction or the addition of a second source of tissue. The reconstructive priorities become very important in this setting and dictate the approach. If the anticipated outcome includes dental implantation for rehabilitation then the bony reconstruction must be planned appropriately. However, the fibula flap will often not provide adequate soft tissue in this situation to complete a complex three-layer repair and will necessitate an additional soft tissue source to close the defect adequately.

In many settings of a three-layer complex defect the reconstruction can be managed with an osteocutaneous free tissue transfer for the intraoral defect combined with a cervico-facial rotation flap, cross lip flap or other local reconstructive technique to manage the external defect.

Another option for very large defects is the combination of several of the methods outlined in this chapter to complete the reconstruction. The combination of an osteocutaneous free flap for the oromandibular reconstruction and a pedicled pectoralis muscle (or myocutaneous) flap covered with a split thickness skin graft to reline an external neck cutaneous defect is fairly straightforward, less time consuming than the combination of two free flaps, and highly reliable (Fig. 11) (82–84).

The sensate radial forearm fasciocutaneous provides the highest quality soft tissue for oral cavity reconstruction and has been successfully combined with iliac crest, fibula and scapula flaps to achieve repairs of large defects of the oromandibular complex (81,85–88). In the case of the fibula flap, the peroneal vascular pedicle has proven to have adequate flow through the flap to allow the anastomosis of the radial vessels to the distal peroneal artery and vein as a "piggy-back" flap (80,81). The obvious disadvantages of using multiple free flaps for a single reconstruction are increased operative time, more anastomoses at risk, multiple donor sites with the associated morbidity and cost. It is uncommon that other acceptable approaches cannot be found to accomplish the needed reconstruction.

In some settings it may be advantageous to plan a second flap as a staged procedure to complete the desired reconstruction provided the patient does well from an

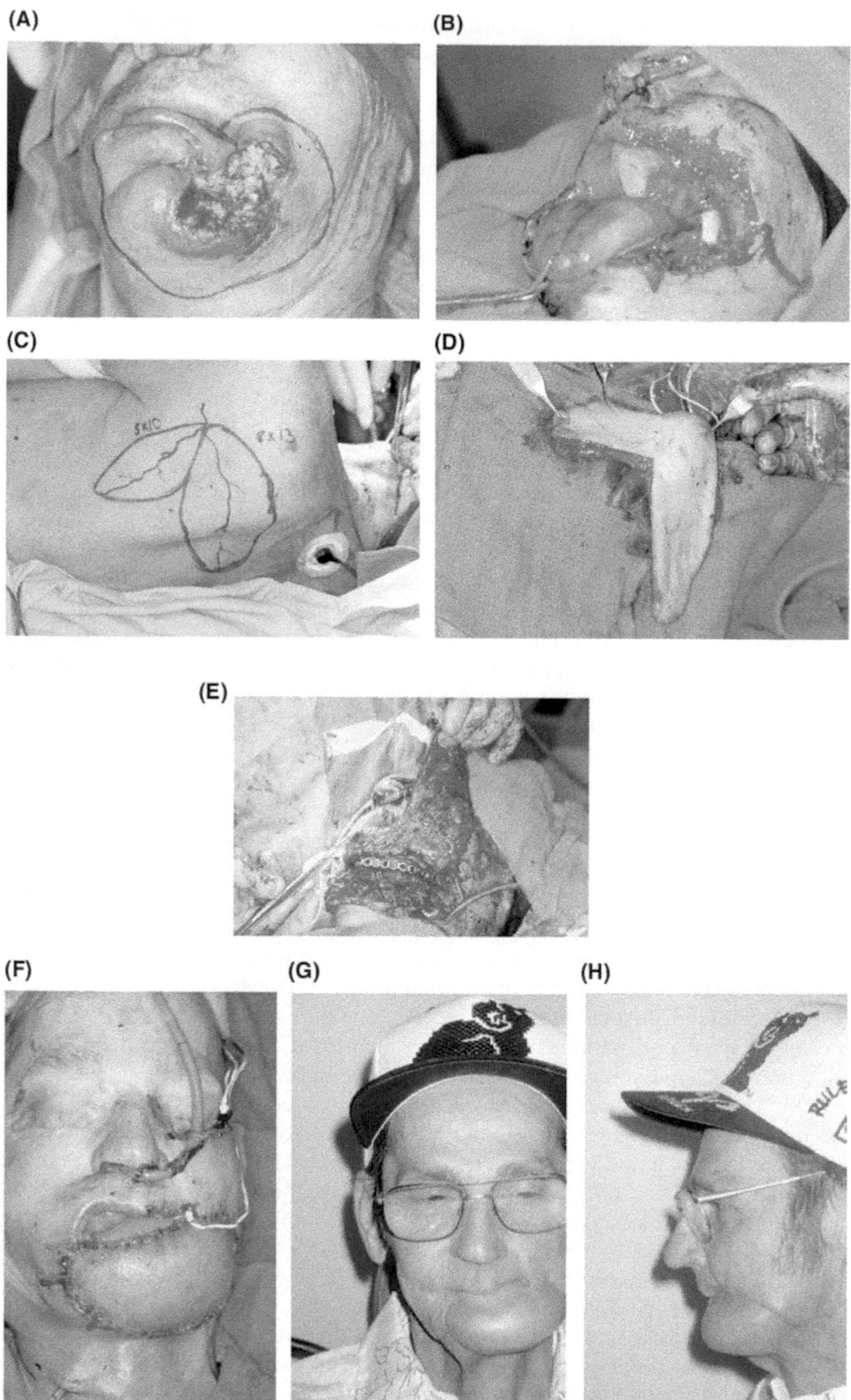

Figure 10 (*Caption on facing page*)

oncological standpoint. For the patient with very advanced local/regional disease (Fig. 12), a reliable and functional, if less than optimal, reconstruction can help get the patient into the much needed adjuvant therapy post-operatively. Once therapy is complete and no recurrence is seen after a reasonable period of time (usually at least one year) further reconstruction can be pursued. Unfortunately, secondary reconstructions are typically much more difficult as a result of extensive post-operative scarring, soft tissue contracture and radiation changes. Reexploration of a previously operated neck may compromise the vascular pedicle of the original flap and there may be fewer options for recipient vessel. Healing problems are certainly more common with secondary reconstructions due to the compromise of the local soft tissues from prior therapy. Most surgeons will attempt to avoid this situation with an appropriate plan for the initial reconstruction if possible, even for patients with advanced disease.

Advantages. The combination of more than one tissue transfer to accomplish a difficult reconstruction allows the surgeon to select the highest quality tissues available for each component (layer) of the reconstruction. In some instances, there may be no other reasonable choice for the closure of massive defects and some combination must be employed.

Disadvantages. This approach adds significant complexity, increases operative time, results in multiple donor sites with the associated morbidity, increases the risk for complications, increases the cost, and reduces future reconstructive options for the patient. For these reasons, most surgeons will reserve the use of multiple flaps for only the most extreme of circumstances.

IMPLANTS AND BIOMATERIALS

There is very little if any role for implants or biomaterials as a primary reconstruction method for large composite defects of the oromandibular complex. However, there are instances where these materials may supplement the reconstruction as discussed in previous chapters.

Mandible Substitutes

A great many materials have been utilized over the years in an attempt to accomplish mandibular reconstruction after ablative therapy. These have included cadaveric rib, mandible and iliac crest, Teflon, and a wide variety of metals in the form of reconstruction plates. Most have not survived the test of time due to wound complications and infection. Reconstruction plates however, have undergone continual evolution

---

Figure 10 Reconstruction of a large recurrent lip and buccal carcinoma 3-layer defect with a scapula osteocutaneous free flap. (**A**) Recurrent carcinoma of the lower lip, chin, mandible and cheek after radiation therapy. (**B**) Defect involving through and through lip and cheek soft tissues and mandible. (**C**) Planned scapula osteocutaneous free flap with both scapular and parascapular skin paddles to provide internal and external soft tissue repair. (**D**) Harvested scapula free flap. (**E**) Inset of flap with mandibular reconstruction with a plate securing the scapula bone to the mandible. (**F**) Completed intra operative appearance. (**G**) Six month post-operative frontal view. Patient reports adequate oral competence and a soft diet. (**H**) Six month postoperative lateral view.

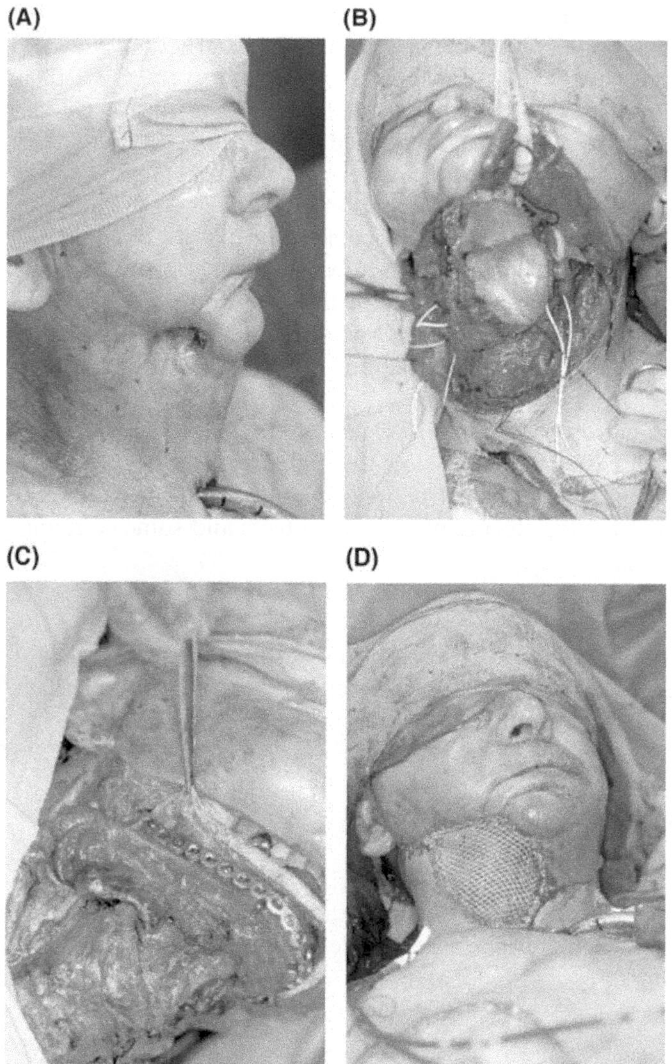

Figure 11 Reconstruction of a large 3 layer defect of the oral cavity and neck with a combination of an OCRFFF and a PMF with a skin graft. (**A**) Pre-operative appearance of a recurrent floor of mouth carcinoma with extensive oral cavity, mandible and neck skin involvement. (**B**) Large 3-layer defect following resection. (**C**) Inset of the OCRFFF to repair the oral cavity soft tissue defect and the lateral and anterior mandible. (**D**) Rotation of a pectoralis muscle flap to reline the neck defect and provide great vessel coverage. A meshed split thickness skin graft is placed on the pectoralis muscle.

of design and materials as discussed previously in this and previous chapters and continue to have an important role in the reconstruction of the mandible. Locking screw plate systems can function as a mandible substitute providing the stability and strength needed for long term reconstruction of lateral and posteriolateral mandibular defects in some settings. Low profile reconstruction plates are ideal for the maintenance of mandibular continuity and fixation of bone grafts with osteocutaneous free flap reconstructions.

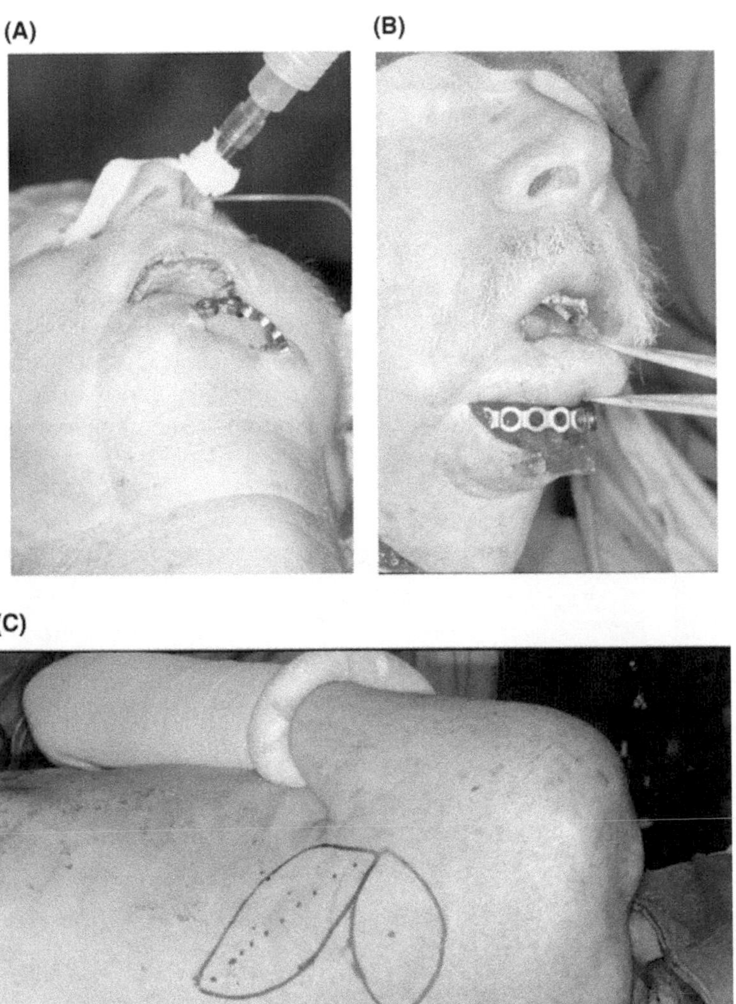

Figure 12 The use of a second free flap for reconstruction of a large 3-layer defect of the oral cavity in a staged (delayed) fashion. (**A**) The same patient seen in Figure 5 with anterior plate exposure one year after completion of therapy and no evidence of cancer. (**B**) The previously placed fasciocutaneous RFFF is divided to preserve the neo-lip from the rest of the flap. (**C**) A large scapula osteocutaneous flap is harvested with both scapular and parascapular skin paddles for internal and external lining. (*Continued*)

Acellular dermis (Alloderm, Lifecell Corp, New Jersey) has proven to be an effective alloplastic material for use in head and neck reconstruction (89–94). It consists of human dermis, which is processed to remove all adnexal structures, and cellular DNA leaving the collagen matrix intact and undisrupted. The collagen matrix (which looks like harvested dermis) can be dehydrated and stored until needed. Upon rehydration and implantation the matrix becomes populated with recipient cells maintaining the matrix as living tissue. Reported uses have included soft tissue augmentation, facial slings for paralysis and parotid coverage to prevent Frey's syndrome (90,94–99). Acellular dermis has also proven to be effective as a mucosal graft substitute for oral cavity reconstruction (89–99). As an intraoral graft it rapidly becomes vascularized and muscoalized over one to two weeks resulting in less contracture than is seen with split thickness skin grafting. It is uncommon, however, that acelluar dermis will be of much benefit in the repair of complex oromandibular defects.

DECISION-MAKING TIPS

As described in the early chapters of this text, success in oromandibular reconstruction is entirely dependent on appropriate anticipation of the functional and cosmetic impact of the defect and the thoughtful review of the required tissue components.

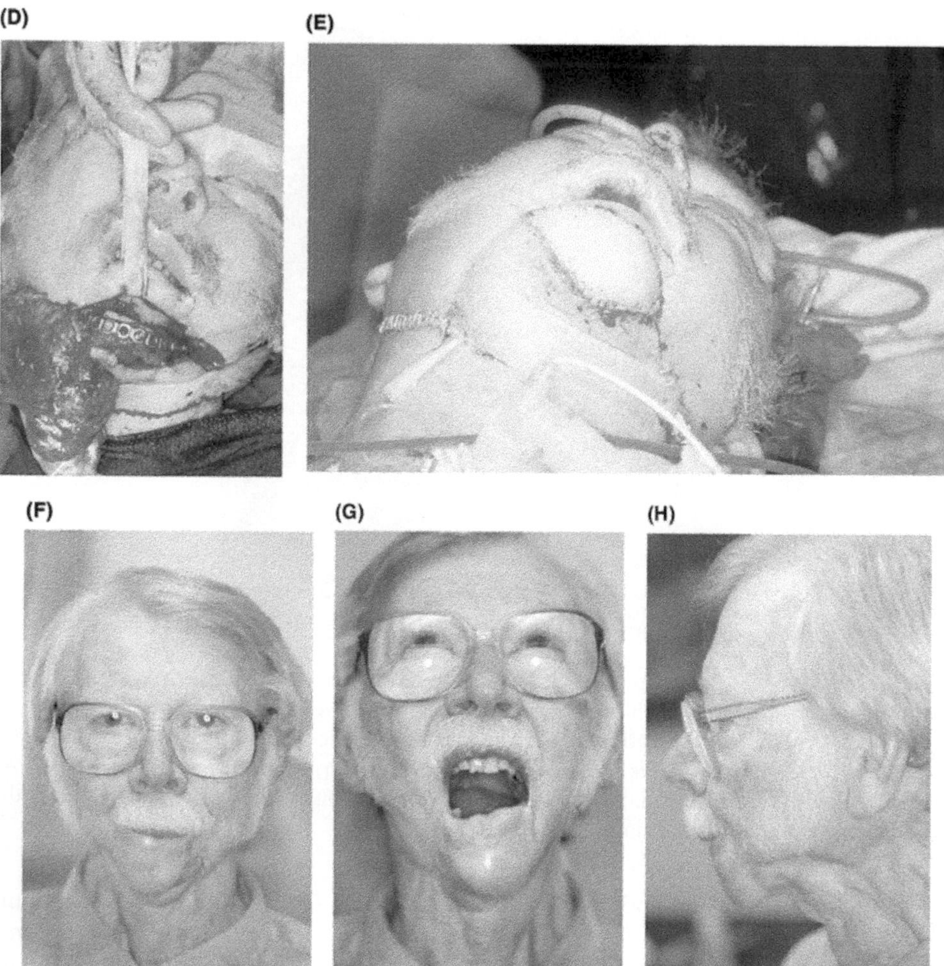

Figure 12 (**D**) Inset of the scapula bone to the existing exposed reconstruction plate. (**E**) Appearance of reconstruction at completion. (**F**) Frontal view eight years after second free flap with good oral competence. (**G**) Mandibular mobility maintained long-term. (**H**) Long-term lateral view.

Table 2

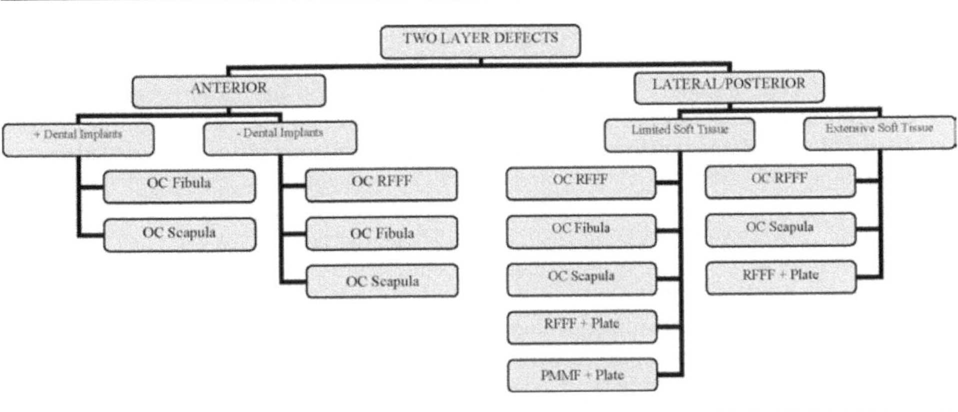

These required components are then prioritized based on the anticipated long-term goals of the patient and surgeon. It is imperative that the patient (and their family) be actively involved in this process to ensure that the reconstructive goals are inline with patient and family expectations.

The thought process and preference for reconstructive options certainly varies by surgeon based on training and experience. The algorhythm for both two-layer and three-layer defects employed most commonly by the authors are outlined in Tables 2 and 3, respectively.

Once the primary reconstructive plan has been identified and confirmed by the necessary medical and vascular studies, thought must be given to an acceptable, if less optimal, alternative. Despite the "best laid plan," the unexpected occurs all too frequently for a multitude of reasons. Therefore, it is always prudent to have a "plan B" in the event the original plan must be aborted.

Table 3

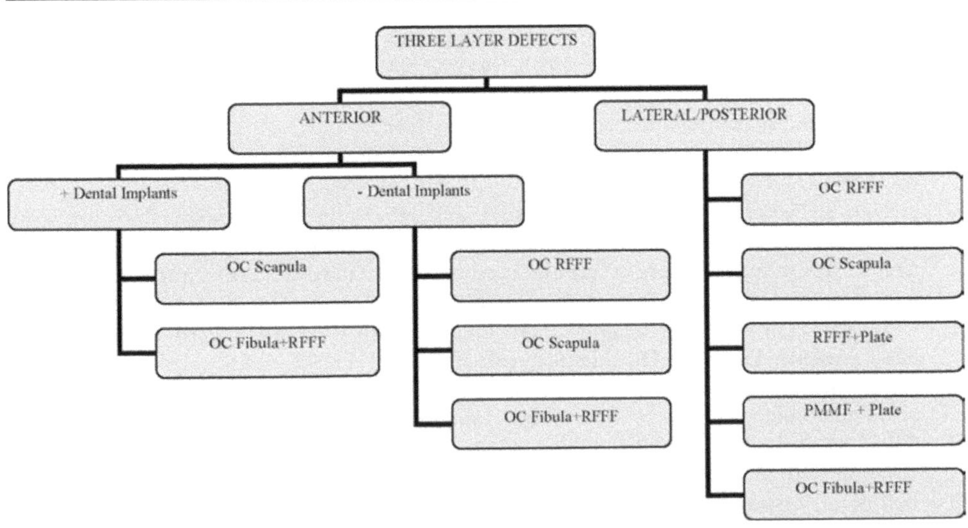

REFERENCES

1. Rhee JS, et al. Intraoperative mapping of sensate flaps. Electrophysiologic techniques and neurosomal boundaries. Arch Otolaryngol Head Neck Surg 1997; 123(8):823–829.
2. Vriens JP, et al. Recovery of sensation in the radial forearm free flap in oral reconstruction. Plast Reconstr Surg 1996; 98(4):649–656.
3. Mah SM, et al. Functional results in oral cavity reconstruction using reinnervated versus nonreinnervated free fasciocutaneous grafts. J Otolaryngol 1996; 25(2):75–81.
4. Dubner S, Heller KS. Reinnervated radial forearm free flaps in head and neck reconstruction. J Reconstr Microsurg 1992; 8(6):467–468; discussion 469–470.
5. Hentz VR, et al. The radial forearm flap: a versatile source of composite tissue. Ann Plast Surg 1987; 19(6):485–498.
6. Urken ML, et al. The neurofasciocutaneous radial forearm flap in head and neck reconstruction: a preliminary report. Laryngoscope 1990; 100(2 Pt 1):161–173.
7. Ozdemir R, et al. Total lower lip reconstruction using sensate composite radial forearm flap. J Craniofac Surg 2003; 14(3):393–405.
8. Huang R, Blackwell KE. Microvascular reconstruction of composite defects of the mandible and lip: aesthetic and functional considerations. Laryngoscope 2000; 110(6): 1066–1069.
9. Carroll CM, et al. Reconstruction of total lower lip and chin defects using the composite radial forearm–palmaris longus tendon free flap. Arch Facial Plast Surg 2000; 2(1):53–56.
10. Orringer JS, et al. Total mandibular and lower lip reconstruction with a prefabricated osteocutaneous free flap. Plast Reconstr Surg 1999; 104(3):793–797.
11. Yuen JC, Zhou A, Shewmake K. Staged sequential reconstruction of a total lower lip, chin, and anterior mandibular defect. Ann Plast Surg 1998; 40(3):297–301.
12. Granick MS, Newton ED, Hanna DC. Scapular free flap for repair of massive lower facial composite defects. Head Neck Surg 1986; 8(6):436–441.
13. Moscoso JF, et al. Vascularized bone flaps in oromandibular reconstruction. A comparative anatomic study of bone stock from various donor sites to assess suitability for enosseous dental implants. Arch Otolaryngol Head Neck Surg 1994; 120(1):36–43.
14. Frodel JL Jr, et al. Osseointegrated implants: a comparative study of bone thickness in four vascularized bone flaps. Plast Reconstr Surg 1993; 92(3):449–455; discussion 456–458.
15. Buchbinder D, et al. Functional mandibular reconstruction of patients with oral cancer. Oral Surg Oral Med Oral Pathol 1989; 68(4 Pt 2):499–503; discussion 503–504.
16. Urken ML, et al. Primary placement of osseointegrated implants in microvascular mandibular reconstruction. Otolaryngol Head Neck Surg 1989; 101(1):56–73.
17. Baek SM, et al. The pectoralis major myocutaneous island flap for reconstruction of the head and neck. Head Neck Surg 1979; 1(4):293–300.
18. Ariyan S. The pectoralis major myocutaneous flap. A versatile flap for reconstruction in the head and neck. Plast Reconstr Surg 1979; 63(1):73–81.
19. Maruyama Y, et al. One stage reconstruction of oral cavity by use of pectoralis major myocutaneous island flap. Keio J Med 1978; 27(2):47–52.
20. Ariyan S. Pectoralis major, sternomastoid, and other musculocutaneous flaps for head and neck reconstruction. Clin Plast Surg 1980; 7(1):89–109.
21. Magee WP Jr, et al. Pectoralis "paddle" myocutaneous flaps. The workhorse of head and neck reconstruction. Am J Surg 1980; 140(4):507–513.
22. Castelli ML, et al. Pectoralis major myocutaneous flap: analysis of complications in difficult patients. Eur Arch Otorhinolaryngol 2001; 258(10):542–545.
23. Bhaya MH, Harel G. Resident training in head and neck flap reconstruction in U.S. academic otolaryngology programmes. J Laryngol Otol 2001; 115(2):119–121.
24. CB IJ, et al. Is the pectoralis myocutaneous flap in intraoral and oropharyngeal reconstruction outdated? Am J Surg 1996; 172(3):259–262.
25. Bell MS, Barron PT. The rib-pectoralis major osteomyocutaneous flap. Ann Plast Surg 1981; 6(5):347–353.

26. Schusterman MA, et al. Use of the AO plate for immediate mandibular reconstruction in cancer patients. Plast Reconstr Surg 1991; 88(4):588–593.
27. Buchbinder D, et al. Bone contouring and fixation in functional, primary microvascular mandibular reconstruction. Head Neck 1991; 13(3):191–199.
28. Lavertu P, et al. The AO system for primary mandibular reconstruction. Am J Surg 1994; 168(5):503–507.
29. Savant D, Bhathena H, Kavarana N. The pectoralis major osteomyocutaneous flap in mandibular reconstruction. Br J Plast Surg 1996; 49(3):191.
30. Margarino G, et al. Mandible reconstruction with metallic endoprosthesis following Commando's operation for advanced head and neck cancer. Personal experience. Eur J Surg Oncol 1993; 19(4):320–326.
31. Boyd JB, et al. The through-and-through oromandibular defect: rationale for aggressive reconstruction. Plast Reconstr Surg 1994; 93(1):44–53.
32. Blackwell KE, Buchbinder D, Urken ML. Lateral mandibular reconstruction using soft-tissue free flaps and plates. Arch Otolaryngol Head Neck Surg 1996; 122(6):672–678.
33. Blackwell KE, Lacombe V. The bridging lateral mandibular reconstruction plate revisited. Arch Otolaryngol Head Neck Surg 1999; 125(9):988–993.
34. Girod DA, et al. Risk factors for complications in clean-contaminated head and neck surgical procedures. Head Neck 1995; 17(1):7–13.
35. Johnson JT, et al. Prophylactic antibiotics for head and neck surgery with flap reconstruction. Arch Otolaryngol Head Neck Surg 1992; 118(5):488–490.
36. Brown MR, et al. Resource utilization and patient morbidity in head and neck reconstruction. Laryngoscope 1997; 107(8):1028–1031.
37. Davidson J, et al. A comparison of the results following oromandibular reconstruction using a radial forearm flap with either radial bone or a reconstruction plate. Plast Reconstr Surg 1991; 88(2):201–208.
38. Tsue TT, et al. Comparison of cost and function in reconstruction of the posterior oral cavity and oropharynx. Free vs pedicled soft tissue transfer. Arch Otolaryngol Head Neck Surg 1997; 123(7):731–737.
39. Kroll SS, et al. A comparison of resource costs for head and neck reconstruction with free and pectoralis major flaps. Plast Reconstr Surg 1997; 99(5):1282–1286.
40. Funk GF, et al. Free tissue transfer versus pedicled flap cost in head and neck cancer. Otolaryngol Head Neck Surg 2002; 127(3):205–212.
41. Yang G, Gao Y, et al. Forearm free skin flap transplantation. Natl Med J China 1981; 61:139.
42. Cordeiro PG, et al. A comparison of donor and recipient site sensation in free tissue reconstruction of the oral cavity. Ann Plast Surg 1997; 39(5):461–468.
43. Muldowney JB, et al. Oral cavity reconstruction using the free radial forearm flap. Arch Otolaryngol Head Neck Surg 1987; 113(11):1219–1224.
44. Soutar DS, McGregor IA. The radial forearm flap in intraoral reconstruction: the experience of 60 consecutive cases. Plast Reconstr Surg 1986; 78(1):1–8.
45. Su WF, et al. Functional comparison after reconstruction with a radial forearm free flap or a pectoralis major flap for cancer of the tongue. Otolaryngol Head Neck Surg 2003; 128(3):412–418.
46. Timmons MJ. The vascular basis of the radial forearm flap. Plast Reconstr Surg 1986; 77(1):80–92.
47. Ryan MW, Hochman M. Length of stay after free flap reconstruction of the head and neck. Laryngoscope 2000; 110(2 Pt 1):210–216.
48. Singh B, et al. Factors associated with complications in microvascular reconstruction of head and neck defects. Plast Reconstr Surg 1999; 103(2):403–411.
49. Blackwell KE. Unsurpassed reliability of free flaps for head and neck reconstruction. Arch Otolaryngol Head Neck Surg 1999; 125(3):295–299.

50. Hidalgo DA, et al. A review of 716 consecutive free flaps for oncologic surgical defects: refinement in donor-site selection and technique. Plast Reconstr Surg 1998; 102(3): 722–732; discussion 733–734.
51. Schusterman MA, et al. The osteocutaneous free fibula flap: is the skin paddle reliable? Plast Reconstr Surg 1992; 90(5):787–793; discussion 794–798.
52. Wei FC, et al. Fibular osteoseptocutaneous flap: anatomic study and clinical application. Plast Reconstr Surg 1986; 78(2):191–200.
53. Shindo M, et al. The fibula osteocutaneous flap in head and neck reconstruction: a critical evaluation of donor site morbidity. Arch Otolaryngol Head Neck Surg 2000; 126(12):1467–1472.
54. O'Leary MJ, Martin PJ, Hayden RE. The neurocutaneous free fibula flap in mandibular reconstruction. Otolaryngol Clin North Am 1994; 27(6):1081–1096.
55. Zimmermann CE, et al. Donor site morbidity after microvascular fibula transfer. Clin Oral Investig 2001; 5(4):214–219.
56. Soutar DS, Widdowson WP. Immediate reconstruction of the mandible using a vascularized segment of radius. Head Neck Surg 1986; 8(4):232–246.
57. Soutar DS, et al. The radial forearm flap: a versatile method for intra-oral reconstruction. Br J Plast Surg 1983; 36(1):1–8.
58. Swanson E, Boyd JB, Mulholland RS. The radial forearm flap: a biomechanical study of the osteotomized radius. Plast Reconstr Surg 1990; 85(2):267–272.
59. Meland NB, et al. The radial forearm flap: a biomechanical study of donor-site morbidity utilizing sheep tibia. Plast Reconstr Surg 1992; 90(5):763–773.
60. Bardsley AF, et al. Reducing morbidity in the radial forearm flap donor site. Plast Reconstr Surg 1990; 86(2):287–292; discussion 293–294.
61. Timmons MJ, et al. Complications of radial forearm flap donor sites. Br J Plast Surg 1986; 39(2):176–178.
62. Boorman JG, Brown JA, Sykes PJ. Morbidity in the forearm flap donor arm. Br J Plast Surg 1987; 40(2):207–212.
63. Swanson E, Boyd JB, Manktelow RT. The radial forearm flap: reconstructive applications and donor-site defects in 35 consecutive patients. Plast Reconstr Surg 1990; 85(2): 258–266.
64. Thoma A, et al. Oromandibular reconstruction with the radial-forearm osteocutaneous flap: experience with 60 consecutive cases. Plast Reconstr Surg 1999; 104(2):368–378; discussion 379–380.
65. Werle AH, et al. Osteocutaneous radial forearm free flap: its use without significant donor site morbidity. Otolaryngol Head Neck Surg 2000; 123(6):711–717.
66. Edmonds JL, et al. Torsional strength of the radius after osteofasciocutaneous free flap harvest with and without primary bone plating. Otolaryngol Head Neck Surg 2000; 123(4):400–408.
67. Bowers KW, et al. Osteocutaneous radial forearm free flaps. The necessity of internal fixation of the donor-site defect to prevent pathological fracture. J Bone Joint Surg Am 2000; 82(5):694–704.
68. Tsue TT, Girod DA. Osteocutaneous radial forearm flap. In: Branham GEA, ed. Otolaryngology and Facial Plastic Surgery/Reconstructive Surgery, 2001. eMedicine.com, Inc.
69. Urken ML, et al. The scapular osteofasciocutaneous flap: a 12-year experience. Arch Otolaryngol Head Neck Surg 2001; 127(7):862–869.
70. Cordeiro PG, et al. Reconstruction of the mandible with osseous free flaps: a 10-year experience with 150 consecutive patients. Plast Reconstr Surg 1999; 104(5):1314–1320.
71. Funk GF. Scapular and parascapular free flaps. Facial Plast Surg 1996; 12(1):57–63.
72. Gopinath KS, et al. The scapular fasciocutaneous flap: a new flap for reconstruction of the posterior neck. Br J Plast Surg 1993; 46(6):508–510.
73. Thoma A, et al. The free medial scapular osteofasciocutaneous flap for head and neck reconstruction. Br J Plast Surg 1991; 44(7):477–482.

74. Sullivan MJ, et al. The free scapular flap for head and neck reconstruction. Am J Otolaryngol 1990; 11(5):318–327.
75. Chandrasekhar B, Lorant JA, Terz JJ. Parascapular free flaps for head and neck reconstruction. Am J Surg 1990; 160(4):450–453.
76. Sullivan MJ, Carroll WR, Baker SR. The cutaneous scapular free flap in head and neck reconstruction. Arch Otolaryngol Head Neck Surg 1990; 116(5):600–603.
77. Yamamoto Y, et al. The combined flap based on a single vascular source: a clinical experience with 32 cases. Plast Reconstr Surg 1996; 97(7):1385–1390.
78. Aviv JE, et al. The combined latissimus dorsi-scapular free flap in head and neck reconstruction. Arch Otolaryngol Head Neck Surg 1991; 117(11):1242–1250.
79. Wooden WA, et al. Liposuction-assisted revision and recontouring of free microvascular tissue transfers. Aesthetic Plast Surg 1993; 17(2):103–107.
80. Wells MD, et al. Sequentially linked free flaps in head and neck reconstruction. Clin Plast Surg 1994; 21(1):59–67.
81. Sanger JR, Matloub HS, Yousif NJ. Sequential connection of flaps: a logical approach to customized mandibular reconstruction. Am J Surg 1990; 160(4):402–404.
82. Edmonds JL, Woodroof JM, Girod DA. Venous valves in the neck: implications for microvascular free flap reconstruction. Arch Otolaryngol Head Neck Surg 1999; 125(10): 1151–1153.
83. Chen HC, et al. Free fibula osteoseptocutaneous-pedicled pectoralis major myocutaneous flap combination in reconstruction of extensive composite mandibular defects. Plast Reconstr Surg 1999; 103(3):839–845.
84. Choi JO, et al. Combined use of pectoralis major myocutaneous and free radial forearm flaps for reconstruction of through-and-through defects from excision of head and neck cancers. J Otolaryngol 1999; 28(6):332–336.
85. Wei FC, et al. Combined anterolateral thigh flap and vascularized fibula osteoseptocutaneous flap in reconstruction of extensive composite mandibular defects. Plast Reconstr Surg 2002; 109(1):45–52.
86. Wei FC, et al. Double free flaps in reconstruction of extensive composite mandibular defects in head and neck cancer. Plast Reconstr Surg 1999; 103(1):39–47.
87. Koshima I, et al. Three-dimensional combined flaps for reconstruction of complex facial defects following cancer ablation. J Reconstr Microsurg 1997; 13(2):73–80; discussion 80–81.
88. Urken ML, et al. The combined sensate radical forearm and iliac crest free flaps for reconstruction of significant glossectomy-mandibulectomy defects. Laryngoscope 1992; 102(5):543–558.
89. Wagshall E, et al. Acellular dermal matrix allograft in the treatment of mucogingival defects in children: illustrative case report. ASDC J Dent Child 2002; 69(1):39–43, 11.
90. Sinha UK, Chang KE, Shih CW. Reconstruction of pharyngeal defects using AlloDerm and sternocleidomastoid muscle flap. Laryngoscope 2001; 111(11 Pt 1):1910–1916.
91. Batista EL Jr, Batista FC. Managing soft tissue fenestrations in bone grafting surgery with an acellular dermal matrix: a case report. Int J Oral Maxillofac Implants 2001; 16(6):875–879.
92. Sclafani AP, Jacono AA, Dolitsky JN. Grafting of the peritonsillar fossa with an acellular dermal graft to reduce posttonsillectomy pain. Am J Otolaryngol 2001; 22(6):409–414.
93. Sinha UK, et al. Use of AlloDerm implant to prevent frey syndrome after parotidectomy. Arch Facial Plast Surg 2003; 5(1):109–112.
94. Govindaraj S, et al. The use of acellular dermis in the prevention of Frey's syndrome. Laryngoscope 2001; 111(11 Pt 1):1993–1998.
95. Clayman MA, Clayman LZ. Use of AlloDerm as a barrier to treat chronic Frey's syndrome. Otolaryngol Head Neck Surg 2001; 124(6):687.
96. Costantino PD, et al. Acellular dermis for facial soft tissue augmentation: preliminary report. Arch Facial Plast Surg 2001; 3(1):38–43.

97. Sclafani AP, et al. Evaluation of acellular dermal graft (AlloDerm) sheet for soft tissue augmentation: a 1-year follow-up of clinical observations and histological findings. Arch Facial Plast Surg 2001; 3(2):101–103.
98. Terino EO. Alloderm acellular dermal graft: applications in aesthetic soft-tissue augmentation. Clin Plast Surg 2001; 28(1):83–99.
99. Kridel RW. Acellular human dermis for facial soft tissue augmentation. Facial Plast Surg Clin N Am 2001; 9(3):413–437.

19

Secondary Oral Cavity Reconstruction

Theodoros N. Teknos, Douglas B. Chepeha, and Steven J. Wang
Department of Otolaryngology—Head and Neck Surgery, University of Michigan, Ann Arbor, Michigan, U.S.A.

INTRODUCTION

Immediate, single-stage reconstruction of the oral cavity is the preferred method of restoration in this functionally critical region of the head and neck. If primary reconstruction is not performed, or if it is performed but is not successful, delayed reconstruction will be undertaken in the presence of scarring, contracture, and tissue atrophy, resulting in diminished capacity for effective speech and swallowing rehabilitation and increased risk for complications (1). Nevertheless, certain clinical situations may arise which mandate secondary oral cavity reconstruction, and such cases will be the focus of this chapter.

EVALUATION AND PLANNING

The principles of oral cavity reconstruction are similar whether performed primarily or secondarily, and are dictated by the anatomy and normal function of the organ being resected. First, we will discuss soft-tissue defects, such as oral tongue, floor of mouth (FOM), and buccal mucosa, as well as composite defects, such as mandible and hard palate. For oral tongue reconstruction, the key components to a successful result are volume restoration and mobility and sensation maintenance (2). To this end, the neotongue must have enough bulk to contact the palate in order to enable food bolus transit to the pharynx, and it must have enough mobility for the tip of the tongue to reach the premaxilla, allowing for speech articulation and food manipulation. Maintenance of sensation may also facilitate swallowing rehabilitation, although this point is controversial. Reconstruction of the FOM, or buccal mucosa should result in a thin, pliable surface that does not tether the tongue or lip.

For composite defects of the hard palate, the primary goal in reconstruction is to separate the oral cavity from the nasal cavity, provide a platform for dentures or dental implants, and maintain premaxillary projection. To optimize the rehabilitation of patients with an oral palate defect, the complementary nature of tissue reconstruction and prosthetics in this site must be considered. On the other hand, most mandibular defects are best reconstructed with vascularized bone. Vascularized bone is mandatory for anterior defects of the mandible. Non-reconstructed anterior mandibular defects lead to an unacceptable functional and cosmetic result, and plates, used alone as spacers for an anterior mandible defect, have a high extrusion rate (3). The reconstruction of lateral defects is more controversial. Several studies have suggested that free, vascularized bone is superior to plate and soft-tissue reconstruction when comparing long-term results (3–5). However, in edentulous patients, adequate functional and cosmetic reconstruction can be achieved without bone for lateral mandibular defects provided adequate restoration of the defect volume.

Secondary reconstruction of soft-tissue defects of the oral cavity is indicated when the result of the primary reconstruction is inadequate. Typically patients present with poor speech and swallowing, because the initial reconstruction did not provide adequate volume or surface area to reconstruct the defect. Often the anatomy of the sulci within the oral cavity has not been respected with the initial reconstruction, resulting in tethering of the tongue to the buccal mucosa, FOM, or lip. Wound-healing problems such as partial or complete flap loss are also common etiologic factors that can necessitate secondary reconstruction. Improved speech and swallowing and decreased aspiration are the goals of secondary reconstruction, and these goals are achieved by restoring volume and adding surface area to the non-reconstructed anatomic subunits.

The indication for secondary reconstruction of composite defects involving the hard palate is usually related to failed prosthetic rehabilitation. A prosthesis is usually involved in initial oral rehabilitation after resection of the hard palate. This traditional form of rehabilitation not only restores function but also facilitates tumor surveillance. However, there may be an inadequate platform to secure the prosthesis, resulting in mobility of the prosthesis, poor masticatory force, and inadequate oral-nasal separation. This results in poor oral hygiene, an inability to chew food effectively, and a hyponasal voice. Secondary reconstruction, usually combining tissue reconstruction and a dental prosthesis, can effectively resolve these issues.

Secondary oromandibular reconstruction is indicated when no primary mandibular reconstruction was performed, or, more often, because the primary reconstructive efforts have failed. Reconstructive plates may fracture or become exposed, or bone may become exposed due to osteoradionecrosis. Several studies have shown that when the primary mandibular reconstruction involved a plate and soft-tissue-only flap, there is a significant long-term incidence of plate exposure or plate fracture (3–6). Additional secondary reconstructive surgery is generally required, usually with a free, vascularized bone flap.

RECONSTRUCTIVE OPTIONS

Local flaps. Soft-tissue defects of the oral cavity may involve the FOM, tongue, or buccal mucosa. For limited secondary soft-tissue defects, such as tethering from scar contracture or small-volume tissue loss, a variety of local flaps for oral cavity reconstruction have been described. The facial artery myomucosal (FAMM) flap provides non-hair-bearing "like" tissue, and has been used to reconstruct a variety of defects of the hard palate, alveolus, FOM, and upper and lower lips (7,8). In addition, the melolabial flap has been described for intra-oral reconstruction, and can provide up to 15 cm^2 of surface area for reconstruction of the FOM, buccal mucosa, and alveolus (9). Reports of sensory recovery with melolabial flaps, especial in FOM reconstruction, are an additional benefit with this flap (10).

The local flap of choice for secondary reconstruction of soft tissue oral cavity defects depends upon the specific subsite being reconstructed as well as the volume requirements. For the oral tongue, with the exception of cases of scar contracture that may improve with local tissue rearrangement, there are no good local flap options. For limited FOM defects, either the inferiorly based FAMM flap or the melolabial flap can be used with equal efficacy. For small buccal mucosal defects, on the other hand, the melolabial flap is the flap of choice.

Regional flaps. Often, local tissue flaps are unable to provide enough volume and surface area to optimally reconstruct large oral cavity defects. In such instances, regional pedicled tissue transfer techniques may be a more appropriate reconstructive option. The most commonly described regional flaps for oral cavity reconstruction include the platysma myocutaneous flap, pectoralis myocutaneous flap, latissimus dorsi myocutaneous flap, temporalis muscle flap, deltopectoral flap and temporoparietal flap. The platysma myocutaneous flap is thin and pliable and may be useful for FOM defects and small- to moderate-volume defects of the lateral tongue, inferior buccal mucosa, or retromolar trigone (11,12). However, previous neck surgery and radiation may preclude use of this flap. The pectoralis myocutaneous flap has historically been the workhorse flap because of its ease of harvest, reduction of wound complications, and volume of well-vascularized, non-radiated tissue. It has been used for a multitude of defects in the oral cavity (13). Although it can provide a large amount of tissue volume for reconstruction, the gravitational pull on the flap and scar contracture along the vector of the pedicle can severely effect the final reconstructive result and work against the goal of achieving sufficient tongue height and mobility. Similarly, the latissimus dorsi myocutaneous flap is a regional flap that can be transferred on its pedicle to reconstruct a variety of defects in the oral cavity; This flap provides greater surface area, is more pliable, and is better vascularized than the pectoralis flap (14). The temporalis muscle flap has been described for oral cavity reconstructive defects, including the tongue, buccal mucosa, and palate (15). Its main limitations result from the limited volume and surface area which can be transferred, a poor arc of rotation, and the creation of an unsightly donor-site defect. The deltopectoral flap may be used when the pectoralis flap is not available or previously used. It often requires delay when applied superior to the mandible but provides an alternative to distant soft tissue flaps in certain situations (16–18). Finally, the temporo-parietal flap has been used for buccal mucosa or palatal defects (19). Although its donor site deformity is more acceptable than the temporalis muscle flap, it provides minimal volume and surface area for adequate reconstruction.

With respect to the various subsites of the oral cavity to be reconstructed, each of these regional flaps has its strengths and weaknesses based on the goals of reconstruction outlined previously. For the FOM, the platysma, pectoralis, and latissimus dorsi flaps are equally effective options. For oral tongue reconstruction, the platysma flap is best suited for very small-volume, lateral defects. The pectoralis or latissimus dorsi flaps have been utilized for larger volume, posteriorly located reconstructions. The pectoralis, deltopectoral and the platysma flaps rarely extend superiorly enough for reconstructing oral tongue defects involving the anterior one-third of the tongue, so it is difficult to conceive how these flaps could be useful in the context of a secondary reconstruction. The latissimus dorsi flap would fare better in the anterior two-thirds of the tongue, as long as the defect was not complex and was limited to the tongue and FOM. Although the temporalis muscle flap has been described for tongue reconstruction, it is a poor reconstructive option for this subsite. For the buccal mucosa, large-volume defects are optimally reconstructed with pectoralis or latissimus dorsi flaps, and smaller volume defects can be reconstructed with temporalis muscle, temporo-parietal flaps or occasionally, cervicofacial rotation flaps.

Distant flaps. Free-tissue transfer offers the most versatile reconstructive options for secondary soft-tissue augmentation of the oral cavity. The radial forearm free flap is sensate, and its thin, pliable quality makes it the most common free flap used for oral cavity reconstruction (20). When additional volume is required, the lateral arm or anterolateral thigh flap can be used (21,22). For large-volume oral cavity reconstruction, one should consider rectus abdominis, scapula, or latissimus dorsi free-tissue transfers (2,23). These free flaps, however, offer less sensory rehabilitative capability than those mentioned previously.

The choice of free flap for soft-tissue secondary reconstruction should be determined by subsite and volume requirements. For the FOM, the radial forearm flap is the optimal choice because of its thin, pliable surface which will not displace or tether the tongue. Similarly, for small-volume defects of the oral tongue, the radial forearm is the best choice. If more volume is needed for the tongue reconstruction, the lateral arm or anterolateral thigh flap can be used. For massive subtotal or total tongue defects, the rectus abdominis or latissimus dorsi flap will provide the necessary volume and height. Through-and-through buccal and cheek defects are best reconstructed with a folded anterolateral thigh or scapula fasciocutaneous flap.

When free-tissue transfer is performed for secondary reconstruction, the surgery is frequently carried out in a previously dissected neck with potentially limited recipient vessels for anastamosis. The surgeon should be familiar with the previous operative report and be prepared for possible exploration of the contralateral neck (24,25). Preoperative angiography of the external carotid and thoracodorsal trunk is helpful in making the vessel exploration more directed and efficient. In addition, a CT-scan with contrast can describe important venous anatomy. Vein grafts may be necessary, although careful flap choice and placement allows the surgeon to avoid vein grafting in many cases. The saphenous vein is a good donor site for arterial grafting as this vein has more rigid walls, whereas venous vein grafting with larger more pliable veins such as the brachial vein may be more desirable. If the saphenous is to be used for the venous vein graft, care must be taken to have a recipient vein of adequate diameter. Alternative arterial recipient sites are the ascending cervical, transverse cervical, or inferior thyroid arteries. Alternative venous sites are the stump of the internal or external jugular vein, the ascending cervical, or the visceral veins around the hypoglossal nerve. When exploration of the contralateral neck is required and the pedicle must be brought across from the other side, a great deal of additional length of the recipient vessels can be obtained if the facial artery and vein are dissected to the angle of the mandible.

Reconstructive Options for Secondary Composite Defects

Local flaps. Composite, secondary oral-cavity defects include those involving the mandible or hard palate. Under most circumstances, local-flap reconstructive options are inadequate; however, for small, composite palate defects, up to 7 cm^2, the palatal island flap has been described (26). The dual layer of mucosa and periosteum of this flap provides adequate separation of the oral and nasal cavity. The FAMM flap has also been described for very small alveolar defects, typically less than 2 cm^2 in size (20). In contrast, for composite segmental mandible defects, there are no good local tissue options. In cases of mandibular bone or reconstructive plate exposure, coverage with local tissue alone is unlikely to lead to a successful outcome.

Regional flaps. Unlike local tissue rearrangement, regional flaps can provide significant volume, sufficient surface area, and in some instances, vascularized bone. Regional-flap reconstruction of composite-palate defects that have been reported include the pectoralis, temporo-parietal, and temporalis muscle flaps (13,15,19). The bulkiness of the flap and the significant distance of the defect from the donor site make the pectoralis flap a suboptimal choice for palate reconstruction. The temporalis muscle and temporo-parietal flaps may be acceptable for smaller palatal defects, but cannot provide bulk or bone.

For composite mandibular defects, the pectoralis, deltopectoral, latissimus dorsi, and trapezius flaps have been described (6,13,14,27). Secondary reconstruction of the mandible is typically indicated because of primary reconstructive failure including flap failure, plate exposure or plate fracture. The goals of reconstruction with a pedicled, regional flap when bone is not being transferred include volume replacement and soft-tissue coverage of the defect. The pectoralis myocutaneous flap has been utilized with moderate success for soft-tissue coverage and volume replacement following mandibular reconstructive plate exposure. Factors limiting its utility, however, are the gradual loss of flap volume secondary to muscle atrophy and the frequent utilization of the distal thin, random portion of the flap to cover the defect and provide volume. Several studies have shown a significantly higher failure rate with pectoralis flap plate coverage when compared to vascularized, free soft-tissue transfer (4,6,28). When plates are exposed or fractured, the best chance for a complication-free outcome is the replacement of volume using vascularized bone and reliable soft tissue coverage. Regional vascularized bone flaps have been described, including pectoralis with rib, trapezius with scapula spine, and latissimus dorsi with rib, but are no longer used due to their lack of reliability and the overall superiority of free, vascularized bone flaps (29–31).

Distant flaps. When vascularized bone is indicated for secondary oral cavity reconstruction, there are no regional flap options that can compare to vascularized bone-containing free flaps. A number of different vascularized bone-containing flaps can be utilized, including fibula, iliac crest, and scapula osseocutaneous free tissue transfers. These flaps differ in the quality of bone stock and the characteristics of their associated soft tissue component. All of these flaps have been used for composite mandible reconstruction, and the choice of flap for a patient depends on the defect as well as an appropriate pre-operative assessment of the available donor sites (28). The fibula offers the longest bone available, is relatively easy to harvest, and provides sufficient bone stock for osseointegrated implants. However, its associated cutaneous paddle is not always reliable and may be insufficient when significant soft-tissue reconstruction is also required. Also, patients having certain anomalies of their lower extremity, peripheral vascular anatomy or those with significant peripheral vascular disease may not be candidates for fibular free flaps. The iliac crest, on the other hand, offers the best available bone stock and is the only flap that can restore similar anterior mandibular height in the dentate patient. However, it has the drawback of a shorter pedicle as well as the limited flexibility of its associated soft-tissue component, particularly if the intraoral defect is more complex than alveolus and FOM. The scapula is most useful when independent, complex soft-tissue reconstruction is also required. The bone stock is not as significant as the other flap choices, and patient positioning for scapula harvest limits the widespread use of this flap.

A variety of flaps, including iliac crest, scapula, fibula, and osseocutaneous radial forearm, have been described for palatal composite defects (32). For large-volume, combined palate and maxillary defects, several authors have described the effective use of the iliac crest and internal oblique muscle free flap (33,34). The iliac bone is used to reconstruct the palate and bony prominence of the midface while the internal oblique muscle is used to obliterate the maxilla and re-surface the hard palate. If only a small amount of bone is needed and there is not a significant volume defect, an osseocutaneous radial forearm flap is another useful option, providing a thin, pliable soft-tissue surface for the neopalate. Large premaxillary defects, commonly encountered following gunshot wounds, can be secondarily reconstructed to improve midface projection. The fibular free flap has been used with success in such instances (35).

DECISION-MAKING TIPS

Definitive, immediate reconstruction of oral-cavity defects is usually preferred over secondary reconstruction. However, when primary reconstruction was not performed, or when it has failed, secondary reconstruction may be indicated. Patients with large palatal defects who desire a more permanent reconstruction than that provided by a dental prosthesis can expect good results with free, composite soft-tissue and bone flaps, achieving separation of the oral and nasal cavity and allowing the use of conventional dentures or osseointegrated implants. Another example of successful secondary reconstruction can be the case of the patient with mandibular plate fracture or exposure. The use of free vascularized bone to achieve mandibular continuity can improve both function and cosmesis.

Successful secondary reconstruction of soft-tissue defects of the oral cavity, however, is not as readily achieved, particularly if improved speech and swallowing function is the surgical indication. Very little appears in the literature on this subject; in one small series of five patients who underwent secondary tongue reconstruction, only one patient was able to successfully transition from gastrostomy tube feedings, and no patients demonstrated improved speech (1).

Despite aggressive attempts to release tongue tethering and maintain volume and tongue height, these authors postulated that progressive scarring and fibrosis occurring over time led to damage to residual tongue muscle function. Immediate reconstruction may allow maintenance of certain functions of normal swallowing that are very difficult to restore with late reconstruction. Speech function is also difficult to improve with secondary reconstruction, due to well-established, compensatory articulating strategies that develop after primary resection. Thus, before undertaking surgery to improve speech or swallowing, both surgeon and patient should be cognizant of the limitations of delayed reconstructive surgery.

Another factor complicating secondary reconstructive surgery is the fact that these procedures are typically performed in the setting of a previously operated surgical field. Frequently, the patient has had a previous free or pedicled flap. Knowledge of the details of the prior surgery, including what initial recipient vessels were used, are critically important when a second free flap surgery is planned. Despite these challenges, secondary reconstructive surgery that includes second free flaps can be successfully performed. A recent study showed the success rate for a second free flap to be similar to that of initial free-flap surgery (24). Another study showed a 100% success rate with free flaps performed after previous neck dissection, although exploration of the contralateral neck was often necessary to attain sufficient recipient vessels (25). These authors recommended the use of flaps with long vascular pedicles in the re-operative setting, to avoid the use of vein grafts.

CONCLUSION

In summary, although primary oral-cavity reconstruction usually offers superior results, secondary reconstruction can achieve improved cosmesis and function in select patients. The principles of secondary oral-cavity reconstruction are similar to those for primary reconstruction. Although secondary reconstructive surgery is more difficult because it is performed in a previously surgically modified area, it can be immensely successful with proper planning and flap selection.

REFERENCES

1. Salibian AH, Allison GR, Strelzow VV, Krugman ME, Rappaport I, McMicken BL, Etchepare TL. Secondary microvascular tongue reconstruction: functional results. Head Neck 1993; 15:389–397.
2. Urken ML, Moscoso JF, Lawson W, Biller HF. A systematic approach to functional reconstruction of the oral cavity following partial and total glossectomy. Arch Otolaryngol Head Neck Surg 1994; 120:589–601.
3. Urken ML, Buchbinder D, Costantino PD, Sinha U, Okay D, Lawson W, Biller HF. Oromandibular reconstruction using microvascular composite flaps: report of 210 cases. Arch Otolaryngol Head Neck Surg 1998; 124:46–55.
4. Shpitzer T, Gullane PJ, Neligan PC, Irish JC, Freeman JE, Van den Brekel M, Gur E. The free vascularized flap and the flap plate options: comparative results of reconstruction of lateral mandibular defects. Laryngoscope 2000; 110:2056–2060.
5. Blackwell KE, Buchbinder D, Urken ML. Lateral mandibular reconstruction using soft-tissue free flaps and plates. Arch Otolaryngol Head Neck Surg 1996; 122:672–678.
6. Cordeiro PG, Hidalgo DA. Soft tissue coverage of mandibular reconstruction plates. Head Neck 1994; 16:112–115.
7. Pribaz J, Stephens W, Crespo L, Gifford G. A new intraoral flap: facial artery musculo-mucosal (famm) flap. Plast Reconstr Surg 1992; 90:421–429.
8. Zhao Z, Li S, Yan Y, Li Y, Yang M, Mu L, Huang W, Liu Y, Zhai H, Jin J, et al. New buccinator myomucosal island flap: anatomic study and clinical application. Plast Reconstr Surg 1999; 104:55–64.
9. Roth J, Patete M, Goodwin WJ. Use of the melolabial flap in intraoral reconstruction. Otolaryngol Head Neck Surg 1996; 114:12–17.
10. Civantos FJ, Roth J, Goodwin WJ, Weed DT. Sensory recovery in melolabial flaps used for oral cavity reconstruction. Otolaryngol Head Neck Surg 2000; 122:509–513.
11. Esclamado RM, Burkey BB, Carroll WR, Bradford CR. The platysma myocutaneous flap: indications and caveats. Arch Otolaryngol Head Neck Surg 1994; 120:32–35.
12. Koch WM. The platysma myocutaneous flap: underused alternative for head and neck reconstruction. Laryngoscope 2002; 112:1204–1208.
13. Liu R, Gullane P, Brown D, Irish J. Pectoralis major myocutaneous pedicled flap in head and neck reconstruction: retrospective review of indications and results in 244 consecutive cases at the Toronto General Hospital. J Otolaryngol 2001; 30:34–40.
14. Sabatier RE, Bakamjian VY. Transaxillary latissimus dorsi flap reconstruction in head and neck cancer. Limitations and refinements in 56 cases. Am J Surg 1985; 150: 427–434.
15. Thomson CJ, Allison RS. The temporalis muscle flap in intraoral reconstruction. Aust N Z J Surg 1997; 67:878–882.

16. Panje WR, Morris MR. The temporoparietal fascia flap in head and neck reconstruction. Ear Nose Throat J 1991; 70:311–317.
17. Soutar DS, McGregor IA. The radial forearm flap in intraoral reconstruction: the experience of 60 consecutive cases. Plast Reconstr Surg 1986; 78:1–8.
18. Civantos FJ Jr, Burkey B, Lu FL, Armstrong W. Lateral arm microvascular flap in head and neck reconstruction. Arch Otolaryngol Head Neck Surg 1997; 123:830–836.
19. Wei FC, Jain V, Celik N, Chen HC, Chuang DC, Lin CH. Have we found an ideal soft-tissue flap? An experience with 672 anterolateral thigh flaps. Plast Reconstr Surg 2002; 109:2219–2226; discussion 2227–2230.
20. Lyos AT, Evans GR, Perez D, Schusterman MA. Tongue reconstruction: outcomes with the rectus abdominis flap. Plast Reconstr Surg 1999; 103:442–447; discussion 448–449.
21. Amin AA, Baldwin BJ, Gurlek A, Miller MJ, Kroll SS, Reece GP, Evans GR, Robb GR, Schusterman MA. Second free flaps in head and neck reconstruction. J Reconstr Microsurg 1998; 14:365–368; discussion 368–369.
22. Head C, Sercarz JA, Abemayor E, Calcaterra TC, Rawnsley JD, Blackwell KE. Microvascular reconstruction after previous neck dissection. Arch Otolaryngol Head Neck Surg 2002; 128:328–331.
23. Genden EM, Lee BB, Urken ML. The Palatal Island flap for reconstruction of palatal and retromolar trigone defects revisited. Arch Otolaryngol Head Neck Surg 2001; 127:837–841.
24. Shapiro MJ. Use of trapezius myocutaneous flaps in the reconstruction of head and neck defects. Arch Otolaryngol 1981; 107:333–336.
25. Moscoso JF, Keller J, Genden E, Weinberg H, Biller HF, Buchbinder D, Urken ML. Vascularized bone flaps in oromandibular reconstruction. A comparative anatomic study of bone stock from various donor sites to assess suitability for enosseous dental implants. Arch Otolaryngol Head Neck Surg 1994; 120:36–43.
26. Bell MS, Barron PT. The rib-pectoralis major osteomyocutaneous flap. Ann Plast Surg 1981; 6:347–353.
27. Maves MD, Philippsen LP. Surgical anatomy of the scapular spine in the trapezius-osteomuscular flap. Arch Otolaryngol Head Neck Surg 1986; 112:173–175.
28. Richards MA, Poole MD, Godfrey AM. The serratus anterior/rib composite flap in mandibular reconstruction. Br J Plast Surg 1985; 38:466–477.
29. Futran ND, Haller JR. Considerations for free-flap reconstruction of the hard palate. Arch Otolaryngol Head Neck Surg 1999; 125:665–669.
30. Genden EM, Wallace D, Buchbinder D, Okay D, Urken ML. Iliac crest internal oblique osteomusculocutaneous free flap reconstruction of the postablative palatomaxillary defect. Arch Otolaryngol Head Neck Surg 2001; 127:854–861.
31. Brown JS. Deep circumflex iliac artery free flap with internal oblique muscle as a new method of immediate reconstruction of maxillectomy defect. Head Neck 1996; 18: 412–421.
32. Futran ND, Wadsworth JT, Villaret D, Farwell DG. Midface reconstruction with the fibula free flap. Arch Otolaryngol Head Neck Surg 2002; 128:161–166.
33. Genden EM, Wallace D, Buchbinder D, Okay D, Urken M. Iliac crest internal oblique osteomusculocutaneous free flap reconstruction of the postablative palatomaxillary defect. Arch Otolaryngol Head Neck Surg 2001; 127(7):854–861.
34. Brown JS. Deep circumflex iliac artery free flap with internal oblique muscle as a new method of immediate reconstruction of maxillectomy defect. Head Neck 1996; 18(5):412–421.
35. Futran ND, Wadsworth JT, Villaret D, Farwell DG. Midface reconstruction with the fibula free flap. Arch Otolaryngol Head Neck Surg 2002; 128(2):161–166.

20
Speech and Swallowing Rehabilitation

Bonnie Martin-Harris and Julie Blair
MUSC Evelyn Trammell Institute for Voice and Swallowing, Charleston, South Carolina, U.S.A.

INTRODUCTION

Speech and swallowing are highly complex physiologic activities essential to human survival and a reasonable quality of life. These functions are refined through development to adulthood, and become highly predictable and reliable. The complexity and importance of these functions are best appreciated by knowing, studying, and treating cancer survivors who have suffered significant disruption to the vocal and speech subsystems and upper aerodigestive tract. The authors' intentions in this chapter include sharing of clinical experience and evidenced-based evaluation and treatment methods from years of practice with patients prior to and following oncologic treatments for oral cancers. Due to the paucity of controlled, prospective studies related to outcomes following oral cavity cancers and associated reconstruction, much of the information provided may be related to oropharyngeal cancer treatment and reconstruction. To fully comprehend the potential dysfunction in these situations, it is important to begin with a functional, physiologic perspective on the voice, speech, and swallowing anatomy that was explained in earlier chapters of this text.

VOCAL SUBSYSTEMS

The primary subsystems of voice and speech production include: respiration, phonation, resonance, and articulation. These subsystems are highly dependent on one another for audible, aesthetic and intelligible oral communication. Any disruption to one or more of these subsystems through surgical ablation, invasion or other adjuvant oncologic treatments will result in a functional maladaptive compensation of one or more of the remaining subsystems, creating increased labor of vocalization and speech production.

The respiratory system drives the onset and efficiency of vocal fold vibration. Decreases in respiratory drive decrease the quality of the vocal signal and contribute to vocal fatigue. Examples of disruptions to pulmonary function that may impact the voice and speech functional outcome of the patient are listed in Table 1. For example, the presence of an indwelling tracheostomy tube, temporary or permanent, requires training to produce a timely and efficient voice for functional oral communication. The type of training will depend in part on the type of tracheostomy tube and/or speaking valve, a topic that goes beyond the scope of this discussion. Further, coexisting chronic pulmonary disease may result in restricted or obstructed airflow with inadequate flow volumes to effect periodic phonation.

Phonation refers to the outcome of tone generation through the vibratory activity of the true vocal folds. If the vocal folds present with characteristics such as, increased viscosity and poor hydration, are constantly bathed in pooled secretions that enter the laryngeal inlet, or have been surgically disrupted, the perceived vocal characteristics of pitch and quality will be disturbed (Table 1). Further, decreased vocal fold hydration may result in increases in phonatory effort (1). High doses of radiation may result in extreme tissue dryness and laryngeal edema, both of which have a significant impact on vocal quality. Alterations in the voice impact the listeners' perception of the total disability of the individual and can lead to

Table 1 Factors Impacting the Vocal Subsystems Following Treatments for Oropharyngeal Cancer

Respiration
Indwelling tracheostomy tubes
Obstructive lung disease
Restrictive lung disease
Decreased elasticity of chest wall
Physical deconditioning
Chronic aspiration
Phonation
Poorly hydrated vocal fold tissues
Pooled pharyngeal secretions
Edema
Chronic coughing, throat clearing
Surgical ablation of vocal fold tissue
Scarring
Resonance
Tongue resection
Mandibular resections
Soft palate resection
Diminished contraction of pharyngeal musculature related to surgery or radiation treatment
Articulation
Partial or total tongue resection
Teeth extraction
Mandibular resections
Palatal resections
Labial resections

significant functional and emotional consequences for patients treated for oral and pharyngeal cancers (2).

The aspects of vocalization that give the voice character and richness are produced by the shaping the fundamental tone via alterations in configuration of the vocal tract chambers or resonators: pharynx, oral and nasal cavity. The fundamental vibration produced at the level of the vocal folds is shaped by these structures and results in a normal, human male or female quality to the voice (2). Resonance has a direct impact on the quality of the voice, and is often altered following surgeries that change the shape of the cavities. In the cases of some tongue resections, a patient's voice will be characterized by aberrations in oral resonance secondary to changes in the shape of the oral chamber and compensate by assuming a predominate pharyngeal resonance to the voice. Even though the vocal folds may not be directly involved in the surgical resection or radiation beam, the altered shape of the pharynx and oral cavities significantly impact the sound quality that is perceived by the listener (Table 1). An explanation of the impact of resonance on voice production used in the clinic includes that of a bell with a designated gong size (i.e., true vocal folds) and characteristic shape (i.e., resonating chamber). The patient is provided with an explanation that even though the gong is spared, changes in the shape of the bell along any dimension will result in a difference from the pre-treatment voice. This scenario is analogous to surgical resection and reconstruction of the oral, nasal and pharyngeal cavities, and the impact of that intervention on resonance.

This refinement of the articulated sound generated in the vocal tract is a highly human trait and one that may be significantly altered by surgical resection or radiation therapy. As the glottic pulse is resonated through the vocal tract, the motions of the intrinsic and extrinsic muscles of the tongue, soft palate and the coupling of these mobile structures to the stable alveolus, teeth and pharyngeal walls produces the placements and manner of speech production that yield intelligible articulated speech. Any invasion to the tissues of these mobile structures or stable framework will impact the precision and manner of the articulated sound. The severity of this disruption, like all aspects of oral communication, will be in part dependent on the extent of the surgical resection and radiation dose, and the nature of the reconstruction.

With any cancer of the oropharyngeal mechanism, disruption of the vocal tract structures will often have an associated impact on the act of swallowing. Though not as refined an action as voice or speech production, swallowing is extremely complex and highly dependent on the coordinated and effective movements of the structures of the upper aerodigestive tract.

SWALLOWING

Swallowing, or deglutition, is the physiologic act that is responsible for secretion management and ingestion of foods and liquids for primary nutrition. This act or process requires complex neural integration and engagement of overlapping movements of muscles and structures in the functional anatomic regions of the oral cavity, pharynx, larynx and esophagus (Table 2) (3–6). The material that is swallowed must be pushed through the upper aerodigestive tract by application of positive pressure to the posterior edge of the bolus in order to safely and efficiently clear the upper airway. Not only is the bolus "pushed," but it is channeled through pockets and pathways formed by oropharyngeal and laryngeal structures, while valves simultaneously open or close to facilitate safe passage through the upper airway and into

Table 2 Physiologic Components of Normal Swallowing in Adults

- Bolus containment
- Stabilization of the floor of mouth
- Bolus preparation, mastication and formation
- Superior and posterior tongue propulsion
- Initiation of the pharyngeal swallow
    - Elevation and retraction of the soft palate
    - Relaxation of the cricopharyngeus
    - Widening and shortening of pharyngeal chamber
    - Superior and anterior hyolaryngeal excursion
    - Closure of the extrinsic and intrinsic laryngeal valves
    - Retraction of the tongue base
    - Opening of the pharyngoesophageal segment
    - Stripping action of the pharyngeal musculature
- Peristaltic contraction of esophageal musculature
- Opening of the lower esophageal segment

the esophagus. There exists a tight temporal and somewhat reciprocal relationship between respiration and swallowing activity, with an apneic event imposed just prior to and during the height of the swallow. Expiration has been shown to bracket swallow activity in the adult human and is often integrated into the latter stages of swallowing (7–9).

Pre-swallowing activity begins prior to placement of food or liquid into the oral cavity. An individual anticipates the upcoming swallow, and makes judgments regarding the types of foods he or she will eat or drink, and selects appropriate volumes of foods and liquids. Therefore, if a patient presents with significant cognitive impairment, is unable to anticipate the consequences of behavior, of experiences problems with upper extremity strength and coordination, their swallow may be compromised because the materials that enter the oral cavity are of inadequate or excessive size to permit a safe and efficient swallow. Once the material is placed into the oral cavity, the floor of mouth stabilizes through contraction of the myohyoid/geniohyoid muscle complex, and is prepared for progressive ingestion. The manner of this preparation will depend on patient preference and characteristics of the bolus (10–13). Liquids free fall rapidly and do not require significant oral preparation or mastication. However, the extent of motor control to temporally manage a liquid bolus requires greater fine motor control than semisolid or solid foods. Therefore, if the tongue is surgically ablated, the patient's ability to contain the bolus in the oral cavity for adequate duration to allow sufficient temporal coordination of laryngeal closure, may be impaired. Semisolids and solids require varying degrees of preparation and mastication. When the bolus is in a ready state for swallowing, the tongue pushes against the hard palate and applies positive pressure to the tail of the bolus (14,15).

When the bolus head contacts the areas of the posterior oral cavity, oropharynx and in some cases, the superior hypopharynx (i.e., depending on the volume and texture of the bolus) a complex series of sequential and simultaneous events begin that are outlined in Table 2 (16). In early literature, this aspect of swallowing was referred to as a swallowing "reflex." However, the pharyngeal components of swallowing have been observed to lack the predictability and necessary brevity of response to be termed a true reflex (3). Rather, swallowing appears to be triggered by a multiplicity of sensory inputs that include pressure or tactile sensation, taste and to a lesser degree temperature. Though the exact neurophysiologic properties of pharyngeal swallow initiation are far from understood, it has been shown that tongue upward and posterior progression of tongue movement and characteristics of the bolus impact the timing of pharyngeal swallow initiation (10–15). Initiation of the pharyngeal swallow is characterized by brisk elevation and retraction of the soft palate that applies a small pressure to the bolus tail (17) and prevents regurgitation of ingested materials into the nasal cavity. Nearly simultaneously there is superior and anterior displacement of the hyoid bone and larynx, that moves as a functional compartment during swallow and termed, the hyolaryngeal complex. The timely movement of this complex during swallowing is critical for airway protection and passage of the bolus into the esophagus. As the larynx begins to move in an upward direction at the start of pharyngeal swallow initiation, the arytenoids cartilages and true vocal folds progress medially, and the epiglottis assumes a horizontal position (8,9). However, it is not until the hyolaryngeal complex moves briskly forward at the height of the swallow that the extrinsic and intrinsic laryngeal valves progress to a tight seal. If the larynx moves only in a superior direction, without full anterior excursion with the hyoid bone, there will be some glottic closure and some degree of laryngeal entry by the ingested material. This extreme anterior displacement of the hyolaryngeal complex results in apposition of the epiglottic base to the anteriorly and forwardly displaced arytenoid cartilages further shielding the laryngeal inlet during bolus passage. The anterior motion of the hyoid and larynx effects a shield for the laryngeal inlet underneath the posteriorward progression of the tongue base, further contributing to airway protection during the swallow. These critical biomechanical events can not be accurately assessed during a clinical or bedside examination, and must be directly observed with visualization instrumentation to ensure accurate diagnosis and the appropriate applications of swallowing treatments. This becomes vitally important in large oral cavity, mandible, and floor of mouth surgeries related to cancer extirpation or to self-inflicted gun shot wounds in which the hyomandibular complex, and therefore the hyolaryngeal complex, may be severely disrupted.

The cricopharyngeal muscle, the primary component of the pharyngoesophageal segment (PES), is tonically contracted at rest to prevent ingestion of air into the lower gastrointestinal tract with basal breathing. However, apparently early in the dynamics of the pharyngeal swallow, this muscle relaxes and becomes compliant (4,10,16,17). The compliant muscle facilitates opening of the cervical esophageal region as the cricoid cartilage is pulled away from the posterior pharyngeal wall with superior and anterior traction applied by the action of the hyolaryngeal complex. Also during this time, the tongue base moves progressively in retracted motion and has been shown to be the highest generator of positive pressure applied to the bolus tail during the swallow allowing for complete pharyngeal clearance of the ingested material or sections (15,17). The entire functional process of oropharyngeal swallowing may be severely disrupted if inadequate tissue bulk exists in the tongue base region or if the muscle function in this region is comprised.

As the bolus is propelled through the pharynx by action of the tongue base, a stripping-like action by sequential contraction of the pharyngeal musculature is applied to the bolus tail. The final muscle contraction in the sequence meets the collapsing cricopharyngeal sphincter as the tail of bolus passes completely from the pharynx and enters the cervical esophagus (17). Once the bolus has cleared the pharynx and enters the esophagus, a sequential peristaltic contractile wave pushes the bolus tail through the esophageal body ending with eventual relaxation of the lower esophageal sphincter and bolus passage into the stomach. This sphincteric mechanism may be disrupted during neck dissection, lingual release approaches to the oral cavity and during oropharyngectomy when the constrictor musculature and associated neurovascular supply is sacrificed.

The functional interdependence of structures required during normal swallowing highlights the primary reason why surgical resection of only one structure may impact several aspects of oropharyngeal swallow ability. This dependency of one structural motion on the other highlights the surgical rehabilitation challenges faced by the surgeon and swallowing clinician. Rehabilitative surgical attempts such as cricopharyngeal myotomy to effect PES opening, or thyroplasty to improve vocal fold closure, have a uni-dimensional impact on the multidimensional oropharyngeal swallow. Though these methods have clinical utility in carefully selected patients, they rarely result in returning the patient to normal or in some cases even functional swallowing ability.

EVALUATION METHODS AND OBSERVATIONS

Preoperative Clinical Assessment and Counseling: Prior to any oncologic treatment applied to the head or neck, the patient's premorbid voice, speech and swallowing function should be evaluated clinically by observation of function and visual examination (18,19). Further, the patient and the individuals involved in the support system and care of the patient should be advised and counseled regarding the potential impact(s) of the oncologic treatments on voice and speech production and swallowing ability. Though case dependent, the patient and caregivers may also benefit from visitations from a trained survivor of head and neck cancer. A clinical evaluation of voice and speech includes obtaining a careful medical and social history, and perceptual assessments of voice and resonance, and articulation. Swallowing is observed with liquid and food textures and clinicial signs of swallowing difficulty and aspiration are recorded (5). During the clinical evaluation, the clinician also observes the patient's general emotional affect, ability to process and retain information, level of independence, and family dynamics. These factors highly impact the success of the rehabilitation program and functional outcome of the patient (20,21). Instrumental evaluations of voice, speech and swallowing may not always be indicated in the standard of care of the patient with head and neck cancer facing surgery, however, these measures are often beneficial to provide the patient, surgeon and speech pathologist (i.e., speech and swallowing specialist) with anticipation of post-treatment impacts on their baseline function. It is crucial for the expirative surgeon to provide the speech and swallowing specialist with an assessment of the expected structures that will likely be involved in the oral cavity resection to facilitate post-operative speech and swallowing treatment planning. Further, information regarding the planned reconstruction approach by the reconstructive will allow the speech pathologist to anticipate post-operative function and treatment options. This pre-operative didactic between the surgeon and speech pathologist assists the latter in understanding the potential neurologic compromise that may involve structures such as, the motor branches of the muscles of mastication, lingual nerve, hypoglossal nerve, glossopharyngeal nerve, and the superior and recurrent laryngeal nerves. Additionally, the muscles that may require resection and/or reconstruction will ultimately play a direct role in swallowing function. Also, edema of the oral, pharyngeal and laryngeal structures following various extirpative surgeries and neck dissections related to removal or ligation of various venous structures (i.e., jugular vein) may play a role in the post-operative approach to evaluation and treatment of the patient's swallowing impairment.

Though this interdisciplinary pretreatment planning greatly assists in anticipating the functional consequences of the surgery on speech, voice and swallowing functions and treatment planning, there will be unknown and sometimes unanticipated changes in these functions and post-operative sequelae that will depend on the extent and nature of the surgical resection and reconstruction, medical and emotional condition of the patient. The functional consequences of primary and post-operative radiation and chemotherapy fit in this category of unpredictable outcomes, because they have not been systematically studied in controlled clinical trials. Reports do suggest sometimes very severe effects of radiation and chemotherapy treatments on voice, speech and swallowing ability (22–26), however, clinical experience reveals that many intervening variables appear to be related to the patient's speech,voice and swallowing disorder(s) and functional recovery. Common complications associated with radiation and chemotherapy include tissue fibrosis with reduction in range of movement during swallowing by critical oropharyngeal structures, xerostomia, and discomfort associated with mucositis. Speech pathologists often assist the surgeon in management of the functional manifestations of these complications. Patients are trained and encouraged to swallow frequently and to engage in routine isometric exercises to prevent or lessen these functional mordities (27,28).

Instrumental Examination of Voice, Speech, and Swallowing

Voice, speech, and swallowing problems often co-occur in patients treated for head and neck cancer, therefore, these functions are most efficiently evaluated in the same clinical session whenever possible. Instrumental examinations are very useful in assisting the extirpative surgeon, reconstructive surgeon, and prosthodontist regarding the evaluation of effectiveness of various restorative surgeries and and devices such as, flap reconstruction (29–34), palatal appliances (35–41), laryngeal advancement (42), cricopharyngeal myotomy (43–45), and vocal fold augmentation and medialization (46–48).

Computerized instruments and software programs are helpful in the generation of clinically meaningful information regarding the acoustic and aerodynamic aspects voice and speech production (49). Pre- and post-operative measures of phonatory efficiency and endurance, signal perturbation, frequency, and intensity may be helpful in anticipating post-operative function and treatment planning. Further, measures of airflow volume, airflow rate, glottal resistance, and nasalance may also assist the surgeon and prosthodontist with judging the functional impact of reconstructive techniques and in the fabrication and refinement of oral appliances. A standard articulation battery that includes co-articulation information in contextual speech is often applied and assists in determining pre- and post-operative changes in speech intelligibility and assists in measuring progressive improvement during the rehabilitation period (49–51).

Direct visualization of laryngeal and vocal tract function with rigid and flexible fiberoptic endoscopy are highly useful techniques for describing maladaptive compensations of these structures that a patient may employ in attempt to adapt to the surgical changes that have occurred. If vibratory characteristics and glottic closure patterns are the functional areas of study, videostroboscopy with a rigid intraoral fiberoptic scope is the desired method for observing this detail during sustained voicing. A secondary benefit of this frequent visual monitoring of function by the speech pathologist and surgeon, is addition opportunity for surveillance of recurrent disease (52,53). Unlike videostroboscopy that permits magnified images of the larynx during sustained voicing, flexible nasopharyngeal laryngoscopy permits visualization of the entire vocal tract dynamics during connected speech. Therefore, this method is particularly effective in assessing the potential effectiveness of surgical flap restoration or prosthetic management of patients with velopharyngeal incompetence.

Flexible endoscopic evaluation of swallowing (FEES) may also be used to assess components of swallowing function (54–57). Endoscopic visualization provides observation of swallowing dynamics that occur early and late in the pharyngeal swallow. The impact of swallowing dysfunction evaluated with this evaluation method are based on the presence of pharyngeal or laryngeal residue and tracheal aspiration observed after the swallow. A limitation of flexible endoscopy is that swallowing dynamics are obscured by obliteration of the view as the endoscope tip opposes pharyngeal and laryngeal structures during hyolaryngeal excursion. Further, the clinician is not able to observe the oral cavity with the distal tip of the scope in the hypopharyx, and is thereby unable to determine the potential interdependent impact of oral dynamics on the pharyngeal components of swallow. Nonetheless, FEES does have a role in the assessment of clinical function, and is often used as an initial screening device to determine patient's airway protection ability and candidacy for further biomechanical study. The selection of this and all methods of swallowing assessment will be dependent on the nature of the patient, the intent of the examination and on the clinical setting. In addition to swallowing mechanics, there has been recent attention placed on the role of sensory input to swallowing initiation, safety and efficiency. This attention is reflected in the development and application of a swallowing evaluation method that combines fiberoptic endoscopic viewing with sensory threshold testing (Flexible Endoscopic Evaluation of Swallowing with Sensory Testing, FEEST) (58,59). This technique establishes a sensory threshold to puffs of air delivered to the laryngeal structures and has been associated with the risk of aspiration in patients with neurologic insults. Though the importance of a patient's ability to feel foods or liquids in the laryngeal inlet would seem to have impact on their initiation of an expectorative attempt, however, the value of the additional sensory testing and the meaning of the sensory threshold in patients treated for head and neck cancer has not been studied in large clinical trials.

The modified barium swallowing evaluation, a videofluoroscopic procedure conducted by a speech pathologist and radiologist, employs video or digital radiographic imaging of upper aerodigestive tract dynamics during orophparyngeal and cervical esophageal swallowing (4,5). This examination permits viewing of the relation of bolus flow to structural movements throughout the upper aerodigestive tract as the bolus passes through the cervical esophagus. Because the physiologic mechanisms of swallow are clearly visualized at the height of swallowing, the clinician can accurately determine the biomechanical nature of the swallowing disorder and the cause of aspiration (4,5,60–62). Therapeutic maneuvers and compensatory postures are introduced during the examination, and the functional impact of these strategies is visualized at the time of the exam (4,5,62,63). This type of information is essential to effective treatment planning, and in expediting the course of functional recovery (61,62). Even though the esophagus is not the major focus of a functional swallowing evaluation in patients with oral and pharyngeal cancers by the speech pathologist, observations of esophageal clearance in the upright position has prognostic nutritional implications by determining a realistic eating and drinking rate for safe and efficient oral intake.

VOICE, RESONANCE, AND SPEECH DISORDERS

Voice and resonance disorders are common following oncologic treatments for oral and pharyngeal cancers. The vibratory characteristics of the vocal folds are highly susceptible to added mass associated with post-surgical swelling secondary to intubation or to edema as a temporary or permanent sequela to radiation therapy or surgical treatment of cancer in the head and neck region. Increased vocal fold mass will often result in a lowered vocal pitch, and edema of the supraglottic structures may alter the resonant frequencies futher leading to the perception of lowered pitch. On the other hand, scarring of the vocal folds can lead to tissue stiffness with the perception of elevated pitch. Further, changes in the glottic closure pattern and periodicity of vocal fold vibration will change the perceived vocal signal. It has been mentioned that alteration to the shape of the vocal tract in any of the resonating cavities may impact the resonance and quality of the voice, and that the severity of the perceptual impairment will depend on the nature and extent of the resection and reconstruction. For example, patient's who have a narrowed pharynx as a result of sacrificed malignant pharyngeal tissue or radiation fibrosis, will often have a voice that is perceived as slightly higher in pitch. Also, the resonant frequencies may be altered by interposition of a tissue graft for reconstruction, or by pharyngeal shortening as in the case of a laryngeal surgical suspension that may be used following a supraglottic laryngectomy (42). These alterations in structural shape lead to consequent changes in the perceived sound. Oral cavity resections that involve significant sections of the tongue may result in a compensatory cul-de-sac resonance that is clearly perceived as abnormal by the patient and listener. Disruption of the hard or soft palate yield varied degrees of hypernasal resonance, with or without nasal emission.

As with voice and resonance, speech production or the articulation of sounds, is affected to varying degrees depending on the size of the surgical resection and type of the reconstruction. The tongue, the primary mobile articulator, is responsible for shaping the breath stream during vowel and consonant production. Surgical ablation of the tongue will result in varied degrees of speech sound distortions (49–51). In the cases of anterior tongue resection, the patient will experience primary difficulty on sounds requiring elevation of the tongue tip and blade to the anterior alveolar ridge. Light articulatory contacts are common following this type of surgery and may be easily compensated for by "overshooting" the target with exaggerated or compensatory articulation placement. Involvement of the lateral tongue will impact tongue shaping ability and likely result in some distortion of sibilant sounds such as, /s/ and /z/, and of fricative productions like, "sh" /ʃ/, "ch" /ʧ/ or "j" /ʤ/. When the back of the tongue is involved in the surgical resection or reconstruction, the result will be variable degrees of distortions on productions requiring tongue back to soft palate contact such as, /k/ or /g/. Much attention is typically given to the distorted consonant phonemes characteristic of patient's speech following oral cavity resections. However, any change in the tongue structure or in the shape of the oral cavity or oropharynx will also result in varying patterns of vowel distortions. Commonly, speech pathologists overlook this important contribution to speech intelligibility. Even though consonants are critical to perceiving word boundaries, the vowels are extremely important to the overall intelligibility of speech and perception of normalcy of speech production (49).

In addition to a discussion of surgical changes that disrupt articulation, fibrosis of oral and pharyngeal cavity structures secondary to primary or post-operative radiotherapy can have a devastating impact on the range and precision of movement of muscles and structures essential for normal articulation and resonance (64). The tongue may loose its degrees of freedom of movement, and consequently become tight with poor agility during oral communication attempts. Finally, extreme xerostomia interferes with the fluidity of co-articulatory movements and the precision of articulatory placements during attempted speech production.

Treatments for Disorders of Voice, Resonance, and Articulation

Voice and Resonance: Voice is rarely treated in isolation in patients treated for oral and pharyngeal cancers. Rather, all subsystems of the vocal tract are treated in unison because of their overlapping influences on one another. Much of what is done in post-treatment rehabilitation is directed toward improvement of the patient's understanding regarding the importance of each subsystem to effect optimal oral communication, and toward teaching the patient strategies for functional compensation of their oral communication impairment(s). The importance of respiratory drive to efficient and audible voice production must be stressed, yet is often difficult challenge to the patient, primarily to those with pre-existing pulmonary diseases or conditions. The patient must be trained to produce voice to their maximum physiologic potential with as little physiologic load as possible. Examples of minimizing the load include the provision and training of one-way speaking valves in the tracheostomized patient. Also, encouraging a patient to increase their voice volume and exaggerate mouth opening often facilitate improved airflow volumes for functional voice production.

Vocal hygiene regimes that include suggestions for adequate vocal tract hydration by oral or non-oral intake of non-caffeinated fluids, and prescribed pharmacologic agents are often included in the patient's interdisciplinary treatment program. In patients with extreme glottic edema, care should be taken to instruct the patient in prevention of further injury to laryngeal tissues by avoiding the urge for chronic throat clearing or other expectorative maneuvers. Unfortunately, the primary goal of safe swallowing may involve some of these vocally abusive expectorative maneuvers to facilitate pharyngeal clearance and airway protection during swallowing of saliva, liquids and foods (16,42,65). If patients have incomplete laryngeal valving secondary to weakness or deconditioning of the intrinsic laryngeal musculature, isometric exercises or high effort phonatory tasks may be applied to effect improve glottic muscle tone and closure patterns (16,66). Improved closure will also assist in generating adequate subglottic pressures for audible vocal production. Teaching the patient balanced resonance techniques can result in a more efficient "placement" of the voice with an overall impact on perceived quality and volume (2).

Following oral cavity surgeries, patients sometimes develop habitual restriction of mouth opening because they are highly self-conscious about their altered facial cosmesis. They may also chronically place their hands in front of their mouth during speech production in an attempt to mask their altered appearance. The clinician must bring these maladaptive habits to the patient's attention with an explanation of how they contribute to a further reduction in listener intelligibility and heightened attention to their speech impairment. Increasing mouth opening often facilitates normalization of oral resonance following such counseling, and visual and auditory feedback are helpful with patient's monitoring of the learned behavior. However, increases in mouth opening during speech production is an unrealistic immediate goal for patients with significant trismus, and a rigorous hierarchy of exercises involving the temporomandibular musculature may be warranted prior to attempting to achieve increased mouth opening during speech (67). Further, instructing the patient to increase the overall affect and prosodic variation of their communication with gesture, eye contact and varied intonation often improve the listener's perception of the total communication effectiveness of the speaker.

Articulation: The motion of the tongue required for precise articulation may be restricted by surgical removal of tissue, connective tissue fibrosis, scar contracture or anchoring related to the necessary surgical closure or reconstruction. Following a complete assessment or inventory of the patient's articulation ability, including manner and placement errors, the patient should be placed on an intensive program of tongue and mandible range of motion and isometric strengthening exercises. These exercises are similar to exercises employed for swallowing therapy, and must become the patient's life-long routine to ensure maintenance of function over time. In conjunction with these physiotherapeutic exercises, the patient is instructed in over-targeting the articulatory placement and in compensatory placement during a hierarchy of speech production tasks to effect optimal speech intelligibility. In addition to isolated speech drills, clinical experience has shown a positive impact of improvements in respiratory drive, vocalization and resonance on the overall articulation ability of the patient and on overall intelligibility. When the patient implements the optimal vocalization and resonance strategies, he or she often takes additional time to target the articulation placement. Focusing on all aspects of voice and speech production reduces the tedium and sometimes the discouraging nature of drill-like speech therapy. The patient should be trained in the ability to implement visual, auditory and tactile feedback techniques into their speech productions such as "tasting and feeling" the movements of their tongue, lips and palate. This may be a particular challenge for patients with intra-oral sensory disruption related to surgical ablation of the hard or soft palate and require an intra-oral prosthesis to redefine the oral and nasal cavities. Though the appliance provides a new point of contact for the tongue in order to achieve more precise articulation during speech and bolus propulsion during swallowing, the patient looses the important tactile information in speech production that is typically provided by the palatal sensory receptive fields (35–41).

SWALLOWING DISORDERS

As is the case with voice, resonance and speech, treatments necessary to treat and cure cancers of the head and neck often lead to devastating impacts on swallowing function (68–76). The nature and severity of the swallowing disorder will be related to the size of the lesion, size of the resection and type of reconstruction (18,21,29,30). Though an experienced clinician may be able to reasonably predict the type of swallowing disorder associated with a given surgery or oncologic treatment, there is normal variability in swallowing function in healthy adults (77,78) as well as in patients treated for cancers to the head and neck. Delineation of the severity and functional impact of the swallowing disorder, as well as the impact of various compensatory behavioral treatments, must be gleaned through an instrumental assessment that permits visualization of the upper aerodigestive tract during swallowing activity (60–62). Appendix A highlights the functional swallowing abnormalities associated with common surgical oral and pharyngeal cavity resections. The following explanation represents a summary of common swallowing problems associated with oncologic treatments to the head and neck, and emphasizes that swallowing treatment must be based on the nature of the swallowing abnormality, the cause of aspiration, and the physical and emotional needs of the patient.

Disturbed Lingual Motility

Surgical ablation of the tongue may lead to slowness, restriction of range, weakness, and discoordination of tongue movements, and cause overlapping oropharyngeal swallowing disturbances. Impairment of the tongue leads to a reduced proficiency with oral bolus containment and preparation, with nutritional and airway protective implications. Inadequate decomposition of the bolus may lead to pharyngeal lodging of bolus fragments or even to airway obstruction. The latter is likely in the case of corresponding disruption of the pharyngeal musculature and inadequate laryngeal valving. A tight seal is required between the tongue circumference and palatal alveolus, and between the back of the tongue and inferiorly/anteriorly displaced soft palate. This valving serves to prevent premature entry of the ingested material into the oro- and hypopharynx. It has been explained that in addition to bolus preparation and oral containment, the tongue also plays a significant role in pharyngeal bolus clearance and airway protection (14,15,17). Disturbances in the range and strength of tongue base retraction lead to the accumulation of pharyngeal residue and to incomplete airway protection with the ultimate threat of airway penetration and aspiration. Slow and disturbed lingual motility also leads to a delay in the triggering of pharyngeal, laryngeal, and cervical esophageal swallowing activity (5). The reconstructive surgeon should consider these issues when providing a functional reconstruction in the oral cavity and oropharynx.

Delayed Initiation of the Pharyngeal Swallow

Disturbances in oropharyngeal sensation and lingual motility are often associated with delayed initiation of pharyngeal swallowing dynamics such as, delayed laryngeal closure and opening of the cervical esophagus (5). The leading edge of the bolus falls into the oropharyx and hypopharynx prior to the initiation of hyolaryngeal excursion and laryngeal valving. This temporal disruption of critical swallowing events enhances the threat of laryngeal entry and aspiration.

Incomplete Hyolaryngeal Excursion

Vigorous contraction of the suprahyoid and suprathyroid musculature lead to the upward and forward movement of the hyolaryngeal complex during normal deglutition. Impairment of these movements will likely lead to incomplete laryngeal closure of the intrinsic and extrinsic laryngeal valves. Further, the cricoid cartilage will not be amply pulled away from the posterior pharyngeal wall, and result in decreased extent and duration of cervical esophageal sphincter opening. Aspiration and incomplete pharyngeal clearance are often the consequences of this swallowing disorder.

Paretic/Paralytic/Partial Intrinsic Laryngeal Valving

Surgeries or treatments that disrupt the neural inervation of the larynx may result in paresis or paralysis of the laryngeal valving mechanism(s). Further, partial resections of the extrinsic and intrinsic laryngeal valves, or radiation fibrosis and edema may result in functional laryngeal impairment and significant aspiration threat. Incomplete medialization of the arytenoid-true vocal fold complex may result in laryngeal penetration (i.e., entry of bolus fragments into the laryngeal inlet above the level of the true vocal folds) or aspiration (i.e., progression of the bolus inferior to the true vocal folds) during the swallow (5). However, if all other physiologic swallowing mechanisms remain in tact, particularly the structure and function of the contralateral arytenoid-true vocal fold complex, hyolaryngeal excursion and tongue base retraction, the patient is usually able to compensate quite well for the altered laryngeal valving using bolus modification or postural techniques (10–13). Typically, if penetration or aspiration occur, it occurs primarily with thin liquids, and the degree of penetration/aspiration will increase with increasing bolus volume.

Pharyngeal Paresis/Paralysis

Surgery or radiation treatments applied to nervous structures innervating the pharyngeal cavity may result in slight or significant weakness of the pharyngeal wall musculature. The functional consequence of this weakness may be minor and easily compensated for with altered positioning or bolus modification. On the other hand, the consequences may be devastating yielding incomplete clearance of the pharynx by a flaccid pharyngeal tube, and gross aspiration, the degree of which increases with increasing bolus volume and viscosity.

SWALLOWING TREATMENT STRATEGIES

Swallowing treatment must be based on the clearly identified nature of the swallowing disorder from instrumented visual examinations. Further, swallowing treatments should be based firmly on empirical evidence derived from clinical studies. Unfortunately, practicing clinicians employ non-evidenced based methods in the swallowing treatment arena, and these methods should be strongly discouraged without empirical data to supporting their use. Further, the selection of efficacious swallowing treatment methods should be dependent on the cognitive and physical capabilities of the individual. The authors group swallowing treatments into six therapeutic categories: cognitive stimulation; modification of bolus variables; compensatory postures, and positions; sensitization techniques; compensatory maneuvers; and isometric exercises of upper aerodigestive tract musculature. In addition to the importance of selecting swallowing treatment method(s) based on visual observation of the swallowing mechanism, the clinician should seek visual confirmation of the effectiveness of the treatment strategy on the instrumental examination. The following discussion presents a summary of commonly observed swallowing impairments, and treatment methods shown to be effective in improving swallowing physiology (11–13,79–92).

Cognitive Stimulation

In order for a patient to participate and benefit from swallowing treatment by a speech-language pathologist, he or she must be able to understand and carry out simple directives. Some treatment strategies require significant retention and follow-through, and are inappropriate for employment in patients with severe communication-cognitive impairment. A speech-language pathologist is trained in communication processes, and should be able to quickly identify the candidacy of the patient for potential swallowing treatment methods. The initiation of swallowing may require significant cognitive cueing and retraining for some patients. Placing a bolus or any type of stimulation into the oral cavity and expecting a timely and safe swallow is likely to be a disappointing event for the treating clinician. Patients often warranted reminders to manipulate the intraoral material and to move their tongue to initiate productive swallowing activity. Cognitive input and some degree of processing are necessary for participation in swallowing therapy and for functional swallowing initiation.

Modification of Bolus Variables

Decreasing, and sometimes increasing the volume and texture of the ingested material may improve the temporal coordination and efficiency of swallowing. It has been observed that thin liquids, primarily in larger boluses, are more likely to be aspirated in patients exhibiting delayed initiation of pharyngeal swallowing (11,12). The non-textured bolus progresses rapidly from the mouth into the pharynx, and the patient's physiologic mechanism can not temporally coordinate laryngeal closure, cervical esophageal segment opening and pharyngeal contraction during this prematurely and rapidly flowing bolus. It has been observed that the increased viscosity of a textured bolus enhances sensory enervation, and hence results in a more timely initiation of pharyngeal and laryngeal swallowing activity (12). Clinical reports (11,12) and experience shows that increasing the viscosity of the bolus will often decrease the likelihood of aspiration because of its slowed progression through the oral cavity and pharynx. However, the use of thickened liquids for aspiration prevention must be employed with caution and assessed for their value during the initial objective swallowing evaluation. For example, when there is a coexisting disruption in pharyngeal contraction or in hyolaryngeal excursion with limited opening to the cervical esophagus, a textured bolus may increase the risk of aspiration of the resulting pharyngeal residue. Also, the hydration needs of the patient may not be met with thickened liquids, and the patient's hydration status must be frequently monitored with thin liquid restrictions.

Other examples of bolus modification include altering the taste and temperature of the bolus. Taste and temperature effects do tend to vary depending on the preferences of the individual, but there is some evidence to support that the presentation of sour boluses enhances the timing of pharyngeal swallow initiation (13). Modifications in bolus volume are simple and highly effective methods for controlling aspiration and improving pharyngeal clearance in many patients. In most instances, patients will demonstrate a safe and efficient swallow with small and isolated boluses because of the decreased neuromuscular integrity required for their control and transport through the upper aerodigestive tract. Further, preliminary data have shown that increased coordination is required between the breathing and swallowing mechanics for large volume cup or straw drinking (8,9). If increased challenges to breathing and swallowing coordination are found to exist in large numbers of healthy subjects, this method of drinking may go beyond the physiologic potential of some patients treated for head and neck cancer.

Compensatory Postures/Positions

Changes in the alignment of the head, neck and trunk have been shown to be highly effective, and often temporary means of ensuring safe and efficient swallowing. These postures and positions have been studied and include:

Chin Tuck (Fig. 1). A chin tuck posture is used for a specific type of swallowing impairment namely, delayed initiation of the pharyngeal swallow (5,79). The chin tuck posture tucks the laryngeal inlet underneath the tongue base protection the

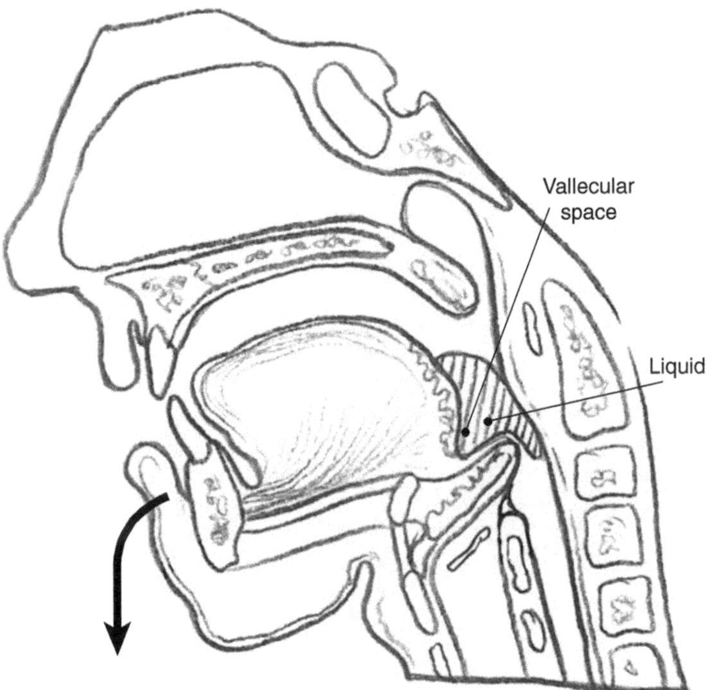

Figure 1 The chin tuck maneuver is appropriate for some patients with delayed initiation of the pharyngeal swallow. The vallecular space widens to maintain the hesitated bolus, and the larynx is shielded under the tongue.

airway during the delay. It has also been observed clinically, though not empirically tested by these authors, that the space between the posterior pharyngeal wall and tongue base decreases when using this posture in some patients, and appears to effect improved bolus clearance from the vallecular region This posture may only be effective when bolus volume is minimized and should be applied with caution, and its effectiveness should be confirmed during a visual instrumental examination. For example, when the head of a larger volume bolus progresses beyond the valleculae and hesitates in the pyriform sinuses during the delay, the bolus may misdirect into the laryngeal inlet when the hyolaryngeal complex begins its upward and forward displacement.

Head Turn (Fig. 2). A left or right rotation of the head facilitates bolus flow through the pharynx . This directional approach is aimed at deflecting the bolus to and through the side of the least impaired pharyngeal musculature (5,63,80,81). A right head turn deflects the bolus through the left side, and a left head turn has the opposite effect. There is some evidence to suggest that a head turn may also result in decreased pressure in and opening of the PESs facilitating bolus passage into the cervical esophagus (81).

Semi-recline. If a patient presents with a chronic and relatively constant degree of pharyngeal retention following an initial swallow, placing the thorax in a semi-reclined position may facilitate safe and efficient bolus passage. Gravity may work in the patient's favor when using this compensatory posture, and prevents the anterior misdirection of the remaining bolus in the pharyngeal recesses and/or

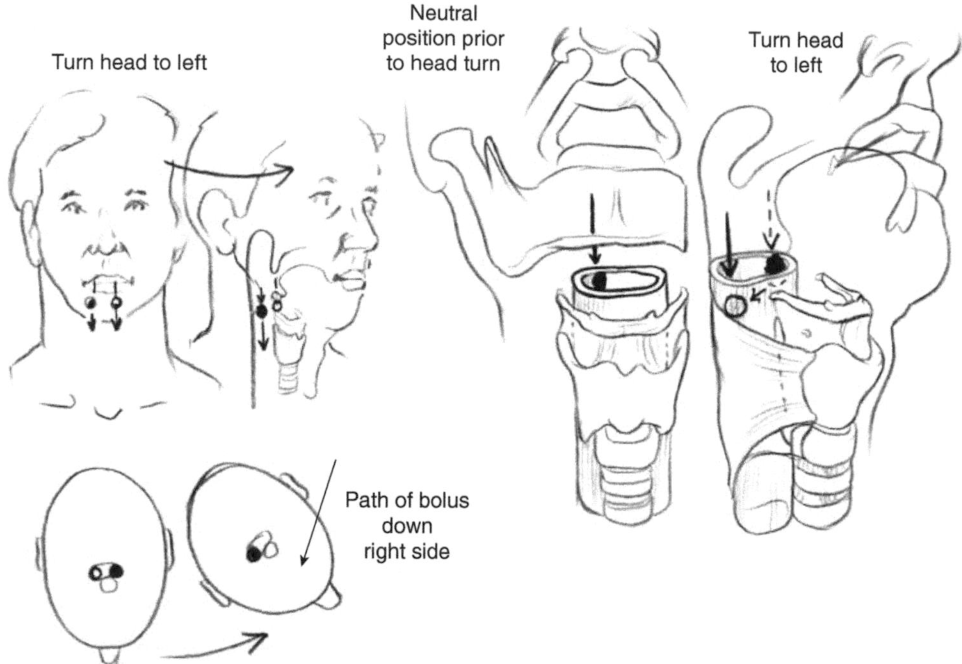

Figure 2 A complete left or right head turn directs the bolus through the opposite side of the pharynx, and facilitates opening of the pharyngoesophageal segment. This maneuver may also improve approximation of the laryngeal valves during swallow.

on the pharyngeal walls into the laryngeal inlet. Cueing the patient to swallow twice per bolus, and minimizing bolus volume further increases the likelihood of pharyngeal clearance and minimizes the threat of aspiration.

Sensitization Techniques

Intra-oral sensitization techniques are used in the treatment of swallowing disorders, but remain somewhat controversial. Thermal stimulation, or application, has been shown to enhance the timing of pharyngeal swallow initiation in patients with pharyngeal swallow delays. The theory behind this technique is that stimulation of the sensory receptive fields in the posterior oral cavity facilitates afferent input to the brainstem swallowing center in the medulla, and thereby enhances the initiation of swallowing activity (Fig. 3) (82). It has been shown that afferent pathways exist between the sensory receptive fields innervated by branches of the IXth and Xth cranial nerves that progress to the nucleus of the solitary tract (nTS) in the dorsal medulla (3). Internuncial communication has been shown between the nTS, a primary sensory swallowing nucleus, and the nucleus ambiguus (nA). nA houses motorneurons that give rise to critical swallowing efferents involved in laryngeal and pharyngeal muscle contraction during swallowing (3). Therefore, based on some studies, and clinical deduction, the application of a mechanical stimulus to the sensory receptive fields of the posterior oral cavity, combined with cognitive stimulation or verbal cueing, may result in the central facilitation and initiation of swallowing activity (82–85).

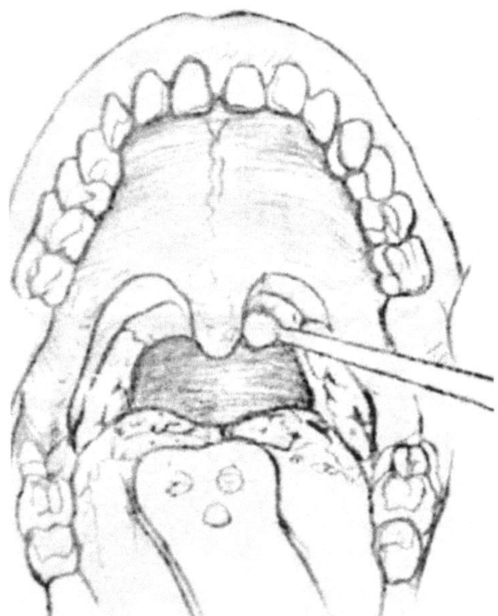

Figure 3 Thermal stimulation involves the application of an iced laryngeal mirror to the anterior faucial pillars.

Compensatory Maneuvers

Acute and chronic swallowing problems associated with head and neck surgery has been shown to improve when patients engage in compensatory maneuvers during eating and drinking. These maneuvers are directed toward either improving airway protection and/or enhancing oropharyngeal clearance. These methods are aimed at bringing the otherwise non-volitional aspects of swallowing under volitional control. Those that have been described and shown to be effective in some patient groups are illustrated in Figures 1–5 and include: intra-oral bolus hold (Fig. 4) (16); supraglottic and super-supraglottic swallow (Figs. 5 and 6) (16,86,88); effortful swallow (Fig. 7) (16); double swallow (16); and Mendelsohn Maneuver (Fig. 8) (16,17,89). While these maneuvers can be highly effective in improving specific physiologic swallowing components, their appropriateness must be based on the cognitive and physical capabilities of the patient, an on visual confirmation of the effectiveness of their application.

Isometric Exercise

Clinical studies demonstrating the potential for muscle retraining and strengthening of the striated musculature of the upper aerodigestive tract are emerging (27,28). Data are beginning to support the use of resistive or isometric training in the habilitation of the upper aerodigestive tract function following neurologic insult (27,28,89,91,92). The primary muscle groups that have been studied include the musculature of the tongue body, suprahyoid musculature, intrinsic laryngeal, and pharyngeal wall musculature. In cases of decreased tongue base retraction, an exercise has been tested and shown to increase anterior pharyngeal wall displacement. The tongue hold or Masako maneuver shown in Figure 9 employs fixating the anterior tongue between the teeth, and immobilizing the tongue during swallowing. It has

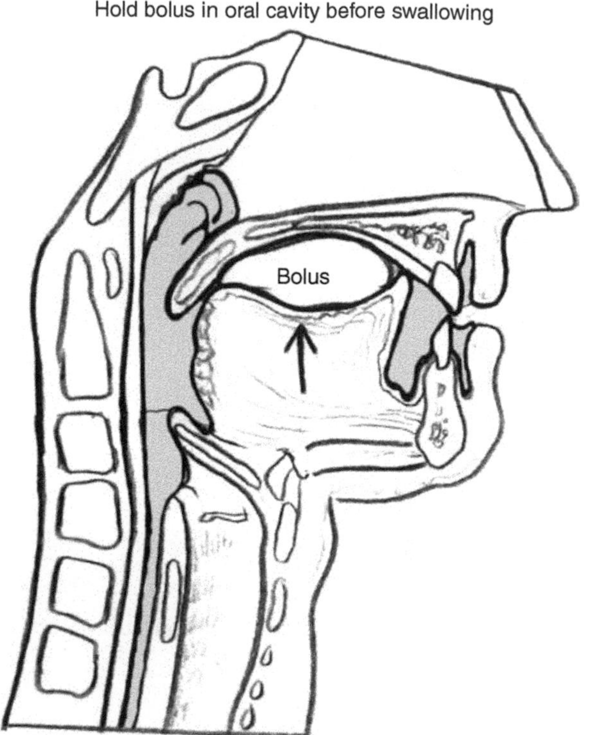

Figure 4 Training a patient to hold a bolus firmly in the oral cavity for a few seconds prior to swallowing heightens awareness and reduces the threat of premature entry of the bolus head into the pharynx.

been shown that implementation of this tongue fixation results in a seemingly compensatory increase in anterior displacement of the posterior pharyngeal wall during swallow (92). Based on these observations in clinical studies, immobilizing the tongue during repetitive exercise swallows in the absence of food or liquid, may result in the development of increased pharyngeal wall contraction to compensate for the impaired tongue driving force in patients following tongue base resections or in cases of radiation fibrosis to this functional region. Another example of isometric exercise impacting improvement in the functional mobility of swallowing structures is the Shaker exercise. This exercise was tested in chronically dysphagic patients, and is directing toward improving hyolaryngeal mechanics. Patients using this exercise are trained in a series of sustained and repetitive chin lifts that have been empirically tested against a sham exercise. Patients who routinely performed the exercise over a period of weeks demonstrated radiographic confirmation of improvements in hyolaryngeal function and PES opening with eventual return to oral intake (27). Novel and exciting work has also shown that tongue muscle mass and driving pressures during swallows can be increased with isometric tongue exercises in healthy aging adults (93). If similar results could be demonstrated in patients treated for oral cancers, there would appear to be wide application of this treatment methodology.

These types of isometric training often incorporate visual feedback methods to assist the patient in achieving target muscle contractions, and permits objective measurement of improvement over time (91). The application of tongue pressure

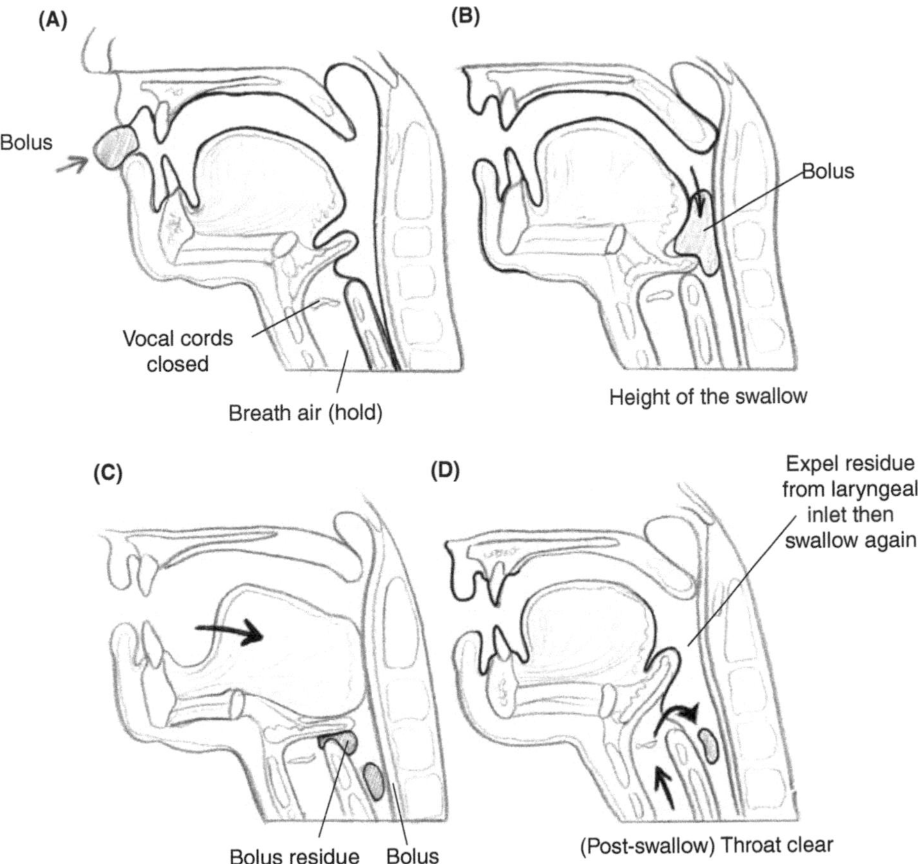

Figure 5 The supraglottic swallow facilitates airway closure and supralaryngeal and pharyngeal clearance. The true vocal folds are closed during a breath hold prior to the swallow. An expectorative maneuver follows the initial swallow, and a second swallow clears the potential laryngeal or pharyngeal residue.

transducers and electromyography with visual display have practically enhanced the effecteness of these noninvasive treatments applied by speech pathologists for the treatment of swallowing disorders in patients treated for oral and pharyngeal cancer.

SUMMARY

The multidimensionality and overlap of speech, voice, and swallowing functions in adult humans is highlighted by the complexity and variety of their overlapping disorders following oncologic treatments to the head and neck. The clinical approach to evaluation and treatment of these functions involves careful collaboration between the speech-language pathologist, extirpative surgeon, reconstructive surgeon, maxillofacial prosthodontist, oncologist, radiation oncologist, members of the medical team, physical therapist, and nutritionist. Perceptual, acoustic and visual assessments of speech, voice, and swallowing function are highly contributory to the differential

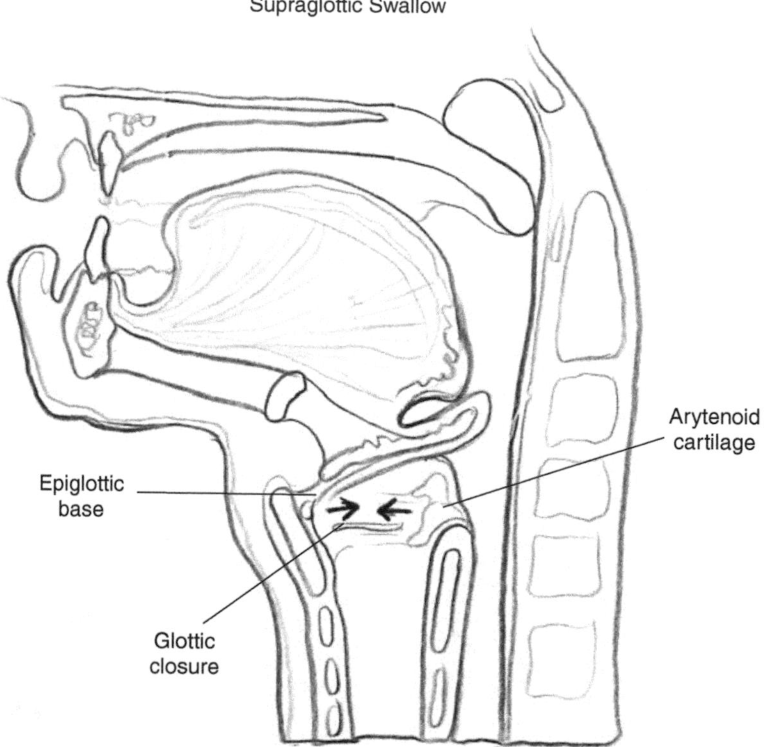

Figure 6 This maneuver is similar the supraglottic swallow maneuver, but is modified using an effortful breath-hold. This has been shown to facilitate closure of true vocal folds, ventricular folds and varied degrees of opposition of the arytenoid cartilages to the epiglottic petiole.

diagnosis of speech, voice, resonance, and swallowing disorders, to expedient and appropriate treatment planning and to confirmation of functional progress over the course of the functional rehabilitation and recovery period. However, though studies have shown positive impacts of specific treatments on speech and voice function, and in the physiology of swallowing mechanics in cross-sectional, cohort and case study reports, controlled clinical trials in large numbers of patients are greatly needed to determine the widespread impact of these treatments on the long term functional outcomes of patients treated for oral and pharyngeal cancers. The outcome studies should include distal outcomes of the treatment such as prevention of aspiration, return to oral intake, and nutritional status (94). The patient's ability to return to acceptable volumes and textures of foods and liquids, prevention of pulmonary complications, and ability to eat in public need to be addressed. Studies are needed that examine the impact of swallowing treatments on hospital re-admission rates, reduction of infection and antibiotic usage. Proximal outcomes that include broader areas incorporating life experience such as quality of life, functional and health status also warrant investigation (94). Finally, the economic outcomes of voice, speech and swallowing treatment have yet to be determined. In the absence of these long term outcome data, the standard of care in the treatment of speech, voice, resonance and swallowing disorders following head and neck cancer treatments is based on the evidence described in clinical reports, related trials and clinical experience. This care plan generally includes patient and caregiver

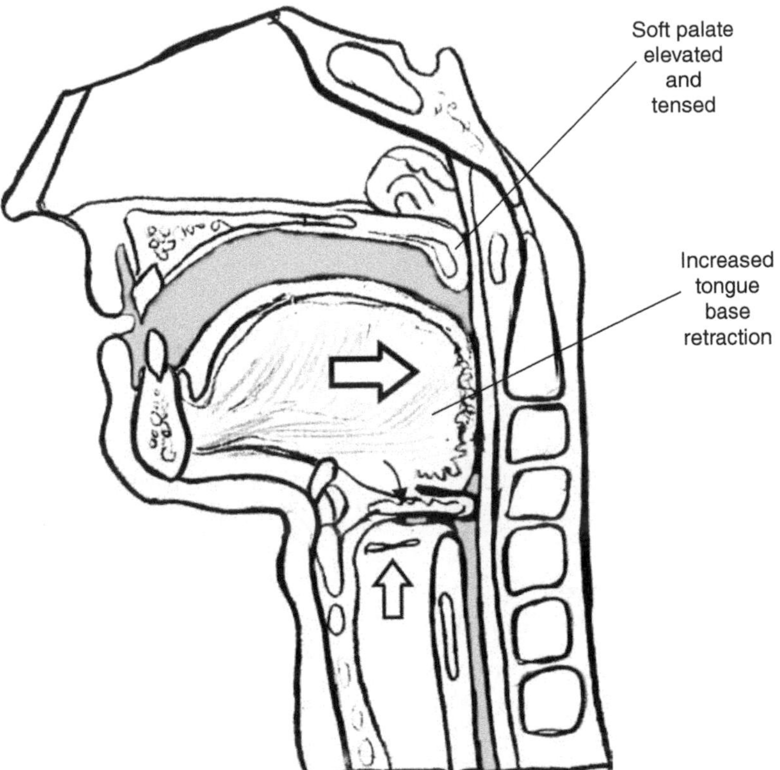

Figure 7 A patient is instructed to swallow hard or with effort. This resulsts in increased tongue base retraction with improved pharyngeal clearance.

education, functional habilitation of residual sensorimotor, structures using sensitization, compensatory and exercise strategies.

APPENDIX A

Swallowing Abnormalities Commonly Associated with Oral and Pharyngeal Cancer Resections

Anterior Tongue – Sensorimotor Deficits

- diminished sensation to surrounding tongue
- decreased integrity of tongue strength and range
- decreased swallow frequency

Anterior Tongue – Clinical/Radiographic Manifestations

- incomplete tongue to palate contact
- pooled saliva (FOM) and potential drooling
- labored bolus manipulation, preparation and mastication
- residue on anterior tongue, FOM, and palate

Hemiglossectomy – Sensorimotor Deficits

- diminished sensation to surrounding tongue, oral cavity and face
- limited strength and range of residual tongue (laterialization, elevation, and retraction)

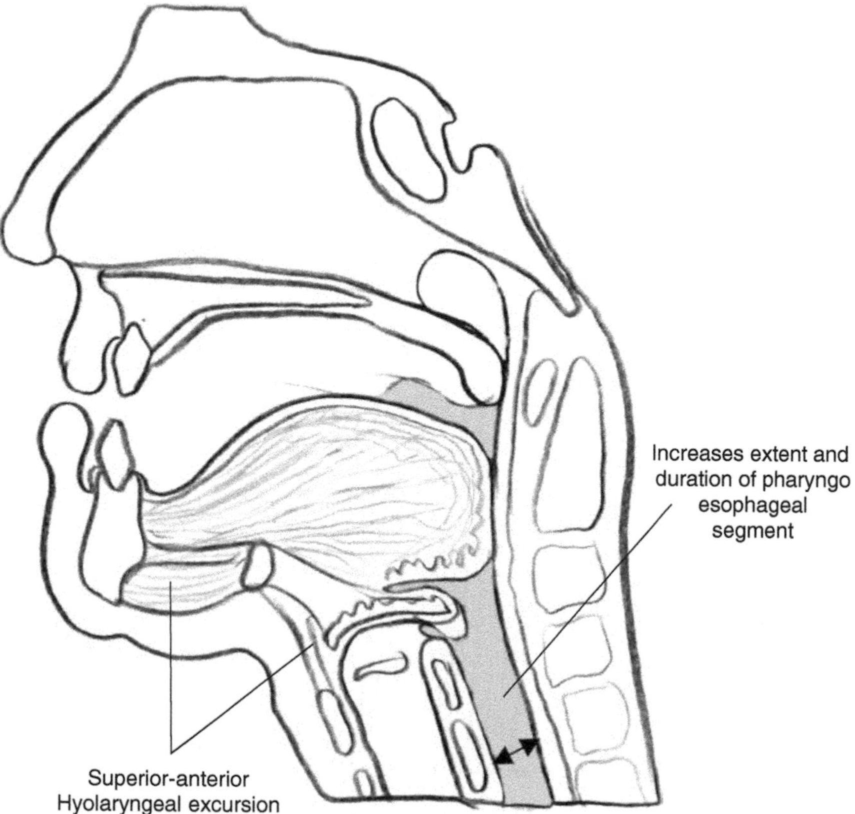

Figure 8 The Mendelsohn maneuver may be used during the swallow to enhance the extent and duration of pharyngoesophageal segment opening or as therapeutic maneuver designed to increase the strength of suprahyoid musculature.

- decreased swallow frequency
- reduced range of mandibular movement/jaw opening
- +/− restricted hyolaryngeal excursion → decreased PES opening

Hemiglossectomy – Clinical/Radiographic Manifestations

- incomplete tongue to palate contact → premature pharyngeal entry
- slow, labored bolus preparation → piecemeal deglutition
- slow, labored and inefficient lingual motility
- laryngeal penetration prior to pharyngeal swallow initiation
- delayed initiation of pharyngeal swallow/airway closure
- oropharyngeal residue: tongue dorsum, FOM, palate, valleculae, posterior pharyngeal wall
- +/− pyriform sinus
- +/− aspiration

Base of Tongue Resection – Sensorimotor Deficits

- diminished oropharyngeal, facial sensation
- decreased swallow frequency
- reduced range of mandibular movement/jaw opening

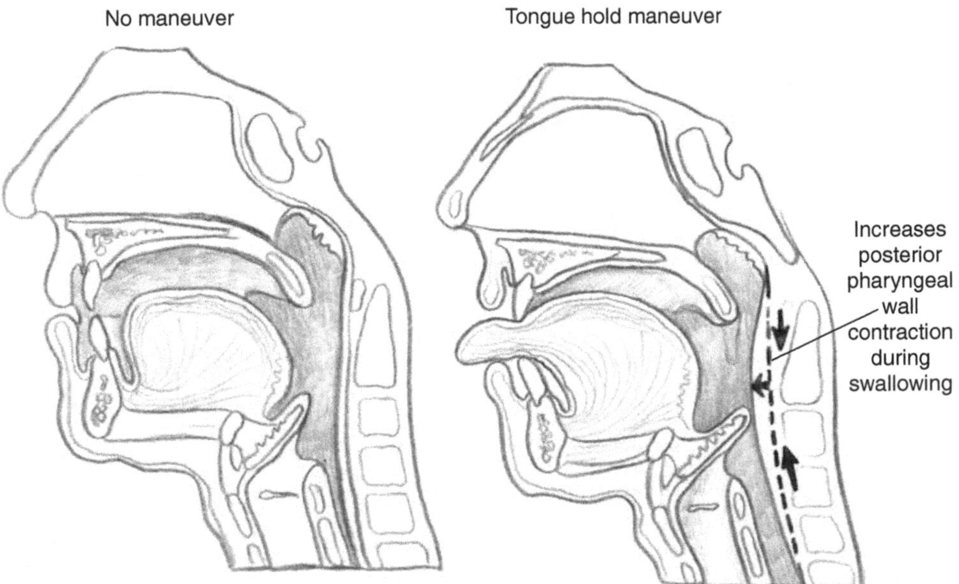

Figure 9 The tongue is held between the central incisors during the tongue hold exercise. Stabilization of the tongue has been shown to increase the contraction of the posterior pharyngeal wall.

- limited strength, range of residual tongue (anterior displacement, retraction)
- decreased supralaryngeal valving
- restricted hyolaryngeal elevation → decreased PES opening

Base of Tongue Resection – Clinical/Radiographic Manifestations

- excessive oropharyngeal secretions
- slow, labored and inefficient lingual motility
- delayed initiation of pharyngeal swallow
- laryngeal penetration prior to pharyngeal swallow initiation
- incomplete tongue base contact to posterior pharyngeal wall
- oropharyngeal residue: mid-tongue, tongue back, palate, posterior pharyngeal wall,
- valleculae, laryngeal vestibule, pyriform sinus
- aspiration

Near Total/Total Glossectomy – Sensorimotor Deficits

- diminished oropharyngeal, facial sensation
- decreased swallow frequency
- reduced range of mandibular movement/jaw opening
- limited strength, range of residual tongue (retraction)
- decreased supralaryngeal valving
- restricted hyolaryngeal excursion → decreased PES opening

Near Total/Total Glossectomy – Clinical/Radiographic Manifestations

- excessive oropharyngeal secretions

- absent oral bolus preparation and propulsion delayed initiation of pharyngeal swallow
- laryngeal penetration prior to pharyngeal swallow initiation aspiration
- oropharyngeal residue: oral cavity, valleculae, posterior pharyngeal wall, laryngeal vestibule, pyriform sinus

Composite Resection – Sensorimotor Deficits

- diminished oropharyngeal, facial sensation
- reduced range and strength of lip movement decreased swallow frequency
- limited range of mandibular movement/jaw opening and lateralization
- limited strength, "range of residual tongue (elevation, lateralization, and retraction)
- +/– restricted hyolaryngeal excursion → PES opening

Composite Resection – Clinical/Radiographic Manifestations

- incomplete labial seal
- excessive oropharyngeal. secretions
- slow, labored bolus preparation → piecemeal deglutition
- slow, labored and inefficient lingual motility
- laryngeal penetration prior to pharyngeal swallow initiation
- delayed pharyngeal swallow/airway closure
- oropharyngeal residue: tongue dorsum, FOM, palate, valleculae, posterior pharyngeal wall
- +/– pyriform sinus
- +/– aspiration

Supraglottic Laryngectomy – Sensorimotor Deficits

- diminished pharyngeal/laryngeal sensation
- decreased swallow frequency
- restricted hyolaryngeal excursion → decreased PES opening
- reduced strength of pharyngeal contraction
- decreased laryngeal closure/valving

Supraglottic Laryngectomy – Clinical/Radiographic Manifestations

- excessive oropharyngeal secretions
- delayed initiation of pharyngeal swallow/airway closure
- reduced pharyngeal shortening and decreased stripping wave
- laryngeal penetration
- oropharyngeal. residue: tongue base, posterior pharyngeal wall, laryngeal vestibule, arytenoids
- aspiration

Partial Pharyngectomy – Sensorimotor Deficits

- diminished pharyngeal sensation
- decreased swallow frequency
- impaired pharyngeal contraction
- limited hyolaryngeal elevation → incomplete PES opening

Partial Pharyngectomy – Clinical/Radiographic Manifestations

- excessive secretions
- delayed initiation of pharyngeal swallow

- delayed airway closure
- laryngeal penetration
- incomplete tongue base to pharyngeal wall contact
- pharyngeal retention
- +/− aspiration

Maxillectomy – Sensorimotor Deficits

- diminished palatal and superior oral cavity sensation
- diminished range/strength of soft palate elevation and retraction
- decreased swallow frequency

Maxillectomy – Clinical/Radiographic Manifestations

- labored bolus preparation and oral bolus transport
- nasoregurgitation
- oropharyngeal residue: palate, nasopharynx, oropharynx

REFERENCES

1. Verdolini K, Titze IR, Fennell A. Dependence of phonatory effort on hydration level. J Speech Hearing Res 1994; 37(5):1001–1007.
2. Colton R, Casper JK. Understanding Voice Problems: A Physiological Perspective for Diagnosis and Treatment. Second Ed. Baltimore MD: Williams & Wilkins, 1996.
3. Doty R. Neural organization of deglutition. In: Code CF, ed. Handbook of Physiology. Motility: Alimentary Canal, 1968:1861–1902.
4. Dodds WJ, Logemann JA, Stewart ET. Physiology and radiology of normal oral and pharyngeal phases of swallowing. Am J Roentgenol 1990; 154:953–963.
5. Logemann JA. Evaluation and treatment of swallowing disorders. Austin: ProEd, 1998.
6. Zald DH, Pardo JV. The functional neuroanatomy of voluntary swallowing. Ann Neurol 1999; 46:281–286.
7. Selley WG, Flack FC, Ellis RE, Brooks WA. Respiratory patterns associated with swallowing: part 2. Neurologically impaired dysphagic patients. Age Ageing 1989; 18: 173–176.
8. Martin BJ, Logemann J, Shaker R, Dodds W. The coordination between respiration and swallow: respiratory phase relationships and temporal integration. J Appl Physiol 1994; 76:714–723.
9. Martin BMH. The Relationship Between Respiratory and Laryngeal Dynamics During Swallow. Presented before. Dysphagia Research Society; Burlington, VT, 1999.
10. Dantas RO, Kern MK, Massey BT, Dodds WJ, Kahrilas PJ, Brasseur JG, Cook IJ, Lang IM. Effects of swallowed bolus variables on oral and pharyngeal phases of swallowing. Am J Physiol 1990; 258(5 pt 1):G675–G681.
11. Lazarus CL, Logemann JA, Rademaker AW, Kahrilas PJ, Pajak T, Lazar R, Halper A. Effects of volume, viscosity, and repeated swallows in nonstroke subjects and stroke patients. Arch Phys Med Rehabil 1993; 74(10):1066–1070.
12. Bisch EM, Logemann JA, Rademaker AW, Kahrilas PJ, Lazarus C. Pharyngeal effects of bolus volume, viscosity, and temperature in patients with dysphagia resulting from neurological impairment and in normal subjects. J Speech Hearing Res 1994; 37: 1041–1049.
13. Logemann JA, Pauloski BR, Colangelo L, Lazarus C, Fugiu M, Kahrilas PJ. Effects of sour bolus on oropharyngeal swallowing measures in patients with neurogenic dysphagia. J Speech Hearing Res 1995; 38(3):556–563.
14. Pouderoux P, Kahrilas PJ. Deglutitive tongue force modulation by volition, volume, and viscosity in humans. Gastroenterology 1995; 108(5):1418–1426.

15. Kahrilas PJ, Lin S, Logemann JA, Ergun GA, Facchini F. Deglutitive tongue action: volume accommodation and bolus propulsion. Gastroenterology 1993; 104(1):152–162.
16. Logemann JA. Evaluation and Treatment of Swallowing Disorders. Austin, TX: ProEd, 1998.
17. McConnel FMS, Cerenko D, Mendelsohn MS. Manoflourographic analysis of swallowing. Otolaryngol Clin N Am 1988; 21:625–637.
18. Colangelo LA, Logemann JA, Rademaker AW. Tumor size and pretreatment speech and swallowing in patients with resectable tumors. Otolaryngol Head Neck Surg 2000; 122(5):653–661.
19. Pauloski BR, Rademaker AW, Logemann JA, Stein D, Beery Q, Newman L, Hanchette C, Tusant S, McCracken E. Pretreatment swallowing function in patients with head and neck cancer. Head Neck 2000; 22(5):474–482.
20. De Graeff A, de Leeuw JR, Ros WJ, Hordijk GJ, Blijham GH, Wimubst JA. Pretreatment factors predicting quality of life after treatment for head and neck cancer. Head Neck 2000; 22(4):398–407.
21. Colangelo LA, Logemann JA, Pauloski BR, Pelzer JR, Rademaker AW. T stage and functional outcomes in oral and oropharyngeal cancer patients. Head Neck 1996; 18(3):259–268.
22. Lazarus CL, Logemann JA, Pauloski BR, Colangelo LA, Kahrilas PJ, Mittal BB, Pierce M. Swallowing disorders in head and neck cancer patients treated with radiotherapy and adjuvant chemotherapy. Laryngoscope 1996; 106(9 pt 1):1157–1166.
23. Kendall KA, McKensie SW, Leonard RL, Jones GU. Timing of swallow events after single modality treatment of head and neck carcinomas with radiotherapy. Ann Otolaryngol Rhinol Laryngol 2000; 109(8):767–775.
24. Mantorani G, Maccio A, Massa E, Mulas C, Mudu MC, Massidda S, Massa S, Murgia V, Ferrelli L, Succu G, et al. Phase II study of induction chemotherapy followed by concomitant chemoradiation in advanced head and neck cancer: clinical response and organ function preservation. Oncol Rep 1999; 6(6):1425–1430.
25. Pauloski BR, Logemann JA. Impact of tongue base and posterior pharyngeal wall biomechanics on pharyngeal clearance in irradiated post–surgical oral and oropharyngeal cancer patients. Head Neck 2000; 22(2):120–131.
26. Pauloski BR, Rademaker AW, Logemann JA, Colangelo LA. Speech and swallowing in irradiated and non–irradiated post–surgical oral cancer patients. Otolaryngol Head Neck Surg 1998; 188(5):616–624.
27. Shaker R, Kern M, Bardan E, et al. Augmentation of deglutitive upper esophageal sphincter opening in the elderly by exercise. Am J Physiol 1997; G1518–G1522.
28. Ferdjallah M, Wertsch JJ, Shaker R. Spectral analysis of surface electromyography (EMG) of upper esophageal sphincter opening muscles during head lift exercises. J Rehabil Res Develop 2000; 37(3):335–340.
29. McConnel FM, Pauloski BR, Logemann JA, Rademaker AW, Colangelo L, Shedd D, Carroll W, Lewin J, Johnson J. Functional results of primary closure vs. flaps in oropharyngeal reconstruction: a prospective study of speech and swallowing. Arch Otolaryngol Head Neck Surg 1998; 124(6):625–630.
30. McConnel FM, Logemann JA, Rademaker AW, Pauloski BR, Baker SR, Lewin J, Shedd D, Heiser MA, Cardinale S, Collins S, et al. Surgical variables affecting post–operative swallowing efficiency in oral cancer patients: a pilot study. Laryngoscope. 1994; 104(1pt1):87–90.
31. Pauloski BR, Logemann JA, Colangelo LA, Rademaker, AW, McConnel FM, Heiser MA, Cardinale S, Shedd D, Stein D, Beery Q, et al. Surgical variables affecting speech in patients treated with oral and pharyngeal cancer. Laryngoscope. 1998; 180(6):908–916.
32. Pauloski BR, Logemann JA, Rademaker AW, McConnel FM, Heiser MA, Cardinale S, Shedd D, Lewin J, Baker SR, Graner D. et al. Speech and swallowing function after anterior and floor of mouth resection with distal flap reconstruction. Journal of Speech and Hearing Research. 1993; 36(2): 267–76.

33. Pauloski BR, Logemann JA, Fox JL, Colangelo LA. Biomechanical analysis of the pharyngeal swallow post–surgical patients with anterior tongue and floor of mouth resection and distal flap reconstruction. Journal of Speech and Hearing Research. 1995; 38(1): 110–123.
34. Urken ML, Buchbinder D, Weinberg H, Vickery C, Sheiner A, Parker R, Schaefer J, Som P, Shapiro A, Lawson W. et al. Functional evaluation following microvascular oromandibular reconstruction of the oral cancer patient: a comparative study of reconstructed and unreconstructed patients. Laryngoscope. 1991; 101(9):935–950.
35. Davis JW, Lazarus C, Logemann JA, Hurst PS. Effect of a maxillary glossectomy prosthesis on articulation and swallowing. Journal of Prosthetic Dentistry. 1987; 57(6): 715–719.
36. Leonard RJ, Gillis R. Effects of prosthetic tongue on vowel intelligibility and food management in a patient with a total glossectomy. Journal of Speech and Hearing Disorders. 1982; 47:25–30.
37. Leonard RJ, Gillis R. Effects of prosthetic tongue on vowel formant and isovowel lines in a patient with total glossectomy (an addendum to Leonard and Gillis, 1982). Journal of Speech and Hearing Disorders. 1983; 48:423–426.
38. Leonard RJ, Gillis R. Differential effects of a speech prostheses in glossectomy patients. Journal of Prosthetic Dentistry. 1990; 64:701–708.
39. Robbins RT, Bowman JB, Jacob RF. Post–glossectomy deglutitory and articulatory rehabilitation with palatal augmentation prostheses. Archives of Otolaryngology Head and Neck Surgery 1987; 113:1214–1218.
40. Wheeler RL, Logemann JA, Rosen MS. Maxillary reshaping prosthesis: Effectiveness in improving speech and swallowing of post-surgical oral cancer patients. Journal of Prosthetic Dentistry. 1980; 43(3):313–319.
41. Logemann JA, Kahrilas PJ, Hurst P, Davis J, Krugler C. Effects of intraoral prosthesis on swallowing in patients with oral cancer. Dysphagia. 1989; 4(2):188–120.
42. Martin BJM, Schleicher MA, O'Conner A. Management of dysphagia following supraglottic laryngectomy. Clinical Communication Disorders. 1993; 3(4):27–36.
43. Jacobs JR, Logemann J, Pajak TF, Pauloski BR, Collins S, Casiano RR, Schuller DE. Failure of cricopharyngeal myotomy to improve dysphagia following head and neck cancer surgery. Archives of Otolaryngology-Head and Neck Surgery. 1999; 125(9): 942–946.
44. Buchholz DW, Neumann S. Pharyngeal swallowing disorders: selection for and outcome after myotomy. Dysphagia. 1999; 14(3):184–185.
45. Mason RJ, Bremmer CG, DeMeester TR, Crookes PF, Peters JH, Hagen JA, Memeester SR. Pharyngeal swallowing disorders: selection for and outcome after myotomy. Annals of Surgery. 1998; 228(4):598–608.
46. Carrau RL, Pou A, Eibling DE, Murry T, Ferguson BJ. Laryngeal framework surgery for the management of aspiration. Head and Neck. 1999; 21(2):139–145.
47. Hensel M, Haake K, Vogel S, Flugel W, Krausch D, Kox WJ. Management of swallowing disorders and chronic aspiration by glottic closure procedure. Journal of Neurosurgical Anesthesiology. 1997; 9(3):273–276.
48. Wisdom G, Blitzer A. Surgical therapy for swallowing disorders. Otolaryngologic Clinic of North America 1998; 31(3):537–560.
49. Morrish ECE. Compensatory vowel articulation of the glossectomy: acoustic and videofluoroscopic evidence. British Journal of Disorders of Communication. 1984; 19:125–134.
50. Georgian DA, Logemann JA, Fisher HB. Compensatory patterns of a surgically treated oral cancer patient. Journal of Speech and Hearing Disorders. 1982; 47(2):154–159.
51. Greven AJ, Meijer MF, Tiwari RM. Articulation after total glossectomy: A clinical study of speech in six patients. European Journal of Disorders in Communication. 1994; 29(1):85–93.
52. Hirano M, Bless DM. Videostroboscopic examination of the larynx. San Diego: Singular Publishing Group, 1993.

53. Woo P, Colton RH, Casper JK, Brewer DW. Diagnostic value of stroboscopic evaluation in hoarse patients. Journal of Voice. 1991; 5:231–238.
54. Kidder TM, Langemore SE, Martin BJ. Indications and techniques of endoscopy in evaluation of cervical dysphagia: Comparison with radiographic techniques. Dysphagia. 1994; 9:256–261.
55. Sonies BC. Instrumental procedures for dysphagia diagnosis. Seminars in Speech and Language: Swallowing Disorders. 1991; 12:185–199.
56. Langemore SE, Schatz K, Olsen N. Fiberoptic endoscopic examination of swallowing safety: a new procedure. Dysphagia. 1988; 2:216–219.
57. Aviv JE. Prospective randomized outcome study of endoscopy versus modified barium swallow in patients with dysphagia. Laryngoscope. 2000; 110(4):564–574.
58. Aviv JE, Kim T, Thompson JE, Sunshine S, Kaplan S, Close LG. Fiberoptic endoscopic evaluation of swallowing with sensory testing (FEESST) in healthy controls. Dysphagia. 1998; 13:87–92.
59. Aviv JE, Martin JH, Kim T, Sacco RL, Thomson JE, Diamond B, Close LG. Laryngopharyngeal sensory discrimination testing and laryngeal adductor reflex. Annals of Otology, Rhinology, and Laryngology. 1999; 108(8):725–30.
60. Ekberg O, Hillarp B. Radiologic evaluation of oral stage of swallowing. Acta Radiologica: Diagnosis. 1986; 27(5):533–537.
61. Logemann JA, Roa Pauloski B, Rademaker A, Cook B, Graner D, Milianti F, Beery Q, Stein D, Bowman J, Lazarus C. Impact of diagnostic procedure on outcome measures of swallowing rehabilitation in head and neck cancer patients. Dysphagia. 1992; 7(4): 179–186.
62. Martin BM, Logemann JA, McMahon S, Schleicher MA, Sandidge J. Clinical utility of the modified barium swallow. Dysphagia. 2000; 15(3):136–141.
63. Rasley A, Logemann JA, Kahrilas PJ, Rademaker AW, Pauloski BR, Dodds WJ. Prevention of barium aspiration during videofluoroscopic swallow studies: Value of change of posture. American Journal of Roentgenology. 1993; 160:1005–1009.
64. Konstaninovic VS, Dimic ND. Articulatory function and tongue mobility after surgery followed by radiotherapy for tongue and floor of mouth cancer patients. British Journal of Plastic Surgery. 1998; 51(8):589–593.
65. Schweinfurth JM, Silver SM. Patterns of swallowing after supraglottic laryngectomy. Laryngoscope 2000; 100(8):1266–1270.
66. Blair JA. Application of the Lee Silverman Voice Treatment technique to vocal fold paresis. Presented before. Pacific Voice Conference; November, 2000. San Francisco CA.
67. Takahashi M, Hideshima M, Park I, Taniguchi H, Ohyama T. Study of mandibular movement in mandibulectomy patients-border movements and functional movements during mastication, deglutition and speech. Journal of Medical and Dental Sciences. 1999; 46(2):93–103.
68. Hirano M, Kuroiwa Y, Tanaka S, Matsuoka H, Sato K, Yoshida T. Dysphagia following various degrees of surgical resection for oral cancer. Annals of Otology, Rhinology, and Laryngology. 1992; 101(2 pt 1):138–141.
69. Lazarus CL, Logemann JA, Kahrilas PJ, Mittal BB. Swallowing recovery in an oral cancer patient following surgery, radiotherapy, and hyperthermia. Head and Neck. 1994; 16(3):259–265.
70. Logemann JA, Pauloski BR, Rademaker AW, McConnel FM, Heiser MA, Cardinale S, Shedd D, Stein D, Beery Q, Johnson J, et al. Speech and swallow function after tonsil/base of tongue resection with primary closure. Journal of Speech and Hearing Research. 1993; 36(5):918–926.
71. Logemann JA, Bytell DE. Swallowing disorders in three types of head and neck cancer surgical patients. Cancer. 1979; 44(3):1095–1105.
72. Pauloski BR, Logemann JA, Rademaker QW, McConnel FM, Stein D, Beery Q, Johnson J, Heiser MA, Cardinale S, Shedd D. et al. Speech and swallowing function after

oral and oropharyngeal resections: one-year follow-up. Head and Neck. 1994; 16(4): 313–322.
73. Allison GR, Rappaport I, Salibian AH, McMicken B, Shoup JE, Etchepare TL, Krugman ME. Adaptive mechanisms of speech and swallowing following after combined jaw and tongue reconstruction in long-term survivors. American Journal of Surgery. 1987; 154:419–422.
74. Logemann JA. Aspiration in head and neck surgical patients. Annals of Otology, Rhinology, and Laryngology. 1985; 94(4):373–376.
75. Lundy DS, Smith C, Colangelo l, Sullivan PA, Logemann JA, Lazarus CL, Newman LA, Murry T, Lombard L, Gaziano J. Aspiration: Cause and Implications. Otolaryngology - Head and Neck Surgery. 1999; 120(4):474–478.
76. Martin BM, Corlew MN, Wood H. et al. The association of swallowing dysfunction and aspiration pneumonia. Dysphagia 1994; 9:1–6.
77. Lof G, Robbins J. Test-retest variability in normal swallowing. Dysphagia 1990; 4: 236–242.
78. Tracy JF, Logemann JA, Kahrilas PJ, Jacob P, Kobara M, Krugler C. Preliminary observations on the effects of age on oropharyngeal deglutition. Dysphagia 1989; 4:90–94.
79. Shanahan TK, Logemann JA, Rademaker AW, Pauloski BR, Kahrilas PJ. Chin-down posture effect on aspiration in dysphagic patients. Arch Phys Med Rehabil 1993; 74:736–739.
80. Logemann JA, Kahrilas PJ. Relearning swallow post CVA: application of maneuvers and indirect biofeedback. A case study. Neurology 1990; 40:1136–1138.
81. Logemann JA, Kahrilas PJ, Kobara M, Vakil B. The benefit of head rotation on pharyngoesophageal dysphagia. Arch Phys Med Rehabil 1989; 70:767–771.
82. Fujiu M, Toleikis JR, Logemann JA, Larson CR. Glossopharyngeal evoked potentials in normal subjects following mechanical stimulation of the anterior faucial pillar. Electroencephal Clin Neurophysiol 1994; 92:183–195.
83. Rosenbek JC, Robbins J, Fishback B, Levine R. Effects of thermal application on dysphagia after stroke. J Speech Hearing Res 1991; 34:1257–1267.
84. Rosenbek JC, Roecker EB, Wood JL, Robbins J. Thermal application reduces the duration of stage transition in dysphagia after stroke. Dysphagia 1996; 11:225–233.
85. Lazzara G, Lazarus C, Logemann J. Impact of thermal stimulation on the triggering of the swallow reflex. Dysphagia 1986; 1:73–77.
86. Lazarus C, Logemann JA, Gibbons P. Effects of maneuvers on swallowing in dysphagic oral cancer patients. Head Neck 1993; 15(5):419–424.
87. Logemann JA, Rademaker AW, Pauloski BR, Kahrilas PJ. Effects of postural changes on aspiration in head and neck cancer patients. Otolaryngol Head Neck Surg 1994; 110(2):222–227.
88. Logemann JA, Pauloski BR, Rademaker AW, Colangelo LA. Super-supraglottic swallow in irradiated head and neck cancer patients. Head Neck 1997; 19(6):535–540.
89. Kahrilas PJ, Logemann JA, Krugler C, Flanagan E. Volitional augmentation of upper esophageal sphincter opening during swallowing. Am J Physiol 1991; 260:6450–6456.
90. Kahrilas PJ, Logemann JA, Gibbons P. Food intake by maneuver; and extreme compensation for impaired swallowing. Dysphagia 1992; 7(3):155–159.
91. Bryant M. Biofeedback in the treatment of a selected dysphagic patient. Dysphagia 1996; 6:140–144.
92. Fujiu M, Logemann JA. Effect of a tongue holding maneuver on posterior pharyngeal wall movement during deglutition. Am J Speech-Language Pathol 1996; 5:23–20.
93. Robbins J, Hamilton JW, Lof GL, Kempster GB. Oropharyngeal swallowing in normal adults of different ages. Gastroenterology 1992; 103(3):823–829.
94. Brenner MH, Curbow B, Legro MW. The proximal–distal continuum of multiple health outcome measures: the case of cataract surgery. Med Care 1995; 33:AS236–AS244.

21 Outcomes Research in Oral Cavity Reconstruction

Michael G. Stewart
Department of Otorhinolaryngology, Weill Medical College of Cornell University, New York, New York, U.S.A.

INTRODUCTION

Outcomes research is the scientific study of the outcomes of disease therapies used for a particular disease, condition, or illness (1). The term outcomes research also refers to the study of a broad range of subjects: the status of the patient or population at entry into the healthcare system, the costs and financing of the healthcare given, or the status of the patient or population after treatment, and these types of outcomes research may be further described by the methods that are used to conduct the studies. For example, record-based outcomes research encompasses administrative or financial records that are studied to retrieve information on costs or outcomes of care. Record-based research can also involve systematic review (meta-analysis) in which results of several studies are considered and analyzed together. Other types of outcomes research such as patient-based outcomes research use data gathered from patients. In this discipline, the researcher may be interested in the patient's perception of their outcome. Although traditional clinical outcomes—such as mortality, complication rate, etc.—remain important, outcomes research uses expanded measures such as quality of life (QOL), and disease-specific health status.

Outcomes research is usually performed in real world settings using larger groups of patients as opposed to traditional clinical research, in which typically smaller numbers of patients are studied under highly-controlled environments with strict entry and exclusion criteria (2). In addition, outcomes research often uses an observational prospective design rather than an experimental prospective design. In observational outcomes research, all patients with a disease are included, and they are studied in the actual setting of them receiving their healthcare. This naturally introduces multiple additional factors that may influence post-treatment outcome, such as patient compliance, co-morbid diseases, and potential selection biases for different treatments. However, many would argue that results from large-scale outcome studies are more applicable to the general population because of their setting and scope. Furthermore, in addition to their real world setting, the expanded outcomes measured (QOL, etc.) might be more important to patients than other clinical or biological outcomes. In contrast to the treatment efficacy measured by clinical trials, outcome studies measure treatment effectiveness (3).

Defining the outcomes to be assessed is a crucial step in outcomes research. The patient-based outcomes usually measured are QOL, health status, and/or functional status. Although there are no standard definitions, outcomes researchers agree that QOL has two characteristics: it is more than merely the absence of disease; and it is both subjective, from the patient's perspective, and multidimensional (4). A person's overall QOL depends on many things not directly disease-related, such as financial or environmental status, so most researchers studying treatment outcomes assess the patient's health-related QOL. Health status is self-explanatory, and must be measured from the patient's perspective. Functional status refers to the patient's ability to perform daily activities. In most circumstances, only the disease-specific functional status is measured because researchers are only interested in the effect of a particular state or disease (1).

To measure health status, functional status, or QOL, the patient must answer several questions (items) in the form of a questionnaire (instrument) that have been validated for measurement.

Since these outcomes instruments measure concepts that are subjective and difficult to quantify, they must be validated using the scientific principles of psychometrics. Briefly, a health status or QOL instrument should be reliable, valid, and sensitive. Reliability means that the results will be similar if the status of the patient has not changed. Validity means that the instrument measures what it is supposed to measure. The presence of validity is confirmed by measuring different types of validity, including content validity, criterion validity, and construct validity (5,6). Sensitivity refers to the numerical score on the instrument that responds to a change in clinical status; sensitivity is assessed using statistical techniques (7).

Hundreds of QOL and health status instruments are available in the literature, and many of those instruments have been rigorously validated. Before using a QOL or health status instrument, one should first decide if that instrument is appropriate for use in a given clinical situation. Another important issue is whether to choose a general (or global or generic) QOL/health-status instrument, or a disease-specific instrument (8). Global instruments offer the advantage of being comparable across disease states, and allowing comparisons among the relative impacts of certain diseases. For example, researchers could compare the global QOL impact caused by head and neck cancer with that of lung cancer. Furthermore, if the relative QOL impact of a given disease state is known, then the decrement caused by another disease could be calibrated to the known state. For example, one might describe the physical functioning status of patients with pulmonary metastases as equivalent to the loss of physical functioning caused by being wheel chair dependent. The problem with many global health-status instruments, however, is that they are relatively insensitive to the influence of more limited disease states which nevertheless cause significant worsening of the patients' QOL (8). In contrast, some global instruments are very sensitive to the effect of isolated disease. Thus, not all health status instruments have the same performance characteristics.

For circumstances in which a global instrument is not sensitive enough, the use of a disease-specific instrument is appropriate. An advantage of disease-specific instruments is that they are usually quite sensitive to the impact of treatment on health status, and therefore allow meaningful comparisons among patients or treatments. A flaw of the global instrument is that it does not allow comparisons across disease states, a distinct disadvantage if the overall effect of a given disease state is in question. Therefore, the use of both a global and a disease-specific instrument may be appropriate (8).

GLOBAL QOL INSTRUMENTS

Interest in QOL assessment has increased dramatically in recent years, and there are now well over 1000 QOL instruments currently available in the literature. The Medical Outcomes Trust in Boston, a nonprofit organization with worldwide membership, has developed an instrument review process using a Scientific Advisory Committee of noted experts in outcomes research. Using strict criteria for instrument content, reliability, validity, responsiveness, interpretability, and respondent burden, the Trust has released a list of "approved" global QOL instruments, which include the Sickness Impact Profile, Medical Outcomes Study Short Form-36 items (MOS SF-36), Short Form-12 items (MOS SF-12), and Quality of Well-Being Scale (QWB). The criteria used for evaluation by the Scientific Advisory Committee have also been published (9).

The SF-36 is one of the most widely used global QOL instruments in the United States (10). It is divided into eight multi-item subscales: physical functioning, social functioning, general health, mental health, role functioning due to physical problems, role functioning due to emotional problems, vitality, and bodily pain. The SF-36 was designed for self-administration, telephone administration, or administration with a personal interview. The SF-36 is reliable and valid for comparisons of group data (rather than individual patient data), and its responsiveness (sensitivity) is adequate. There is no overall sum-total score for the SF-36; instead, each subscale is scored individually. This has definite advantages, because creating a total score would require proportional scaling of individual aspects of QOL toward a total score. Instead, the individual subscale scores are more appropriately used for comparisons. In addition, the SF-36 is relatively easy for patients to complete. The SF-36 has been used to assess the QOL of patients with several chronic medical conditions as well as otolaryngologic diseases (11,12), and baseline data exist for multiple disease processes. In fact, much of the appeal of the SF-36 lies in the availability of comparison data.

HEAD AND NECK INSTRUMENTS

Several disease-specific instruments have been designed for use in patients with head and neck cancer. Before using a particular instrument, an investigator should check with the instrument designer to see if permission is needed.

The University of Washington Quality of Life (UWQOL) instrument originally contained nine questions to assess nine separate areas important to patients with head and neck cancer: pain, disfigurement, activity, recreation/entertainment, employment, eating-chewing, eating-swallowing, speech, and shoulder disability (13). Since its introduction, the UWQOL has been modified twice by adding importance scores for which patients rank each item on its importance to them, adding items covering other constructs affected by head and neck cancer, and adding global QOL items (14,15). The authors currently recommend using the UWQOL-Revised (UWQOL-R) instrument which has ten individual items, an importance-ranking item, and three global QOL items (15). Items are scored from 0 (worst possible) to 100 (best possible) on a four- or five-point Likert scale; each item represents an individual domain. The average of the ten domain scores represents the composite score on the instrument. The UWQOL instrument was found by the developers to be valid, reliable, and responsive, and the UWQOL has been successfully used in head and neck outcome studies, both at the University of Washington and at other centers.

The Functional Assessment of Cancer Therapy (FACT) instrument was designed to assess global QOL in cancer patients (4). The FACT-G (FACT —General) instrument has 29 items that can be used for any patients with cancer. In addition, there are several disease-specific modules that gather information to assess specific cancer sites, for example the FACT-B assesses breast cancer and the FACT-L is used for patients with lung cancer. The FACT-H&N assesses head and neck cancer, and has 11 additional items for a total of 40 items (including the general items). The additional items cover eating (solid food, swallowing, quantity, quality), breathing, voice quality, ability to communicate, and physical appearance. In addition, the FACT-H&N instrument has been appropriately validated by the authors.

The Performance Status Scale-Head and Neck (PSS-HN) was designed to be administered by the clinician, not the patient (16). The clinician rates the patient on three areas: normalcy of diet, speech, and eating in public. Each subscale generates a separate score. There have been some problems with the applicability of the scale to diverse groups of patients, and the scoring algorithm has been questioned, but the instrument has been used successfully in head and neck outcomes studies.

The European Organization for Research and Treatment of Cancer (EORTC) has developed and validated a set of QOL instruments with disease-specific subscales, based on a similar model as the FACT instrument. The organization named the instruments after itself, and has developed a 30-item global (or core) QOL instrument, the EORTC-Quality of Life Questionnaire (EORTC-QLQ30). This global instrument demonstrated good reliability, validity, and responsiveness (17). The Organization then developed a 21-item addendum to the EORTC-QLQ30 for use with head and neck cancer patients. No subscales were created, but items covered breathing, swallowing, pain, mucus production, and related subjects. Therefore, there is only a total score for the H&N addition. In addition, the EORTC-H&N is fairly lengthy; the authors reported that 40% of subjects required greater than 30 minutes to complete the instrument, and 39% required assistance to complete it (17). However, the EORTC instruments have been used successfully in outcomes studies, primarily in European populations.

Another available head and neck-specific instrument is the Head and Neck Quality of Life (HNQOL) questionnaire (18). This instrument contains 20 items, which are scored into four subscales: communication, pain, eating, and emotion. The authors designed the HNQOL to overlap with the content of existing, validated head and neck instruments (UWQOL, EORTC, etc.) and to add additional depth to the evaluation of pain and emotional impact of head and neck cancer. The instrument is appropriately reliable, valid, and responsive, and respondent burden seemed relatively low.

An additional available instrument is the Head and Neck Survey (HNS) (19). This 11-item instrument was designed to measure disease-specific QOL in patients with head and neck cancer. During validation, the developers identified three subscales represented: appearance, speech/communication, and eating/swallowing. In addition, the authors developed and tested two other items measuring head and neck pain, but did not consider those as part of the HNS instrument. The HNS was found to be reliable and valid. In addition, the developers noted that subscale scores were poorly correlated with global QOL scores, indicating that the HNS instrument was identifying aspects of the patient's QOL that were not adequately assessed using global instruments.

In summary, there are several validated instruments to assess disease-specific QOL in patients with head and neck cancer. These instruments all assess aspects of QOL and disability that are somewhat unique to head and neck cancer, and provide additional discriminative power over global instruments in assessing the head and neck cancer patient's perspective of QOL.

FUNCTIONAL STATUS AFTER RECONSTRUCTION

Several studies have evaluated particular aspects of function after free-flap reconstruction. For instance, studies have shown that innervated free flaps develop sensory function but also that some non-innervated free flaps develop sensory function over time (20–23).

Urken has developed a comprehensive classification system for classifying bony, soft-tissue and neurologic defects in patients requiring oromandibular reconstruction (24). This system was not designed to predict post-surgery outcome, rather it was to be comprehensive for classifying lesions and planning reconstruction. Toward that end, it is a very effective and well-designed system, and has been widely used.

Other investigators have compared functional results after different types of oromandibular reconstruction, typically using some combination of self-developed questionnaires, self-rating scales completed by clinicians and patients, formal or informal speech evaluation, radiologic swallowing evaluation, mastication force, or interincisal opening (20,24–30). Most studies found very similar results: in general, flap reconstruction is well tolerated, has low complication rates, and offers good functional restoration with adequate swallowing, good quality of speech, and good cosmetic results in most patients (20,21,24,28,30–32). However, one study found that flap reconstruction was not beneficial compared to primary closure (25) and another found that functional outcomes were not significantly different between innervated and non-innervated flaps (27). Another study found that patients treated with flap reconstruction had poorer speech outcomes than patients treated with primary closure, but that seemed to be due more to the large impact of resection (particularly of the tongue) on speech rather than a negative impact of the flap itself (29).

Most of these studies, however, were retrospective reviews of patients treated using similar reconstructive techniques. The patient's perspective of outcome was often assessed, but rarely by using validated instruments. Furthermore, few were comparative studies using control groups or similar groups treated using different techniques. Of course, very few centers have a large enough volume of patients undergoing flap reconstructions to be able to accrue a statistically significant sample of patients for analysis. In addition, as comprehensive staging systems have shown, the defects caused by trauma, cancer, and resection are extremely variable, so identifying groups of similar patients for study is very difficult. Furthermore, the standard of care changes over time and it becomes difficult if not impossible to randomize patients away from expected treatments. Also, clinical and anatomic factors sometimes preclude several options for reconstruction, which is another factor contributing to the difficulty of controlled trials in this area. Thus, evolving standards and slow accrual of patients at most centers complicate or make impossible randomized or controlled comparative trials to compare outcomes.

QOL AFTER RECONSTRUCTION

In one study of QOL in oral cancer patients, the authors evaluated 135 patients who had been treated with resection of an oral tumor (33). The study used the Functional Living Index-Cancer (FLIC) as the instrument to assess QOL. Overall FLIC scores were lower in patients with higher stage tumors, and in patients with both midline and lateral mandibular defects, or bilateral lateral mandible defects. Patients who had undergone myocutaneous flap reconstruction had lower scores than patients reconstructed with local tissue closure only, but these patients probably initially had larger tumors. Patients with a discontinuous segment of mandible also had lower FLIC scores than patients who had either been reconstructed or had no mandible resection.

A multivariate analysis revealed that the single factor most responsible for poor QOL was resection of the mandible. However, a separate analysis of patients with mandible resection revealed that the group without reconstruction did not have different scores from the group with reconstruction. So, the authors concluded that restoration of the shape of the mandible alone was inadequate to restore QOL.

A few other authors have reported QOL outcomes in study abstracts or summaries (21,27,34), but in most cases standardized techniques or instruments for assessing QOL instruments were not used. Thus, comparisons with other disease states, or between different types of reconstruction cannot be performed.

COST-EFFECTIVENESS ISSUES

Cost-effectiveness research is a type of outcomes research in which costs of treatment are associated with the effectiveness of treatment, in an attempt to maximize effectiveness relative to cost. There are many ways to measure effectiveness, but one unit used frequently is the quality-adjusted life-year (QALY). Briefly, a unit of years of life is combined with a unit of QOL, or life utility in which the utility of perfect health is defined as 1.0, death is defined as utility of 0.0, a mild illness or deformity might result in life utility of 0.90, and severe illness might be 0.40. Thus, if an average patient lives three years after Treatment A with an average life utility of 0.90, whereas after Treatment B, an average patient lives four years but with life utility of 0.50, you could calculate that the QALY after Treatment A is 2.70 (3×0.90) and the QALY after treatment B is lower at 2.0 (4×0.50) even though Treatment B yields one more year of life. Then, in a cost-effectiveness analysis, the costs of Treatments A and B could be compared against those life-utility outcomes. Therefore, even if a treatment has a higher cost, improvements in effectiveness will make the cost-effectiveness ratio smaller, which would make it the desired treatment in the analysis.

Noticeably absent in the study of oral-cavity reconstruction are data on life-utility or QOL after different types of treatment. However, even though the data on effectiveness or utility of treatment are incomplete, there have been several studies that evaluated cost issues surrounding oral-cavity reconstruction.

One study retrospectively compared 14 patients who underwent reconstruction using free-tissue reconstruction with 21 other patients who underwent pedicled myocutaneous flap reconstruction without mandibular bony continuity (34). The patients were not randomized. Outcomes assessed included hospital charges, length of stay, readmission, complications, operative blood loss, demographic data, tumor stage, physician's assessment of aesthetic outcome and speech, and the patient's perception of outcome using a self-designed questionnaire. At the time of the study, there were no disease-specific QOL instruments available for use in patients with head and neck cancer, although global QOL instruments were available. Costs were noted to be higher in the free-flap group, but aesthetic outcome was rated as higher by patients and physicians. The authors noted that differences in the treatment groups (for example, a higher proportion of anterior mandible defects in the free-flap group) made direct comparisons difficult; furthermore, the lack of a validated outcome instrument is also problematic.

Another retrospective study of 53 patients with posterior oral cavity and oropharyngeal reconstruction included 24 patients treated with a pedicled myocutaneous flap, and 29 patients treated using a fasciocutaneous free flap (35). The authors found that inpatient costs (using charges as a proxy for cost) were slightly higher for free-flap patients, but almost all of the increase was due to higher professional charges for those cases. Complications were slightly higher in the pedicled-flap group, but hospital length of stay, decannulation before discharge, and other clinical outcomes were similar in both groups. However, patients with pedicled flaps were significantly more likely to require long-term feeding tubes to maintain adequate enteral intake than were free-flap patients. The authors discussed direct, indirect, and intangible costs in the economic analysis, but they did not have the data from this retrospective study to perform complete analyses. Furthermore, QOL was not assessed, although the authors did note that a prospective study assessing QOL was underway at their institution.

Another group reported a retrospective study of 127 patients who underwent free-flap reconstruction after resection of oral or oropharyngeal cancer (36). The authors assessed operative time, other clinical variables such as ICU length of stay, re-admission rate, and costs in three groups of patients: 64 patients with no mandibulectomy and only soft-tissue reconstruction (group 1), and 63 patients with partial mandibulectomy: 30 with plate and soft-tissue reconstruction (group 2) and 33 with bone-containing free flaps (group 3). Although patients were not randomized, and the three groups were not comparable (i.e. some did not have a bony defect), nevertheless the authors found no significant differences in cost or other clinical variables between the groups, and recommended that perceived additional expense or complexity should not deter the use of the most appropriate reconstruction because overall costs were not significantly different. They also noted that although "quality of life is, apart from survival, probably the most important outcome of any cancer treatment," the retrospective design of their study did not allow for analysis of QOL after treatment.

Another retrospective study evaluated post-operative length of stay in 100 consecutive free-flap reconstructions, of which 41 were oral cavity/mandible, and 12 were glossectomy reconstructions (37). The authors found that the average post-operative stay was 11 days, but in patients with no complications (69% of all patients) the mean length-of-stay was nine days, and in patients with any complication (31% of patients) the mean length-of-stay was 16 days. For the subset of patients with flap-related complications (9% of all patients), the mean length-of-stay was 20 days. The authors also noted a very low re-admission rate after discharge, and noted that all major complications occurred within the first seven post-operative days. Therefore, they recommend early discharge in patients who have had no post-operative problems because in their series it was safe and less costly.

A final cost-related study retrospectively evaluated a group of 73 patients with oral cavity cancer to identify treatment- and patient-related factors which were associated with increased costs (38). They found that the majority of costs (about 70%) during the first year were associated with the treatment (rather than evaluation or follow-up costs), and that the single largest contributing factor was the tumor stage. The second largest contributing factor was treatment type, with combined modality (surgery with radiation) treatment costing significantly more. The other factor significantly associated with cost was the presence of co-morbid disease. The study did not address the costs of reconstruction techniques. The authors concluded that cost reduction schemes should focus on identifying cancers at earlier stages because this appeared to be the largest predictor of the overall cost of care.

SUMMARY

There has been a significant amount of work reported on clinical outcomes after oral cavity reconstruction. Overall, outcomes after reconstruction are very good, with high success rates, good functional recovery, good cosmesis, and minimal increased costs. Although some types of reconstruction are more costly and have a higher complication rate, it is likely that their increased effectiveness for certain types of reconstruction would make these cost differences worthwhile over time. However, QOL and effectiveness data are currently not available to prove this hypothesis. Future outcomes studies should address this important issue.

REFERENCES

1. Piccirillo JF. Outcomes research and obstructive sleep apnea. Laryngoscope 2000; 110: 16–20.
2. Foundation for Health Services Research. Health Outcomes Research: A Primer. Washington, D.C.: Foundation for Health Services Research, 1993.
3. Stewart M. Patient-based outcomes research. In: Rosenfeld R, Bluestone C, eds. Evidence-Based Otitis Media. Hamilton, B.C.: Decker and Company, 1999.
4. Cella D. Manual for the functional assessment of cancer therapy (fact) scales and the functional assessment of HIV (Fahi) Scale. Chicago: Rush-Presbyterian-St. Luke's Medical Center, 1994.
5. Aday L. Designing and Conducting Health Surveys. San Francisco, California: Jossey-Bass Publishers, 1996.
6. DeVellis R. Scale Development: Theory and Applications. Newbury Park: Sage Publications, 1991.
7. Gliklich RE, Hilinski JM. Longitudinal sensitivity of generic and specific health measures in chronic sinusitis. Qual Life Res 1995; 4:27–32.
8. Patrick DL, Deyo RA. Generic and disease-specific measures in assessing health status and quality of life. Med Care 1989; 27:S217–S232.
9. Perrin E. Sac instrument review process. Med Outcomes Trust Bull 1995; 3:I–IV.
10. Ware JE Jr, Sherbourne CD. The Mos 36-item short-form health survey (Sf-36). I. Conceptual framework and item selection. Med Care 1992; 30:473–483.
11. Stewart AL, Greenfield S, Hays RD, Wells K, Rogers WH, Berry SD, McGlynn EA, Ware JE, Jr. Functional status and well-being of patients with chronic conditions. Results from the Medical Outcomes Study. J Am Med Assoc 1989; 262:907–913.
12. Gliklich RE, Metson R. The health impact of chronic sinusitis in patients seeking otolaryngologic care. Otolaryngol Head Neck Surg 1995; 113:104–109.
13. Hassan SJ, Weymuller EA Jr. Assessment of quality of life in head and neck cancer patients. Head Neck 1993; 15:485–496.

14. Deleyiannis FW, Weymuller EA Jr, Coltrera MD. Quality of life of disease-free survivors of advanced (Stage III or IV) Oropharyngeal Cancer. Head Neck 1997; 19:466–473.
15. Weymuller EA Jr, Alsarraf R, Yueh B, Deleyiannis FW, Coltrera MD. Analysis of the performance characteristics of the University of Washington Quality of life instrument and its modification (Uw-Qol-R). Arch Otolaryngol Head Neck Surg 2001; 127: 489–493.
16. List MA, Ritter-Sterr C, Lansky SB. A performance status scale for head and neck cancer patients. Cancer 1990; 66:564–569.
17. Bjordal K, Kaasa S. Psychometric validation of the eortc core quality of life questionnaire, 30-Item Version and a Diagnosis-Specific Module for Head and Neck Cancer Patients. Acta Oncol 1992; 31:311–321.
18. Terrell JE, Nanavati KA, Esclamado RM, Bishop JK, Bradford CR, Wolf GT. Head and neck cancer-specific quality of life: instrument validation. Arch Otolaryngol Head Neck Surg 1997; 123:1125–1132.
19. Gliklich RE, Goldsmith TA, Funk GF. Are head and neck specific quality of life measures necessary? Head Neck 1997; 19:474–480.
20. Close LG, Truelson JM, Milledge RA, Schweitzer C. Sensory recovery in noninnervated flaps used for oral cavity and oropharyngeal reconstruction. Arch Otolaryngol Head Neck Surg 1995; 121:967–972.
21. Urken ML, Weinberg H, Buchbinder D, Moscoso JF, Lawson W, Catalano PJ, Biller HF. Microvascular free flaps in head and neck reconstruction. Report of 200 Cases and Review of Complications. Arch Otolaryngol Head Neck Surg 1994; 120:633–640.
22. Katou F, Shirai N, Kamakura S, Ohki H, Motegi K, Andoh N, Date F, Nagura H. Intraoral reconstruction with innervated forearm flap: a comparison of sensibility and reinnervation in innervated versus noninnervated forearm flap. Oral Surg Oral Med Oral Pathol Oral Radiol Endod 1995; 80:638–644.
23. Shindo ML, Sinha UK, Rice DH. Sensory recovery in noninnervated free flaps for head and neck reconstruction. Laryngoscope 1995; 105:1290–1293.
24. Urken ML, Weinberg H, Vickery C, Buchbinder D, Lawson W, Biller HF. Oromandibular reconstruction using microvascular composite free flaps. Report of 71 Cases and a New Classification Scheme for Bony, Soft-Tissue, and Neurologic Defects. Arch Otolaryngol Head Neck Surg 1991; 117:733–744.
25. McConnel FM, Pauloski BR, Logemann JA, Rademaker AW, Colangelo L, Shedd D, Carroll W, Lewin J, Johnson J. Functional results of primary closure vs flaps in oropharyngeal reconstruction: a prospective study of speech and swallowing. Arch Otolaryngol Head Neck Surg 1998; 124:625–630.
26. Jacobson MC, Franssen E, Fliss DM, Birt BD, Gilbert RW. Free forearm flap in oral reconstruction. Functional outcome. Arch Otolaryngol Head Neck Surg 1995; 121:959–964.
27. Mah SM, Durham JS, Anderson DW, Irvine RA, Chow C, Fache JS, Weir I, Coupland DB. Functional results in oral cavity reconstruction using reinnervated versus nonreinnervated free fasciocutaneous grafts. J Otolaryngol 1996; 25:75–81.
28. Shpitzer T, Neligan PC, Gullane PJ, Boyd BJ, Gur E, Rotstein LE, Brown DH, Irish JC, Freeman JE. The free iliac crest and fibula flaps in vascularized oromandibular reconstruction: comparison and long-term evaluation. Head Neck 1999; 21:639–647.
29. Pauloski BR, Logemann JA, Colangelo LA, Rademaker AW, McConnel FM, Heiser MA, Cardinale S, Shedd D, Stein D, Beery Q, et al. Surgical variables affecting speech in treated patients with oral and oropharyngeal cancer. Laryngoscope 1998; 108:908–916.
30. Wagner JD, Coleman JJ 3rd, Weisberger E, Righi PD, Radpour S, McGarvey S, Bayler A, Chen J, Crow H. Predictive factors for functional recovery after free tissue transfer oromandibular reconstruction. Am J Surg 1998; 176:430–435.
31. Salibian AH, Allison GR, Armstrong WB, Krugman ME, Strelzow VV, Kelly T, Brugman JJ, Hoerauf P, McMicken BL. Functional Hemitongue reconstruction with the microvascular ulnar forearm flap. Plast Reconstr Surg 1999; 104:654–660.

32. Azizzadeh B, Yafai S, Rawnsley JD, Abemayor E, Sercarz JA, Calcaterra TC, Berke GS, Blackwell KE. Radial forearm free flap pharyngoesophageal reconstruction. Laryngoscope 2001; 111:807–810.
33. Schliephake H, Neukam FW, Schmelzeisen R, Varoga B, Schneller H. Long-term quality of life after ablative intraoral tumour surgery. J Craniomaxillofac Surg 1995; 23:243–249.
34. Talesnik A, Markowitz B, Calcaterra T, Ahn C, Shaw W. Cost and outcome of osteocutaneous free-tissue transfer versus pedicled soft-tissue reconstruction for composite mandibular defects. Plast Reconstr Surg 1996; 97:1167–1178.
35. Tsue TT, Desyatnikova SS, Deleyiannis FW, Futran ND, Stack BC Jr, Weymuller EA Jr, Glenn MG. Comparison of cost and function in reconstruction of the posterior oral cavity and oropharynx. Free vs. pedicled soft tissue transfer. Arch Otolaryngol Head Neck Surg 1997; 123:731–737.
36. Smeele LE, Irish JC, Gullane PJ, Neligan P, Brown DH, Rotstein LE. A retrospective comparison of the morbidity and cost of different reconstructive strategies in oral and oropharyngeal carcinoma. Laryngoscope 1999; 109:800–804.
37. Ryan MW, Hochman M. Length of stay after free flap reconstruction of the head and neck. Laryngoscope 2000; 110:210–216.
38. Funk GF, Hoffman HT, Karnell LH, Ricks JM, Zimmerman MB, Corbae DP, Hussey DH, McCulloch TM, Graham SM, Dawson CJ, et al. Cost-identification analysis in oral cavity cancer management. Otolaryngol Head Neck Surg 1998; 118:211–220.

22
New Horizons in Oral Cavity Reconstruction

Ahmed S. Ismail and Peter D. Costantino
Department of Otolaryngology—Head and Neck Surgery, St. Luke's—Roosevelt Hospital Centers, New York, New York, U.S.A.

David H. Hiltzik
Department of Otolaryngology—Head and Neck Surgery, Columbia University, New York, New York, U.S.A.

Jason Moche
Department of Otorhinolaryngology, University of Maryland, Baltimore, Maryland, U.S.A.

Craig D. Friedman
Facial Plastic and Reconstructive Surgery, New Haven Hospital, New Haven, Connecticut and Biomerix, Inc., New York, New York, U.S.A.

INTRODUCTION

For almost a century, the reconstructive surgeon has struggled to find the best method for repairing oral cavity defects. Early on, surgeons attempted to use simple compounds such as gold, steel, and glass wool to repair major defects resulting from trauma, tumor, and infection. As industrial, chemical, and scientific techniques progressed, so have the available material and methods. The advances in material science, improved surgical techniques, and tissue engineering have allowed for major strides in the field of oral cavity reconstruction.

Presently, surgeons largely depend on autogenous or autologous grafts for the repair and reconstruction of soft tissue, and both non-stress bearing and stress bearing facial skeletal defects. The availability of microvascular transfer of osseomyocutaneous free flaps and alloplastic materials have greatly improved the surgeon's ability to repair large defects. However, these autogenous grafting techniques and alloplasts also have many disadvantages. One of the complicating factors for all types of head and neck reconstruction is the potential for salivary contamination and the difficulty with reconstructing previously radiated tissue beds.

Microsurgical techniques are both complex and time consuming, and may only be performed by a surgeon with special training. In addition to their limited availability and quantity, autogenous grafts have donor site morbidity, are difficult to contour, and suffer from infection and graft resorption (1,2). While much improved over previous options such as pedicled and free non-vascularized grafts, vascularized osseous tissue transfers such as fibular or iliac crest flaps and radial forearm flaps are technically difficult to perform and, depending on the donor site, may supply an insufficient amount of bone or soft tissue replacement for oromandibular rehabilitation especially in the cases needing dental implants (3). Furthermore, the bone provided is rectilinear and is not readily contoured for reconstruction.

Current synthetic materials address some of these concerns but leave others unanswered. Synthetic materials such as carbon-based polymers or hydroxyapatite have proven useful in aesthetic augmentation but frequently lack the structural stability necessary for major head and neck reconstruction. Conversely, titanium reconstruction plates provide excellent temporary stability but act only as a bridge of the defect and are not a substitute for bone. As a result, there can be exposure of the appliance, infection, structural instability, plate fracture and eventual facial deformity. Oftentimes, many patients gain substantial cosmetic benefit with little functional improvement. New and improved methods are needed to restore function as well as appearance.

It is clear that as technology advances many new alternatives are becoming available to improve on the techniques of past and present. In this chapter, a few of these technical and scientific feats will be described. We believe that distraction osteogenesis (DO), bone growth factors, oral mucosal equivalents, and resorbable alloplasts have the potential to change the face of oral cavity reconstruction. Specifically, these new methods of reconstruction must allow for: (i) the reestablishment of adequate masticatory function, (ii) the creation of a supportive surface for dental fixtures or implants, and (iii) the restoration of a symmetrical appearance to the lower third of the face. DO and bone growth factors are two new methods that can potentially meet these demands and therefore hold significant promise for mandibular reconstruction.

DISTRACTION OSTEOGENESIS

DO defines the technique of growing new bone by stretching pre-existing bone. Cordivilla (4) first reported DO in orthopedic medicine in 1905. The current concepts evolved, however, from the ideas of Dr. Gavriel Ilizarov, a Soviet orthopedic surgeon who pioneered this technique in the 1950s. Dr. Ilizarov, with a deep understanding of the biophysiology of bone, developed techniques to move bone fragments in controlled vectors using a system of wires and fixed rings joined together with threaded rods and hinges. These techniques allowed slow transport of bone segments without invasive surgery. To quote Dr. Ilizarov (6) from a lecture given as the 1987 Sir Jones Lecturer of the Hospital for Joint Diseases Orthopaedic Institute, London, England, "This new method has given us the opportunity to ... replace extensive bone and soft tissue [loss] ... to elongate limb segments by 30 cm and more; to thicken and reshape thin shanks; to correct and align severe bone and foot deformities; and to grow missing parts of limbs such as fingers and toes." Ilizarov's technique (5) was introduced for the treatment of orthopedic injuries and conditions, and proved especially useful in the treatment of pediatric fractures and in the lengthening of unsymmetrical lower limb long bones.

Currently, the basic concept of DO involves creating an osteotomy while preserving the periosteum across the osteotomy site. A reparative callous is then permitted to form within this osteotomy site for a period of 7–10 days. At that point, the bones on either side of the osteotomy are slowly distracted or stretched apart. This distraction can proceed at approximately 1.0 mm per day. As the distraction progresses, osteoid tissue is laid down between the ends of the bone that abut the osteotomy site.

The three types of DO performed are monofocal, bifocal, and trifocal distraction. Many early studies were monofocal and involved the placement of a single osteotomy through a continuous length of mandible with subsequent distraction across the site to stimulate bone growth. Monofocal DO is only appropriate for the lengthening of linear bone and is not applicable for reconstruction of substantial segmental defects, which require the use of bifocal or trifocal DO (Fig. 1). The stumps of bone on either side of a segmental defect do not need to be brought in direct contact with bifocal or trifocal distraction, as is required by the monofocal type. Instead, these types of distraction utilize a transport disk of bone that is cut from one or both ends of a segmental skeletal defect. The vascular supply to the transport disk is preserved by maintaining the continuity of the periosteum across the osteotomy that was used to create the transport disk of bone. The movement of that vascularized transport disk across the segmental defect leaves a regenerative callus in its wake at a rate of 1 mm per day per transport disk (6,7).

In essence, the process of DO involves the mobilization, transport, and fixation of a healthy segment of bone adjacent the deficient site. A mechanical distraction device is used to provide gradual, controlled transport of a mobilized mandibular segment. When the desired repositioning of the bone segment is achieved, the distraction device is left in a static mode to act as a fixation device. Displacement of the osseous segment results in positioning of a healthy portion of bone into a previously deficient site. Because the soft tissue is left attached to the transport segment, the movement of the bone also results in expansion of the soft tissue adjacent the bone segment. At the original location of the segment is left a regeneration chamber that has a natural capacity to heal by filling with bone. The propensity of the regeneration chamber to heal with bone rather than fibrous tissue is a function of the surrounding, healthy cancellous bone walls and its location within the skeletal functional matrix. As a result of gradual distraction, the osseous and soft tissue components are enlarged in a single, concordant process.

It was not until 1973, that Snyder et al. first applied DO technique to the lengthening of bone in the craniofacial skeleton of the canine model. Since then, a number of experimental and clinical reports have shown DO to be effective in the treatment of various craniofacial deformities due to congenital, traumatic, and post-resection defects. In its current clinical applications, DO is predominantly used for the correction of various bone deficiencies either in the vertical, transverse, or anteroposterior dimensions. Neonates and infants with congenital defects relating to mandibular deformities such as mandibular and hemifacial hypoplasia have benefited greatly from this advancement (8,9).

DO for reconstruction of mandibular segmental bone defects from tumor resection and trauma, however, is still in its nascent stages. Costantino et al. (10) was the first to demonstrate that bifocal DO was effective in the reconstruction of a segmental mandibular defect in the dog. Oda et al. (11) showed that DO could be accomplished while being covered by a skin flap. Anino et al. (12) demonstrated the feasibility of curved trifocal osteogenesis for reconstruction of symphyseal defects in the dog. In 1995, Costantino et al. (13) reported the first use of DO for

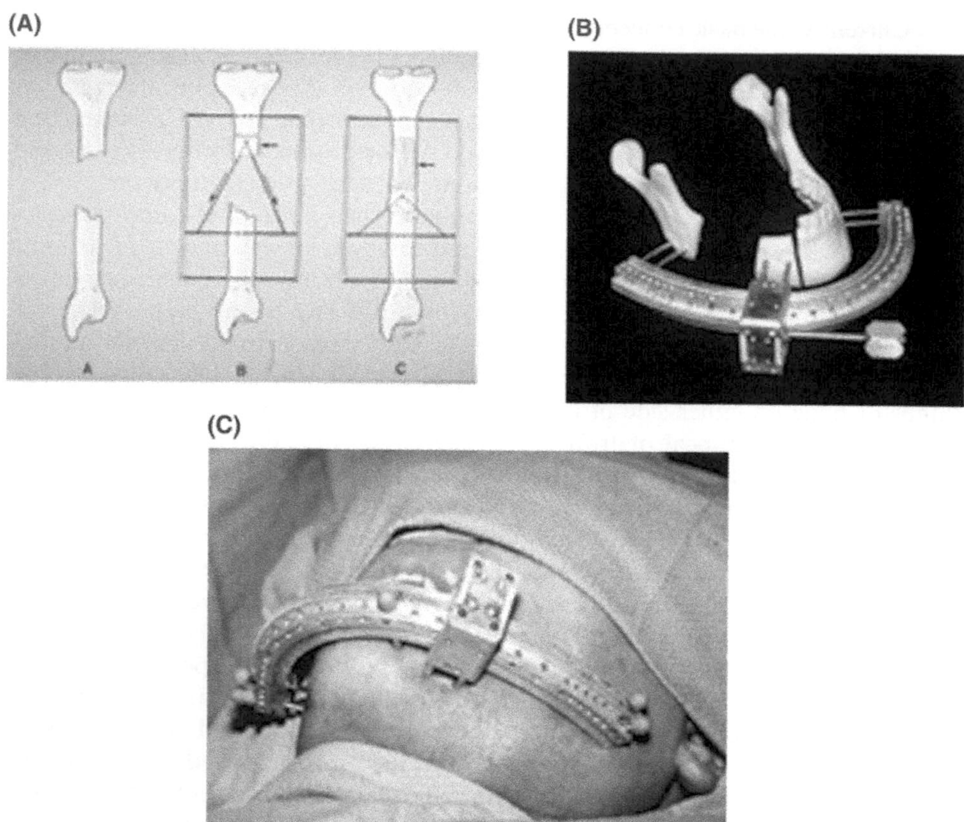

Figure 1 (**A**) General principles of bifocal DO. Segmental tubular bone defect. Center, the transport disk (*arrow*) has been cut from the proximal stump, and the distraction appliance placed. Arrows indicate force vectors that will distract the transport away from the proximal stump. Right, regenerate (*arrow*) is proximal to the transport disk, and the transport disk in compression with the distal segment. The entire segmental defect has been closed without a loss of length. (**B**) External distraction device for the repair of a mandibular segmental defect. Transport disk has been mobilized to promote osteogenesis. (**C**) Example of a patient undergoing distraction osteogenesis with the external distraction device in a place. *Abbreviation*: DO, distraction osteogenesis.

repair of a segmental mandibular defect in a human. Shvyrkov et al. (14) reported the application of DO in gunshot defects of the mandible and Sawaki et al. (15) reported a case in which an irradiated mandible was reconstructed by trifocal DO both however with some assistance from small free flaps.

DO is a true advancement in the correction of segmental mandibular defect repair for several reasons. By stretching the callous and replacing the defect with native bone, DO obviates the need for both alloplastic materials and autogenous free flaps and their respective complications of extrusion, infection, donor site morbidity, and functional impairment. This is particularly important considering the older age of many of these patients. Additionally, the creation of intraoral distractors allow for the resumption of normal daily activities and improve the quality of life during the course of the treatment without damage to the inferior alveolar nerve and the dental follicles.

(A)

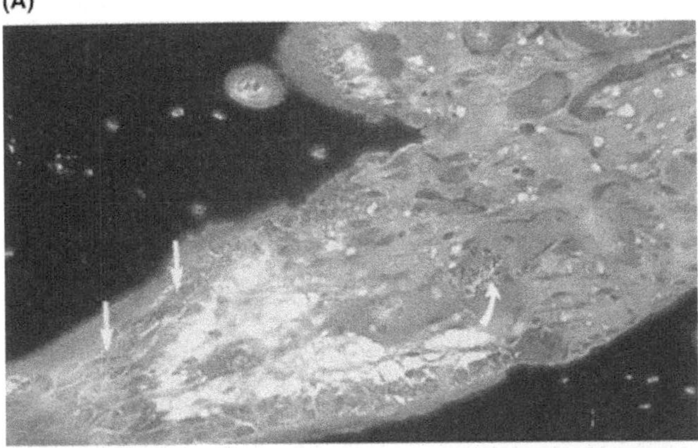

(B)

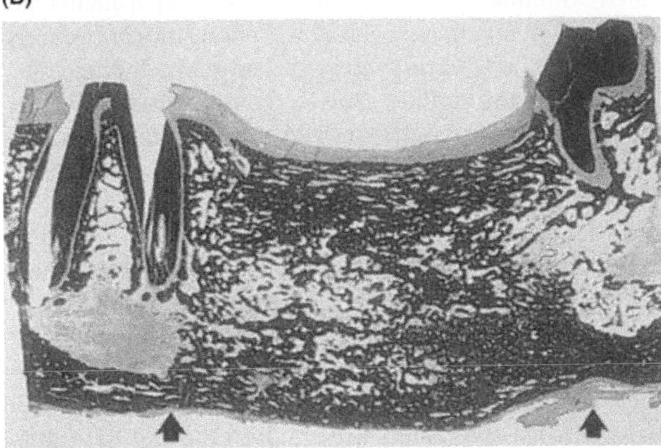

Figure 2 (**A**) Inactive bone matrix and human recombinant bone morphogenetic protein-2 (*rhBMP-2*) used to reconstruct a canine segmental mandibular defect. Active bone formation with large osteoblasts (*arrows*), osteoid, and blood vessels (*curved arrows*) indicate new bone growth. B indicates mineralized bone (*modified von Kassa's stain*). (**B**) Interface between original bone and BMP-2 repaired mandibular defect. Arrows indicate the transition from the new bone to the old bone, demonstrating the excellent degree of integration of the new bone.

There are however several issues that still need to be resolved. Because the mandible is a three-dimensional curved structure, DO may not be suitable for the reconstruction of the ramus and or condyle. A curved distractor may be necessary. It is also questionable as to what type and strength of bone will develop in elderly patients or in those patients who have pre or post-operative irradiated mandibles. The effects of bone aging and radiotherapy on the regenerative process are unknown. In the external devices, "tract" scars are an aesthetic problem that result from the piercing of the bicortical pins through the skin of the face. More importantly, some studies report difficulties with equipment such as bent or broken rods and screws, thereby allowing for the rotation of the bony fragment (16). Undoubtedly, some of the equipment must be further tested and studies must be undertaken to perfect the technique in order for DO to be a fully reliable treatment option for the repair of mandibular segmental defects. Although success is evident in congential anomalies, given current limitations, the role of DO in head and neck oncologic and traumatic including mandibular reconstruction is yet to be established.

BONE GROWTH FACTORS

Another technique for mandibular defect reconstruction that bodes well for the future is injectable bone growth factor that allows for native bony tissue growth. In order to understand the origins of this advancement, one must remember that bone maintains the ability to repair and regenerate after injury and to remodel in response to physical stress. Once initiated, bone formation is promoted and modulated by growth and differentiation factors that proceed through a complex physiologic process. Urist's first description of these "osseoinductive" properties of demineralized bone matrix in the mid 1960s were discovered from his experiments using bone fragment implantation subcutaneously or intramuscularly to induce bone formation. These experiments led to the elucidation of the variety of growth factors associated with bone morphogenesis (17,18). Bone matrix in the marrow contains various growth factors including tranforming growth factor-beta (TGF-beta), insulin-like growth factors I and II (IGF-I and IGF-II), fibroblast growth factors, and platelet derived growth factors. These factors help moderate cellular proliferation, differentiation, chemotaxis, and protein synthesis (19,20). It is believed that these local bone growth factors act in an autocrine or paracrine manner on regional osteoblasts and osteoclasts thereby affecting cellullar proliferation and biosynthetic activity (21). Growth factors are in essence tissue–specific polypeptides that act as local regulators of cellullar activity. They bind to large, cell surface transmembrane receptors on the target cell that through an intracellullar domain initiate the activation of a protein kinase cascade that results in the transcription of various proteins that act both intra and extracellullarly (22).

Bone morphogenic proteins (BMPs) specifically are a subdivision of the transforming growth factor-B (TGF-B) superfamily which play a crucial role in this process of cell growth and differentiation (23). There are eight classes of BMPs that have been identified as osteogenic regulatory molecules, BMP-2 through BMP-9 (BMP-1 is not part of the TGF-B family; it is a proteinase and possesses different properties). These have been further subdivided into three subsets based upon similarities in their amino acid sequences. BMP-3 is the sole member of its subset; BMP-5, BMP-6, and BMP-7 form a second set; and finally BMP-2 and BMP-4 are categorized together and are the two most closely related BMPs. (25). Clinical interest has focused on the application of BMPs in bone engineering therapies to initiate and promote osteogenesis. Bone morphogenetic protein-3 (osteogenin) has been localized in perichondrium, cartilage, periosteum, and bone, but also in the membranous bones of the craniofacial skeleton. It has been shown to have the highest bone inductive activity of all the BMPs (25). This was confirmed in a study by Khouri et al. (26) and tested in irradiated skull defects in the rat. When the defects were treated with both the bone morphogenetic protein-3 and a microvascular non-irradiated muscle flap, there was 96% healing at four months and 100% healing at eight months. The transplanted muscle was entirely formed into bone and was indistinguishable from the surrounding calvarial tissue. BMP-3, or osteogenin, has also been combined with tricalcium phosphate, a resorbable ceramic alloplast, as an onlay bone graft implant in a rabbit calvarial model (25). At six months, the osteogenin–treated implants showed a statistically significant increase in bone ingrowth and a decrease in tricalcium phosphate. Furthermore, they contained predominantly mature lamellar bone compared to the immature woven bone in the controls. All implants maintained their original volume at intervals of one, three, and six months after implantation. Further studies comparing the use of resorbable hydroxyapatite cement, which is more easily contoured than tricalcium phosphate, with osteogenin would be of interest with regard to the determination of long-term implant volume and shape.

Recent studies have shown increased expression of BMPs 2, 4 and 7 in primitive mesenchymal and osteoprogenitor cells present at fracture sites (27). In addition, these three BMPs were present in newly formed trabecular bone and osteoclast-type cells, leading to the conclusion that they work synergistically to promote fracture healing and bone regeneration. BMP-2 and 4 have been shown to increase dramatically during ossification at fracture sites after injury, particularly in osteoblasts (27). BMP-2 also has been shown to promote undifferentiated mesenchymal cells into osteoblasts (28). Based on this property, recombinant human bone morphogenic protein-2 (rhBMP-2) has been successfully used in the regeneration of calvaria and critical-sized radial defects in animal studies (29,30). RhBMP-2 has also been added to porous ceramic hydroxyapatite as a combined implant in a rabbit skull model (31). After one month, the subperiosteal placement of the composite implant demonstrated an enhanced osseointegration at the host-bone interface compared to HA alone. Given that the extent and rate of bone induction determines the overall clinical outcome of the implant, the early osseous fixation of the BMP-2 embedded implants serves to prevent host bone resorption as well as decrease the risk of implant extrusion (31). It is important that the delivery matrix allow for angiogenesis and bone ingrowth, either from osseoconduction (skeletal contact) or osseoinduction (extra-skeletal sources) and that it must be malleable so that it may be contoured, and it should have an average pore size of 200 μm and 400 μm in order to allow bony and fibrovascular ingrowth. Another study attempted to prefabricate a vascularized bone flap in the immature rabbit using the auricularis oris muscle as a pedicle (32). The subperiosteal HA/BMP implant showed 17.1% ingrowth versus HA alone at 11.3% ingrowth under the electron microscopic imaging at four weeks. Supraperiosteal HA/BMP showed a mean 19.33% versus HA alone at 0% bone growth. Histologically, woven bone appeared within the HA/BMP implant while the HA alone implant demonstrated only fibrovascular ingrowth and no bone formation. The results demonstrate the potential for prefabrication of vascular bony parts for reconstruction. Further studies continue to elucidate the ideal carrier and delivery system for embedded BMPs, including absorbable collagen sponge (33–35), poly-alpha-hydroxy acids (36).

With regard to oral cavity reconstruction specifically, rhBMP-2 has been implemented in two animal studies involving reconstruction of the mandible with differing delivery systems with high degree of success. In 1999, Yoshida et al. (37) evaluated bone formation in surgically created defects of rabbit mandibles by a combination of rhBMP-2, with porous hydroxyapatite and atelopeptide type I collagen used as the carrier for rhBMP-2. They found that at 21 days trabecular bone lined some pore walls and the external portion of the carrier disk. Angioid tissue and bone marrow was observed in the central portion. The control composed of HA demonstrated minor mesenchymal cell infiltration and some osseoconduction on the surface. Additionally, the rhBMP-2/HA had a significant increase in alkaline phosphatase activity, an osteoblast function marker, over the control. The study confirmed the rhBMP promoted bone growth/osteoblastic activity in a segmental defect in an animal mandible.

In 1991, Toriumi et al. (38) used dog bone matrix implants containing human recombinant BMP-2 to reconstruct 3-cm full thickness segmental defects in the dog mandible. They evaluated the ability of the implants to form host bone and to restore mandibular continuity and to provide mechanical stability by measuring the amount of mineralized formation, the dimensions of the bone character, and the strength of the segment as compared to the contralateral control segment. At three and six months there was "extensive bone formation" across the defect without violation of the defect margins. Eighty-six percent of the vertical height was restored. 50% of the volume mineralized and was "almost as dense" as bone. Biomechanically, the rhBMP-2 had enough strength such that the dogs could sustain a solid food diet, i.e., the forces of mastication. The rhBMP-2 induced bone, however, still only had 26% of the mechanical strength. Although, it is a very encouraging experiment, the amount of BMP-2 used in the study was never reported. In the study reporting long-term follow-up of Toriumi's canines, using poly lactide-co-glycolide as a carrier, similar success in bone formation and functionality was achieved at up to 30 months. Interestingly, this experiment revealed that, after initial bone formation, there was a period of resorption that stabilized at 11 months. More importantly, the rhBMP-2 induced bone increased to a density of 56.5% as compared to 41% at three months (39). The bone density continuously increased and was mainly trabecular bone without a distinct medullary cavity and without any regrowth of the inferior alveolar nerve or artery. The roentgenographic and histomophometric evaluation concurred with the earlier study.

Overall, rhBMP-2 bone formation for mandibular segmental defect reconstruction performed sufficiently well to warrant continued research and clinical studies in this area. Already, preclinical studies evaluating BMP-2 in radiated bone have yielded positive results (40). Further research must also include applying osseointegrated dental implants to preserve the strength of the bone and pursue better carrier materials to allow for a more uniform delivery as well as to determine the optimal dosing and delivery timing.

Resorbable Implants

An alternative strategy for the reconstruction of the oromandibular cavity that represents the combination of cutting edge technology and technique is the use of bioresorbable implants. Since Kulkarni (41) first proposed polylactide as a resorbable biomaterial for use in surgery in 1966, much study and research has been done to fully assess and apply the potential of these biomaterials. Although most commonly used as suture material, since the 1960s and increasingly in the last fifteen years, resorbable biomaterials have also been implemented for various reconstructive, orthopedic and craniofacial applications. They have found particular use in replacing permanent metallic implants, i.e., titanium, for fixation in a variety of fractures and defect repairs (42–44).

Due to the resorptive and biocompatible properties, bioresorbable materials offer several clinical benefits over the use of metallic implants for oral cavity repair and reconstruction. In addition to being osseoconductive and allowing for effective new bone growth, resorbable implants also reduce the theoretical risk of stress shielding, i.e., the weakening of healing bone resulting from excessively rigid fixation. Moreover, the resorption time of the implant not only assists in providing a gradual transition of forces to the regenerating bone or bone transplant, thereby strengthening the new bone, but the presence of the implant also protects the bone from external forces until it is able to withstand them on its own (4,6). As compared to metallic implants, this resorbable temporary structure eliminates the need for secondary operations for removal of permanent metallic implants, the possibility of corrosion, and carcinogenic potential. In addition, the polymer presents with clear radiographic scans of the reconstructed region due to the absence of radiographic scatter (42,48,49).

After implantation into the body, all polymers are hydrolyzed over time into carbon dioxide (CO_2) and water (H_2O). More specifically, the resorption process includes (i) hydrolysis of the implant by aqueous body fluids that may be autocatalyzed by carboxylic endgroups of degradation products and unspecified tissue enzymes, and (ii) fragmental metabolization of the implant polymer into single molecules (50). These single molecules are then metabolized in the liver into CO_2 and H_2O via the Krebs cycle and finally excreted by the lungs and kidney (42). The specific material's monomer makeup, crystallinity, melting temperature, glass transition temperature, initial molecular weight, and location of placement are all factors that dictate the degradation rate of the resorbable polymer (47,48,51). The higher the crystallinity and the higher the initial molecular weight, the longer the degradation time and the greater the strength persists (52). Resorption rate is also proportionate to external factors such as mechanical wear and blood supply. Plates should be carefully placed within surrounding vascularized tissue in order to allow for local tissue tolerance and transportation mechanisms to properly dispose of the degradation products. Although the intrinsic properties cannot be directly manipulated by the surgeon, careful placement and choice of location can be used to influence rate of resorption.

Currently, the most common resorbable substances include polylactic acid (PLA), polyglycolic acid (PGA), (both alpha esters) and polydiaxanone and various combinations and proportions therein. While the biocompatibility and osseoconductivity of both PLA and PGA is equal, PGA exhibits a greater inflammatory tissue reaction at the implantation site and weaker mechanical properties. Currently available resorbable implants are composed of some combination of poly-L-lactide (PLLA), poly-D-lactide (PLDA), and PGA comprise . Poly-L-lactide is the most mechanically strong polymer with the least tissue reaction and bulk although not as resorbable, and poly-D-lactide is a weaker polymer that degrades rapidly. This alloy of PLLA and PLDA can potentially achieve an effective balance between strength, lack of bulkiness, and optimal resorption rate.

Emerging products on the market employ a combination of each of these polymers. Macropore (Medtronics, San Diego, California) has a 70:30 ratio of PLLA: PDLA, Lactosorb (Walter Lorenz, Jacksonville, Florida) is a copolymer of PLLA and PGA, and the Delta System (Stryker-Leibinger, Kalamazoo, Michigan) is a tripolymer of L-lactide, D-lactide, and glycolide in a 85:5:10 proportion. The proper blend of PLLA and PLDA can potentially achieve an effective balance between strength, contourability, and optimal resorption rate. Add other companies i.e., synthes, KLS, etc.

In animal and human trials, PLLA, PLDA, and PGA implants have performed well in craniofacial and oromandibular applications. Include reference here. An in vivo study of polylactide plates in sheep mandibular osteotomy repair over the course of five years demonstrated that the plates were discernible after one year, although disintegration had already begun (53). There was minimal inflammatory response and resorption lacunae with osteoclasts could be seen. After two years, the plates were clearly seen but the disintegration had significantly progressed. A thin connective tissue capsule surrounded the implants and multinucleated cells were seen in close contact with the plates. Compared with two years, after three years very little implant remained and lamellar bone had replaced it. However, in some marrow spaces, fragments of the implant were still present. After four and five years, the implant was difficult to find, although with polarized light small angular and rounded fragments could be detected. Though the implants theoretically resorb completely by 36–48 months, they lose their mechanical strength long before this point from anywhere between 6 and 32 months, depending on the specific polymer composite (54,55).

In one clinical report of 20 patients ranging in ages from four months to sixty-seven years old, a PLLA/PGA copolymer was used for rigid fixation and reconstruction of the upper and middle third of the face (56). The conditions treated included craniosynostosis, facial bipartition, and Lefort fractures. With approximately six months follow-up, only one soft tissue infection occurred that was managed with antibiotics and drainage. Removal of plates was not required. Overall, the PLLA/PGA was effective.

In 1987, ten patients with unstable zygomatic fractures were treated with resorbable poly(L-lactide) (PLLA) plates and screws. The results show that this method of fixation provided adequate stability over a sufficiently long period to enable undisturbed fracture healing (57). The long term results, published in a second article, reported that three years postoperatively, four patients returned because of intermittent swelling at the site of implantation. Six of the ten were operated on again and the tissue swelling revealed a non-specific foreign body reaction. There was an internalization of crystal like PLLA material in the cytoplasm of predominantly macrophages. Increased osmotic pressure in the subcutaneous tissue, increase in volume of the disintegrated implant, and development of fibrous tissue are possible explanations (58). Another adverse reaction reported using PLLA clinically was the protrusion of plates through the skin of four of 25 patients. In all studies, however, the resorbable implants performed more than adequate fixation and were successful in their implementation. Additionally, it has been suggested, that the plates should be carefully placed within surrounding vascularized tissue in order to allow for local tissue tolerance and transportation mechanisms to properly dispose of the degradation products. Sentence qualifying current use and potential use and problems such as masticatory forces in mandibular application.

TISSUE ENGINEERED ORAL MUCOSAL LINING

Another area of increasing interest and research is the application of tissue engineering techniques to produce mucosal grafts ex vivo for transplant into the oral cavity. Mucosal lining for oral reconstruction after trauma, surgical resection, or pre-prosthetic surgery is highly sought after by surgeons. Wounds created intraoperatively call for protection in order to prevent microbial infection, excessive fluid loss, and foreign material contamination. Routinely, regional and free flaps restore volume while split thickness grafts (STSG) from the upper thigh or a palatal oral mucosal grafts are used to cover the mucosal defect. These grafts promote healing, restore function, and minimize wound contraction (59). However, these grafts have intrinsic disadvantages. Oral mucosa material in the form of grafts is available in short supply, and poses the issue of donor site morbidity. Conventional STSGs are available in ample supply but can develop adnexal structures and have different surface keratinization than the oral mucosa. In essence, the STSG retains its original structure and function without changing into oral mucosa, i.e., STSG can still grow hair and secrete sweat from the skin (60–62). The STSGs may also allow for infection and maceration (secondary to the moist oral environment) (63), skin contracture (due to the lack of dermis), hypertrophic scar formation within the oral cavity, and donor site morbidity. Additionally, STSGs serve as an insufficient base for dentures and leads to hyperplasia around the implants (64). Many attempts to avoid these potential sequelae with the use of allograft donor skin have been limited by their rejection after short periods of incorporation (65). Tissue engineered human oral mucosa equivalents and newer alternative allografts, however, may offer viable solutions.

Tissue engineering techniques for producing large oral mucosal grafts from a punch biopsy by reconstituting them ex vivo for subsequent transplantation has opened up a whole new field in reconstructive surgery of the oral cavity. Current techniques allow for the cell population in a 1 mm^2 biopsy to be amplified by 10,000 in culture and then easily sized, shaped, and transplanted onto oral mucosal defects (66). Since 1975, when Rheinwald and Green (67,68) first introduced a method of growing epithelial cell sheets in vitro using a feeder layer of irradiated fibroblasts and a serum-containing medium of growth, cultured epithelia have been successfully implemented as autografts for treatment of burn wounds (69,70), unepithelialized, mastoid cavities (71,72) and oral mucosa (73).

Oral mucosal composites, originating from a punch biopsy, composed of epithelial sheets and dermal equivalents can be created in one to two months. These tissue engineered grafts allow for an unlimited supply of oral tissue that is similar to native mucosa. There are three basic components to these mucosal equivalents: the superficial dermis, the deep dermis, and the interpositional basement membrane (74). The main function of the epidermis is to serve as a barrier. The dermal component aids in enhancing the quality and time of the wound healing and in promoting epithelial renewal (75,76). Initially, the two principal methods of mucosal equivalent production were either transplanting a stratified epithelial sheet alone or in combination with a condensed dermal equivalent containing fibroblasts to support the epithelium (76). Clinical reports of grafting oral mucosal defects, however, have demonstrated that epithelial sheets alone are very delicate, unmanageable, and thereby result in low engraftment rates (75,77,78). The dermal equivalent gives structural integrity, plays a role in minimizing contracture, but it also promotes the deposition of basement membrane components. The continuous interpositional basement membrane serves to assist in the optimal growth of keratinocytes, as an anchoring zone, and to provide tensile strength that alleviates sheer stresses placed on the graft (79,80).

Throughout the short history experimentation with oral mucosal equivalents, there have been several key advances in the field that have allowed for faster, easier, and safer production for human implantation. Until recently, most protocols utilized a feeder layer for in vitro growth of human keratinocytes composed of irradiated 3T3 murine fibroblasts and a fetal bovine serum containing medium with growth factors. Feeder layers have since become undesirable because of the risk of introducing a high level of xenogenic DNA content onto proliferating cells and the risk of contamination with undefined factors or slow viruses from the irradiated transformed cells (81,82). Furthermore, there have been advances in the types of dermal equivalents. Initially, a single epithelial sheet mucosal graft was attached to vaseline gauze for transfer in to the oral defect. Once the value of the dermal equivalent was appreciated, studies investigated various types of dermal equivalents including a hemostatic collagen sponge made from bovine tendon collagen overlaid by a second bovine collagen solution, a collagen-glycosaminoglycan (GAG)/silastic bilayer membrane, and acellular, non-immunogenic cadaveric human dermis containing a true basal lamina (83,84). The collagen-GAG/silastic bilayer relied on peripheral epithelialization and was antigenic and cytotoxic (84). The acellular dermal matrix or Alloderm (Lifecell, Co, Branchburg, New Jersey), however, has proven to be a highly effective dermal equivalent, allowing for successful seeding of oral keratinocytes. Alloderm contains an intact basement membrane and therefore does not need fibroblasts within its interstices to enhance adherence of the epithelial cells to underlying mesenchymal tissue, it does it by itself (85). Alloderm also allows for ingrowth of fibroblasts and angiogenic cells, consistently integrates into the host tissue, and trims, adapts, and sutures like autologous tissue (86) (Fig. 3). Alloderm fulfills all the previously enumerated qualities of a dermal matrix equivalent and has all the positive attributes of human dermis itself. As a side note, in a recent clinical study of 29 patients, Alloderm was used alone for intraoral resurfacing as an alternative to STSGs (87). Alloderm had a 90% "take" rate and epithelialization was noted in all successful grafts after four weeks. There were only minor complaints of pain in four patients and only one case of wound contracture that was in the setting of tumor recurrence.

Composite human oral mucosal equivalents have been proven to be efficacious in human oral mucosal defect repair. Although there has not been a large scale clinical trial, several patients have been the recipients of mucosal grafts. Raghoebar et al. (73) took punch biopsies of eight patients and cultured 20 cm^2 epithelial sheets, using a feeder layer. The sheets were then transplanted on vaseline gauze into eight patients with mucosal defects secondary to vestibuloplasty. Half the defect was repaired with oral mucosal equivalent and the other half was repaired with a conventional split thickness palatal graft. After three months follow-up, the grafted mucosa of both sites resembled palatal mucosa. Both the cultured and split-thickness grafts were vascularized, showed a smooth graft/lip mucosal junction, and demonstrated minimal wound contraction. Light microscopy and electron microscopy revealed that both types of grafts formed a fully differentiated keratinizing mucosa with a well-developed basement membrane. Lauer and Schwimming (88) produced epithelial sheet mucosal grafts up to 75 cm^2 in six patients for reconstruction of the intraoral

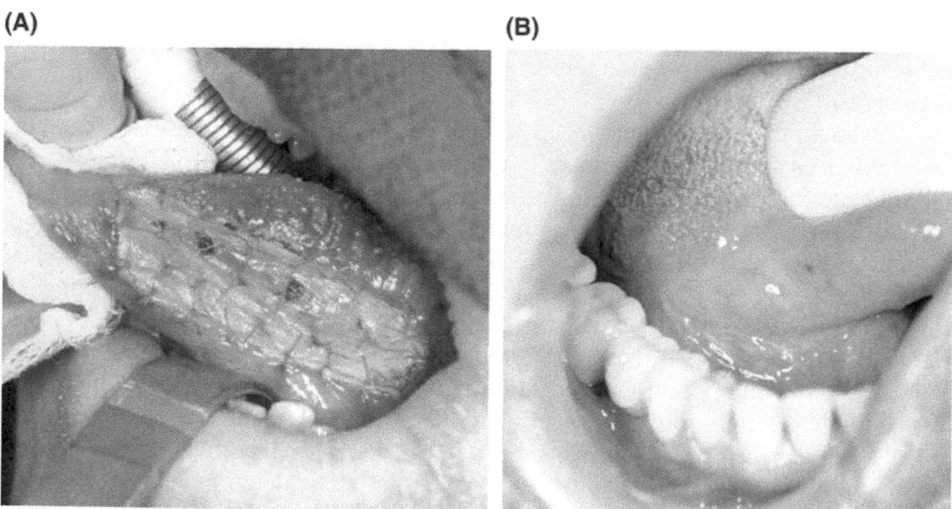

Figure 3 (**A**) Intraoperative suturing of acellular dermal matrix in tongue. (**B**) Six weeks postoperative image demonstrating a fully epithelialized dermal matrix in tongue.

lining after freeing of the tongue. After six-month follow-up, post-operative immunohistochemical staining revealed that the cultured cells integrated into the newly formed mucosal epithelium. Histologically, the mucosal epithelium had differentiated and stratified.

Additional studies using dermal equivalents such as Alloderm are forthcoming and their results are anticipated. If this treatment is to become widespread, the effects of radiation on these grafts must be studied. Although human mucosal equivalents require a large amount of preoperative laboratory preparation and therefore limit patient selection, it is clear from these preliminary studies that tissue engineering of human oral mucosal equivalents has great potential and a bright future.

CONCLUSION

Never before has the surgeon had such a vast array of options for the repair and reconstruction of oral cavity defects. Recent advancements in bone regeneration and healing have produced numerous improvements in the techniques of DO for the repair of oral cavity skeletal elements. Developments in tissue engineering and biomaterials have produced oral mucosal equivalents and resorbable implants for use in the repair of both soft tissue and skeletal defects, further eliminating reliance on autogenous grafts. With current studies focussing on improving the strength, contourability and biointegration of presently available materials, we are steadily developing materials that even more closely mimic autogenous tissue. Through such progress, the dream of eliminating autogenous tissue grafting is slowly becoming reality, making this a very exciting time in head and neck reconstruction.

REFERENCES

1. Oklund SA, Prolo DJ, Gutierrez RV, King SE. Quantitative comparisons of healing in cranial fresh autografts, frozen autografts and processed autografts, and allografts in canine skull defects. Clin Orthop 1986; 205:269–291.
2. Wolfe SA. Autogenous bone grafts versus alloplastic material in maxillofacial surgery. Clin Plast Surg 1982; 9(4):539–540.
3. Riediger D. Restoration of masticatory function by microsurgically revascularized iliac crest bone grafts using endoenosseous implants. Plast Reconstr Surg 1988; 81(6):861–877.
4. Cordivilla A. On the means of lengthening in the lower limbs, the muscle, and tissues which are shortened through deformity. Am J Orthop Surg 1905; 2:353–358.
5. Ilizarov GA. The principles of the Ilizarov method. Bull Hosp Jt Dis 1997; 56(1):49–53.
6. Ilizarov GA, Barabash AP, Imerlishvili IA, Larionov AA, Kochetkov IS. Morphological characteristics of the formation and reconstruction of bone tissue the replacement of extensive bone defects. Ortop Travmatol Protez 1984; 1:16–20.
7. Paley D, Catagni M, Argnani F, Prevot J, Bell D, Armstrong P. Treatment of congenital pseudoarthrosis of the tibia using the Ilizarov. Clin Orthop 1992; 280:81–93.
8. Polley JW, Figueroa AA. Distraction osteogenesis: its application in severe mandibular deformities inhemifacial microsomia. J Craniofac Surg 1997; 8(5):422–430.
9. van Strijen PJ, Perdijk FB, Becking AG, Breuning KH. Distraction osteogenesis for mandibular advancement. Int J Oral Maxillofac Surg 2000; 29(2):81–85.
10. Costantino PD, Shybut G, Friedman CD, Pelzer HJ, Masini M, Shindo ML, Sisson GA. Segmental mandibular regeneration by distraction osteogenesis. An experimental study. Arch Otolaryngol Head Neck Surg 1990; 116(5):535–545.

11. Oda T, Sawaki Y, Fukuta K, Ueda M. Segmental mandibular reconstruction by distraction osteogenesis under skin flaps. Int J Oral Maxillofac Surg 1998; 27(1):9–13.
12. Annino DJ, Goguen LA, Karmody CS. Distraction osteogenesis for reconstruction of mandibular symphyseal defects. Arch Otolaryngol Head Neck Surg 1994; 120(9):911–916.
13. Costantino PD, Johnson CS, Friedman CD, Sisson GA Sr. Bone regeneration within a human segmental mandible defect: a preliminary report. Am J Otolaryngol 1995; 16(1):56–65.
14. Shvyrkov MB, Sumarokov DD, Shamsudinov AH. Osteoplasty of the mandible by local tissues. J Craniomaxillofac Surg 1995; 23(6):377–381.
15. Sawaki Y, Hagino H, Yamamoto H, Ueda M. Trifocal distraction osteogenesis for segmental mandibular defect: a technical innovation. J Craniomaxillofac Surg 1997; 25(6):310–315.
16. Rubio-Bueno P, Padron A, Villa E, Diaz-Gonzalez FJ. Distraction osteogenesis of the ascending ramus for mandibular hypoplasia extraoral or intraoral devices: a report of 8 cases. J Oral Maxillofac Surg 2000; 58(6):593–599.
17. Urist MR. Bone formation by autoinduction. Science 1965; 150:893.
18. Reddi AH. Regulation of cartilage and bone differentiation by bone morphogenetic proteins. Curr Opin Cell Biol 1992; 4:850–855.
19. Bolander ME. Regulation of fracture repair by growth factors. Proc Soc Exp Biol Med 1992; 200(2):165–170.
20. Bourque WT, Gross M, Hall BK. Expression of four growth factors during fracture repair. Int J Dev Biol 1993; 37(4):573–579.
21. Khan SN, Bostrom MP, Lane JM. Bone growth. Orthop Clin North Am 2000; 31(3): 375–388.
22. Solheim E. Growth factors in bone. Int Orthop 1998; 22(6):410–416.
23. Schmitt JM, Hwang K, Winn SR, et al. Bone morphogenetic proteins: an update on basic biology and clinical relevance. J Orthop Res 1999; 17:269.
24. Riley EH, Lane JM, Urist MR, et al. Bone morphogenetic protein-2 biology and applications. Clin Orthop Relat Res 1996; 39.
25. Breitbart AS, Staffenberg DA, Thome CHM, et al. Tricalcium phosphate and osteogenin: a bioactive onlay bone graft substitute. Plast Reconstr Surg 1995; 96:699/biblio-misc>.
26. Khouri RK, Brown DM, Koudsi B, et al. Repair of calvarial defects with flap tissue: role of bone morphogenetics proteins and competent responding tissues. Plast Reconstr Surg 1996; 98:103.
27. Bostrom MPG, Lane JM, Berberian WS, et al. Immunolocalization and expression of bone morphogenetic proteins 2 and 4 in fracture healing. J Orthop Res 1995; 13:357.
28. Thies RS, Bauduy BA, Ashton L, et al. Recombinant human bone morphogenetic protein-2 induces osteoblastic differentiation in W-20-17 stromal cells. Endocrinology 1992; 130:1318.
29. Kenley R, Marden L, Turek T, et al. Osseous regeneration in the rat calvarium using novel delivery systems for recombinant human bone morphogenetic protein-2 (rhBMP-2). J Biomed Mater Res 1994; 28:1139.
30. Younger EM, Chapman MW. Morbidity at bone graft donor sites. J Orthop Trauma 1989; 3:192–195.
31. Koempel JA, Patt BS, O'Grady K, et al. The effect of recombinant human bone morphogenetic protein-2 on the integration of porous hydroxyapatite implants with bone. J Biomed Mater Res 1998; 41:359.
32. Levine JP, Bradley J, Turk AE, Ricci JL, Benedict JJ, Steiner G, Longaker McCarthy JG. Bone morphogenetic protein promotes vascularization and osteoinduction inpreformed hydroxyapatite in the rabbit. Ann Plast Surg 1997; 39(2):158–168.
33. Boyne PJ, Marx RE, Nevins M, et al. A feasibility study evaluating rhBMP-2/absorbable collagen sponge for maxillary sinus floor augmentation. Int J Periodontics Restorative Dent 1997; 17:11.

34. Hanisch O, Tatakis DN, Rohrer MD, et al. Bone formation and reosseointegration in peri-implantitis defects following surgical implantation of rhBMP-2. Int J Oral Maxillofac Implants 1997; 12:604.
35. Howell TH, Riorellini J, Jones A, et al. A feasibility study evaluating rhBMP-2/absorbable collagen sponge device for local alveolar ridge preservation or augmentation. Int J Periodontics Resotrative Dent 1997; 17:124.
36. Hollinger JO, Leong K. Poly (alpha-hydroxy acids): carriers for bone morphongenetic proteins. Biomaterials 1996; 17:187–194.
37. Yoshida K, Bessho K, Fujimura K, Konishi Y, Kusumoto K, Ogawa Y, Iizuka T. Enhancement by recombinant human bone morphogenetic protein-2 of boneformation by means of porous hydroxyapatite in mandibular bone defects. J Dent Res 1999; 78(9):1505–1510.
38. Toriumi DM, Kotler HS, Luxenberg DP, Holtrop ME, Wang EA. Mandibular reconstruction with a recombinant bone-inducing factor. Functional, histologic, and biomechanical evaluation. Arch Otolaryngol Head Neck Surg 1991; 117(10):1101–1112.
39. Toriumi DM, O'Grady K, Horlbeck DM, Desai D, Turek TJ, Wozney J. Mandibular reconstruction using bone morphogenetic protein 2: long-term follow-up in a canine model. Laryngoscope 1999; 109(9):1481–1489.
40. Wurzler KK, DeWeese TL, Sebald W, Reddi AH. Radiation-induced impairment of bone healing can be overcome by recombinant human bone morphogenetic protein-2. J Craniofac Surg 1998; 9(2):131–137.
41. Kulkarni KC, Pani KF, Neuman C, Leonard F. Polylactic acid for surgical implants. Arch Surg 1966; 93(5):839–843.
42. Hollinger JO, Battistone GC. Biodegradable bone repair materials. Synthetic polymers and ceramics. Clin Orthop 1986; 207:290–305.
43. Pensler JM. Role of resorbable plates and screws in craniofacial surgery. J Craniofac Surg 1997; 8(2):129–134.
44. Cordewener FW, Bos RR, Rozema FR, Houtman WA. Poly(L-lactide) implants for repair of human orbital floor defects: clinical and magnetic resonance imaging evaluation of long-term results. J Oral Maxillofac Surg 1996; 54(1):9–13.
45. Bos RM, Rozema FR, Boering G, Pennings AJ. Bioresorbable osteosynthesis in maxillofacial surgery. Oral and Maxillofacial Surgery Clinics of N America 1990; 2:745.
46. van der Elst M, Klein CP, de Blieck-Hogervorst JM, Patka P, Haarman HJ. Bone tissue response to biodegradable polymers used for intra medullary fracture fixation: a long-term in vivo study in sheep femora. Biomaterials 1999; 20(2):121–128.
47. Bergsma JE. Discussion: Reconstruction of mandibular continuity defects in dogs using poly (L-lactide) mesh and autogenic particulate cancellous bone and marrow: preliminary report. J Oral Maxillofac Surg 1997; 55(7):723–724.
48. Suuronen R, Pohjonen T, Hietanen J, Lindqvist C. A 5-year in vitro and in vivo study of the biodegradation of polylactide plates. J Oral Maxillofac Surg 1998; 56(5):604–614.
49. Viljanen J, Kinnunnen J, Bondestam, et al. Bone changes after experimental osteotomies fixed with absorbable self-reinforced poly-L-lactide screws or metallic screws studied by plain radiographs, quantitative computed tomography and magnetic resonance imaging. Biomaterials 1995; 16:1353.
50. Bostman OM. Absorbable implants for the fixation of fractures. J Bone Joint Surg Am 1991; 73(1):148–153.
51. Vert M, Mauduit J, Li S. Biodegradation of PLA/GA polymers: increasing complexity. Biomaterials 1994; 15(15):1209–1213.
52. Goglewski S, Jovanovics M, Perren SM, et al. Tissue response and in vivo degradation of selected polyhydroxyacids: polylactides (PLA), poly(3-hydroxybutyrate) (PHB), and poly(3-hydroxybutyrate-co-3-hydroxyvalerate) (PHB/VA). J Biomed Mater Res 1993; 27:1135.
53. Suuronen R, Pohjonen T, Hietanen J, Lindqvist C. A 5-year in vitro and in vivo study of the biodegradation of polylactide plates. J Oral Maxillofac Surg 1998; 56(5):604–614; discussion 614–615.

54. Claes LE, Ignatius AA, et al. New bioresorbable pin for the reduction of small bony fragments: design, mechanical properties, and in vitro degradation. Biomaterials 1996; 17:1621.
55. Suuronen R, Pohlonen T, Taurio R, et al. New generation biodegradable plate for fracture fixation: comparison of bending strengths of mandibular osteotomies fixed with absorbable self-reinforced multi-layer poly-L-lactide plates and metallic plates–an experimental study in sheep. Clin Mater 1992; 9:77.
56. Edwards RC, Kiely KD, Eppley BL. Fixation of bimaxillary osteotomies with resorbable plates and screws: experience in 20 consecutive cases. J Oral Maxillofac Surg 2001; 59(3):271–276.
57. Bos RR, Boering G, Rozema FR, Leenslag JW. Resorbable poly(L-lactide) plates and screws for the fixation of zygomatic fractures. J Oral Maxillofac Surg 1987; 45(9):751–753.
58. Bergsma EJ, Rozema FR, Bos RR, de Bruijn WC. Foreign body reactions to resorbable poly (L-lactide) bone plates and screws used for the fixation of unstable zygomatic fractures. J Oral Maxillofac Surg 1993; 51(6):666–670.
59. Donoff RB. Biological basis for vestibuloplasty procedures. J Oral Surg 1976; 34(10):890–896.
60. Moller JF, Jolst O. A histologic follow-up study of free autogenous skin grafts to the alveolar ridge humans. Int J Oral Surg 1972; 1(6):283–289.
61. Martis C. Mucosa versus skin grafts in Stoelinga PJW (ed): Proceedings Consensus Conference: The relative roles of vestibulopasty and ridge augmentation in the management of the atrophic mandible. Chicago, Quintessence, 1984:41–44.
62. Ueda M, Kaneda T, Oka T, Torii S. Experimental study of dermal grafts for reconstruction of oral mucosa. J Oral Maxillofac Surg 1984; 42(4):213–223.
63. Donoff RB. Discussion: Ex vivo development of a composite human oral mucosal equivalent. J Oral Maxillofac Surg 1999; 57(5):577–578.
64. Mitchell DL, Synnott SA, VanDercreek JA. Tissue reaction involving an intraoral skin graft and CP titanium abutments: a clinical report. Int J Oral Maxillofac Implants 1990; 5(1):79–84.
65. McCarthy JG. Plastic Surgery. Philadelphia, PA: WB Saunders Co; 1990:221–267.
66. de Luca M, Albanese E, Megna M, Cancedda R, Mangiante PE, Cadoni A, Franzi AT. Evidence that human oral epithelium reconstituted in vitro and transplanted in patients with defects in the oral mucosa retains properties of the original donor site. Transplantation 1990; 50(3):454–459.
67. Rheinwald JG, Green H. Serial cultivation of strains of human epidermal keratinocytes: the formation of keratinizing colonies from single cells. Cell 1975; 6(3):331–343.
68. Rheinwald JG, Green H. Epidermal growth factor and the multiplication of cultured human epidermal keratinocytes. Nature 1977; 265(5593):421–424.
69. Gallico GG, O'Connor NE, Compton CC, Kehinde O, Green H. Permanent coverage of large burn wounds with autologous cultured human epithelium. N Engl J Med 1984; 311(7):448–451.
70. Teepe RG, Ponec M, Kreis RW, Hermans RP. Improved grafting method for treatment of burns with autologous cultured human epithelium. Lancet 1986; 1(8477):385.
71. Premachandra DJ, Woodward BM, Milton CM, Sergeant RJ, Fabre JW. Treatment of postoperative otorrhoea by grafting of mastoid cavities with cultured autologous epidermal cells. Lancet 1990; 335(8686):365–367.
72. Woodward BM, Shotton JC, Helme DM, Premachandra DJ, Milton CM, Sergeant RJ, Green CJ. Long-term results of the use of cultured autologous epithelial cell grafting to mastoid cavities. Clin Otolaryngol 1996; 21(6):490–491.
73. Raghoebar GM, Tomson AM, Scholma J, Blaauw EH, Witjes MJ, Vissink A. Use of cultured mucosal grafts to cover defects caused by vestibuloplasty: an in vivo study. J Oral Maxillofac Surg 1995; 53(8):872–878.
74. Izumi K, Takacs G, Terashi H, Feinberg SE. Ex vivo development of a composite human oral mucosal equivalent. J Oral Maxillofac Surg 1999; 57(5):571–577.

75. Feinberg SE, Krishnan V, Gordillo G, Shuler CF. Intraoral grafting of a canine full-thickness oral mucosal equivalent produced in vitro. J Oral Maxillofac Surg 1989; 47(7):712–718.
76. Leary T, Jones PL, Appleby M, Blight A, Parkinson K, Stanley M. Epidermal keratinocyte self-renewal is dependent upon dermal integrity. J Invest Dermatol 1992; 99(4): 422–430.
77. Ueda M, Ebata K, Kaneda T. In vitro fabrication of bioartificial mucosa for reconstruction of oral mucosa: basic research and clinical application. Ann Plast Surg 1991; 27(6):540–549.
78. Lauer G. Autografting of feeder-cell free cultured gingival epithelium. Method and application. J Craniomaxillofac Surg 1994; 22(1):18–22.
79. Auger FA, Lopez Valle CA, Guignard R, Tremblay N, Noel B, Goulet F, Germain L. Skin equivalent produced with human collagen. In Vitro Cell Dev Biol Anim 1995; 31(6):432–439.
80. Cooper ML, Andree C, Hansbrough JF, Zapata-Sirvent RL, Spielvogel RL. Direct comparison of a cultured composite skin substitute containing human keratinocytes and fibroblasts to an epidermal sheet graft containing human keratinocytes on athymic mice. J Invest Dermatol 1993; 101(6):811–819.
81. Lauer G. Discussion: Use of cultured mucosal grafts to cover defects caused by vestibuloplasty: an in vivo study. J Oral Maxillofac Surg 1995; 53(8):878–879.
82. Parenteau NL, Nolte CM, Bilbo P, Rosenberg M, Wilkins LM, Johnson EW, Watson S, Mason VS, Bell E. Epidermis generated in vitro: practical considerations and applications. J Cell Biochem 1991; 45(3):245–251.
83. Izumi K, Terashi H, Marcelo CL, Feinberg SE. Development and characterization of a tissue-engineered human oral mucosa equivalent produced in a serum-free culture system. J Dent Res 2000; 79(3):798–805.
84. Omura S, Mizuki N, Horimoto S, Kawabe R, Fujita K. A newly developed collagen/silicone bilayer membrane as a mucosal substitute: a preliminary report. Br J Oral Maxillofac Surg 1997; 35(2):85–91.
85. Krejci NC, Cuono CB, Langdon RC, McGuire J. In vitro reconstitution of skin: fibroblasts facilitate keratinocyte growth and differentiation on acellular reticular dermis. J Invest Dermatol 1991; 97(5):843–848.
86. Wainwright DJ. Use of an acellular allograft dermal matrix (AlloDerm) in the management of full-thicknessburns. Burns 1995; 21(4):243–248.
87. Rhee PH, Friedman CD, Ridge JA, Kusiak J. The use of processed allograft dermal matrix for intraoral resurfacing: an alternative to split-thickness skin grafts. Arch Otolaryngol Head Neck Surg 1998; 124(11):1201–1204.
88. Lauer G, Schimming R. Tissue-engineered mucosa graft for reconstruction of the intraoral lining after freeing of the tongue: a clinical and immunohistologic study. J Oral Maxillofac Surg 2001; 59(2):169–175.

Index

Abnormal oral competence, 26–27
ACC. *See* Adenoid cystic carcinoma.
Acellular allograft dermal matrix, in mouth reconstruction, 181
Acellular human collagen matrix, in split thickness skin grafts, 159–162
Adenoid cystic carcinoma (ACC), of salivary gland, 51
Adenomatoid odontogenic tumor, 72
Allograft dermal matrix, in mouth reconstruction, 181
Alveolar mucosa, in oral squamous malignancy, 43–44
Alveolar ridges, in oral cavity, 14
Ameloblastic fibroma, 72–73
Ameloblastoma, 71–72
Anatomy
  alveolar ridges in oral cavity, 14
  buccal mucosa, in cheek, 13–14
  hard palate, 15–16
  lips, 12–13
  mandible, 20
  of the mouth floor, 15
  oral cavity, 11–22
  retromolar trigone, 14
  tongue, 19–20
Anterolateral thigh free flap, in tongue reconstruction, 245

Benign lesions
  bone central giant cell lesion, 64
  cheilitis granulomatosa, 62–63
  cherubism, 65–66
  epulis fissuratum, 63
  exostosis, 68
  fibroid epulis, 60–61
  fibroma, soft tissue traumatic, 59
  fibrous dysplasia, 66–67
  florid osseous dysplasia, 64–65
[Benign lesions]
  giant cell epulis, 50
  gingival hyperplasia, drug-induced, 63
  granular cell tumor, 62
  Langerhans cell granulomatosis, 67–68
  Miescher's cheilitis, 62–63
  mucocele, 61–62
  osteosclerosis, 68
  peripheral giant cell granuloma, 50
  peripheral ossifying fibroma, 60–61
  pyogenic granuloma, 60
  soft tissue traumatic fibroma, 59
  squamous papilloma. 61
  tumors, oral cavity, 59–74
Bilateral cleft lip deformity
  reconstruction options, 296–298
Biomaterials for reconstruction
  implants, 607
  mandible substitutes, 373–376
  oromandibular complex, 373–376
BMP. *See* Bone morphogenic proteins.
Bolus formation and propulsion
  abnormal, 33–35
  normal, 32–33
  physiology, 32–35
Bolus variables modification, swallowing rehabilitation, 404
Bone central giant cell lesion, 64
Bone growth factors, 436
Bone growth factors
  in oral cavity reconstruction, 436–400
  resorbable implants, 438–440
Bone morphogenic proteins (BMP), 436
Buccal fat pad grafts, 163–165
Buccal mucosa reconstruction, 157–173
  buccal fat pad grafts, 163–165
  cervical pedicled flaps, 166–168
  combined flaps, 171
  evaluation and planning, 158–159
  free tissue transfer, 169–171

[Buccal mucosa reconstruction]
local tissue flaps, 162–163
options, 159–173
parotid duct, 171–173
regional myocutaneous flaps, 168–169
split thickness skin grafts, 159–162
temporalis/temporoparietal fascia flaps, 165
Buccal mucosa
of the oral cavity, 13–14
oral squamous malignancy, 42

Carcinoma, adenoid cystic, 51
Cervical based flaps, in lip reconstruction, 148
Cervical pedicled flaps, in buccal mucosa reconstruction, 166–168
Cheek advancement flaps
in lip reconstruction, 144–147
Von Burnow-Bernard flaps, 144–147
Cheeks, buccal mucosa in, 13–14
Cheilitis granulomatosa, 62–63
Chemotherapy
radiation therapy, and dental reconstruction, 309–310
treatment considerations, 310
Cherubism, 65–66
Circumoral advancement flaps
Karapandzic flaps, 136
in lip reconstruction, 136–137
Cleft lip and palate, 283–305
classification systems, 286–287
embryology, 285
epidemiology, 283–285
reconstruction options
bilateral cleft lip deformity, 296–298
palatoplasty, 298
unilateral cleft lip repair, 292–296
repair timing, 289–291
secondary palate, 287–289
unilateral cleft lip deformity, anatomy of, 291–292
Cognitive stimulation, swallowing rehabilitation, 403–404
Combined flaps, in buccal mucosa reconstruction, 171
Compensatory postures/positions, swallowing rehabilitation, 404–406
Condylar defects. *See* Mandibular defects, posterior.
Cross-lip flaps, in lip reconstruction, 138–141
Cysts
dentigerous cyst, 69

[Cysts]
odontogenic keratocyst, 69
periapical cyst, 69
tumors, 69

Degloving, oral cavity surgery, 111–114
Deltopectoral chest flap, in lip reconstruction, 150–151
Dental reconstruction
chemo-/radiation therapy, 309–310
evaluation and planning, 308–309, 324–325
hard palate defects, 311–314
mandible defects, 319–323
midfacial defects, 323–324
prosthetic reconstruction, 307–325
soft palate defects, 314–319
tongue defects, 319–323
Dentigerous cyst, 69
Dermal matrix, allograft, 181
Distant tissue transfer
oromandibular complex, 357
reconstruction options, 5–6
Distraction osteogenesis (DO), oral cavity reconstruction, 432–436
Disturbed lingual motility, swallowing disorders, 402
DO. *See* Distraction osteogenesis.
Double-reversing Z-plasty. *See* Furlow palatoplasty, 301
Dynamic pharyngoplasty/velopharyngeal complex reconstruction, 276–279

Embryology, of the oral cavity, 23–25
Epulis fissuratum, 63
Exostosis, benign lesions and, 68

FD. *See* Fibrous dysplasia.
Fibroid epulis. *See* Peripheral ossifying fibroma.
Fibrous dysplasia (FD), 66–67
Floor of mouth (FOM) lesions
evaluation and planning, 177–178
ventral tongue, 177–200
Floor of mouth (FOM) oral squamous malignancy, 45–46
Floor of mouth (FOM) reconstruction
acellular allograft dermal matrix, 181
case studies, 199–200
common techniques, 178
flap characteristics, comparison of, 198
lateral arm free flap, 196–198

[Floor of mouth (FOM) reconstruction]
nasolabial flap, 190
options, 178–198
platysma myocutaneous flap, 181–185
radial forearm free flap, 194–196
split-thickness skin graft, 178–181
submental island flap, 186–190
Florid osseous dysplasia (FOD), benign lesion, 64–65
FOD. *See* Florid osseous dysplasia, 64–65
FOM. *See* Floor of mouth.
Free bone grafts, non-vascularized, 328–329
Free flaps
characteristics of, 334
vascularized grafts, 332–337
Free tissue transfer, in buccal mucosa reconstruction, 169–171
Furlow palatoplasty
double-reversing Z-plasty, 301
palatoplasty, 301–305

Giant cell epulis. *See* Peripheral giant cell branuloma.
Giant cell reparative granuloma. *See* Bone central giant cell lesion.
Giant cell tumor. *See* Bone central giant cell lesion.
Gillies flap, in lip reconstruction, 141–142
Gingiva, alveolar mucosa, 43–44
Gingival hyperplasia, drug-induced, 63
Glossectomy reconstruction, 248–249
for tongue base reconstruction, 248–249
Gracilis free flap, for tongue base reconstruction, 247–248
Granular cell tumor, 62

Hard palate, anatomy, 15, 18–19
Hard palate defects, reconstruction options, 311–314
Hard palate reconstruction, 253–270
evaluation and planning, 253–254
options, 254–263
preoperative considerations, 269
recommendations, 263–269
special surgical requirements, 269
Head and neck surgical issues, 99
Hemiglossectomy defects, 213–218

Implants
biomaterials for, 6–7
oromandibular complex, 373–376

Incomplete hyolaryngeal excursion, 402
Infrahyoid myocutaneous flaps. *See* Cervical pedicled flaps.
Intrinsic laryngeal valving, 402–403
Irritation fibroma. *See* Soft tissue traumatic fibroma.
Island flaps, in lip reconstruction, 147
Isometric exercise, as swallowing rehabilitation, 407–409

Karapandzic flaps. *See* Circumoral advancement flaps.

Langerhans cell granulomatosis, 67–68
Langerhans cell histocytosis (LCH), 67–68
Lateral arm free flap
advantages anddisadvantages, 197
in floor of mouth reconstruction, 196–198
in tongue base reconstruction, 243–244
Lateral thigh free flap, in tongue base reconstruction, 245–246
Laterally-based forehead flap, in lip reconstruction, 149–150
Latissimus dorsi free flap, in tongue base reconstruction, 247
LCH. *See* Langerhans cell histocytosis.
Lingual release, in oral cavity surgery, 115–116
Lip advancement flaps, 132–136
Lip reconstruction, 119–153
anatomy, 119–122
cervical-based flaps, 148
cheek advancement flaps, 144–147
circumoral advancement flaps, 136–137
cross-lip flaps, 138–141
deltopectoral chest flap, 150–151
evaluation and planning, 122–123
Gillies flap, 141–142
island flaps, 147
laterally-based forehead flap, 149–150
lip advancement flaps, 132–136
melolabila flaps, 142–144
microvascular free flaps, 151–153
primary cutaneous lip repair, 124
skin grafts, 124–125
temporoparietal scalp flap, 148–149
vermilion repair, 125–129
V-lip repair technique, 129–132
Lip/chin split incision
mandibulotomy, 108–111
reconstructive options, 108–111

Lips
  anatomy of, 12–13
  oral squamous malignancy, 40–42
Lobular capillary hemangioma. *See* Pyogenic granuloma.
Local tissue flaps, for buccal mucosa reconstruction, 162–163
Local tissue rearrangement, reconstruction options, 4

Mandible, anatomy of, 20
Mandible defects
  dental reconstruction options, 319–323
  treatment considerations, 320
Mandible substitutes, oromandibular complex, 373–376
Mandible surgery, methods, 343–344
Mandibular defects
  anterior defects, 337–338
  condylar defects, 343
  lateral defects, 337–341
  posterior defects, 343
  reconstruction for, 327–344
Mandibular reconstruction, 327–344
  evaluation and planning, 327–328
  for mandibular defects, 337–343
  non-vascularized grafts, 328–331
  options for, 328–337
  vascularized grafts, 331–337
Mandibulotomy, for lip/chin split incision, 108–111
Mastication
  abnormal, 30–32
  normal, 28–30
  oral cavity, physiology of, 28–32
MEC. *See* Mucoepidermoid carcinoma.
Melanoma, neoplastic disease pathology, 52–53
Melolabial flaps
  lip reconstruction, 142–144
Microvascular free flap lip reconstruction, 151–153
Midface degloving, in oral cavity surgery, 114–115
Midfacial defects, in dental reconstruction, 323–324
Midline glossotomy, reconstructive options, 107–108
Miescher's cheilitis. *See* Cheilitis granulomatosa.
Millard rotation-advancement cleft lip repair. *See* Unilateral cleft lip repair.
Mouth floor, anatomy of, 15
Mucocele, 61–62
Mucoepidermoid carcinoma (MEC), 49
Mucosal flaps, rotation-advancement reference points, 296
Myocutaneous nasolabial flap, 192–194
Myxoma, 73

Nasolabial flap
  advantages and disadvantages, 193
  floor of mouth reconstruction, 190
  myocutaneous, 192–194
  one-stage cutaneous, 192
  random cutaneous, 190–192
  Nasolabial flaps. *See also* Melolabila flaps.
Neoplastic disease pathology
  melanoma, 52–53
  of oral cavity, 39–54
  oral lichen planus, 52
  oral squamous malignancy, 40–51
  osteoradionecrosis, 52
  sarcoma, 53
  tissue procurement, 54
Nevoid basal cell carcinoma syndrome, 70
Non-vascularized grafts, 328–329
  in mandibular reconstruction, 328–331
  reconstruction options, 3
  reconstructive bars/plates, 329–331
Normal oral competence, 25

Odontogenic keratocyst (OKC), cyst, 59
  nevoid basal cell carcinoma syndrome, 70
Odontogenic tumor, 71
Odontoma, 74
OKC. *See* Odontogenic keratocyst, 59
OLP. *See* Oral lichen planus, 52
Omental free flap, in tongue base reconstruction, 246
One-stage cutaneous nasolabial flap, 192
Oral cancer resections, swallowing abnormalities, 411–415
Oral cavity, anatomy
  alveolar ridges, 14
  cheek, buccal mucosa, 13–14
  hard palate, 15–16
  lips, 12–13
  mandible, 20
  mouth floor, 15
  oral tongue, 19–20
  retromolar trigone, 14
Oral cavity, benign lesions, 59–74
Oral cavity, prosthetic reconstruction, 307–325

Oral cavity, function, 20–21
Oral cavity, neoplastic disease pathology, 39–54
Oral cavity, physiology, 23–36
 bolus formation and propulsion, 32–35
 embryology, 23–25
 mastication, 28–32
 oral competence, 25–27
 salivation, 27–28
 taste, 35–36
Oral cavity reconstruction
 bone growth factors, 436–440
 diagnostic evaluation and planning, 2–3, 79–91
 distraction osteogenesis, 432–436
 future techniques, 431–443
 history and principles of, 1–7
 laboratory and radiologic studies, 82–83
 outcome research, 421–428
 patient history and physical examination, 80–82
 primary and neck resection, 85–87
 reconstruction options, 3–7, 87–91
 secondary, 383–389
 surgical planning and incisions, 84–85
 tissue-engineered oral mucosal lining, 440–443
 treatment planning, 83–84
Oral cavity, related structures, 11–22
Oral cavity surgery
 approaches, 95–117
 degloving, 111–114
 evaluation and planning, 98–102
 head and neck surgical issues, 99
 lingual release, 115–116
 midface degloving, 114–115
 reconstructive options, 102–116
 transhyoid approach, 116
Oral competence
 abnormal, 26–27
 normal, 25
 physiology, 25–27
Oral lichen planus (OLP), 52
Oral squamous malignancy
 anatomic sites, 40
 buccal mucosa, 42
 floor of mouth, 45–46
 gingiva, 43–44
 lips, 40–42
 neoplastic disease pathology, 40–51
 palate, 47–48
 retromolar trigone, 44–45
 salivary gland, 49–51
 tongue, 46
Oral tongue, anatomy, 19–20
Oromandibular complex
 biomaterials, for mandible substitutes, 373–376
 composite defects, 347–377
 distant tissue transfer, 357
 evaluation and planning, 348–350
 fasciocutaneous radial forearm free flap, 357–360
 implants, biomaterials for, 373–376
 multiple flaps, 371–373
 osteocutaneous fibula free flap, 360–363
 osteocutaneous radial forearm free flap, 363–369
 pectoralis major myocutaneous pedicled flap, 351–357
 reconstruction methods, 376–377
 reconstruction options, 350–371
 regional tissue transfer, 350–351
 relevant anatomy, 348
 scapula osteocutaneous free flap, 369–371
Oropharyngeal cancer, post-treatment factors, 392
Osteocutaneous fibula free flap, 360–363
Osteocutaneous radial forearm free flap, 363–369
Osteoradionecrosis, 52
Osteosclerosis, 68
Outcomes research
 cost-effectiveness issues, 426–428
 head and neck instruments, 423–425
 oral cavity reconstruction, 421–428
 quality of life, 421

PA. *See* Plenmorphic adenomas.
Palate, oral squamous malignancy of, 47–48
Palatoplasty
 of cleft lip and palate, 298
 Furlow palatoplasty, 301–305
 preferred techniques, 305
 principles of, 299
 repair timing, 299
 three-flap technique, 300–301
 two-flap technique, 301
 von Langenbeck, 299–300
Parascapular free flaps, in tongue base reconstruction, 244
Parotid duct (Stensen's), in buccal mucosa reconstruction, 171–173
Partial glossectomy defects, 213–218, 219
 reconstruction options, 206–219
 subtotal glossectomy defects, 218–219

Partial tongue base defects, reconstruction, 233–234
Pectoralis major myocutaneous pedicled flap (PMMF), 351–357
Pectoralis major regional flap, 237
Pedicled infrahyoid flap, for tongue base reconstruction, 240
Pedicled latissimus dorsi myocutaneous flap, 238–239
Pedicled myocutaneous flap, 237
Pedicled myocutaneous flap, for tongue base reconstruction, 237–238
Pedicled osteomyocutaneous flaps, 331–332
Periapical cyst, 69
Peripheral giant cell branuloma, 50
Peripheral ossifying fibroma, 60–61
Pharyngeal flap, in velopharyngeal complex reconstruction, 279–281
Pharyngeal swallow delayed initiation, 402
Platysma flaps. *See* Cervical pedicled flaps.
Platysma myocutaneous flap
  advantages and disadvantages, 187
  in floor of mouth reconstruction, 181–185
Plenmorphic adenomas (PA), of salivary gland, 49
PMMF. *See* Pectoralis major myocutaneous pedicled flap.
Pregnancy tumor. *See* Pyogenic granuloma.
Primary cutaneous lip repair, options, 124
Prosthetic reconstruction, evaluation and planning, 308–309
Prosthetic therapy, in velopharyngeal complex reconstruction, 275–277
Pyogenic granuloma, 60

QQL. *See* Quality of life, 421
Quality of life (QQL)
  global instruments to measure, 423
  outcomes research, 421

Radial forearm free flap, 357–369
  advantages and disadvantages, 196
  floor of mouth reconstruction, 194–196
  tongue base reconstruction, 240–241
Radiation therapy
  dental reconstruction, 309–310
  treatment considerations, 310
Random cutaneous nasolabial flap, 190–192
Reconstruction options
  local tissue rearrangement, 4
  non-vascularized grafts, 3
  lip/chin split incision, 108–111
[Reconstruction options]
  midline glossotomy, 107–108
  oral cavity surgery, 102–116
  transoral approach, 104–107
  oral cavity reconstruction, 3–7
  regional flap transfer, 4–5
  distant tissue transfer, 5–6
  implants, biomaterials for, 6–7
Rectus abdominis myocutaneous free flap, 246–247
Regional flap transfer, reconstruction options, 4–5
Regional myocutaneous flaps, for buccal mucosa reconstruction, 168–169
Regional tissue transfer, in oromandibular complex reconstruction, 350–351
Resorbable implants, bone growth factors, 438–440
Retromolar trigone
  anatomy of, 14
  oral squamous malignancy, 44–45
Rotation-advancement reference points, 294
  flap design measurement, 295
  skin flaps, mucosal flaps, 296
Rotation-advancement technique
  measurement and flap design, 293–296
  unilateral cleft lip repair, 293–296

Salivary gland
  adenoid cystic carcinoma, 51
  mucoepidermoid carcinoma, 49
  oral squamous malignancy, 49–51
  pleomorphic adenomas, 49
Salivation
  abnormal, 28
  normal, 27–28
  oral cavity physiology, 27–28
Sarcoma, neoplastic disease pathology, 53
Scapular free flaps, parascapular free flaps, 244
Scapular osteocutaneous free flaps, 369–371
Secondary oral cavity reconstruction, 383–389
  evaluation and planning, 383–384, 388–389
  options, 384–386, 388
Sensitization techniques, swallowing rehabilitation, 406
Skin flaps, rotation-advancement reference points, 296
Skin grafts, in lip reconstruction, 124–125
Small tongue base defects, reconstruction options, 229–232

Soft palate defects
reconstruction options, 314–319
treatment considerations, 320
Soft palate reconstruction, velopharyngeal complex, 273–281
Soft tissue traumatic fibroma, 59
Speech disorders
post-operative, 399–401
treatment for, 400–401
Speech rehabilitation
evaluation, 396–398
instrumental evaluation, 397–398
swallowing rehabilitation, 391–415
vocal subsystems, 391–393
Split thickness skin grafts (STSC)
acellular human collagen matrix, 159–262
buccal mucosa reconstruction, 159–162
floor of mouth reconstruction, 178–181
Squamous papilloma, 61
Stensen's duct. *See* Parotid duct.
Sternocleidomastoid flaps. *See* Cervical pedicled flaps.
STSG. *See* Split-thickness skin graft.
Submental island flap
advantages and disadvantages, 190
floor of mouth reconstruction, 186–190
Subtotal glossectomy defects
entire tongue, 218–219
partial glossectomy defects, 218–219
Subtotal tongue base defects, 234–235
Surgical planning-incisions, for oral cavity reconstruction, 84–85
Swallowing abnormalities, oral and pharyngeal cancer resections, 411–415
Swallowing disorders, 401–403
disturbed lingual motility, 402
incomplete hyolaryngeal excursion, 402
instrinsic laryngeal valving, 402–403
pharyngeal swallow delayed initiation, 402
Swallowing physiology, 393–396
Swallowing rehabilitation
evaluation, 396–398
physiology, 393–396
speech rehabilitation, 391–415
treatment strategies, 403–409
bolus variables modification, 404
cognitive stimulation, 403–404
compensatory maneuvers, 407
compensatory postures/positions, 404–406
isometric exercise, 407–409
sensitization techniques, 406
Taste
abnormal, 36
normal, 35–36
Temporalis fascia flaps, in buccal mucosa reconstruction, 165
Temporoparietal fascia flaps
in buccal mucosa reconstruction, 165
in lip reconstruction, 148–149
Tensor fascia lata free flap, in tongue base reconstruction, 248
Three-flap technique, in palatoplasty, 300–301
Tissue-engineered mucosal lining, in oral cavity reconstruction, 440–443
Tissue procurement, neoplastic disease pathology, 54
Tongue
anatomy and physiology, 224–225
oral squamous malignancy, 46
Tongue base reconstruction, 248–249
anterolatefal thigh free flap, 245
evaluation and planning, 225–227
glossectomy reconstruction, 248–249
gracilis free flap, 247–248
lateral arm free flap, 243–244
lateral thigh free flap, 245–246
latissimus dorsi free flap, 247
omental free flap, 246
options, 227–249
partial tongue base defects, 233–234
pedicled infrahyoid flap, 240
pedicled latissimus dorsi myocutaneous flap, 238–239
pedicled myocutaneous flap, 237–238
radial forearm free flap, 240–241
rectus abdominis myocutaneous free flap, 246–247
scapular and parascapular free flaps, 244
small tongue base defects, 229–232
subtotal tongue base defects, 234–235
tensor fascia lata free flap, 248
total glossectomy defects, 223–250
total tongue base defects, 234–235
ulnar forearm free flap, 241–243
Tongue defects
dental reconstruction, 319–323
treatment considerations, 320
Total glossectomy defects, 235
Transhyoid approach
oral cavity surgery, 116
reconstructive options, 104–107
Traumatic bone cyst, 70–71

Tumors
adenomatoid odontogenic tumor, 72
ameloblastic fibroma, 72–73
ameloblastoma, 71–72
myxoma, 73
odontogenic 71
odontoma, 74
oral cavity, benign, 59–74
traumatic bone cyst, 70–71
Two-flap technique, palatoplasty, 301

Ulnar forearm free flap, in tongue base reconstruction, 241–243
Unilateral cleft lip deformity, 291–292
Unilateral cleft lip repair
Millard rotation-advancement cleft lip repair, 293
reconstruction options, 292–296
rotation-advancement technique, 293–296

Vascularized grafts
free flaps, 332–337
mandibular reconstruction, 331–337
[Vascularized grafts]
pedicled osteomyocutaneous flaps, 331–332
Velopharyngeal complex reconstruction
asymmetrical pharyngeal flap, 279–281
dynamic pharyngoplasty, 276–279
evaluation and planning, 274–275
options, 275
prosthetic therapy, 275–276
soft palate reconstruction, 273–281
velopharyngeal dysfunction, 273
Velopharyngeal dysfunction, symptoms of, 273–274
Ventral tongue, floor of mouth lesions, 177–200
Vermilion repair, in lip reconstruction, 125–129
V-lip repair technique, 129–132
Vocal subsystems, oropharyngeal cancer
post-treatment factors, 392
speech rehabilitation, 391–393
Von Burnow-Bernard flaps. *See* Cheek advancement flaps.
von Langenbeck, palatoplasty, 299–300

Milton Keynes UK
Ingram Content Group UK Ltd.
UKHW052023071024
449327UK00027B/2402

9 780367 392000